Cutaneous and Cosmetic Laser Surgery

To my patients who allow me to improve my skills daily

To my staff for providing outstanding patient care

To my colleagues for their teaching

To my Fellows for their inspiration

To my wife for her support

Art + Science = Rejuvenation

In memory of my father, Arnold Leonard Goldman, 1930–2004.
His enthusiasm for science and education along with his unconditional and unwavering support led to my development.

Commissioning Editor: Belinda Kuhn
Development Editor: Claire Bonnett
Project Manager: Jane Dingwall
Design Manager: Andy Chapman
Illustration Manager: Mick Ruddy
Illustrator: Danny Pyne
Marketing Managers (UK/USA): Amy Hey/Laura Meiskey

Cutaneous and Cosmetic Laser Surgery

Edited by

Mitchel P. Goldman MD

Volunteer Associate Clinical Professor, Department of Medicine Division of Dermatology, University of California, San Diego; and Medical Director, La Jolla SpaMD, La Jolla, California, USA

MOSBY

ELSEVIER

MOSBY
ELSEVIER

First published 2006

ISBN 0-323-03312-1

British Library Cataloguing in Publication Data
A catalogue record for this book is available from the British Library

Library of Congress Cataloging in Publication Data
A catalog record for this book is available from the Library of Congress

EAD/13digit
ISBN: 9780323 033121

Notice

Medical knowledge is constantly changing. Standard safety precautions must be followed, but as new research and clinical experience broaden our knowledge, changes in treatment and drug therapy may become necessary or appropriate. Readers are advised to check the most current product information provided by the manufacturer of each drug to be administered to verify the recommended dose, the method and duration of administration, and contraindications. It is the responsibility of the practitioner, relying on experience and knowledge of the patient, to determine dosages and the best treatment for each individual patient. Neither the Publisher nor the author assume any liability for any injury and/or damage to persons or property arising from this publication.

The Publisher

Printed in China

Contents

video footage available for this chapter.

List of Contributors

Tina Alster MD
Director and Clinical Associate Professor, Georgetown University, Washington Institute of Dermatologic Laser Surgery, Washington DC, USA

R. Rox Anderson MD
Professor of Dermatology, Harvard Medical School; and Director, Wellman Center for Photomedicine, Massachusetts General Hospital, Boston, MA, USA

Alex S. Carcamo MD
American Academy of Cosmetic Surgery Fellow, La Jolla SpaMD, La Jolla, CA, USA

Christine C. Dierickx MD
Visiting Scientist, Wellman Laboratories of Photomedicine, Massachusetts General Hospital, Harvard Medical School, Boston, MA, USA; Director Laser Clinic, Boom, Belgium

Michelle Ehrlich MD
Attending Dermatologist and Clinical Instructor, Harbor-University of California, Los Angeles; and American Academy of Cosmetic Surgery Fellow, La Jolla SpaMD, La Jolla, CA, USA

Michael Gold MD
Medical Director, Gold Skin Care Center, Tennessee Clinical Research Center, Nashville, TN, USA

Mitchel P. Goldman MD
Volunteer Associate Clinical Professor, Department of Medicine, Division of Dermatology, University of California, San Diego; and Medical Director, La Jolla SpaMD, La Jolla, CA, USA

George J. Hruza MD
Clinical Associate Professor of Dermatology, St Louis University, St Louis, MO, USA

Suzanne L. Kilmer MD
Assistant Clinical Professor, Department of Dermatology, University of California, Davis Medical Center; and Director, Laser and Skin Surgery Center of Northern California, Sacramento, CA, USA

Woraphong Manuskiatti MD
Associate Professor of Dermatology, Department of Dermatology, Siriraj Hospital, Mahidol University, Bangkok, Thailand

Brent R. Moody MD
Assistant Professor of Dermatology and Director of Cosmetic Surgery, Department of Medicine, Division of Dermatology, Vanderbilt University Medical Center, Nashville, TN, USA

Anju Pabby MD
Board Certified Dermatologist, Laguna Niguel, CA, USA

Nina Pabby MD
Dermatology Resident, Harvard–Beth Israel Deaconess Medical Center, USA

Divya Railan MD
Dermatologist, San Francisco, CA, USA

Jaggi Rao MD
Associate Clinical Professor of Medicine, Division of Dermatology and Cutaneous Sciences, University of Alberta, Edmonton, Alberta, Canada

E. Victor Ross Jr MD
Residency Program Director, Dermatology Department, Naval Hospital, San Diego, CA, USA

Javier Ruiz-Esparza MD
Associate Clinical Professor, University of California, San Diego, CA, USA

Penny J. Smalley RN CMLSO
Technology Concepts International, Chicago, IL, USA

Margaret A. Weiss
Assistant Professor of Dermatology, Johns Hopkins School of Medicine, Maryland Laser Skin and Vein Institute, Hunt Valley, MD, USA

Robert A. Weiss MD
Professor of Dermatology, Johns Hopkins School of Medicine, Maryland Laser Skin and Vein Institute, Hunt Valley, MD, USA

Robert Willard MD
Advanced Skin & Laser Center, Brentwood, TN; West Kentucky Dermatology, Madisonville, KY, USA

Preface

Laser medicine and surgery continues to evolve on multiple fronts: from continued improvement in laser technology to the addition of photodynamic therapy, postoperative and topical anesthetic techniques.

A number of outstanding textbooks on laser surgery precede the production of this text. The last two textbooks that I co-authored and co-edited with Richard Fitzpatrick, MD, on laser therapy in 1999 and 2000 provide the foundation for this text.[1,2] This text will update the reader on advances in the use of lasers for the treatment of cosmetic concerns. I have asked a variety of leaders in laser medicine and surgery to put their experience on paper and we are privileged that they have taken the time and effort to do so. What this text represents, therefore, is the combined experience of the true leaders in this field.

The multiple authors who have contributed chapters to this edition have expanded on the past editions with an additional 5 years of development in laser surgery. Yet the authors have kept their chapters concise for easy reading by the laser expert and understanding by the laser novice. Case reports have been added to this text to better illustrate treatment modalities.

I hope that this volume proves useful to all laser physicians and surgeons in the treatment of cosmetic conditions with minimally invasive procedures. As the patient is the focus of the art and science of laser medicine and surgery, when detailed information on the variety of procedures available is obtained, patients will be best served.

As medicine is not a static science, I am hopeful that this textbook will serve as a stimulus to further the development of this exciting field of medicine.

Mitchel P. Goldman

References

1. Goldman MP, Fitzpatrick RE 1999 Cutaneous laser surgery, 2nd edn. Mosby, St Louis.
2. Fitzpatrick RE, Goldman MP 2000 Cosmetic laser surgery. Harcourt Health Sciences, St Louis.

Acknowledgments

This page is always a difficult one to write as it is never possible to acknowledge all those that have helped contribute to this textbook.

From the production side at Elsevier, although she is not mentioned on the dedication page, I am indebted to the friendship of Sue Hodgson, who believed that another comprehensive laser textbook was needed to combine and add to the two previous textbooks I published with Mosby in 1999 and 2000 along with my former partner, Richard E. Fitzpatrick. Although 'Fitz' is not a named author on any of the following chapters, his past contributions have been noted and are reflected in this new volume. The rest of the production team have been a joy to work with. I appreciate their dedication and professionalism to this project. From the time of chapter submission to production occurred in record time (less than 6 months) guaranteeing that this volume is the most up-to-date textbook available in this rapidly expanding field.

Because of the rapidly growing field of ***Cutaneous and Cosmetic Laser Surgery*** it was necessary to enlist the help of many experts to complete this text. No one person could have brought together this volume of information in such a timely manner. I am honored and thankful that so many of my friends, who are renowned experts in their field, agreed to take time out of their busy schedules and personal lives to organize their thoughts on these pages. In fact, the list of contributors reads like a 'who's who' of laser experts.

The reader will also note that many of the chapters have been co-authored by a variety of young dermatologic and cosmetic laser surgeons. These future experts, most of whom recently completed advanced fellowship training in various, private laser fellowship programs as well as recognized American Academy of Cosmetic Surgery and American College of Moh's Surgery fellowship training programs, added enthusiasm to this project.

Finally, the true stimulus that pushed this work to fruition is the curiosity and interest of young dermatologic surgeons who have rotated through our clinic at La Jolla SpaMD. Their sometimes 'nagging' curiosity and lust for knowledge pushed me into this project. It really was started to aid me in teaching our future colleagues the art and science of medicine. My only wish is that it succeeded to do so.

Mitchel P. Goldman

Abbreviations

5-ALA: 5-aminolevulinic acid
μs: microsecond
ABNOMs: acquired bilateral nevus of Ota-like macules
ADM: acquired dermal melanosis
AK: actinic keratoses
AL: argon laser
ALA: 5-aminolevulinic acid
ALA-PDT: photodynamic therapy with 5-aminolevulinic acid
ASR: ablative skin resurfacing
ATDL: argon-pumped tunable dye laser
BCC: basal cell carcinoma
CALMs: café-au-lait macules
CO_2: carbon dioxide
CPF: cooling protection factor
CPG: computer pattern generator
CSC: cryogen spray cooling
CVL: copper vapor laser
CW: continuous wave
DCD: dynamic cooling device
DE: dermis–epidermis
deoxyHb: deoxyhemoglobin
Diode: long pulsed diode laser (810 nm to ms range)
ECM: extracellular matrix
EMR: electromagnetic radiation
Er:YAG: erbium: yttrium-aluminium-garnet
ET: endotracheal
EU: European Union
FD: frequency-doubled
FDA: Food and Drug Administration
FIR: far infrared
FLPD: flashlamp-pumped pulsed dye
FP: fractional photothermolysis
GY: green–yellow
HbO_2: oxyhemoglobin
HEPA: high efficiency particulate air filter
HS: hydradenitis supporitiva
HSP: heat shock protein
IM: intramuscular
IPL: intense pulsed light
IR: infrared
IV: intravenous
KTP: potassium-titanyl-phosphate laser (532 nm to ms range)
KTPO: KTP (532 nm) laser
LED: light-emitting diode
LES: Lancer ethnicity scale
LEV: local exhaust ventilator
LHR: laser hair reduction
LMA: laryngeal mask airway
LSO: laser safety officer
LSR: laser skin resurfacing
LTI: laser–tissue interaction
MD: medical doctor
Metvix: methyl-ester cream derivative of 5-ALA
MIR: medium infrared
MMP: matrix metalloproteinases
MPE: maximum permissible exposure
ms: millisecond
MTZ: microscopic treatment zone
MTZ: microthermal zone
MW: microwave
Nd: neodymium
Nd:YAG: neodynium: yttrium-aluminium-garnet
NDR: nonablative dermal remodeling
NHZ: nominal hazard zone
NIR: near infrared
NMRL: normal-mode ruby laser
ns: nanosecond

OD: optical density
PDL: pulsed dye laser
PDT: photodynamic therapy
PFE: perifollicular edema
PIH: postinflammatory hyperpigmentation
PLDL: pigmented lesion dye laser (510 nm to 400 ns)
PO: per oral (by mouth)
PpIX: protoporphyrin IX
PS: photosensitizer
pw: pulse width
PWS: port-wine stains
QS: quality-switched
QS alex: Q-switched alexandrite
QS alexandriteL: Q-switched alexandrite laser (755 nm to 50–100 ns)
QS FD Nd:YAG: Q-switched frequency doubled Nd:YAG laser (532/1064 nm to 5–10 ns)
QS ruby: Q-switched ruby laser (694 nm to 25–40 ns)
QSRL: Q-switched ruby laser
Q-switched: quality-switched
RBC: red blood cell
RF: radiofrequency
RTD: residual thermal damage
SC: subcutaneous
SCC: squamous cell carcinoma
SGH: sebaceous gland hyperplasia
SPT: selective photothermolysis
TCA: trichloroacetic acid
TDT: thermal damage time
TKS: thermokinetic selectivity
ULPA: ultra low penetrating air filter
UV: ultraviolet
VIS: visible
VP: variable pulse width frequency doubled
XeCl: excimer laser
YAG: yttrium-aluminum-garnet laser

Chapter 1

Laser–Tissue Interactions

E. Victor Ross and R. Rox Anderson

The reader should note that although the title of this chapter is 'Laser–tissue interactions', the introduction of many new and diverse technologies makes this term somewhat obsolete. Although the term will be used in this chapter, one more appropriate is 'electromagnetic radiation (EMR)–tissue interactions'; both terms are used interchangeably in the remainder of the text.

Introduction

When using a light source, many physicians dial in 'suggested' settings and proceed, using identifiable endpoints to determine if the parameters are appropriate. For example, when treating a port-wine stain (PWS) with the pulsed dye laser (PDL), physicians look for immediate purpura and are vigilant to ensure that no surface whitening occurs. Although this is a good way (perhaps the best) to ensure that a favorable outcome is secured, it is instructive for operators to know from first principles how the clinical endpoint was achieved. This will allow physicians to expand their laser repertoire and optimize the use of this very expensive equipment. For example, armed with an education in laser–tissue interactions (LTIs), one can cajole the PDL to treat pigmented lesions without purpura by compressing the lesions with a clear plastic piece (Fig. 1.1). This removes blood as a chromophore and increases the ratio of melanin to vascular heating.[1] There are many other creative ways to use light-based technologies but without a basic understanding of LTIs one is reduced to treating skin ailments like one microwaves popcorn (according only to the instructions and with no license to do it better). In short, an understanding of light–tissue and electrical–tissue interactions optimizes clinical outcomes in cutaneous laser surgery.

Macroscopic Basis of Laser–Tissue Interactions

For our purposes, light can be divided into the UV (200–400 nm), visual (VIS; 400–760 nm), near infrared (NIR; 760–1400 nm), mid-infrared (MIR; 1.4–3 microns), and far infrared (FIR; 3 microns and beyond). These are the important wavelength ranges in laser dermatology.[2] Light demonstrates both wave and particle properties. Normally, wave behavior accurately characterizes the behavior of light in space and at large interfaces (i.e. skin and air).[2] However, the particle properties (and quantum physics) are more useful in characterizing EMR–tissue interactions on a molecular level (see below).[3] On a macroscopic level, light behavior conforms to various laws and equations that are consistent with our 'eyeball' observations in nature. For example, we are familiar with refraction and reflection. The surface of a pond is a partial mirror (reflection); a fish seen in the pond is actually closer than it appears (refraction).[4] Normally, the percentage of incident light reflected from the skin surface is determined by the index of refraction mismatch between the skin surface (stratum corneum n = 1.55) and air (n = 1).[2]

The Fresnel equations can be used to describe how much light will be reflected from the skin.[5] Depending on the angle between the light beam and the skin surface, this value varies considerably. More light is reflected at 'grazing' angles of incidence. It follows that, in most laser applications, we want to deliver light approximately perpendicular to the skin to minimize reflective losses.[6,7] This regular reflectance is about 4–7% for light incident at right-angles to the skin (Fig. 1.2). One can reduce interface losses by applying an alcohol solution (n = 1.4) or even water (n = 1.33). This allows for optical coupling (see below). On the

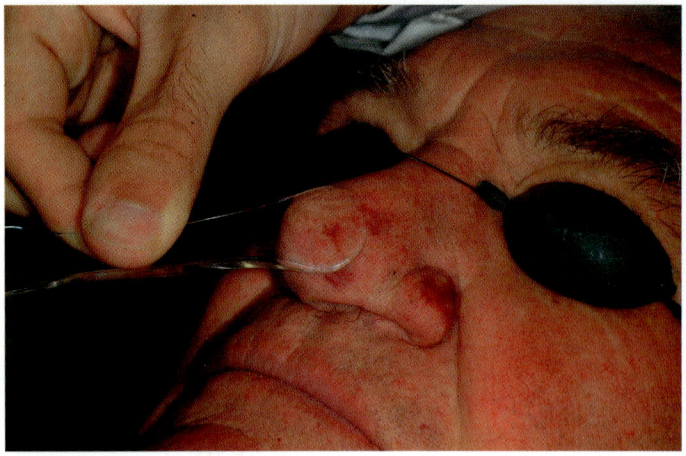

Figure 1.1 Example of compression technique. The plastic piece is used to 'remove' blood so that lentigo can be treated with 1.5 ms pulsed dye laser without purpura.

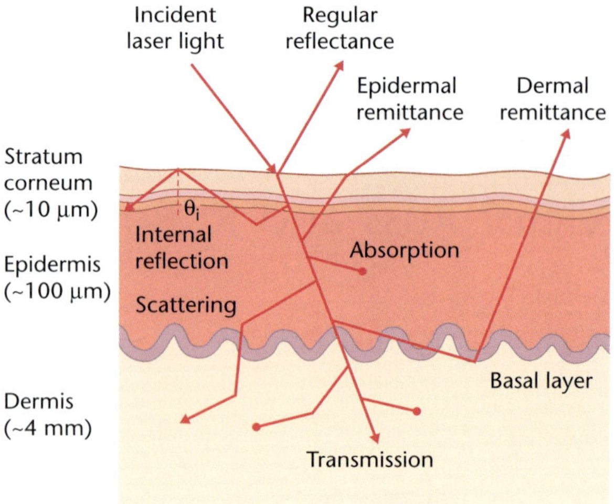

Figure 1.2 The behavior of light at skin surface.

other hand, the surface of dry skin reflects more light because of the higher index. If scale is present, reflectance is very high because of multiple skin–air interfaces (hence the white appearance of a psoriasis plaque). Light not reflected at the skin surface penetrates into the epidermis. At this point, further light propagation in skin is determined by wavelength-dependent localized absorption and scattering (see below).[5] Overall, because of scattering, much incident light is remitted (remittance refers to the total light returned to the environment due to multiple scattering in the epidermis and dermis, as well as the regular reflection from the surface (see Fig. 1.2)). From a therapeutic point of view, light reflected from the surface is 'wasted' energy. The amount of light wasted because of remittance varies from 15% to as much as 70%, depending on wavelength and skin type. For example, for 1064 nm, 60% of an incident laser beam may be remitted. One can easily verify this by holding a finger just adjacent to the beam near the skin surface. Considerable warmth will be felt with higher fluences, all of which is due to a remitted portion of the beam.

Types of Lasers and Properties of Lasers

Lasers as light sources to generate heat are very useful because they can, depending on parameters, allow for exquisite control of where and how much one heats. However, biological reactions are not intrinsically specific to the heating source. In principle, a very large number of nonlaser devices could be used for heating skin.[3] What are the advantages of lasers? For the most part, the properties of laser light (i.e. coherence) are irrelevant in so far as the way light interacts with skin in therapeutic applications. This contention is supported by the increasing use of filtered flashlamps in dermatology. Four properties are common to all laser types: (1) beam directionality; (2) narrow beam divergence; (3) spatial and temporal coherence of the beam; and (4) high intensity of the beam.[8]

The greatest advantages of laser light are intensity and monochromaticity, which allow a degree of precision that is hard or impossible to reproduce with nonlaser sources. The beam of the laser is easy to manipulate. The beam can, for example, be expanded or focused quite easily. On the other hand, with nonlaser sources like flashlamps, it is physically impossible for the brightness at the skin surface to exceed the brightness of the source lamp. By contrast, lasers can create extremely high-intensity light because of the property of stimulated emission. With many lasers, a lamp similar to the intense pulsed light (IPL) flashlamp pumps the laser cavity. The amplification of the light within the cavity sets laser light apart from other sources.

Laser is really a fancy way to convert lamplight to a more powerful monochromatic form.[9] The high power possible with lasers (especially 'peak power') is not attainable with other sources. For many dermatology applications requiring millisecond (ms) or longer pulse deliveries to large skin areas, IPLs are either adequate or preferable to lasers. The ability to focus the laser beam is an important contributor to the peak power density of the laser. Very small beam angles, which are not possible with intrinsically divergent nonlaser light sources (i.e. IPL),[10] can be obtained with laser.

With respect to lasing media, there are diode lasers, solid-state lasers, and gas lasers. An example of a solid-state laser is the neodymium (Nd) laser. These lasers typically have a solid rod that is pumped by a flashlamp (Fig. 1.3). Miniaturized diode and diode-pumped Nd lasers have become more powerful and popular. Some diode lasers are housed separate from the handpiece and delivered by fiber optics (Fig. 1.4). Others are configured with the laser diodes in the handpiece (Fig. 1.5). Modern diode lasers are capable of much higher powers than in past years but their peak powers are still limited compared to most pulsed solid-state lasers.[11]

Intense pulsed light devices are becoming increasingly popular and increasingly comparable to lasers that emit ms domain pulses.[12–18] Absorption spectra of skin chromophores are broad and therefore a broadband light source is a logical approach for cosmetic applications. Rather than using a xenon flashlamp to pump a laser, these devices use

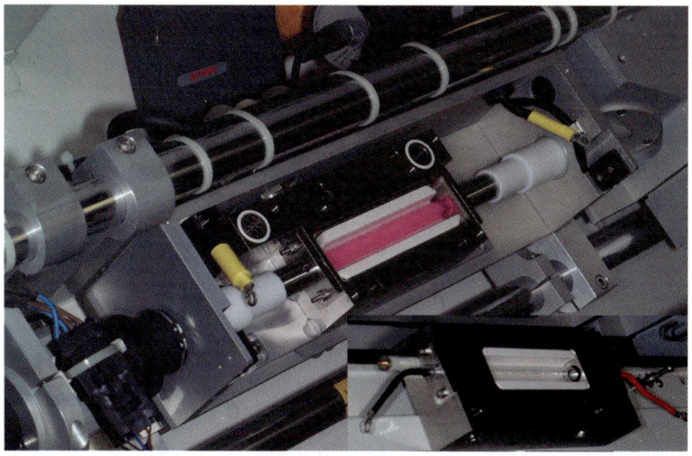

Figure 1.3 Ruby rod attached to high-power voltage. Flashlamp assembly is adjacent to rod. Normally the lamp is attached atop the rod assembly. Mirror allows the rod to be excited circumferentially.

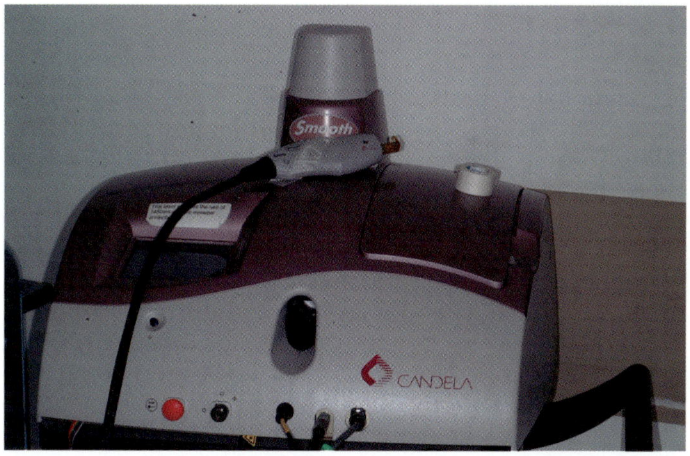

Figure 1.4 Diode laser where the diode light is coupled into fiber that is attached to the handpiece.

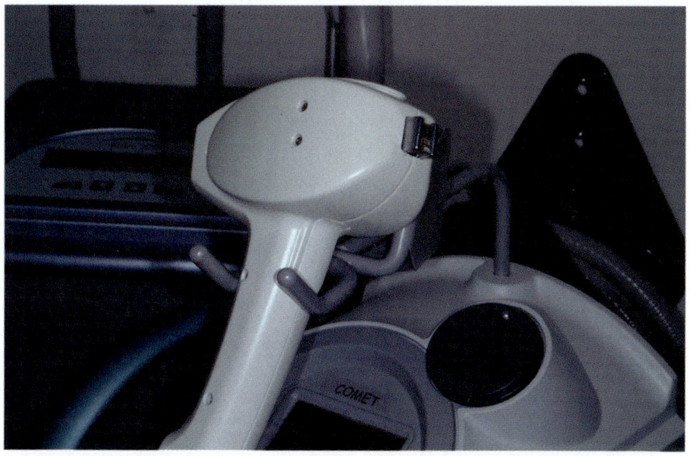

Figure 1.5 Another diode laser; in this case the diodes are in the handpiece. This configuration allows for more direct application of laser light. However, placement of diodes in the handpiece requires that 'high voltage' and laser cooling be attached to the handpiece by larger 'umbilical' cord.

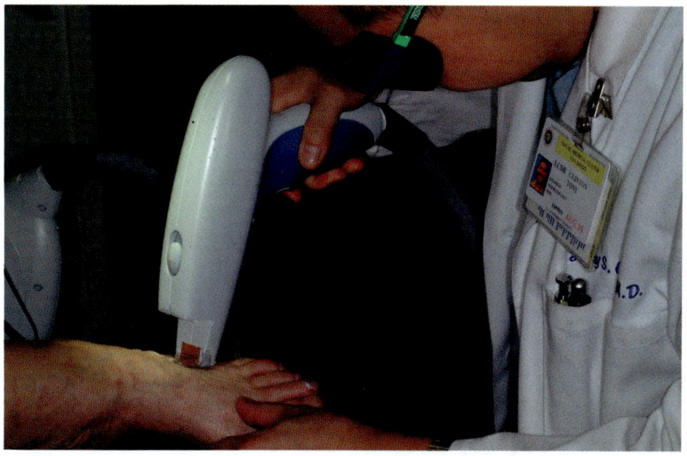

Figure 1.6 Q-switched laser pumped by flashlamp in IPL device. The laser rod is in the handpiece.

the lamp directly. Appropriate filtration creates a desired output spectrum for a particular application. Much like a slide projector with a specific color slide, these bright lamps produce spectra that overlap the absorption spectra of melanin, hemoglobin, and/or water. The advantages of these devices are their flexibility; a disadvantage is that one must hold the lamp, cooling apparatus, and the high-voltage wires all in one's hand. This creates a larger 'umbilical cord' and heavy handpiece compared with most laser devices. Also, the beam diverges quickly and is not optically as easily manipulated as laser beams. High-energy short pulses (Q-switched ns pulses, for example) are not possible with flashlamps. They can, however, be used to pump a Q-switched laser and newer IPLs have featured a Q-switched laser attachment (Fig. 1.6). In general, the size, weight, and cost of both laser and flashlamp technology are steadily decreasing.

Basic parameters for any procedure using EMR are power, time, and spot size for continuous wave (CW) lasers; for pulsed lasers they are the energy per pulse, pulse duration, spot size, fluence, repetition rate, and the total number of pulses.[19] Energy is measured in joules (J) The amount of energy delivered per unit area is the fluence, sometimes called the dose or radiant exposure, given usually in J/cm^2. The rate of energy delivery is called power, measured in watts (W). One watt is one joule per second (W = J/s). The power delivered per unit area is called the irradiance or power density, usually given in W/cm^2. Laser exposure duration (called pulsewidth for pulsed lasers) is the time over which energy is delivered. Dermatology uses EMR exposures ranging from many seconds to nanoseconds. Fluence is equal to the irradiance times the exposure duration.[20] Power density is one of the most important parameters, for it often determines the action mechanism in cutaneous applications (Fig. 1.7). For example, a very low irradiance (typical range of 2–10 mW/cm^2) does not markedly increase tissue temperature and is associated with diagnostic applications, photochemical processes, and biostimulation. On the other extreme, a very short nanosecond (ns) pulse can generate high peak power densities associated with photomechanical effects and even

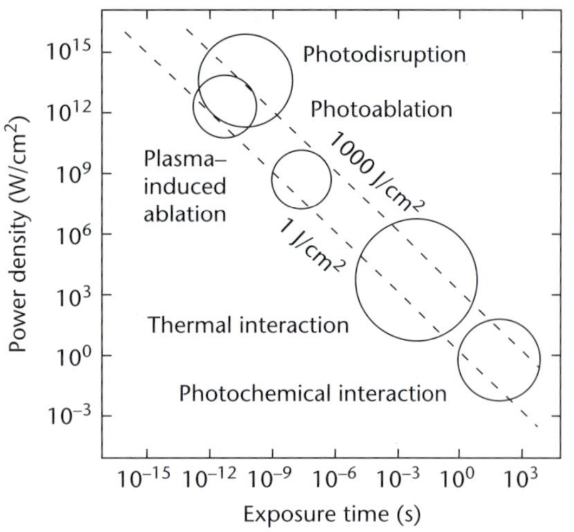

Figure 1.7 The relative mechanisms of action as a function of power density ranges. (Modified from Boulnois JL et al, Photophysical processes in recent medical developments. Lasers in Medical Science 1986; 1:47–66. With kind permission of Springer Science and Business Media.)

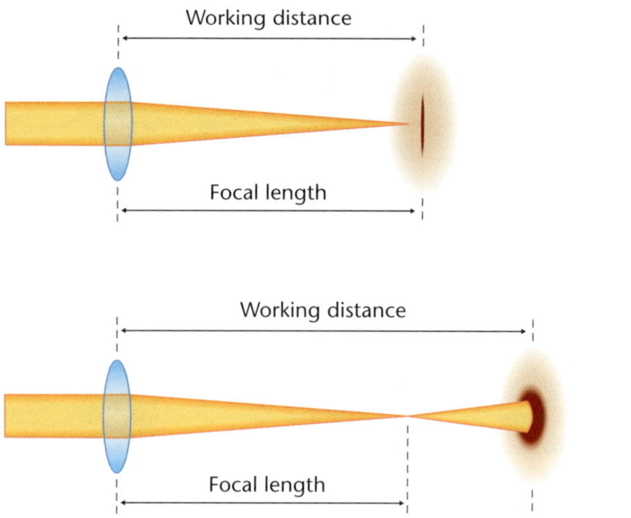

Figure 1.9 A focusing handpiece like that typically used with continuous wave CO_2 laser. Operator can vary spot size and therefore power density 'on the fly' simply by moving the handpiece away and toward the skin surface.

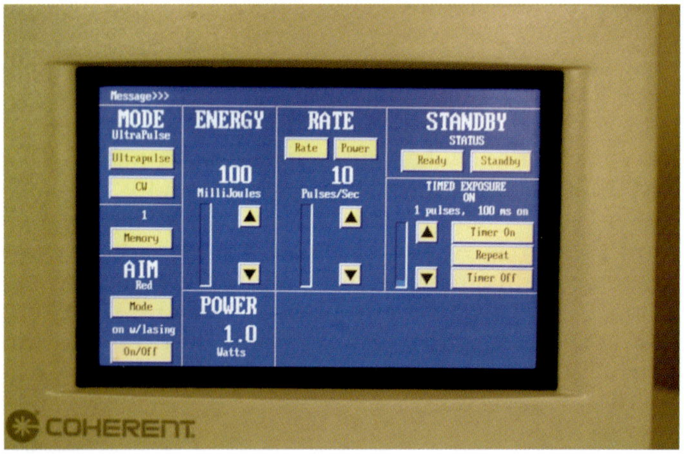

Figure 1.8 Instrument panel of a common CO_2 laser. The panel is intuitive once the operator is experienced.

plasma formation.[21] Plasma is a 'spark' due to ionization of matter. Other important factors are the laser spot size (which greatly affects intensity inside the skin), whether the incident light is convergent, divergent, or diffuse, and the uniformity of irradiance over the exposure area (spatial beam profile). The pulse profile, that is, the character of the pulse shape in time (instantaneous power versus time) is another feature that can impact the tissue response.[19]

One of the challenges is understanding all these terms within the context of a specific device and specific clinical situation. When the novice confronts a laser instrument panel, there is often a grimace born of confusion. The staggering array of options on some user interfaces can be overwhelming (Fig. 1.8). Many physicians would prefer to have fewer options and a simpler display, especially early on in their use of a particular laser. However, like the driver who feels confined by an automatic transmission, the experienced laser surgeon usually wants the flexibility of adjusting many parameters. Some manufacturers have accommodated both types of users, providing preset parameter sets (and 'go-bys') while still allowing for experienced physicians to choose parameter configurations of their liking. Those who *only* use preset parameters are unlikely to provide optimum safety *and* efficacy.

Most lasers in modern skin surgery are pulsed, and the instrument panel fields are given in terms of pulse duration and fluence. Also, the spot size is often adjustable and displayed. Multi-wavelength or tunable wavelength lasers are also available. However, some lasers, for example a popular CO_2 laser, provide only the pulse energy on the panel, or in CW mode, the number of watts. Likewise, our photodynamic therapy (PDT) system (a potassium-titanyl-phosphate (KTP)-pumped 630-nm dye laser) gives the display in 'watts'. In these cases one uses the exposure area and exposure time to calculate the total light dose (fluence).

$$\text{Fluence} = \left(\frac{Power \times time}{area}\right)$$

It is helpful in these cases to attach a dosimetry table on the side of the laser showing different fluences for the various spot sizes and exposure times.

With CW sources, the user must know the spot size, exposure time, and power density to determine the fluence. In many CW applications (i.e. wart treatment with a CO_2 laser), the fluence is not too helpful in characterizing the overall tissue effect. One normally observes tissue vaporization and coagulation in real-time and suspends the procedure when an appropriate endpoint is reached. On the other hand, in PDT applications with CW light, the total fluence and power density are very important in predicting tissue responses.

For CW mode, CO_2 lasers are typically used with a focusing (noncollimated) handpiece. This allows the operator to control spot size and tissue effects simply by moving the handpiece tip toward or away from the skin (Fig. 1.9). For the accomplished laser surgeon, particularly in ablative

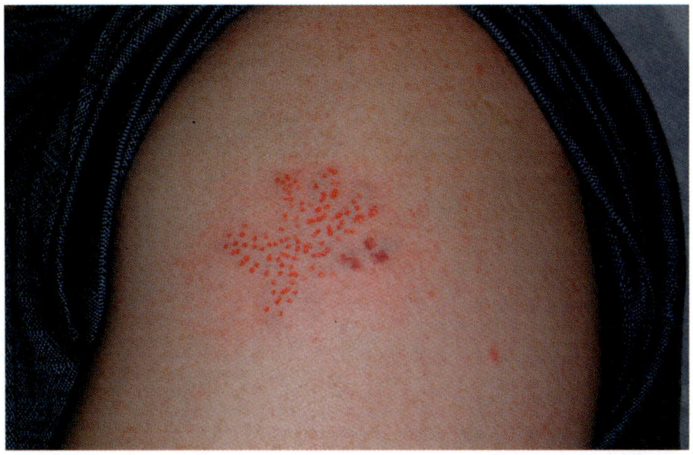

Figure 1.10 Immediate postoperative result on tattoo on shoulder. In this case the operator inadvertently moved the toggle 'spot size' switch from 4 to 2 mm. Fluence in 532 Q-switched mode increased from 3 to 12 J/cm^2 (fourfold increase). This resulted in loud snap and punctate bleeding.

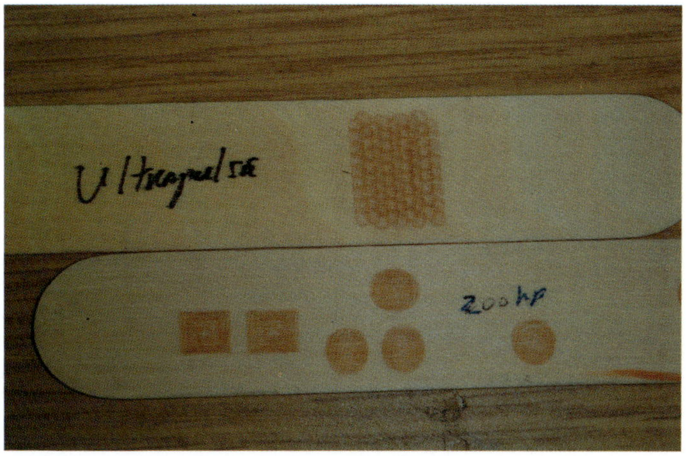

Figure 1.11 Scan pattern with two CO_2 lasers. Both patterns show uniform coverage. Scanners appear to be working properly.

applications for small lesions, this classic CO_2 laser configuration offers 'on the fly' flexibility and control not available with more modern locked-in spot sizes and fluences.

'Enlightened' laser practitioners should know their particular devices in detail. For example, some lasers 'know' what spot size is being used (e.g. insertion of the handpiece into the calibration port will signal the spot size to the laser), whereas with others you select the spot size on the display and the laser calculates the fluence accordingly. For example, one of our Q-switched lasers has a toggle that allows us to choose 2, 4, or 6 mm spots. However, the handpiece does not communicate the spot size to the laser control system. The user 'tells' the laser what spot size is to be used and the laser calculates the fluence based on this user input. In this case, if one mis-sets or inadvertently changes the spot size (for example, by accidentally moving the toggle to the 2 mm from the 4 mm spot), the laser still 'thinks' the 4 mm spot is being used, so that the actual surface fluence is now 4 × fluence on the panel. The resulting small spot, which impacts the skin with a loud snap and punctate bleeding, should alert the savvy operator that something is amiss (Fig. 1.10). The operator can then examine the device and ensure that all the knobs are in the proper position before proceeding. The reader should note that if the tissue response looks unusual there is probably a problem and the physician should do a laser 'walkaround' before proceeding (akin to the pilot who dutifully checks the exterior of his plane before taking off). Most newer lasers allow for calibration through the end of the handpiece. This configuration allows for interrogation of the entire system, from the lamps to the fiber to the handpiece optics. This setup ensures that any problem is identified before patient care. For example, if a fiber is damaged, the laser will be unable to 'make' calibration, and a failure message appears on the panel.

There are some quick and dirty, but not infallible, ways to check for system integrity. One can examine the aiming beam as it illuminates a piece of white paper, checking that the beam edges are sharp (usually the aiming beam and treatment beam are following the same optical path). This suggests that the treatment beam is also sharp and the profile is according to the manufacturer's specifications. Also, burn paper can be used – here the laser is used with a low energy and the spot is checked for uniformity from beam edge to edge. With FIR lasers (erbium:yttrium-aluminum-garnet (Er:YAG) and CO_2), a tongue depressor can be used. This is especially useful for Er:YAG and CO_2 lasers, where calibration is typically carried out only internally. It follows that by checking the impact pattern on wood, one can uncover damaged mirrors in the knuckle of the articulated arm, or a bad focusing lens that renders the laser unstable or unsafe. Likewise, for scanners, it is wise to check the tongue depressor with FIR lasers to ensure that skin coverage will be uniform (Fig. 1.11).

Beam Profiles: Top Hat Versus Gaussian

Laser beam profiles can be of various shapes: the Gaussian profile is common. This has the shape of a bell curve and is the fundamental mode of most lasers (Fig. 1.12). One often sees this shape when the beam has been delivered through an articulated arm (with mirrors at the knuckles). For some wavelengths, this is still the most effective way to deliver energy (CO_2 and erbium). The disadvantage of the arm is the limited motion and the counterweight of the arm pulling against the surgeon's hand.[11] The Gaussian profile is often disparaged as an inferior profile for lasers. In many applications, the criticism is well founded. For example, in treating a lentigo with a typical Q-switched ruby laser, one will often observe complete ablation of the epidermis at the center of the 'spot' but only whitening at the periphery. On the other hand, sometimes a bell-shaped profile is desirable, for example, when applying a small spot FIR beam with a scanner. In this scenario, the wings of the beam allows for some overlap without delivering 'too much' energy at points of overlap (see Fig. 1.11).

In most applications, a flat top profile is desirable, and with many fiber delivery systems this is the case, as the beam is mixed by the multiple internal reflections within

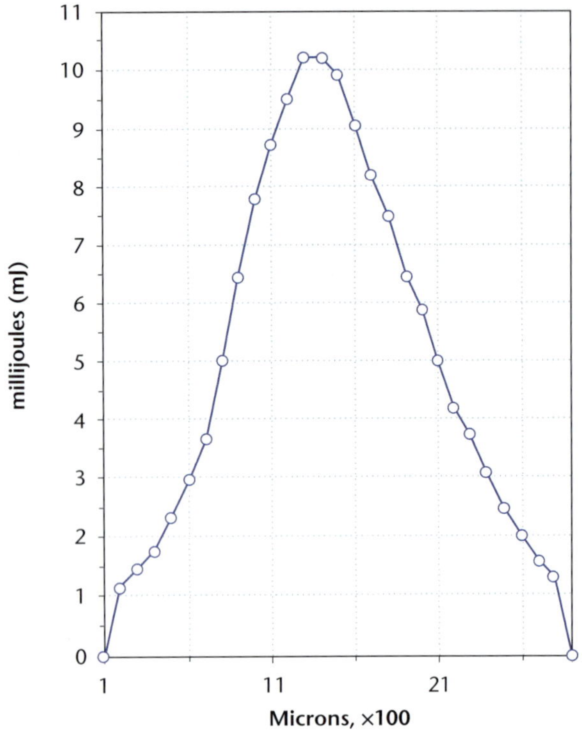

Figure 1.12 Gaussian beam profile of a popular CO_2 laser, as measured by author.

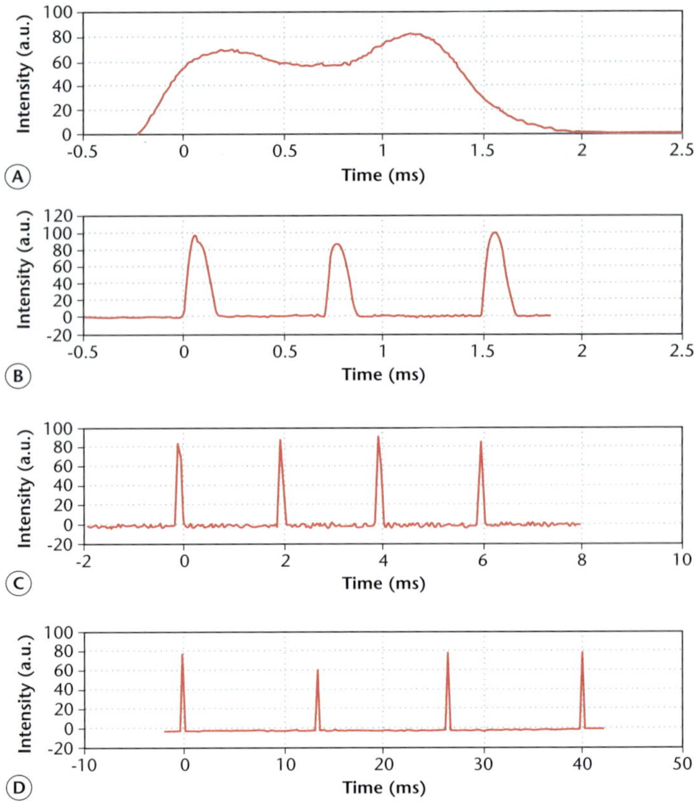

Figure 1.13 Various pulse profiles for pulsed dye laser. A. Scleropus 1.5 ms; B. V-Beam 1.5 ms; C. V-Beam 6 ms; D. V-Beam 40 ms. a.u. = Arbitrary units.

the fiber. Fibers have become increasingly popular with VIS, NIR lasers and MIR lasers. Some high peak power Q-switched lasers exceed fiber damage thresholds such that articulated arms are still required.

Pulse Profiles: Square Versus Spiky

The pulse profile is the temporal shape of the laser pulse (Fig. 1.13).[22] Many laser physicians assume that, for example, a 10 ms pulse with a pulse dye laser comprises a single burst of energy. In fact, in many pulsed laser applications, and particularly the pulse dye laser, the 'macro pulse' is composed of several smaller pulses.[23] Depending on the application, the temporal pulse profile may impact the tissue effect. For example, we recently evaluated various pulse durations in the treatment of leg veins with a neodymium YAG laser. We found, for example, that when applying a 40-ms macropulse, where the micropulses were delivered in four 'installments' versus 14 installments, the purpura threshold did not change. However, a very different response was observed in the application of green–yellow light. Purpura thresholds in this wavelength range are much lower, making the tissue response more susceptible to subtle changes in the pulse structure. For example, in our own experience and that of others,[24] even with longer pulse PDLs, purpura (both inside the vessel and extending throughout the spot) are more likely after PDL than KTP lasers. Although both lasers generate pulse trains, the PDL delivers the energy in very energetic narrow spikes whereas the long pulse KTP lasers deliver a smoother temporal pulse profile.[22] The spiky pulse profile is more likely to cause immediate thrombosis and vessel rupture versus the smooth pulse profile, which is more likely to contract the vessel wall. We have observed that even by extension of the macropulse duration with the PDL (125 μs micropulse width) up to 20 ms, fluences sufficient to achieve vessel contraction or persistent bluing (two typical endpoints for effective vessel reduction), there is still a risk for immediate or delayed purpura. On the other hand, with the IPL, even when configured with pulse trains, the micropulses are usually over 2 ms long (macropulse width about 20–30 ms), and the IPL is not normally associated with purpura. This suggests that there is a critical difference in purpura threshold for this wavelength range (500–600 nm) between 125 and 2000 μs micropulse durations, regardless of the total macropulse length.

Molecular Basis of Laser–Tissue Interactions

Most devices that have been developed for cosmetic rejuvenation are based on photothermal or 'electrothermal' mechanisms, that is, the conversion of light or electrical energy to heat. Two fundamental processes govern all interactions of light with matter: absorption and scattering. Besides scattering and absorption, photons can be totally internally reflected at a tissue–air interface, or they can be remitted out of the tissue (Fig. 1.14).[5,19] Absorption and excitation are necessary for all photobiologic effects and laser–tissue interactions. Plank's law describes how much energy is invested in one photon as a function of

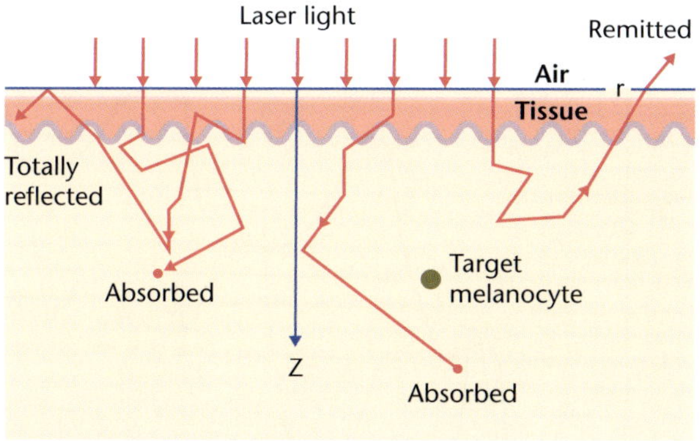

Figure 1.14 The behavior of light at and just below skin surface.

wavelength. Energy is proportional to frequency and inversely proportional to wavelength. Thus a 532nm photon (532nm is the distance between two of the transverse waves in a stream of light) is twice as energetic as a 1064nm photon.[6,25,26] When absorption occurs, the photon loses its energy to an atom or molecule, known as a chromophore. Upon absorption, the photon ceases to exist and the chromophore becomes excited; it may undergo photochemistry or may dissipate the energy as either heat or reemission of light (e.g. fluorescence). The probability that absorption will occur depends on specific transitions between allowed electron orbitals or molecular vibration modes. Thus chromophore molecules exhibit characteristic bands of absorption around certain wavelengths.[20]

The molecular basis of LTIs is based on electronic transitions for the UV and VIS wavelengths. However, NIR wavelengths and beyond are absorbed via rotational and vibrational excitations in biomolecules (all of which are hydrocarbons with the exception of pigments). The reactions can be considered a two-step process. In the first, the molecule is brought to an excited state. Then, through a process known as nonradiative decay, there are inelastic collisions with nearby molecules, giving rise to an increase in kinetic energy and therefore temperature. The temperature rise results from the transfer of photon energy to kinetic energy. In most biological systems, tissue constituents show broad absorption bands with only a few distinct absorption peaks. Leon Goldman[27] noted years ago that the biggest difference between tissue necrosis with laser and nonlaser devices, such as high-frequency electrical current, was the specificity of the reaction for color. For example, unlike the electric needle, only the darkly pigmented areas strongly absorb laser radiation in the VIS and NIR range. Thus the heterogeneity of the skin (in this case, melanin in small concentrations in tissue water) allows for selective heating with chromophore-specific wavelengths.[28]

From 200 to 290nm (UVC), light is absorbed by all cellular constituents[2] and all biological objects (cells and tissue) absorb energy very strongly. From 290 to 320 (UVB) nm, only a limited number of biomolecules show absorption (aromatic amino acids and nucleic acids). For UVA (near UV) 320–400nm, light is weakly absorbed by colorless skin parts. From 400nm to 1000nm only very few

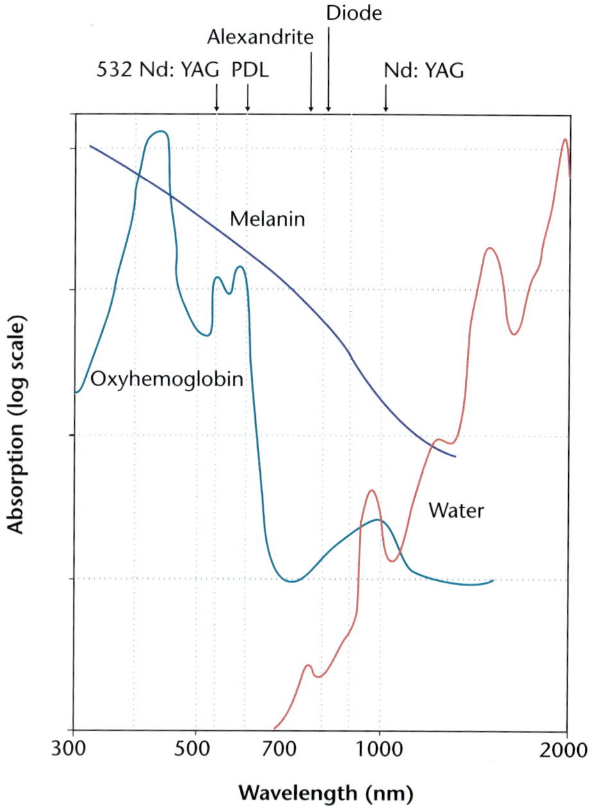

Figure 1.15 Absorption spectra of three major skin chromophores.

biomolecules absorb (mainly pigments – bilirubin, blood, melanin). But it is over this wavelength range that the heterogeneity of the skin allows for discrete heating and therefore most of the magical properties of laser. For >1100nm, all biomolecules have specific strong vibrational absorption bands. The principal absorber is tissue water, and all processes are guided by absorption of tissue water.

The absorption spectra of major skin chromophores dominate laser tissue interactions in dermatology. The absorption coefficient (μ_a) is the probability per unit path length that a photon at a particular wavelength will be absorbed. It is therefore measured in units of 1/distance and is typically designated μ_a, given as cm^{-1}. The absorption coefficient depends on the concentration of chromophores present. Skin contains pigments and distinct microscopic structures that have different absorption spectra[5] (Fig. 1.15).

If tissues were clear, then only absorption would be required to characterize light propagation in skin. However, the dermis is white because of light scatter. Scattering is responsible for much of the light's behavior in the skin (beam dispersion, spot size effects, etc). The main scattering wavelengths are between 400 and 1200nm, where the average distance a photon travels between two scattering events is between 0.05 and 0.2mm. Whereas absorption occurs where the frequencies of the wavelength equal the natural frequency of the free vibrations of the particles (absorption is associated with resonance),[4] scattering takes place at frequencies not corresponding to those natural frequencies of particles.[4] The resulting oscillation is

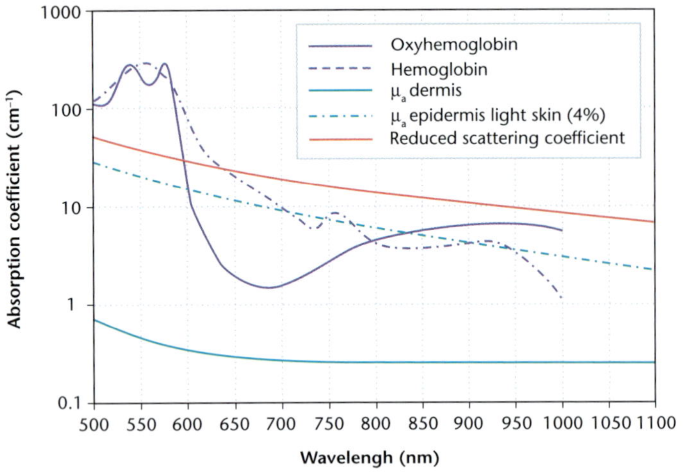

Figure 1.16 Hemoglobin (Hb) absorption versus bloodless dermis. Note that Hb absorption always exceeds bloodless dermis. μ_a, absorption coefficient.

determined by forced vibration. Scattering is decreased as wavelength increases. In most biological tissues it has been found that photons are preferably scattered in the forward direction.

There are three chromophores of interest (water, blood, and melanin). Water makes up about 65% of the dermis and lower epidermis. There is some water absorption in the UV. Between 400 and 800 nm, water absorption is quite small (which is consistent with our real-world experience that light propagates quite readily through a glass of water). Beyond 800 nm, there is a small peak at 980 nm, followed by larger peaks at 1480 nm and 1060 nm. The water maximum is 2940 nm (Er:YAG).

Hemoglobin

There is a large HbO_2 (oxyhemoglobin) peak at 415 nm, followed by smaller peaks at 540 and 577 nm. An even smaller peak is found at 940 nm. For deoxyhemoglobin (deoxyHb), the peaks are at 430 and 555 nm. Because of the discrete peaks of hemoglobin absorption, the laser physician can optimize heating of the vessel with excellent protection of the surrounding structures. Figure 1.16 illustrates the multiple opportunities for selectively heating blood vessels. Conjugated double bonds in their structure are responsible for the absorption of deoxyHb and HbO_2 by VIS light.[3]

Melanin

Most pigmented lesions result from 'too' much melanin in the epidermis. By choosing almost any wavelength (<800 nm), one can preferentially heat epidermal melanin (see Fig. 1.15). Shorter wavelengths will tend to create very high superficial epidermal temperatures, whereas longer wavelengths tend to bypass epidermal melanin (i.e. 1064 nm).

Fat

Fat shows strong absorption at 1200 and 1700 nm (Fig. 1.17). Although the ratios of fat to water absorption are small, the small differences could be exploited with the proper choice of parameters (or possibly through interstitial therapy).

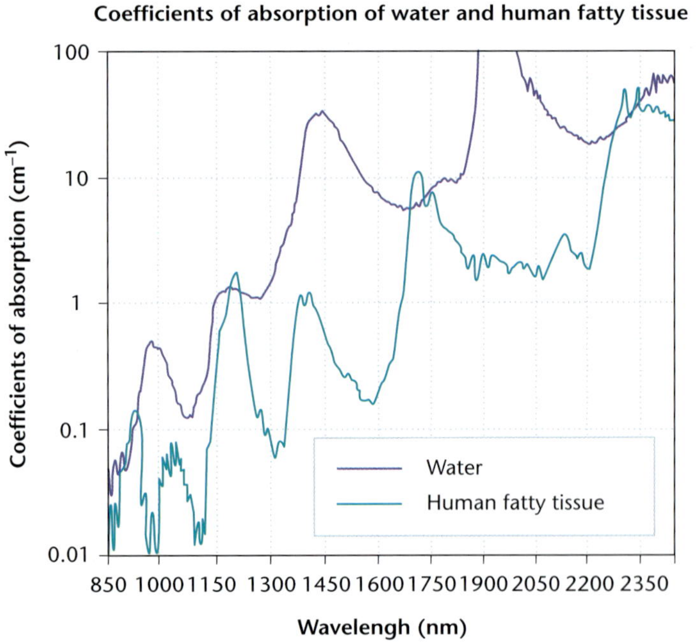

Figure 1.17 Water and fat absorption curves.

Carbon

Carbon is not *per se* a chromophore but rather a product of prolonged skin heating. Once carbon is formed at the skin surface, the skin become 'opaque' to most laser wavelengths (that is, most energy will be absorbed very superficially). It follows that the dynamics of surface heating changes immediately once carbon is formed. This can be used creatively as an advantage. For example, one could use a layer of carbon paper to convert a deeply penetrating laser to one that would only affect the surface. If the pulse were short enough, a 694 nm laser, for example, could optically act as a CO_2 laser![29]

Collagen

Dry collagen shows absorption peaks near 6 and 7 μm. With a free electron laser, these peaks can be exploited for selective molecular targeting. In this manner, collagen is directly heated rather than relying on heat conduction due to its close bonds to tissue water (where Er:YAG and CO_2 lasers work). Ellis et al found that this approach provided more efficient resurfacing and might allow for less tissue irradiation and less thermal damage than CO_2 laser.[30]

Selective Photothermolysis

With the exception of water, heating in the skin is based on discrete heating by chromophores of relatively low concentration (i.e. melanin, hemoglobin). Dr R Anderson described the concept of selective photothermolysis more than 20 years ago.[25] Although Dr Leon Goldman argued for color as a means to selectively damage dermal targets as early as 1963, selective photothermolysis (SPT) offered an elegant and mathematically rigorous rationale for developing different tissue-selective lasers. As described by Dr Anderson, extreme localized heating achieved with selective photothermolysis relies on: (1) a wavelength that reaches and is preferentially absorbed by the desired target structures; (2) an exposure duration less than or equal to the time necessary for cooling of the target structures; and (3) sufficient energy to damage the target. The heterogeneity of the skin allows for very selective injury in thousands of microscopic targets. Unlike tracing out blood vessels with an electric needle (or using a CO_2 laser on a wart), the laser surgeon can apply a large light beam without the need to aim at the target. The effect is like the legendary 'magic bullet', which seeks only the desired target. In contrast to gross thermal injury, selective photothermolysis (with discrete targets, i.e. melanin and Hb) allows for focal heating with large volumes of undamaged skin between chromophores. The focal nature of the heating decreases the likelihood of catastrophic pancutaneous thermal damage. Because temperature elevations are localized, there is often less pain than with devices targeting tissue water.

Thermal Relaxation Time

In simple terms, the thermal relaxation time (τ) is the time it takes for a target to cool to a certain percentage of its peak temperature.[25] We know from experience that larger volumes require longer times than smaller volumes to cool. For example, a tubful of warm bathwater requires about 1 hour to cool to room temperature, whereas a thimbleful requires only a few minutes. In laser scenarios, we assume instantaneous heating of the target, so that τ is usually thought of as the time for cooling *after* the pulse. However, if the pulse is long, the target can cool during the pulse, akin to one pouring water into a leaky bucket. If the water represents heat, one observes that the bucket never fills (akin to a target never becoming very hot). If one wants to spatially confine heating one chooses a short pulse that coincides roughly with the τ of the chromophore. For the same volume, a sphere will cool faster than a cylinder, which will cool faster than a slab. When defining thermal relaxation time, one should consider the immediate target and the boundaries of the target. Normally, it is defined by:

$$\delta^2/g\kappa \qquad \text{(Eq. 1)}$$

where δ is the optical penetration depth for homogeneously absorbing layers (such as tissue water for IR applications). For discrete absorbers, i.e. the melanosome, τ is defined in terms of the particle size, and δ represents the diameter of the particle. κ is the thermal diffusivity, a quantity based on the thermal conductivity and specific heat of the medium, and 'g' is a constant based on the geometry of the target (slab, cylinder, or sphere).[31] See Table 1.1 for sample thermal relaxation times for common targets in skin.

The optical penetration depth of laser irradiation is defined as the depth where fluence is attenuated to 37% of

Table 1.1 *Thermal Relaxation Time of Some Potential Targets*

Target	Thermal Relaxation Time
Erythrocyte	2 μs
200 μm hair follicle	40 ms
0.5 μm melanosome	0.25 μs
10 μm nevus call	0.1 ms
0.1 mm diameter vessel	10 ms
0.4 mm diameter vessel	80 ms
0.8 mm diameter vessel	300 ms

its incident value. The often-used term 'thermal relaxation time of the skin' is meaningful only when used for specific wavelengths (or specific skin structures, i.e. the epidermis). For example, with a ubiquitous absorber such as tissue water, τ should be considered within the context of δ, not the dimensions of the skin constituents. For example, if one uses the 1540 nm laser, the entire epidermis and large portions of the dermis are heated, and τ is on the order of seconds, because δ is several hundred μm. So even though τ of the epidermis is about 10 ms on a dimensional basis, because a thick slab of skin is heated at 1540 nm, the 10 ms value is somewhat irrelevant. In this case, the epidermis will take several seconds to cool because there is no real gradient between its temperature and the dermis.

On the other hand, when establishing τ of the epidermis with the melanosome as the immediate chromophore, one can consider either the entire epidermis as the target (thickness of 80–100 μm), or the dermal epidermal junction (10 μm), or finally, the melanosome itself (1 μm diameter) when using melanin as chromophore. Each skin 'unit' will have its own respective τ. A Q-switched laser pulse will confine high temperatures to the melanosome. The upper epidermis is heated only after post pulse heat conduction away from the dermis–epidermis (DE) junction. On the other hand, in treating with a 10 ms 532 nm pulse, heat will diffuse freely from the melanosome during the pulse, resulting in more uniform epidermal heating. This diffuse and gentle epidermal heating may be desirable or undesirable depending on the specific clinical indication. Most importantly, the physician can titrate the degree of epidermal heating by manipulation of the pulse duration (Fig. 1.18).

When the pulse width (pw) is too short, pulses 'violently' vaporize targets, leading to substantial immediate or delayed vessel wall damage and hemorrhage in the treatment of vascular lesions.[26] With longer pulses, one can more gently heat targets without causing rupture of the vessels. On the other hand, the shortcoming with a long pulsed ruby laser for nevus of Ota is that the pigmented nevus cells cool off too fast during the delivery of the pulses; also, the very high fluence can damage the pigmented pidermis.[9]

For most tissue targets, a simple rule of thumb can be used: the thermal relaxation time in seconds is about equal

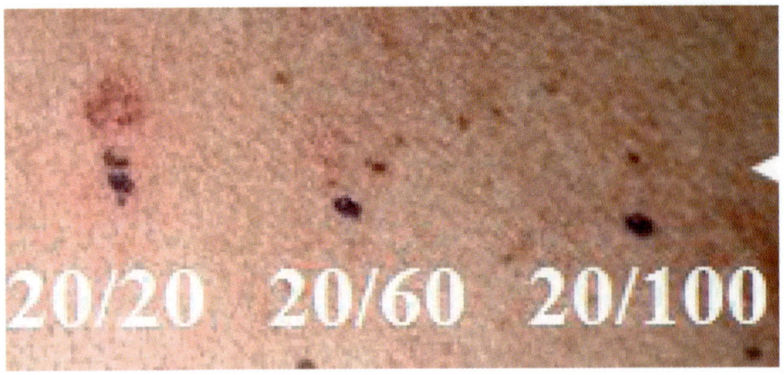

Figure 1.18 The impact of pulse duration on epidermis. The fluence was 20 J/cm^2 for all sites with an IPL. The second number at each site represents the pulsewidth in milliseconds. Note the decrease in epidermal damage as pulse duration increases.

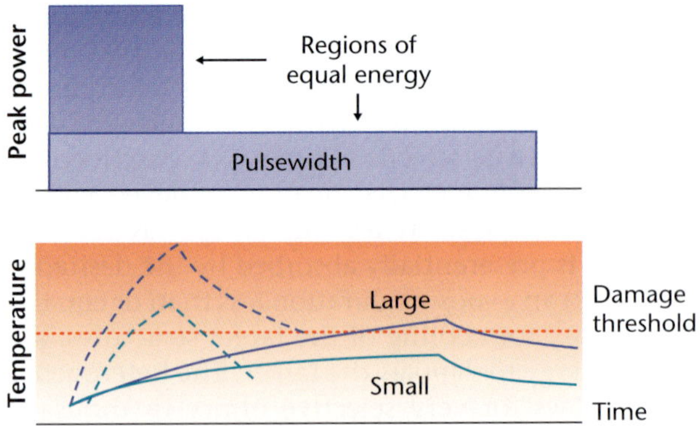

Figure 1.19 Relationship between size of target and pulse duration to peak temperature. The longer pulse favors heating of the larger target (blood vessel) versus the smaller melanosome.

to the square of the target dimension in millimeters. Thus a 0.5 μm melanosome (5×10^{-4} mm) should cool in about 25×10^{-8} second, or 250 ns, whereas a 0.1 mm PWS vessel should cool in about 10^{-2} second, or 10 ms. The natural variation of target sizes in tissue leads to an even greater variation in thermal relaxation times, such that much more precise calculations, although certainly possible, are probably unnecessary.[25] This is a feature that should be noted well by the reader. The τ is derived from a solution of the general heat equation. It follows that these values are not absolute cooling times but rather provide ballpark figures of pulse durations that achieve varying degrees of thermal confinement. Also remember that perfect thermal confinement is not always desirable, as gentle heating sometimes is a preferred method in cutaneous laser applications.

Two 'offshoots' of SPT are the concepts of thermal damage time and thermokinetic selectivity (TKS).

Thermal Damage Time

In some applications, the immediate chromophore and the final target are not collocated (i.e. hair shaft and hair bulb/bulge). In this case, thermal damage time is defined as the time required for irreversible target damage with sparing of the surrounding tissue. For a nonuniformly absorbing target structure, the thermal damage time is the time when the outermost part of the target reaches the target damage temperature through heat diffusion from the heater. In this case the eventual target and the heater (for example, hair shaft) are different and at a considerable distance from each other.[32] Using this model, the thermal damage time can be many times longer than the thermal relaxation time.

Thermal Kinetic Selectivity

Along the same lines is the concept of thermal kinetic selectivity (TKS). In this model, one selects larger or smaller targets based on pulse duration (Fig. 1.19). For example, if one wants to heat larger targets while sparing relatively smaller ones, the pulse duration is extended beyond the thermal relaxation time of the smaller target. In this manner, for example, a melanosome will be heated to a lower temperature than the subjacent vessel.

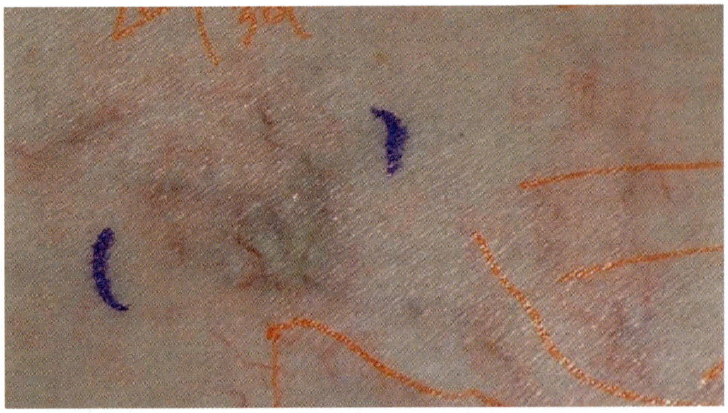

Figure 1.20 The effect of pulse stacking on skin overlying leg vein. Two previous pulses caused no effect, then immediate whitening was noted. Biopsy would show full thickness necrosis (treatment was with Nd:YAG laser).

Reaction Types

Photothermal

Most laser applications in dermatology rely on heating. Temperature is directly related to the average kinetic energy of molecules; as temperature is raised, tissue coagulates.[20] A familiar example of denaturation and coagulation is the cooking of an egg white. Thermal denaturation is both temperature and time dependent, yet it often shows an all-or-none like behavior. For a given heating time there is usually a narrow temperature region above which complete denaturation occurs; this is readily evident in Fig. 1.20. As a rule, for denaturation of most proteins, one must increase the temperature by about 10°C for every decade of decrease in the heating time to achieve the same amount of thermal coagulation.[20]

Photothermal processes depend on type and degree of heating, from coagulation to vaporization. A mild to moderate temperature increase results in breakage of hydrogen bonds and van der Waals bonds leading to denaturation of enzymes and function. If the heating is very fast, a phase change occurs.[28] Depending on the rate of energy delivery, photovaporization occurs with or without inertial confinement (see below), where time is short compared to the time for pressure relaxation. Here the laser induced pressure causes compressive stresses in tissue. Microcracks in the tissue are the result of these large stress gradients.[28]

Thermal Injury to Cells

There is a range of measurable effects on skin based on temperature. Below 43°C, the skin remains unharmed, even for very long exposures.[4] Thus one can exceed body temperature by about 5°C without a measurable change in the skin. The first change is a conformational change in the molecular structure. These typically occur at temperatures from 43 to 50°C. After several minutes, there will be tissue necrosis as described by the Arrhenius equation (an equation that quantitatively describes conversion of tissue from a native to denatured state). Thermal denaturation is a rate process: heat increases the rate at which molecules denature, depending on the specific molecule. For example, at 45°C, cultured human fibroblasts die after about 20 minutes. However, the same cells can withstand over 100°C for 10^{-3} seconds.[33] In general, a temperature of >60°C lasting for at least six seconds leads to irreversible damage.[4]

Coagulation

This is normally the first heating step that is identifiable on routine light microscopy. An absolute temperature for coagulation–denaturation does not exist. It appears that for very short times, higher temperatures than the oft-quoted '62–65°C' would be required. It is not known to what extent the Arrhenius formulation holds for very short heating times (less than 1 s).[34] In most scenarios of light–tissue interaction, tissues and cells may be reversibly or irreversibly damaged. Normally, pathologists examine tissue for changes such as vacuolization, hyperchromasia and protein denaturation (birefringence loss). Moderate temperature-induced damage phenomena in tissue have been difficult to assess with conventional methods of detection such as light microscopy. However, particularly in light of newer large volume low intensity heating devices for rejuvenation, more sensitive tools might be required to characterize subtle thermal effects. Beckham et al[34] found that over a narrow temperature range, heat shock protein (HSP) expression correlated with laser induced heat stress, and that the HSP production followed the Arrhenius integral. Thus HSP expression (in addition to tissue ultrastructure, i.e. EM) might be an excellent tool to examine low-intensity, high-volume heat injury.

Vaporization

At a certain threshold power density, coagulation gives way to vaporization. Often, this process is referred to as ablation and is an important component of laser skin resurfacing (LSR). At this higher power density (and higher fluence), water expands as it is converted to steam. Vaporization is beneficial in that much of the heat is carried away from the skin during the process.[4] The vaporization energy for water is approximately 2.4 kJ/cm^3. When there is vaporization there is also increasing pressure as the water tries to expand in volume. The expansion leads to localized microexplosions. At temperatures beyond 100°C (without further vaporization), carbonization takes place, which is obvious by blackening of adjacent tissue and the escape of smoke. Carbon is the ultimate end product of all living tissues being heated and carbon temperatures often reach up to 300°C.[35] Normally, this should be avoided, because the depth of tissue injury will extend well beyond the blackened skin surface. This is particularly true, for example, when treating a rhinophyma or performing LSR.

Photomechanical

With even more rapid heating, there is insufficient time for pressure relaxation. In this scenario there will be disassembly and microcracks in the tissue. On the other hand, with slow energy deposition, there will be no pressure increase. Mechanical damage plays an important role in selective photothermolysis with high-energy, submicrosecond lasers for tattoo and pigmented lesion removal. Inertially confined ablation occurs when there is high pressure at constant volume. In a very short pulse, the energy is invested so quickly one that there is no time for the pressure to be relieved. Under these conditions of inertial confinement, there is not enough time for material to move – this can lead to the generation of tremendous pressures.

Photochemical

Photochemical reactions are governed by specific reaction pathways, and are becoming increasingly important in dermatology.[4] The most common type of photodynamic action in dermatology is one where singlet oxygen is created. In the reaction, a photosensitizer is excited by a certain wavelength of light. In the presence of oxygen, oxygen is transformed from its triplet state, which is its normal ground state, to an excited singlet state. The excited singlet state oxygen reacts with biological molecules and often attacks plasma and intracellular membranes. The most common photosensitizer (PS) in dermatology is PpIX. This PS is formed by skin cells by the pro-drug, aminolevulinic acid (ALA). The proper combination of wavelength and power density will achieve the best results. Overall, most photochemical reactions proceed more efficiently with lower power densities, such that for example, the Blu-U light (DUSA, Vahalla, NY) will normally outperform a pulsed source (IPL, KTP, or PDL) for AKs with one treatment.[36] However, pulse light sources can theoretically also be used, and have proven useful in a range of skin disorders.[37,38] There is little endogenous photochemistry beyond 319 nm. Some exceptions are homoisomerization of bilirubin (450 nm) and singlet O_2 production by *P. acnes* porphyrins (similar absorption peaks as PpIX). Beyond 800 nm, photochemistry, even with exogenous photosensitizers or pro-drugs, is unlikely.

Pulsed Light Sources and PDT

It has been shown that lower irradiances demonstrate a more marked PDT effect for equivalent total light doses.[39] Although pulsed light sources have been shown to be as effective as CW sources in some experiments, the PDT effect was only equivalent if the light doses and average irradiances were similar. Most pulsed light sources in dermatology do not meet the theoretical PDT saturation threshold ($4 \times 10^8\,W/m^2$).[40] All of this suggests that an optimal pulsed light PDT configuration might require multiple passes with blue, green, yellow, or red light. The interval between passes should be designed such that the average irradiance is similar to that of CW devices with similar emission spectra.

Excimer Laser (308 nm)

The mechanism of action for the excimer laser (XeCl) is thought to be the same as narrow band UV therapy. There is an erythema action spectrum determined by plotting a reciprocal of the minimal erythema dose against wavelength. It appears a reduction in cellular proliferation most likely plays a part in ultraviolet radiation shorter than 320 nm. This range has a profound influence on epidermal cellular DNA synthesis and mitosis. In Parrish's original study in 1981, he showed that wavelengths between 300 and 313 nm were most effective.[41] It appears that the excimer laser works through an immunomodulatory way much like UVB. The precise chromophore is unknown. There may be a thermal component as well at fluences >800 mJ/cm^2.[42]

Biostimulation

Biostimulation is thought to belong to the group of photochemical interactions. However, the term 'biostimulation' has not been scientifically well defined. Most biostimulation studies involve low power lasers and have been a subject of controversy for decades. Typical fluences are in the range of one to 10 J/cm^2, and normally there is no acute temperature elevation. Some scientists define biostimulation by the absence of any thermal mechanism.[4] The most vexing problem about many biostimulation studies is the difficulty in assessing what is occurring at a clinical level (beyond the cell culture model). It is unknown if any features of laser light, coherence, monochromaticity, polarization, are really relevant for biostimulation.[4] One example of a recent 'biostimulation' device in dermatology is the Gentlewaves LED Photomodulation unit (Light BioScience, LLC, Virginia Beach, VA). This device uses 590 nm light in a high repetition rate and low power density to purportedly increase collagen synthesis and enhance facial tone. Cell culture work supports this concept.[43] However, more work clearly needs to be done in this arena of biostimulation. Is it really plausible to unlock the code for subcellular processes through low-level irradiation?

Plasma-induced Ablation

With very high power densities exceeding $10^8\,W/cm^2$, a phenomenon called optical breakdown occurs. With plasma-induced ablation, very clean and well-defined removal of tissue without evidence of mechanical or thermal damage can be achieved when choosing appropriate parameters. Plasmas are sometimes produced by laser tattoo removal, where one can observe a spark.[20,28] Also, there is a new resurfacing system that uses this fourth state of matter to target the skin surface. The plasma is created by an RF-excited nitrogen (N_2) gas, which is directed toward the skin. The plasma is above the surface, creating very high but superficially confined temperatures. The goal is to achieve damage to the skin surface with minimal residual thermal damage (RTD).

Skin Optics

The optical properties of human skin determine the penetration, absorption, and internal dosimetry of laser light in skin. The cosmetic surgeon can divide the skin into two main components: (1) the epidermis (primarily an absorber of visible light due to melanin); and (2) the dermis (which can be envisioned as a carton of milk with red dots in it). When one uses a laser, one should envision where the photons and/or electrical energy are going and where the primary heating is. The laser surgeon should memorize the absorption spectra of the main chromophores in planning the procedure and should remember that the optical properties of the skin are not static. For example, just a positional change in the arm will change the dermal blood fraction. Also, just a few minutes in the sun will increase the pigmentation index. Light–tissue interactions can be broken down into: (1) The transport of light in tissue; (2) absorption of light and heat generation in tissue; (3) localized temperature elevation in the target tissue (and denaturation of proteins); and (4) heat diffusion away from the target (Fig. 1.21).

The optical properties of the skin mimic those of a turbid medium intermixed with focal discrete visible and infrared light absorbers (blood, melanin, bilirubin, and dry collagen). There is absorption by proteins, nucleic acids, and other compounds in the UV spectrum, but outside of photochemistry, possibly with a blue light source, these light–tissue interactions are probably irrelevant for skin rejuvenation.

In any light–tissue interaction, the thermal or photochemical effects depend on the local energy density at the target. Surface fluence represents the energy per unit area incident on the skin. Once the light penetrates the surface, it undergoes a complex series of absorbing and scattering events. Characterization of the light pathways is best understood by thinking of the incident beam in terms of its constituent photons, where the photons statistically are either scattered or absorbed in a wavelength dependent fashion.[44] The probabilities of absorption or scattering (designated μ_a and μ_s, respectively) are determined by

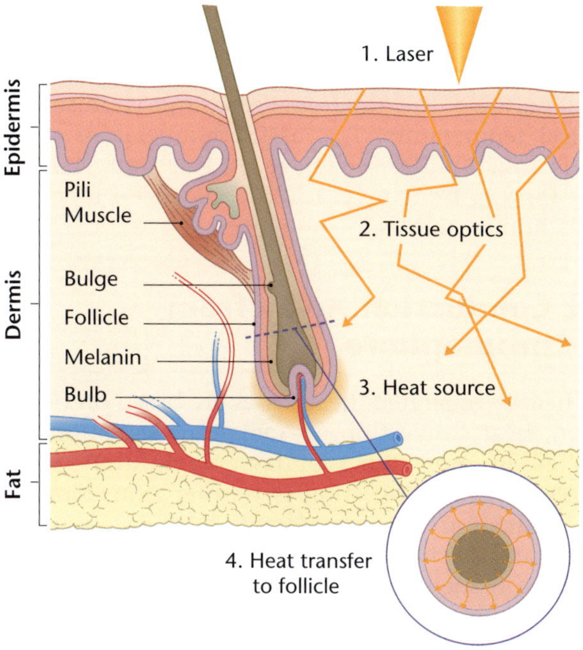

Figure 1.21 The cascade of events in typical laser–tissue interaction with discrete chromophore (in this case the hair follicle).

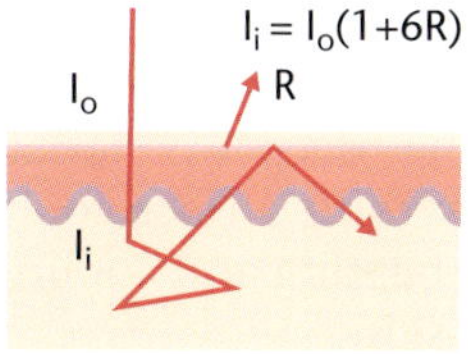

λ (nm)	R	I_i/I_o
585	0.3	2.8
694	0.6	4.6
1064	0.7	5.2

Figure 1.22 How backscattered light can result in subsurface fluence exceeding incident fluence. I_o is the surface fluence. R is the total light reflected from the skin for the respective wavelength. Note that ratio increases with wavelength over this range.

experiment. For a path length, L, the probability that a photon will not be absorbed or scattered is

$$e^{-\mu aL} \quad \text{(Eq. 2)}$$

Jacques notes that a typical bloodless tissue value for μ_a in the visible range is $1\,cm^{-1}$ and the mean free path of a photon is therefore 1 cm.[45] For most visible light, there are typically 100 scattering events before a photon is absorbed. As it turns out, the photon scatters roughly 10 times before it loses its orientation with respect to the initial direction as it migrates in a random walk. With scattering, there is backscattered light that augments the delivered irradiance to yield a higher fluence beneath the tissue than at the tissue surface[45] (Fig. 1.22). An often-used term is 'penetration depth' (δ), which describes the path length that causes light to be reduced to 37% of its surface irradiance. For a clear solution, δ accurately conveys the depth-dependent fluence attenuation. However, for turbid tissue like the dermis, where backscattering can be considerable, the 'real' penetration depth can be >δ. This value may be 2–3 × δ for example, with 1064 nm.[44–46] Different charts show different penetration depths in different bodies of literature. For example, in an article by Reinisch,[11] the optical penetration depths are somewhat larger than those in another article by Dr Rox Anderson.[6] The trends are the same in both articles, and neither chart is 'wrong'. The δ can change based on how it is defined. Therefore one will see a wide range of different values for similar wavelengths.

One should consider the choice of laser within the context of the application and the respective absorption and scattering coefficients. If the absorption coefficient is greater than $200\,cm^{-1}$, one typically is looking at a 'what you see is what you get' laser (examples are Er:YAG and CO_2). Between 1 and $200\,cm^{-1}$, one sees a wavelength range where lasers can sometimes be useful (i.e. PDL, KTP, alexandrite). Finally, when one considers $\mu_a < 1\,cm^{-1}$, we are typically dealing with deeply penetrating light sources where you can injure the skin without obvious surface changes (a 'what you don't see can hurt you' laser (an example is Nd:YAG).[21]

Beyond 600 nm, the increase in penetration and a brisk cut off in Hb absorption makes for a therapeutic window between 600 and 1200 nm. In this range radiation penetrates biological tissues at a lower loss thus enabling treatment of deeper tissue structures.[20] At times, the various skin pigments can play optical 'tricks' on the cutaneous surgeon. For example, poikiloderma appears to be a mix of hyperpigmentation and hypervascularity. In fact, although there is some melanin influence – the red–brown appearance – the dyschromia is by far more a disorder of matted telangiectasia. This is confirmed by the response of the condition to the PDL, even with surface cooling. Additionally, with diascopy, skin often appears no browner than the surrounding apparently normal skin. The explanation is that deoxyHb contributes to a 'pigmented skin appearance'. This finding follows from the absorption spectrum of deoxyHb in the 630–700 nm range, which is very similar to the absorption spectrum of epidermal melanin. The size of the vessels in the superficial venous plexus is such that the transmitted light through these vessels is approximately 50% lower than the incident intensity. These vessels therefore appear dark.[47]

Heat Generation

All laser–tissue interactions are guided by the same energy balance rules that guide all of physics. Heat generation can occur in one of two ways. In one scenario, it occurs at discrete chromophore sites. In this case, there is very precise localized heating consistent with the theory of selective photothermolysis. These hotspots under the skin allow for only the bad guys to be damaged. The good guys (normal skin), so long as the ratio of absorption coefficients (i.e. blood versus bloodless dermis) is high enough (optimally >10), remains unharmed. The primary areas where SPT is helpful in dermatology are the treatment of vascular lesions, tattoos, and pigmented lesions. However, even in applications where water is the chromophore, the principles of SPT are useful.[25] When treating by heating tissue water, the injury is typically from 'top to bottom', the exception being deeper-penetrating NIR and MIR wavelengths coupled with surface cooling. In this scenario, one can coordinate heating and cooling to damage specific slices of subsurface skin.

Once the local subsurface energy density has been determined using models, heat generation can be predicted by energy balance (conservation of energy) and the wavelength specific absorption for that target. Depending on the amount of thermal diffusion during the pulse, the local peak temperature can be determined. The temperature increase of a desired target can be roughly calculated by knowing the absorption and scattering coefficients, surface light dose, size of the target, and the length of the pulse, as follows:

$$\Delta T = \frac{F_z \mu_a}{\rho c}\left(\frac{\tau_r}{\tau_r + \tau_p}\right)^{g/2} \qquad \text{(Eq. 3)}$$

where Fz is the local subsurface fluence, rho is the density, c is the specific heat, g is a geometric factor (1 for planes, 2 for cylinders, and 3 for spheres), τ_p is the laser pulse duration, and τ_r is the thermal relaxation time of the target (time for target to cool to 37% of peak temperature), defined by Eq. 1 (see p. 9). Thus one can perform some quick algebraic calculations to estimate the peak temperatures of local targets in the skin.

Spatially selective temperature elevation is possible when: (1) the absorption coefficient of the target exceeds that of collateral tissue (selective photothermolysis); or (2) when the 'innocent bystander' tissues are cooled so their peak temperatures do not exceed some damage threshold. Localized heating, for example, in telangiectasias and lentigos, follows from the concentrations of blood and melanin there, respectively, such that μ_a is focally increased.

Coagulation

As noted above, denaturation depends on time and temperature and – at least over times greater than 1 s – appear to conform to a rate process as described by the Arrhenius equation (Fig. 1.23). The characteristic behavior of the Arrhenius-type kinetic damage model is that, below a threshold temperature, the rate of damage accumulation is negligible; it increases precipitously when this value is exceeded. This behavior is to be expected from the exponential nature of the function. Pearce and Thomsen define a critical temperature, T_{crit}, as the temperature at which there is roughly 100% damage in 1 second. A range of values for T_{crit} from 60°C to 85°C has been reported for various human tissues.[48]

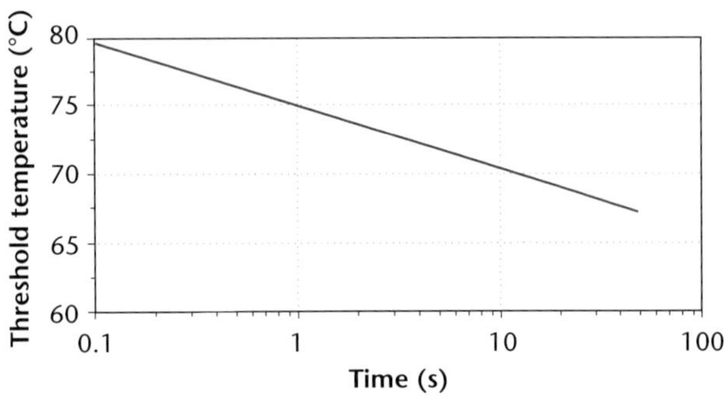

Figure 1.23 Denaturation as a function of t and T. t, time; T, temperature.

Heat Conduction Away from the Chromophore

Once heat is generated, heat losses are based on heat conduction, heat convection, or radiation. Radiation can be neglected in most types of laser applications. A good example of heat convection is transfer from blood flow. Heat conduction is a considerable heat loss term and is the primary mechanism by which heat is transferred to unexposed tissue structures.

Wavelength Ranges Useful for Cutaneous Surgery

UV Laser and Light Sources

UV laser and light sources have been used primarily for treatment of inflammatory skin diseases and/or vitiligo, as well as striae. The presumed action is immunomodulatory. The XeCl excimer laser emits at 308 nm, near the peak action spectrum for psoriasis. Other UV nonlaser sources have also been used for hypopigmentation, striae, and various inflammatory diseases.[49,50]

Violet IPL Spectra and Low-power 410 nm LED and Fluorescent Lamps

Both Violet IPL spectra and low power 410 nm LED and fluorescent lamps are used either alone or with ALA. Alone, the devices take advantage of endogenous porphyrins and kill *P. acnes*.[51–54] After application, of ALA, this wavelength range is highly effective in creating singlet O_2 after absorption by PpIX. Uses include treatment of actinic keratoses, actinic cheilitis, and basal cell carcinomas.[55]

Green-yellow (GY)

These wavelengths are highly absorbed by Hb and melanin and are especially useful in treating epidermal pigmented lesions and superficial vessels.[12,13,24,56–60] The relatively poor penetration in skin (and the even poorer penetration in blood; Table 1.2) make them poor choices for treatment of deeper pigmented lesions or of deeper larger vessels. The effective portions of many IPL spectra include the GY range. There are absorption peaks for PpIX in the green yellow range, making these wavelengths useful for PDT (i.e. sodium lamp, IPL, or PDL).[53,61]

Table 1.2 *Absorption Coefficients (cm^{-1}) for Various Chromophores*

Wavelength (nm)	410	532	595	694	755	810	940	1064
OxyHb (40% Hct)	1990	187	35	1.2	2.3	3.6	5.2	2.2
DeoxyHb	1296	138	96	6.6	5.2	2.7	3.0	0.6
Melanin*	140	56	38	23	17	13	7	5.7
Water	6.7×10^{-5}	0.00044	0.0017	0.005	0.03	0.02	0.27	0.15
Bloodless dermis	10	3	2	1.2	0.8	0.6	0.5	0.4
OPD in skin (μm)	100	350	550	750	1000	1200	1500	1700

*Net epidermis for moderately pigmented adult: 10% melanin volume fraction in epidermis[46,143]
DeoxyHb, deoxyhemoglobin; Hct, hematocrit; OPD, optical penetration depth; OxyHb, oxyhemoglobin

Near Infrared (A) (755–810 nm)

These two popular wavelengths are used primarily in hair reduction but have also been used to treat blood vessels and hyperpigmented lesions. They are positioned in the absorption spectrum for blood and melanin between the GY wavelengths and 1064 nm. They will penetrate deeply enough in blood to coagulate vessels up to 2 mm;[62,63] also, they are reasonably tolerant of epidermal pigment in hair reduction (with surface cooling) so long as very dark skin is not treated.[64]

Near Infrared (B) 940 nm and Nd:YAG

These two wavelengths have been used extensively for various sized vessels on the legs and face.[65–67] They occupy a unique place in the absorption spectrum of our 'big 3' chromophores (i.e. blood, melanin, and water). Because of the depth of penetration (the order of mm), they are especially useful for hair reduction and coagulation of deeper blood vessels. On the other hand, they are not well suited for epidermal pigmented lesions. Also, although water absorption is poor, it exceeds that of the VIS and near VIS wavelengths. The result is that 940 and 1064 nm can cause large volume mild temperature elevation in the skin, and with repeated laser impacts, because of the slow cooling of this volume (large τ), catastrophic pancutaneous thermal damage is possible. We observed this phenomenon when treating a piece of discarded tissue after Moh's surgery. After exposing the tissue to one, three, and six repeated exposures of Nd:YAG laser at 1 Hz, we noted widespread coagulation that occurred as an 'all or none' phenomenon between the 3rd and 6th pulses, consistent with the threshold behavior of protein denaturation (Fig. 1.24). This wavelength (1064 nm) represents the extreme example of a 'what you don't see can hurt you laser'.[21] They are extremely useful, but the user must develop an understanding of where this energy is going to effectively harness it and benefit his patients. One can appreciate firsthand that the neodymium laser penetrates deeply by taking a fingertip on one side of the ear and applying the laser to the opposite side of the lobe. The author promises a hot finger!

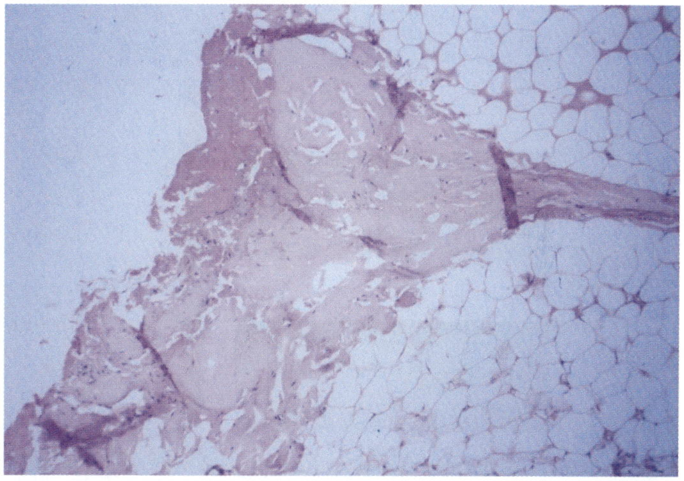

Figure 1.24 Full thickness necrosis in ex vivo sample after multiple pulses of a Nd:YAG laser.

MIR Lasers and Deeply Penetrating Lamps

These lasers and lamps heat tissue water. Depending on where we want to heat, we can 'choreograph' our laser and/or cooling settings to maximize the skin temperature in certain bands. In general, with more deeply penetrating wavelengths, larger volumes are heated. On the other hand, achieving temperature elevations in the volume will require higher fluences than with highly absorbing wavelengths. With more highly absorbing wavelengths, one will heat a tighter band of dermis. This is referred to as selective dermal heating. Accordingly, without surface cooling, unless very small fluences are applied, a top to bottom thermal injury occurs (Fig. 1.25). The absorption coefficients for the 1320, 1450, and 1540 nm systems are ~3, 20, and 8 cm^{-1} respectively,[68,69] while the effective scattering coefficients are about 14, 12, and 11 cm^{-1}. The corresponding penetration depths are ~1500 μm, 300 μm, and 700 μm. It follows that for equal surface cooling and equal fluences, the most superficial heating will occur with the 1450 nm laser, followed by the 1540 and 1320 nm lasers.

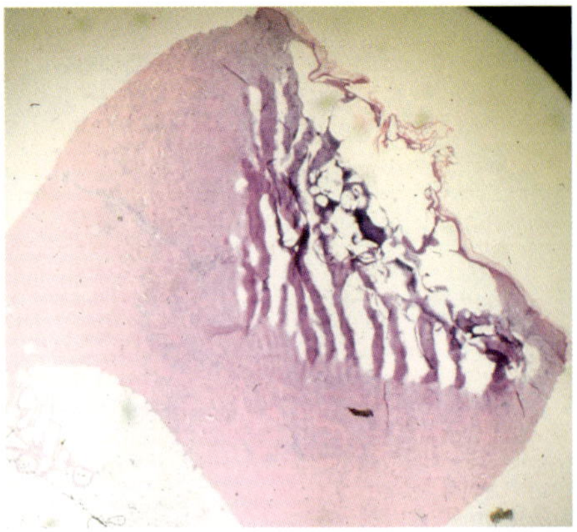

Figure 1.25 Effect in pigskin of a 1540 nm laser with a 2.5 mm spot without cooling and fluence of ~15 J/cm^2.

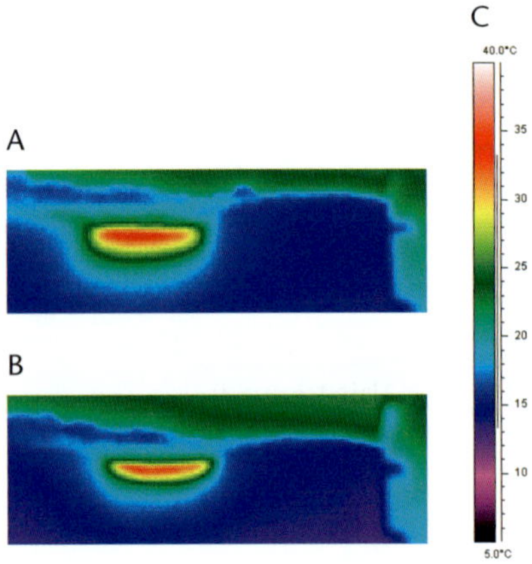

Figure 1.26 Heating bands with a mid-infrared heat lamp (Titan, Cutera, CA). By filtering out water, the depth and thickness of the heated slab increases.

The advantage of deeper penetration (i.e. less absorption) is that surface cooling does not need to be as aggressive. On the other hand, higher fluences must be applied and the peak temperature elevation will tend to be slightly deeper. Newer deeply penetrating lamps have been introduced (Titan, Cutera, Brisbasne, CA). They emit light over a 1–2 µm band with relatively low power densities and long exposures (several seconds). In a typical scenario, the irradiation begins after a roughly two second period of cooling. At this point, a band of tissue from roughly 700 µm to 1.5 mm deep in the skin is heated. By varying the fluence, this relatively large volume can be heated to different peak temperatures (Fig. 1.26). As part of each iteration, post-pulse cooling is included. This is because such a large volume of skin is heated that a 'thermal wake' is created of several seconds. It follows, that if one removes the handpiece too quickly, there is a tendency for heat to build up near the skin surface with the possibility of pain, dermal thermal injury, and scarring. One can make various arguments for large-volume deep subsurface heating versus heating a precise band of dermis more superficially (i.e. the deep papillary or superficial reticular dermis). As one attempts to confine heat superficially, a more highly water-absorbing mid-IR laser is optimal, but the counterpoint is that the cooling must also be confined superficially. It follows that, as one tries to heat superficially and spare the epidermis, the heating-cooling tandem must become ever more synchronized, lest one overheat the epidermis or overcool the dermis. On the other hand, with more penetrating wavelengths, heating will occur in the deeper dermis, often below the level of solar elastosis, the very pathology we presumably are trying to reverse. Despite the various modalities used in selective dermal heating, the degree of rhytid improvement typically seen after Er:YAG and CO_2 LSR has not been observed.[70] Even where fibroplasia is observed histologically, clinical improvement is often modest.[71] Several reasons for this apparent discrepancy are suggested. Although selective dermal heating can be achieved with deeply penetrating mid-IR lasers combined with topical cooling, the zone of heating in the dermis will always be broader and deeper than the fine band of basophilic staining denaturation observed with Er:YAG and far IR lasers. The wounds are quite dissimilar and if one creates a subepidermal zone of injury with the complete denaturation characteristics of the CO_2 laser, pitted scarring will be the likely result. Thus in mid-IR based NSR, one is substituting a larger volume of gentler heating for the precise and complete denaturation observed after typical short pulsed CO_2 LSR.

Far Infrared Systems

The major lasers are the CO_2 and Er:YAG lasers. Using models, as well as experiments, one can determine relative rates of ablation and heating.[31,72,73] Overall, the ratio of ablation to heating is much higher with the Er:YAG laser. However, one can extend the thermal field of the Er:YAG laser by extending the pulse or increasing the repetition rate, and likewise one can decrease the thermal field of CO_2 laser by decreasing pulse width or increasing fluence.[74,75] It follows that for applications where precision is required in ablation, Er:YAG is preferred. On the other hand, depending on settings, the CO_2 laser combines an enviable blend of ablation and heating. The depth of RTD is typically more uniform with CO_2 than the depth of ablation with Er:YAG, such that the CO_2 laser is more useful for global skin improvement (fine or moderate wrinkle without severe contour defects) on the face. The thresholds for ablation for CO_2 and erbium lasers vary inversely with their optical penetration depths in tissue (20 and 1 µm respectively). This assumes thermal confinement. It follows that less surface fluence is required for ablation with the erbium laser. With the CO_2 laser, we are operating at ablation threshold in typical resurfacing applications, so a large fraction of energy is invested in tissue heating. This results in low ablation efficiency, and only a small mass of dermal tissue is ablated. In contrast, the erbium laser operates well above threshold (approximately 8–10 × for a fluence of 5 J/cm^2), resulting in greater ablation and less thermal denaturation. The CO_2 laser at typical operating parameters performs self-limited controlled heating of the skin, whereas the erbium laser operates in an almost purely ablative regime.

Radiofrequency Technology

Radiofrequency (RF) skin interactions are fundamentally different than optical ones. Rather than 'optical' fluence and absorption coefficients, local heat generation depends on the local resistance and the local current density. With most RF systems, there is a rapidly alternating current that, given the impedance of the skin, generates heat. The distribution of the current density is determined by the configuration of the electrodes relative to the skin anatomy. Depending on the type of surface cooling, one can create various zones of heating under the skin. There are two types of electrode deployment:[76,77] In one scenario, bipolar electrodes are combined with either a diode laser or intense pulsed light device (Fig. 1.27). In this configuration, there is so-called synergy between the two applications.[77] With the bipolar electrode configuration, electrical field density is intrinsically confined fairly superficially (the field intensity reaches about as deep as one half the distance between the electrodes).

In monopolar configurations, the dispersive electrode is located at a distant point on the body. Monopolar skin rejuvenation systems tend to create large volumes of heating. They disperse the electrical energy over the breadth of the electrode through a concept known as capacitive coupling. This type of coupling helps to prevent the natural accumulation of electrical energy at the electrode edge.[78] The first nonablative RF device (Therma Cool TC, Thermage, Hayward, CA) uses cryogen spray cooling (CSC), where the spray is started before the RF current. With a large monopolar electrode (>1 × 1 cm), for example, current is deposited diffusely in the dermis and the effects tend to be deep, i.e. large volume of skin is heated. The goal is uniform heating of the deep dermis and fat. Depending on the dose, electrode configuration, time, and local skin structure, one observes various immediate ultrastructural changes.[78]

On the other hand, if both positive and negative electrodes are placed in the contact tip (bipolar electrode), current density tends to flow superficially (path of least resistance from electrode to electrode, and therefore temperature elevation is confined to superficial skin). By placing the electrodes further apart, the current density depth will increase. Otherwise, control of the tissue heating is determined by variations in electrode type, power, and cooling times.[77] If one uses 'rail' metal type electrodes placed next to a flashlamp crystal, EM field theory predicts that there will be a hot spot near the edge of the electrode. These hot spots can be reduced by electrically coupling the energy into the skin (for example, ensuring that the dry stratum corneum, with high intrinsic impedance, is wetted with an electrolyte solution).

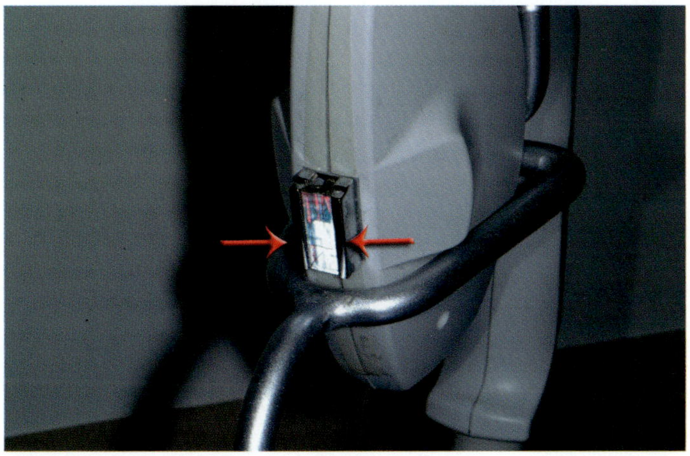

Figure 1.27 Tip of diode-radiofrequency device (metal rails (arrows) are the electrodes in bipolar configuration; Comet, Syneron, Canada).

One device (Aurora SR, Syneron, Richmond Hill, Ontario, Canada) combines RF energy and a flashlamp. The near-simultaneous application of electrical and optical fields is proposed to optimize efficacy and safety. In this configuration, the local optical energy (fluence) increases the discrete chromophore temperature (i.e. hair, vessel). This localized heating reduces impedance (skin is treated as an electrolyte with decreasing impedance as a function of increasing temperature) and therefore in higher localized current densities. Thus, there is 'synergy' between the optical and electrical parts of the device.[77] A purported advantage of the treatment is that lower optical energies can be used to selectively heat subsurface targets than if a light source were used alone (thus enhancing epidermal preservation). There is some evidence that white hairs could be reduced with this technology. The working theory is that although there is little melanin in white hairs, there is higher current density around the follicle (as the current navigates around the high-resistance shaft).[77] The current density in the tissue adjacent to the hair shaft is roughly twice the current density and other parts of the skin this is because the electrical current streams around the hair shaft concentrating in a layer just around the hair. Although certainly promising in principle, and based on sound scientific principles, no study has clearly shown at the time of this writing that the 'synergy', at least in its present configurations, is clinically relevant. That is, for example, no peer-reviewed study has shown that hair removal without RF is more effective than that with RF (with all other parameters held constant). Many studies are pending which may or may not support the role of radio frequency energy and optical energy as good dance partners.

Brief Overview of Applications

Psoriasis

In psoriasis, one can target the microvasculature with vascular specific lasers or, alternatively, vaporize plaques with resurfacing lasers. Due to the size of the vessels, the pulsed dye laser with its shorter pulse is the most logical choice among vascular lasers.[79–81] Laser resurfacing has also been used to remove lesions.[82] The excimer laser has been used. Here photochemistry is the primary mechanism.[83] PDT configurations have also been applied with varying degrees of plaque clearing.[84–86]

Hypopigmentation

The excimer laser and UV lamp sources have been used to restore pigment through photochemical pathways.[49,87]

Postinflammatory Hyperpigmentation

This is typically very resistant to laser therapy. Some exceptions are Q-switched laser therapy for long-standing hyperpigmented areas on the extremities. Also, the pulsed dye laser, in treating certain hyperpigmented hypertrophic scars, can reduce both the pigmentation and vascular aspects of the scar. Finally, long pulsed KTP lasers and IPLs can sometimes reduce postinflammatory hyperpigmentation.

Wrinkle and Scar Reduction

Wrinkle and scar reduction are typically achieved via ablative mechanisms. The CO_2 and Er:YAG lasers are ideally suited for laser skin resurfacing. The CO_2 laser functions more as a heating tool with typical parameters (5–10 J/cm^2 in pulsed mode), whereas the Er:YAG laser acts more as a purely ablative tool. A summary of the mechanisms follows. In brief, when energy deposition occurs rapidly, water does not vaporize at 100°C because the pressure is higher than 1 atm. Energy is deposited isovolumetrically and the temperature may reach 300°C with pressures up to 1000 atm.[20] These high pressure gradients can assist tissue removal because, depending on the mechanical properties of the tissue, the explosive removal process can be more energetically efficient than the 2500 J/cm^3 latent heat of vaporization for water. For example, the heat of ablation for epidermis is small, and portions of the friable cellular epidermis can be observed in the plume. Thus not all of the tissue is actually vaporized but rather forcibly ejected from the surface. For dermis, about 4.3 kJ/cm^3 are required for ablation by many CO_2 lasers, almost twice that needed for water vaporization. It has been suggested that this is related to the high tensile strength of collagen fibers. A large induced pressure is necessary to disrupt the tissue.[88] The erbium laser vaporizes tissue more explosively than with CO_2 LSR, so that at fluences of only 5–10 J/cm^2, there is violent ablation, and particles are ejected at supersonic velocities. There is recoil at the tissue surface – the skin actually appears to be 'pushed down' in real time. Momentum transfer produces stress waves, which combined with the small level of RTD, may contribute to the tendency for bleeding after Er:YAG LSR. In general, in any laser resurfacing procedure, by confining energy both spatially and temporally, more efficient vaporization occurs with less thermal decomposition of proteins and less chance of charring. Nonablative skin remodeling has also been used with water as a chromophore (1320, 1450, and 1540 nm) and is intended to heat a subsurface 'slab' of tissue (without epidermal damage). Both wrinkles and scars have improved with these approaches, but results are normally modest compared to properly applied ablative approaches. Pulsed dye lasers and other visible light modalities have proved effective in scars.[68,89–92] Although there is an indirect effect of visible light technologies on wrinkles in some cases, no visible light modality has achieved the same improvement in fine wrinkling as ablative modalities with traditional fluences.

Acne

There are many EMR-based approaches to acne treatment, which are limited only by our understanding of the pathophysiology of acne. Mechanisms for improving acne include suppression of *P. acnes* (PDT with endogenous and exogenous PS), normalization of the keratinization process through infundibular heating (some mid-infrared lasers), and possible sebaceous gland damage through deep heating with IR lamp, deep MIR, and RF technologies.[93] Of all the techniques, the only one that shows long-term acne reduction with microscopic evidence of marked sebaceous gland damage is red and/or blue light ALA-PDT. This histologic picture has only been observed with long ALA incubation times (>4 hours) coupled with low power density red light sources.[94]

Pigmented Lesions

Melanosome heating conforms well with the basic theory of selective photothermolysis.[20] With very short pulses (ns) one observes immediate frostlike whitening at the surface (Fig. 1.28). Although the exact cause is unknown, it is most certainly related to the formation of gas bubbles that intensely scatter light.[20] Over several minutes, these bubbles dissolve, causing the skin color to return to nearly normal. As the pulse duration increases, melanosome heating becomes more gentle, and there tends to be focal DE junction heating but with considerable diffusion outside the melanosome. Pigmented lesions can be divided into superficial and deep. Static epidermal pigmented lesions such as lentigos tend to be straightforward to treat. In most cases, the most complete removal (with only one treatment session) is achieved via Q-switched technologies. On the other hand, the least invasive and gentlest removal is via long pulse (ms) technologies in the visible light

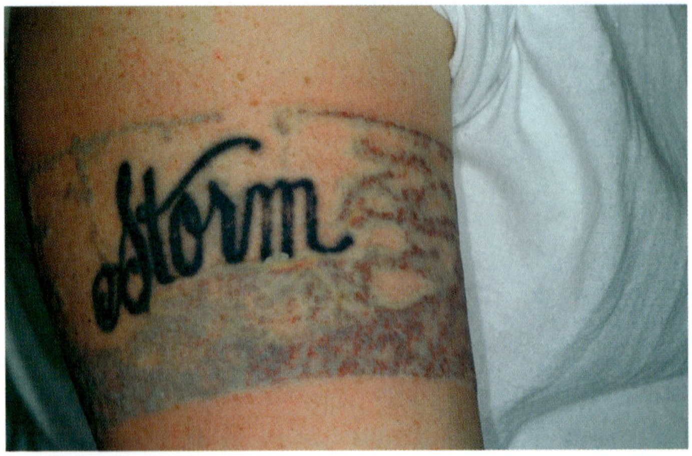

Figure 1.28 Note immediate 'frosty' whitening after alexandrite laser theory. This figure also shows rupture of small vessels. 'Storm' was not treated.

spectrum such as intense pulsed light devices as well is KTP lasers. Recently, long pulse alexandrite lasers have also been employed as well as long pulsed diode lasers to gently heat epidermal static pigmented lesions. 'Dermal' static pigmented lesions such as nevus of Ota respond best to Q-switched lasers.[95] This is consistent with the theory of selective photothermolysis. With longer pulses (ms domain), the dermal melanocytes, which are of relatively low concentration (compared to melanocytic nests in compound nevi or highly pigmented basal cell layers in lentigos), simply do not become hot enough to achieve pigment reduction.[9]

For light lentigos, the contrast between the skin's background color and the lesions may become too small for effective reduction by long pulsed green–yellow (GY) sources. In these cases, the shorter pulses of Q-switched lasers are required for selective heating of pigmented lesions. Melasma is a challenging condition to treat via lasers, most likely due to its dynamic and inflammatory nature (compared to the static nature of lentigos).[96] Ablative lasers can sometimes result in improvement, however the ablation normally has to be carried out deeply, or postinflammatory hyperpigmentation may outweigh any achievement gains. Q-switched lasers typically result in only temporary improvement (followed by post inflammatory hyperpigmentation that worsens the appearance!).[96] On the other hand, longer pulsed visible light laser technologies can sometimes achieve gradual improvement in melasma so long as the settings are not too high.[97,98]

Vascular Lesions

Selective microvascular injury can be achieved well into the penetrating red visible wavelengths. The absorption coefficient of bloodless dermis is only 0.1–0.3 cm^{-1} throughout the red wavelength region, and Hb absorption exceeds bloodless dermis throughout the red and NIR spectrum. It follows that even lasers with relatively poor Hb absorption such as the ruby laser have been used for PWS treatment. Despite competition from melanin, GY wavelength (532–595 nm) laser pulses appear to work well for treating larger vessel (0.1–1 mm diameter) PWSs or telangiectasias, and at the longer pulses appropriate to PWS treatment, pigment cell injury is minimized. By adding a second pass to vascular lesions, the dermal blood fraction will have increased from the first pass, and the blood absorption can increase many-fold. This has been shown to result in more comprehensive vessel heating within a volume of treated tissue.[99] Part of the improvement may also stem from methemoglobin (MetHb) production.[100,101] With GY lasers and IPLs, longer pulses (or pulse sequences) allow for some epidermal cooling between vascular events. The rationale is that the vessel will have a longer τ than the DE junction. It follows that longer pulses should allow for a greater ratio of vascular to epidermal heating; see Fig. 1.19). This is supported by our recent work which shows that longer IPL pulses allowed for greater epidermal sparing (see Fig. 1.18).

Hair

In this application, the target is either the bulge or bulb, and the innocent bystander is the DE junction. The goal is to maximize the ratio of bulb to epidermal heating. The melanin density of the bulb normally exceeds the DE junction (most people have darker hair than skin). The challenge in laser hair reduction (LHR) is that the bulb lies deep in the skin (about 1–3 mm), such that the local fluence at the DE junction will exceed the bulb fluence. However, we can maximize the bulb to epidermal temperature ratio by: (1) extending the pulse; (2) using longer wavelengths; (3) applying epidermal cooling; and (4) compression of the skin (which decreases the bulb to surface distance).[102] In laser hair reduction, the heater (shaft) and the target (bulb or bulge) are not collocated. It follows that pulse widths should be designed that exceed the τ of the shaft but not be so long that the dermis is overheated beyond the bulb.[103] Pulses that are too short provide only temporary hair reduction for the same reasons very short pulses are ineffective in treating vascular lesions – heating is too confined to the immediate chromophore and does not extend to the intended target. Nanosecond pulses result in vaporization, but with or without a carbon suspension, hair reduction is akin to that of laser waxing. Very short ns pulses expel the melanosomes outside the shaft but do not allow for significant heat conduction, and an immediate leukotrichia may be observed (the pulses are so short that the skeleton of the hair shaft remains).[104] With longer pulses (1–3 ms) and high power densities, the entire shaft is often coagulated, and it tends to coil up on the surface. Thus, like the blood vessel, one observes a continuum in the immediate laser-light hair response as a function of pulse duration. What about immediate endpoints and their relationship to the laser tissue interaction? We normally think of perifollicular edema (PFE) as a necessary (and possibly) sufficient condition for semi or permanent hair reduction. However, PFE can be a deceptive endpoint. Most likely it represents peribulbar damage. However, no one has characterized an association between the level of damage and PFE severity. The failure of PDL, for example, to cause PFE despite obvious hair vaporization at the surface, suggests that deeper heating is required for PFE. Shorter pulses, at least in a range from 3 to 100 ms, cause (Fig. 1.29) more PFE than longer ones with other parameters held constant, most likely due to more 'intense' short-term damage to the follicle. It follows that there is no reliable endpoint for permanent reduction. The presence of PFE always signals short-term reduction, but its absence does not preclude delayed LHR. For example, with a very long pulse (200–400 ms) 810 nm diode laser (Super Long Pulse, Palomar, Burlington, MA), we have observed permanent LHR without PFE. What is the optimal wavelength for laser hair reduction? Theory suggests that longer wavelengths (for example 1064 versus 755 nm) will always achieve a greater ratio of dermal to epidermal heating.[102] But studies have not confirmed that longer wavelengths are necessarily more effective in LHR.[105–109] Overall, the greatest limitation in using longer wavelengths is the absolute decrease in melanin absorption. For example, let us take the

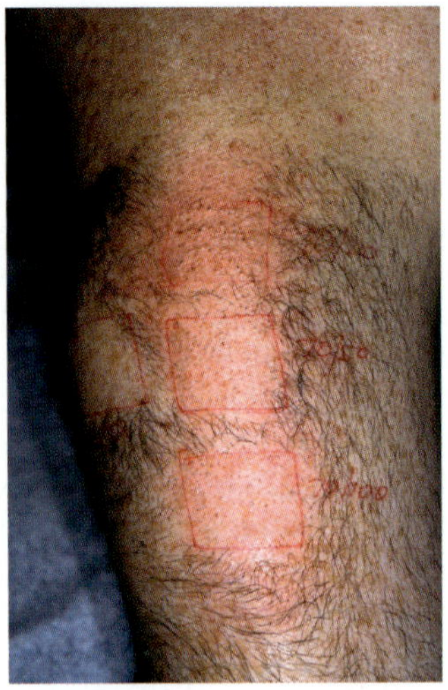

Figure 1.29 Note perifollicular edema increases with decreasing pulsewidth for same fluence with 1064 nm laser.

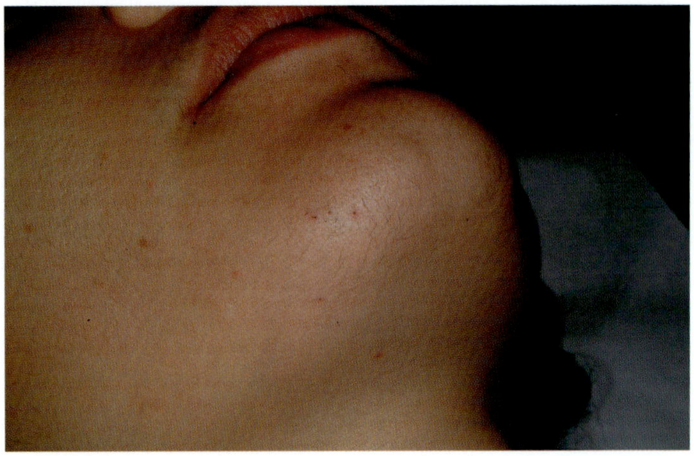

Figure 1.30 Selective heating of thicker black hairs with 1064 nm. The thinner hairs were unchanged on the surface after treatment with 1064 nm laser at 80 J/cm^2 and 40 ms with a 5 mm spot.

typical case of a young type II patient with dark coarse hair on the neck. If one compares the 810 nm diode laser with the 1064 nm laser, for example, treating one side with a 10 mm spot at 810 nm and 44 J/cm^2 and 21 ms, and the other side with identical parameters with the Nd:YAG laser, although both lasers will achieve marked hair reduction, LHR will be better on the 810 nm side. We can use arguments from the 'skin optics' section to support this result. We can also use those same arguments to optimize our parameters to enhance 1064 nm LHR. 810 nm light is absorbed roughly 2.5× that of 1064 nm. It follows that scattering and penetration issues aside, 2.5× the fluence should be required for identical bulb heating for the two wavelengths. However, more 1064 nm light will penetrate 3 mm deep in the skin such that there are about 25% more photons at this depth versus 810 nm.[110] It follows that to achieve identical bulb heating, (assuming all other parameters are held constant), simple algebra suggests that about 2× more fluence must be delivered at the surface for similar bulb heating. Most Nd:YAG lasers, however, do not routinely allow for fluences above 80 J/cm^2 with big spots. Also, with larger spots and high fluences, although the epidermis is preserved, the Nd:YAG laser poses a risk for generalized dermal heating with multiple pulses. It follows that Nd:YAG lasers are ideal when the skin is very dark or the hair is very thick and black (Fig. 1.30). In these scenarios, the bulb/epidermal heating ratio is greater than 1, and even with lower fluences, μ_a of the follicle is so large (~75 cm^{-1} for a thick dark hair versus 10 cm^{-1} for a fine brown hair at 1064 nm) that sufficient heat is generated (the hair is 'saturated' with heat). With lighter finer hairs, one can use very high fluences and shorter pulses and still achieve some degree of permanent LHR with 1064 nm. We were able to see this in a sandy brown haired patient, where a biopsy showed that a combination of 150 J/cm^2 and a 5 mm spot was necessary to see the earliest clearly identifiable heat changes in the bulb. Still, this heating was far less that that seen with a very thick black hair at 50 J/cm^2. For the author's own fine black arm hair, 120 J/cm^2 with 1064 nm achieved the same degree of PFE as 50 J/cm^2 with 810 nm. Hair reduction is a good example of why studies must be carefully examined before proclaiming victory for one laser over another (or at least one wavelength over another!). Often, a study will compare lasers in their commonly deployed parameters (and not the optimal parameters) and then score the results. To the investigators' credit, often the optimal parameters are not available with a particular device. Unfortunately, some Nd:YAG lasers are compromised by too low fluences, and shorter wavelength lasers usually prevail in head to head studies unless the studied hairs are very thick and/or very black. Although the alexandrite and diode lasers can be used in most skin types (so long as effective surface cooling is applied), the one exception is very dark skin (i.e. darkest African American).[105,111] In this case, we have found that no matter how long the pulse and how exquisite the cooling, 1064 nm offers the greatest combination of efficacy and safety. This finding is consistent with our pigment readings with reflectance spectrophotometers, which show that a dark skinned African American is about 1.8× as dark as a light skinned African American, but that the light skinned African American is only about 1.2× as dark as a tanned medium complexion Caucasian. PDT is another potential means for LHR. The major advantage is its non-dependence on pigment. At this time, no system is readily available for ALA-assisted hair reduction, and several obstacles (pain, incubation time of ALA) remain before such a system can be deployed over large areas. A device that combines RF and light has been proposed to work in whitish hairs (vide supra).

Sebum and Fat

Laser lipolysis has been examined but no device has truly exploited the absorption maxima at 1200 and 1700 nm. An RF device selectively heats fat in some applications at some threshold power.

Tattoo Removal by Selective Photothermolysis

Tattoos consist of mainly intracellular, submicrometer-sized insoluble ink particles that have been ingested by phagocytic skin cells after intradermal injection. The stability and longevity of most tattoos shows that many phagocytic skin cells do not traffic or migrate widely, although tattoos do become less distinct over decades.[20] A great variety of inks are used in professional tattoos, which consist mainly of insoluble metal salts, oxides, or organic complexes.[112] Amateur tattoos are almost always carbon in some form – India ink (amorphous carbon), graphite, or ash. Goldman first noted that tattoos were responsive to pulsed laser treatment using normal mode ruby laser pulses.[9] A dose-response and histologic study of Q-switched ruby laser pulses was subsequently performed, which led to widespread interest in Q-switched ruby lasers in the United States, followed by further ultrastructural studies of response.[113] It is now apparent that the Q-switched ruby laser is generally effective and relatively well tolerated in the treatment of black, blue-black and green tattoos. Multiple treatments are required at fluences ranging from 4 to 10 J/cm^2. Typically, four to six treatments given 1-month intervals are needed for amateur tattoos, and six to eight for professional tattoos, although individual response is extremely variable. The risk of scarring is about 5% to 10% for the series of treatments, although over one fourth of patients have transient textural changes. The Q-switched ruby laser causes blistering and hypopigmentation in most patients and permanent depigmentation in about 1–3%.

The mechanisms involved in tattoo removal are largely unknown.[112] It is clear that much of the ink, although apparently removed from the skin, is not removed from the body. All persons with tattoos have tattoo ink pigmentation of the lymph nodes draining the tattooed skin, and it is likely that this is the fate of most of the ink after laser treatment. Lightening of the tattoo occurs gradually about 1 week after each treatment and may go on for months. Occasionally it is clear that ink is present in the scale crust that forms following epidermal injury and sheds 1–2 weeks after treatment, but it is equally apparent that tattoos are removed in cases where no scale crust is formed. Before treatment ink particles are contained in phagolysosomes in fibroblasts, macrophages, and mast cells. After treatment by Q-switched ruby laser, electron microscopy suggests that some ink particles are fractured into 10–100 smaller fragments, which are extracellular, presumably released by rupture of the phagocytic cells.[114] A recent study comparing nanosecond and picosecond 1064 nm pulses showed that carbon black particles became more electron-lucent after irradiation both in vivo and in vitro.[115] The threshold fluences for these changes were less for the shorter pulses. Also, a cuvette of a carbon black suspension was lightened by simply irradiating its contents. The gradual reduction in absorbance has been shown to be due to a well-known steam carbon reaction; this reaction occurs when particles are heated sufficiently to cause a chemical reaction between carbon and surrounding water. The products are H_2 and CO gases.[116] This suggests that changes in optical properties of the particles may play a role in the tattoo lightening process. Observations strongly suggest but do not prove that the primary effects of Q-switched lasers are: (1) fragmentation of ink particles; (2) laser-induced optical property changes; (3) release into the extracellular dermal space; (4) partial elimination of ink in a scale crust if present; (5) probably greater elimination into lymphatics; and (6) rephagocytosis of laser-altered residual tattoo ink particles. Irreversible changes can occur in tattoo inks, especially those used in cosmetic skin-colored tattoos. Photochemical changes may conceivably affect tattoo ink removal for some kinds of ink. This appears to be especially true for tattoos containing red (ferric oxide) and titanium dioxide (see below).[117,118] All of the pulsed lasers used for tattoo removal occasionally cause irreversible immediate darkening of these tattoos, which may be temporarily obscured in part by the immediate whitening reaction, discussed above. It is therefore prudent to perform a small test exposure of cosmetic red, flesh-colored, or white tattoos to see whether immediate darkening occurs. In some cases the darkened ink cannot be removed by subsequent laser treatments and adds to the disfigurement. The mechanism of red tattoo ink darkening is not known but probably involves reduction of ferric oxide (rust color) to ferrous oxide (black). Pure ferric oxide is easily converted in this manner by Q-switched laser pulses in vitro and is present in many cosmetic tattoos.[117] During tattoo treatment there is surface whitening (as in epidermal pigmented lesions; see above). This is accentuated where there is the highest pigment concentration. The proposed causes have already been discussed. In treating black tattoos with 1064 nm (where there is little epidermal effect), one can also see a subsurface transient bright light. This probably represents laser-induced incandescence (Vanderwal) with maximum temperatures around 2000 K. At 4000 K, carbon particles vaporize.[112] There are few controlled studies to understand and optimize tattoo removal. The study cited above addressed the role of pulse duration (nanosecond versus picosecond domain pulses) in tattoo removal.[115] One of the study goals was to examine the role of inertial confinement in laser–tattoo reactions. Somewhat analogous to the concept of thermal confinement, inertial confinement can be achieved when the laser pulse is delivered within the time for which pressure can be relieved from the ink particles. The inertial confinement time is simply the particle diameter divided by the speed of sound, which for tattoo ink particles equals about 1 ns. Because of the high pressures, shock waves (bulk disruption of the material) can occur which should increase the probability of mechanical fracture. It may therefore be that all of the laser pulses being used now are too long. Ross et al[115] showed that the picosecond domain pulses were more effective than nanosecond pulses in black tattoo removal for the same radiant exposures, suggesting that tattoo removal is very sensitive to power density. A theoretical model predicts that the nanosecond pulses would only generate peak temperatures about 3% that of the picosecond pulses, so that photothermal effects alone could explain the more efficient tattoo resolution with shorter pulses. It is unclear if shock waves were generated with the picosecond pulse. Significant details of wavelength-dependent effects are unknown. One study has examined the spectra for most colors and showed absorption peaks for all known colors; however many tattoos are resistant to multiple treatments, especially green tattoos.[119] In a recent study of tattoos at our lab, TiO_2 was detected by X-ray diffraction in four of five resistant green tattoos, and the Q-switched alexandrite laser produced an immediate blue–black discoloration of TIO_2 ink; the ink is often used as a brightener for green and other colors. Paradoxically, with additional treatments, some laser-darkened tattoos can be lightened.[118] It may be that once all the photochemistry has taken place the newly formed products also are capable of absorbing visible or IR radiation. The chemical identity of many tattoo inks, and how they are affected by high-intensity laser pulses, are unknown and – most important – have never been linked to clinical response. Several unresolved issues persist in tattoo removal, only a few of which have been answered: (1) Is a laser induced plasma involved? Possibly, if the generation of surface plasma facilitates ink removal through generation of shock waves. (2) Must the ink particles be fractured? Ink particles need not be fractured for clinical resolution. This has been shown for carbon black, where particles may actually increase in size yet lighten through a change in chemistry. It appears that more crystalline particles are more likely to fracture than relatively amorphous organic substances.[120] (3) Is it the ink or the cells containing it that are the targets? It appears that the ink is the target but that cell death is associated with clearing, since this allows ink release from the cell. (4) How is the ink removed, and where does it go? The ink is removed by the mechanisms cited above; in addition optical property changes in the ink itself may contribute to clearing for some inks. (5) What role might phagocytosis by different cell types play in the retention of ink following treatment, and how can this be optimized? Attempts have been made to modulate the immune response in tattoo removal. Recently imiquimod cream has been used in the interval between laser treatment sessions to augment ink removal.

Cooling

Before the availability of surface cooling, fluence thresholds for efficacy and epidermal damage were often close. Visible light technologies (especially green–yellow light sources such as IPL, KTP laser, and PDL) are popular in cutaneous laser surgery. They are also the wavelength ranges where epidermal damage is most likely. The epidermis is an innocent bystander in cutaneous laser applications where the intended targets, such as hair follicles or blood vessels, are located in the dermis. Specifically, absorption of light by epidermal melanin causes epidermal heating. Melanin is distributed throughout the epidermis but is especially concentrated in the basal cell layer. Melanin absorption of visible light causes heating of melanosomes and through thermal diffusion, subsequent damage to the entire epidermis. This is especially true for green–yellow light, but the risk of selective DE-junction-derived epidermal injury extends to wavelengths as long as 1064 nm. Overall, shorter wavelengths pose a greater risk to the skin surface, because the ratio of epidermal to dermal heating is higher. This ratio derives from: (1) a higher absorption of melanin by shorter wavelengths; and (2) a tendency for photon scatter to limit penetration of shorter wavelengths. This leads to an accumulation of energy near the DE junction.[59,121–123]

Beyond visible light (green, yellow, and red) sources, surface cooling also has been employed in NIR and MIR lasers. With NIR lasers, surface cooling is important, but not only because of DE-junction-derived epidermal heating. In addition, deep beam penetration may cause catastrophic bulk heating. With MIR lasers (1.32, 1.45, and 1.54 μm), the chromophore is water. It follows that with even very low fluences, surface cooling is imperative. Without cooling, the ubiquitous nature of water in the skin causes laser-induced top to bottom injury. There is no discrete heating. All of the techniques are susceptible to operator error and device failure. It follows that as physicians rely more heavily on cooling devices, any lack of their proper deployment unveils the dark side of cooling.

The first goal of surface cooling is preservation of the epidermis. Unintentional heating of the basal cell layer can lead to vesiculation, crusting, and at times, scarring. The second and related goal of surface cooling is to allow for delivery of higher fluences to the intended target (i.e. the hair bulb and/or bulge or a subsurface blood vessel). Often, the highest fluence that can be used in targeting hair and/or subsurface vessels is limited by heating of the epidermis.[124] By cooling the epidermis, higher fluences and therefore higher temperature elevations are possible in the targeted structures in the dermis. Another benefit of surface cooling is analgesia, as almost all cooling strategies will provide some pain relief.[125–131]

The timing of the cooling relative to the laser pulse is important. Cooling can be pre, during the pulse (parallel), or after the pulse (post).[123] All three cooling periods are important. For example, post-cooling may prevent retrograde heating (i.e. from the vessel back to the epidermis) from damaging the skin surface. A cooling protection factor (CPF) has been proposed by Dr R Anderson, who likens it to the sun protection factor concept used in sunscreen assessments. The cooling protection factor is the ratio of fluence, with and without surface cooling, that spares the epidermis. It can be evaluated from the following equation:

$$\mathrm{CPF} = \frac{T_c - T_{ic}}{T_c - T_i}$$

In the above equation, T_{ic} and T_i are basal layer temperatures before laser irradiation with and without cooling, respectively.[124] T_c is the critical temperature at which thermal injury occurs. If the initial skin temperature is 30°C, contact cooling reduces the temperature of the basal layer to about 20°C. If T_c is assumed to be 60°C (it is actually somewhat higher for the brief laser exposure times in this analysis), this would give the CPF as (60 – 20)/(60 – 30) or 1.33. Similarly, cryogen cooling reduces the temperature to about 0°C, thus giving a CPF value as (60 – 0)/(60 – 30) or 2.0. In summary, the CPF values provided by cryogen spray cooling and contact cooling are predicted as 2.0 and 1.33 respectively.

Finally, there is convective air cooling, where cold air is commonly used in skin chilling. The Zimmer (Cyro5, Zimmer MedizinSysteme, Ulm, Germany) directs −10°C air at the skin at a rapid rate (1000L/minute). This system proves for good bulk cooling but spatial localization of the cooling is poor. The CPF, depending on the air temperature and nozzle velocity, is near that of contact cooling.[132]

Besides protection of the DE junction from pigment 'unfriendly' wavelengths, bulk cooling is sometimes required because the volume heated is large and there is a risk for large volume overheating and catastrophic scarring (i.e. with 1064nm). There are some scenarios where cooling is unlikely to prove beneficial: (1) when the absorption of the wavelength is very strong by water (i.e. Er:YAG and CO_2), here the cooling and heating zone are collocated so that preservation of epidermal viability is unfeasible; also (2) when using Q-switched lasers in the range from 532nm to 1064nm, cooling achieves pain reduction but will only modestly reduce the high peak temperatures generated by these ultrashort pulses in melanin and exogenous inks (tattoos).

Some Interesting Concepts and Ideas in Laser–Tissue Interactions

Focusing the Laser Beam

A trick to increase the dermal to epidermal damage ratio is use of a convergent lens. This tool increases the local photon density in the dermis (targeting the hair bulb, a blood vessel, or dermal water). Theoretically, one should be able to use smaller incident fluences, therefore achieving some protection of the epidermis.[133] Because of scattering and subsequent beam broadening, the increased subsurface photon densities that would be predicted in a transparent medium are not realized. Still, there should be a relative increase in deeper photon density versus using a more collimated beam.

Vacuuming the Target in the Laser Beam

Recently a company (Aesthera, Livermore, CA) has proposed a pneumatic device whereby the skin is vacuumed into the light path such that the light penetration in skin is enhanced (Fig. 1.31). In this way more energetic high frequency photons can be delivered, for example, to the hair follicle, with relative epidermal sparing.

Pixilated Injury (aka Fractional Photothermolysis)

One can create a 'pixilated' injury with water as a chromophore in what is called fractional photothermolysis. Roughly 100µm spots have been used with 250–500µm spacing.[134] The tissue can recover form this fractional injury without the widespread epidermal loss observed after traditional resurfacing applications (Fig. 1.32).

Optical Damping

Optically, replacing air (n = 1.0) with a higher-index medium at the skin surface such as glass (n = 1.5) or sapphire (n = 1.7) tends to spare the epidermis. This effect has nothing to do with heat transfer, but rather is a consequence of optical scattering behavior. At wavelengths from about 600 to 1200nm, the majority of light in Caucasian epidermis is actually back-scattered and multiply-scattered light. Indeed, the contribution of scattered light can be

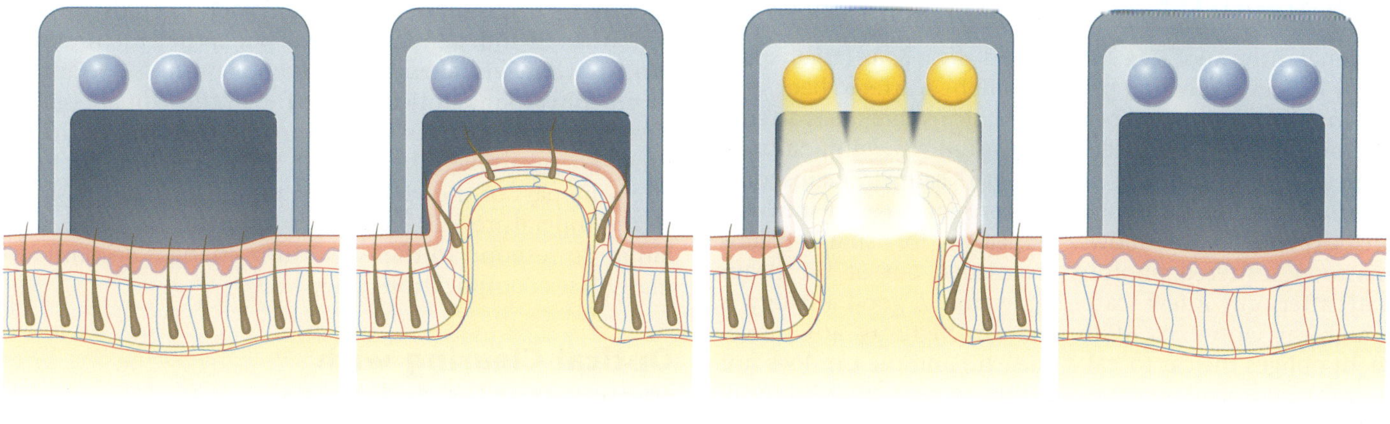

Figure 1.31 Novel device that 'vacuums' skin into the light path. Skin is stretched and thinned, providing enhanced 'relative' penetration of the beam.

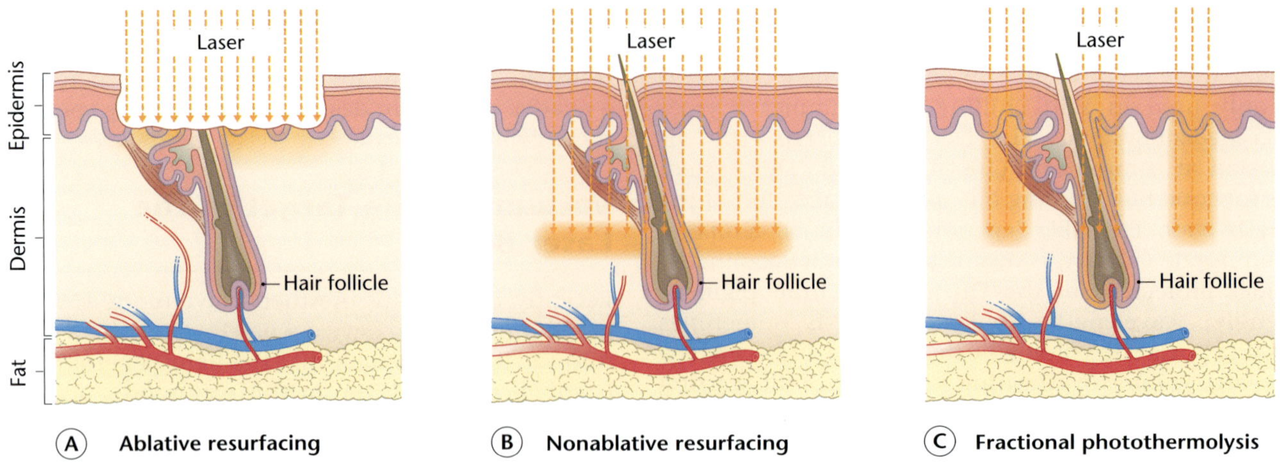

Figure 1.32 Pixilated injury versus traditional nonablative and ablative modalities.

almost an order of magnitude higher than that of the laser beam itself! By providing a closer match to the skin's refractive index, internal reflection of the back-scattered light is greatly reduced, decreasing the natural convergence of photons at the skin surface. This version of optical epidermal sparing requires a physically thick external medium such as a thick layer of gel.

Compacting the Dermis

One can decrease the depth photons must propagate by applying pressure over the treated area. This maneuver may, for example, decrease the relative depth of the bulb and bulge up to 30% relative to the skin surface. Disadvantages might include variability in the amount of pressure, such that adjacent treatment areas are exposed to different subsurface fluences. Also, it is unclear if compacting the dermis might alter its scattering properties. In theory compression should decrease water content and improve dermal transmission.[20]

Spot Diameter

In general the spot size should be 3–4× > δ, as larger spots make it more likely that photons will be scattered back into the incident collimated beam.[102] Photons that are scattered out of the beam are essentially wasted. Traveling 'alone', they carry insufficient energy to cause macroscopic thermal responses in tissue. The consequences of spot size are explained as follows. Basically, for small beams (narrow) scattered photons are carried out of the beam path after only a few scattering events. A good analogy is a highway with exits. With a narrow highway, any movement obliges the car to 'take' the exit, and the car does not return to the road. On the other hand, on a superhighway with many lanes, cars can move about and stay within the original boundary of the thoroughfare. Only cars on the extreme left and right are likely to 'get' off the road. Large spots increase the dermal/epidermal damage ratio as well as the relative penetration depth. However, absolute epidermal damage will be greater with the larger spot with the same fluence as the smaller spot. It follows that it is prudent to reduce the fluence by 20%, for example, if one increases the spot size between treatment sessions in care of a PWS. Also, one should note that for any turbid medium, even if the spot is 'top hat,' there will be an accumulation of photons near the center of the beam such that a greater clinical effect will often be noted at the center of the spot. As a clinical example of the effect of spot size, we have found for 3 mm versus 6 mm spots with the Nd:YAG laser that roughly half the fluence is required with the larger spot for leg vein clearance. For shallow penetrating lasers such as CO_2 and erbium where the δ ≪ spot size, the diameter of the beam does not intrinsically affect the tissue response. That is why equivalent results can be obtained for skin resurfacing, using pulsed CO_2 lasers versus scanned, tightly focused CW CO_2 lasers.[135]

Changing Optical Properties in Real Time

One should always be aware of the changing chromophore concentrations as a function of time during a treatment session. One should never consider each laser–tissue interaction as an independent event, but rather a cumulative process where visual endpoints are the most important ally for the physician. Optical properties of the skin are like the weather[6] and one must accommodate the changes in real time. For example, the dermal blood fraction increases after one pass of the PDL, such that for a second pass, the skin temperature will increase due to the higher μ_a.[136] A failure to respond to these real time changes accounts for many laser complications (Fig. 1.33).

Optical Clearing with Hyperosmolar Solutions

One can increase the transparency of the dermis by topical application or intradermal injection of solutions such as glycerin.[137] The working theory is that water and collagen become less bound such that the effective scattering coefficient of the dermis is reduced. Already this concept has been applied to increase the visibility of blood vessels from

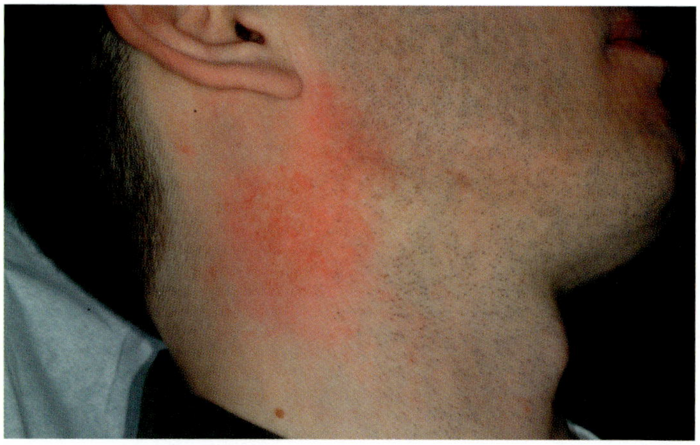

Figure 1.33 Note erythema in poikiloderma patient during KTP laser treatment. One can and should reduce fluence during treatment to decrease risk of overheating.

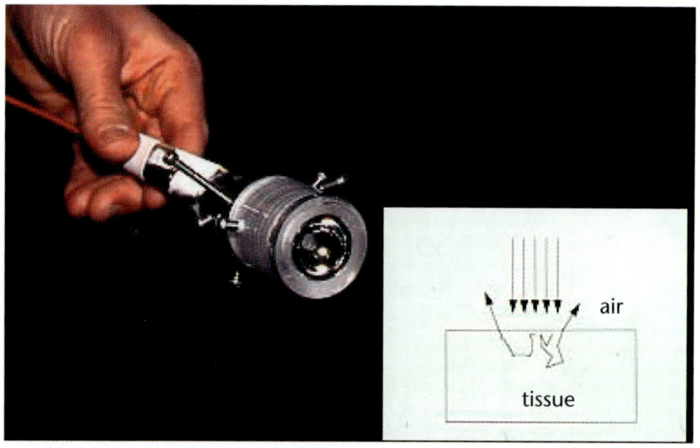

Figure 1.34 Hemispheric mirror that 'sits' over the skin and reflects remitted photons back to the skin surface (so-called 'photon recycling').

Table 1.3 *μ_a for Fine Layer of Carbon on Surface*[144]

Laser	Wavelength (nm)	μ_a (cm^{-1})
Argon ion	488	504
Argon ion	514	463
HeNe	633	317
Diode	805	183
Nd:YAG	1064	80

HeNe, helium neon; Nd:YAG, neodynium:yttrium-aluminum-garnet μ_a, absorption coefficient

the surface. Possible applications include tattoo removal, where particles often are found several mm deep in tissue.

'Carbonization' at the Surface

Carbon will cause all wavelengths to increase absorption such that one can convert a deeply penetrating laser to a more superficially penetrating laser by having a fine carbon layer at the surface. For example, one can 'convert' a 694 nm ruby laser into a laser with CO_2-laser-like effects by applying a fine layer of graphite from a copy machine to the skin surface. In this way the 694 nm laser energy is confined to the surface by the almost 100% absorption by carbon. This fine layer of heated material then cools much like a superficial layer of tissue heated by a CO_2 laser alone (Table 1.3).

Photon Recycling

The remittance of human skin is wavelength dependent and ranges from 15% to 70% through the visible and near-infrared regions of the electromagnetic spectrum. These reflected photons are scattered into the environment and essentially 'wasted' in surgical laser applications. One can (and we did) design a simple hemispherical reflector to return reflected light to the incident spot on the skin (Fig. 1.34). In theory the gain in total energy available to skin is a factor of:

$$\frac{1}{(1 - R_S M_M)}$$

where R_S is the skin reflectance, and R_M is that of a hemispherical mirror. For example, if R_S is 0.7, and R_M is 0.9, a gain of:

$$\frac{1}{(1 - 0.63)}$$

or almost 3-fold, can be achieved.

Plasma for Skin Regeneration

Gas plasmas have been used in surgical devices for many years. Typically, ionized gas acts as a conducting pathway to deliver radiofrequency (RF) energy to achieve superficial tissue coagulation. The plasma energy is relatively small, as the tissue effect is achieved primarily by RF energy. In contrast, the Portrait PSR[3] (Rhytec, UK) uses ultra-high-frequency RF (UHF) energy to ionize a flow of nitrogen gas producing millisecond pulses of plasma. The plasma, characterized by a lilac glow transitioning to a yellowish light called a Lewis–Rayleigh Afterglow as it flows out of the nozzle of the handpiece, produces short-lived rapid elevations in the temperature of the skin's surface. The disruptive effect of energy conversion through an intermediate chromophore found with high-energy lasers is avoided (from Rhytec white paper). The important clinical reason for selecting nitrogen is that it purges oxygen from the skin's surface so that oxidative carbonization is minimized, eliminating unpredictable 'hot-spots' and charring that can produce scarring.

Pigment/Erythema Meters to Assist in Guiding Parameters

Many laser complications stem from a failure of the operator to consider subtle pigmentary differences

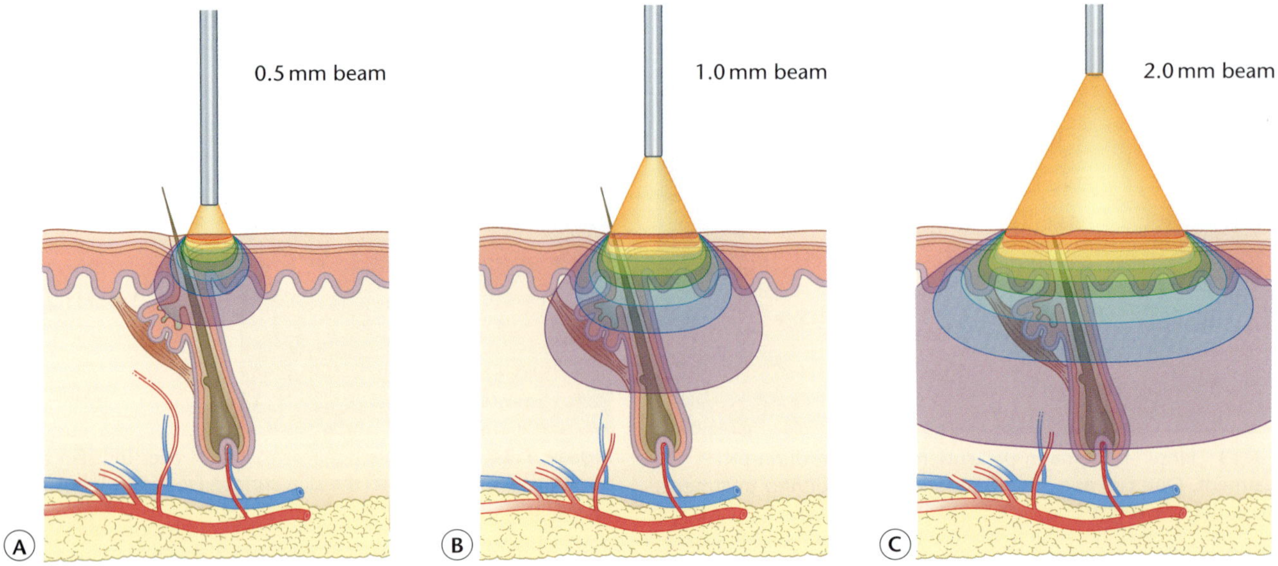

Figure 1.35 Note how spot size changes impact depth of penetration. Shown are the fluence patterns for 1064 nm light with beams (A) 0.5 mm, (B) 1.0 mm, and (C) 2.0 mm in diameter on the skin surface.

between patients as well as the transitory nature of pigmentary status in the same patient. For example, a tanned Caucasian patient may appear to be equally dark as an Asian–American patient who is untanned. However, in laser hair reduction, the patient with the higher constitutive coloration will normally show a greater epidermal tolerance. Tanned skin is injured skin, and newly introduced spectrophotometers can allow the operator to distinguish between levels of coloration within the context of erythema and time. Proper use of these handheld devices allows the astute operator to adjust settings based on absolute pigment levels as well as ratios of pigment to erythema. Also, step-off regions between tanned and untanned areas can be accounted for.[138]

Using a Polarizing Lamp to Enhance Illumination

One can optimize laser treatment by using a polarizing lamp during procedures to enhance the appearance of blood and pigment dyschromias.[139]

Selective Cell Targeting

A process called selected cell targeting has been examined as a way to destroy selected cells. This precise energy deposition is achieved by using laser pulses and light absorbing immunoconjugates tagged to the respective cells. The investigators in one study showed, for example, that lymphocytes could be selectively damaged by attaching iron oxide microparticles absorbing 565 nm radiation at those sites.[140] One can imagine, in the future, using this type of modality to treat T-cell mediated diseases such as atopic dermatitis or psoriasis. In this way, one makes the 'bad guy' more noticeable to the laser.

Scatter-limited Therapy Using Small Microbeams

Reinisch[141] proposed the use of variously sized beams to limit penetration into the dermis. By using the aforementioned spot size arguments, one can exploit the properties of small spots to change the way particular wavelengths behave in the skin. For example, one can tailor a 1064 nm laser to heat progressively larger depths of skin by increasing the spot size (Fig. 1.35).

Two Photon Excitation

We often are limited in dermatology by using visible light laser technologies which are intrinsically nonpenetrating. By using very high power density sources, there is a concept known as 'two photon excitation'.[142] This concept allows for optimal beam penetration while still preserving tissue target selectivity for shorter wavelengths. If, for example, one wants to target a red tattoo deep in the skin with 532 nm light, high fluence 1064 nm light can be applied to the surface. By chance some photons will arrive simultaneously at the target, creating one higher energy photon. Although presently only used in diagnostic applications in the future this sort of technology might overcome some obstacles in our present approaches.

Finally, the reader should note that most of this chapter has dealt with the physical portion of the skin's reaction to light and electricity. However, oftentimes a characterization of the reaction between tissue and the energy source is not as difficult as the subsequent biological sequelae. For example, as Dr Martin van Gemert (an astute PhD!) remarked at a recent meeting, why do DE-junction-derived blisters (after KTP laser) often cause scars but CO_2 laser, even after obvious removal of the epidermis, does not? Obviously, much of the work in the future for scientists will involve a more complete 'mapping' of these complex responses.

Laser, nonlaser light sources, and other physical modalities will undoubtedly play different roles than the traditionally destructive ones that they have played to date. As we further harness and understand EMR, the role of light will expand into real-time bedside diagnostic tools. One day the dermatologist could well diagnose a BCC noninvasively, prep the patient for PDT, and months later rebiopsy the patient with optical coherence tomography for test of cure! All of this would occur without disruption of even the stratum corneum! The future is indeed exciting.

References

1. Kono T, Isago T, Honda T, Nozaki M. Treatment of facial lentigines with the long pulsed dye laser by compression method. Lasers Surg Med 2004; suppl 16 (abstract):33.
2. Grossweiner L. The science of phototherapy. Boca Raton: CRC; 1994:217.
3. Hillenkamp F. Interaction between laser radiation and biological systems. In: Hillenkamp FRP, Sacchi C, eds. Lasers in medicine and biology. Series A. New York: Plenum; 1980:37–68.
4. Neimz M. Laser–tissue interactions, 2nd edn. Berlin: Springer; 2002:303.
5. Welch A, van Gemert MJ, Starr JC, Wilson BC. Definitions and overview of tissue optics. In: Welch AJ, van Gemert MJ, eds. Optical–thermal response of laser-irradiated tissue. New York: Plenum; 1995:15–46.
6. Anderson RR, Parrish JA. The optics of human skin. J Invest Dermatol 1981; 77:13–19.
7. van Gemert MJ, Jacques SL, Sterenborg HJ, Star WM. Skin optics. IEEE Trans Biomed Eng 1989; 36:1146–54.
8. Goldman L, Rockwell R. Laser systems and their applications in medicine and biology. In: Levine S, ed. Advances in biomedical engineering and medical physics. New York: Interscience; 1968:317.
9. Anderson RR. Dermatologic history of the ruby laser: the long story of short pulses. Arch Dermatol 2003; 139:70–4.
10. Knappe V, Frank F, Rohde E. Principles of lasers and biophotonic effects. Photomed Laser Surg 2004; 22:411–17.
11. Reinisch L. Laser physics and tissue interactions. Otolaryngol Clin N Am 1996; 29:893–914.
12. Angermeier MC. Treatment of facial vascular lesions with intense pulsed light. J Cut Laser Ther 1999; 1:95–100.
13. Bitter PH. Noninvasive rejuvenation of photodamaged skin using serial, full-face intense pulsed light treatments. Dermatol Surg 2000; 26:835–42; discussion 843.
14. Cliff S, Misch K. Treatment of mature port wine stains with the PhotoDerm VL. J Cut Laser Ther 1999; 1:101–4.
15. Goldberg DJ, Cutler KB. Nonablative treatment of rhytids with intense pulsed light. Lasers Surg Med 2000; 26:196–200.
16. Raulin C, Greve B, Grema H. IPL technology: a review. Lasers Surg Med 2003; 32:78–87.
17. Sadick NS, Weiss R. Intense pulsed-light photorejuvenation. Semina Cut Med Surg 2002; 21:280–7.
18. Weiss RA, Goldman MP, Weiss MA. Treatment of poikiloderma of Civatte with an intense pulsed light source. Dermatol Surg 2000; 26:823–7; discussion 828.
19. Welch AJ, van Gemert MJ. Overview of optical and thermal interaction and nomenclature. In: Welch AJ, van Gemert MJ, eds. Optical–thermal response of laser-irradiated tissue. New York: Plenum; 1995:1–14.
20. Anderson R, Ross E. Laser–tissue interactions. In: Fitzpatrick R, Goldman M, eds. Cosmetic laser surgery. St Louis: Mosby; 2000:1–30.
21. Fisher JC. Basic biophysical principles of resurfacing of human skin by means of the carbon dioxide laser. J Clin Laser Med Surg 1996; 14:193–210.
22. Kimel S, Svaasand LO, Cao D et al. Vascular response to laser photothermolysis as a function of pulse duration, vessel type, and diameter: Implications for port wine stain laser therapy. Lasers Surg Med 2002; 30:160–9.
23. Tanghetti E, Sierra RA, Sherr EA, Mirkov M. Evaluation of pulse-duration on purpuric threshold using extended pulse pulsed dye laser (cynosure V-star). Lasers Surg Med 2002; 31:363–6.
24. West TB, Alster TS. Comparison of the long-pulse dye (590–595 nm) and KTP (532 nm) lasers in the treatment of facial and leg telangiectasias. Dermatol Surg 1998; 24:221–6.
25. Anderson RR, Parrish JA. Selective photothermolysis: precise microsurgery by selective absorption of pulsed radiation. Science 1983; 220:524–7.
26. Anderson RR, Parrish JA. Microvasculature can be selectively damaged using dye lasers: a basic theory and experimental evidence in human skin. Lasers Surg Med 1981; 1:263–76.
27. Goldman L, Rockwell RJ, Jr. Laser systems and their applications in medicine and biology. Adv Biomed Eng Med Phys 1968;1:317–82.
28. Itzkan I, Izatt J. Medical use of lasers. Encyclopedia of applied physics. Washington, DC: VCH Publishers, Inc. & American Institute of Physics; 1994:33–59.
29. Jacques SL. Spectrum of carbonized tissue. Online. Available: http://omlc.bme.ogi.edu/spectra/carbonizedtissue/index.html [1998].
30. Ellis DL, Weisberg NK, Chen JS et al. Free electron laser infrared wavelength specificity for cutaneous contraction. Lasers Surg Med. 1999;25:1–7.
31. Walsh JT, Jr., Flotte TJ, Anderson RR, Deutsch TF. Pulsed CO_2 laser tissue ablation: effect of tissue type and pulse duration on thermal damage. Lasers Surg Med 1988; 8:108–18.
32. Altshuler GB, Anderson RR, Manstein D et al. Extended theory of selective photothermolysis. Lasers Surg Med 2001; 29:416–32.
33. Polla BS, Anderson RR. Thermal injury by laser pulses: protection by heat shock despite failure to induce heat-shock response. Lasers Surg Med 1987; 7:398–404.
34. Beckham JT, Mackanos MA, Crooke C et al. Assessment of cellular response to thermal laser injury through bioluminescence imaging of heat shock protein 70. Photochem Photobiol 2004; 79:76–85.
35. Verdaasdonk RM, Borst C, van Gemert MJ. Explosive onset of continuous wave laser tissue ablation. Physics Med Biol 1990; 35:1129–44.
36. Smith S, Piacquadio D, Morhenn V et al. Short incubation PDT versus 5-FU in treating actinic keratoses. J Drugs Dermatol 2003; 2:629–35.
37. Alexiades-Armenakas MR, Geronemus RG. Laser-mediated photodynamic therapy of actinic cheilitis. J Drugs Dermatol 2004; 3:548–51.
38. Karrer S, Baumler W, Abels C et al. Long-pulse dye laser for photodynamic therapy: investigations in vitro and in vivo. Lasers Surg Med 1999; 25:51–9.

39. Finlay JC, Conover DL, Hull EL, Foster TH. Porphyrin bleaching and PDT-induced spectral changes are irradiance dependent in ALA-sensitized normal rat skin in vivo. Photochem Photobiol 2001; 73:54–63.
40. Sterenborg HJ, van Gemert MJ. Photodynamic therapy with pulsed light sources: a theoretical analysis. Physics Med Biol 1996; 41:835–49.
41. Parrish JA, Jaenicke KF. Action spectrum for phototherapy of psoriasis. J Invest Dermatol 1981; 76:359–62.
42. Gerber W, Arheilger B, Ha TA et al. Ultraviolet B 308-nm excimer laser treatment of psoriasis: a new phototherapeutic approach. Br J Dermatol 2003; 149:1250–8.
43. Weiss RA, McDaniel DH, Geronemus RG, Weiss MA. Clinical trial of a novel non-thermal LED array for reversal of photoaging: clinical, histologic, and surface profilometric results. Lasers Surg Med 2005; 36:85–91.
44. Jacques SL. Laser–tissue interactions. Photochemical, photothermal, and photomechanical. Surg Clin N Am 1992; 72:531–58.
45. Jacques S. Simple optical theory for light dosimetry during PDT. In: Tuchin V, ed. Selected papers on tissue optics. MS 102 vol. Bellingham: International Society for Optical Engineering (SPIE); 1992:655.
46. Jacques S. Skin optics summary. Online. Available: http://www.omlc.ogi.edu/news/jan98/skinoptics.html [1998].
47. Stamatas GN, Kollias N. Blood stasis contributions to the perception of skin pigmentation. J Biomed Optics 2004; 9:315–22.
48. Pearce J, Thomsen SL. Rate process analysis of thermal damage. In: Welch AJ, van Gemert MJ, eds. Optical thermal response of laser-irradiated tissue. New York: Plenum; 1995: 561–608.
49. Alexiades-Armenakas MR, Bernstein LJ, Friedman PM, Geronemus RG. The safety and efficacy of the 308-nm excimer laser for pigment correction of hypopigmented scars and striae alba. Arch Dermatol 2004; 140:955–60.
50. Raulin C, Greve B, Warncke SH, Gundogan C. [Excimer laser. Treatment of iatrogenic hypopigmentation following skin resurfacing]. Hautarzt 2004; 55:746–8.
51. Gold MH, Rao J, Goldman MP et al. A multicenter clinical evaluation of the treatment of mild to moderate inflammatory acne vulgaris of the face with visible blue light in comparison to topical 1% clindamycin antibiotic solution. J Drugs Dermatol 2005; 4:64–70.
52. Omi T, Bjerring P, Sato S, et al. 420 nm intense continuous light therapy for acne. J Cosmetic Laser Ther 2004; 6:156–62.
53. Gold MH, Bradshaw VL, Boring MM, et al. The use of a novel intense pulsed light and heat source and ALA-PDT in the treatment of moderate to severe inflammatory acne vulgaris. J Drugs Dermatol 2004; 3:Nov–Dec.
54. Tzung TY, Wu KH, Huang ML. Blue light phototherapy in the treatment of acne. Photodermatol, Photoimmunol Photomed 2004; 20:266–9.
55. Itkin A, Gilchrest BA. delta-Aminolevulinic acid and blue light photodynamic therapy for treatment of multiple basal cell carcinomas in two patients with nevoid basal cell carcinoma syndrome. Dermatol Surg 2004; 30:1054–61.
56. Bjerring P, Christiansen K. Intense pulsed light source for treatment of small melanocytic nevi and solar lentigines. J Cut Laser Ther 2000; 2:177–81.
57. Bjerring P, Christiansen K, Troilius A. Intense pulsed light source for treatment of facial telangiectasias. J Cosmetic Laser Ther 2001; 3:169–73.
58. Chan H. The use of lasers and intense pulsed light sources for the treatment of acquired pigmentary lesions in Asians. J Cosmetic Laser Ther 2003; 5:198–200.
59. Kauvar AN, Frew KE, Friedman PM, Geronemus RG. Cooling gel improves pulsed KTP laser treatment of facial telangiectasia. Lasers Surg Med 2002; 30:149–53.
60. Lee MW. Combination 532-nm and 1064-nm lasers for noninvasive skin rejuvenation and toning. Arch Dermatol 2003; 139:1265–76.
61. Avram DK, Goldman MP. Effectiveness and safety of ALA-IPL in treating actinic keratoses and photodamage. J Drugs Dermatol 2004; 3:Jan–Feb.
62. McDaniel DH, Ash K, Lord J et al. Laser therapy of spider leg veins: clinical evaluation of a new long pulsed alexandrite laser. Dermatol Surg 1999; 25:52–8.
63. Dover JS. New approaches to the laser treatment of vascular lesions. Aust J Dermatol 2000; 41:14–18.
64. Eremia S, Li C, Umar SH. A side-by-side comparative study of 1064 nm Nd:YAG, 810 nm diode and 755 nm alexandrite lasers for treatment of 0.3–3 mm leg veins. Dermatol Surg 2002; 28:224–30.
65. Passeron T, Olivier V, Duteil L et al. The new 940-nanometer diode laser: an effective treatment for leg venulectasia. J Am Acad Dermatol 2003; 48:768–74.
66. Kaudewitz P, Klovekorn W, Rother W. Effective treatment of leg vein telangiectasia with a new 940 nm diode laser. Dermatol Surg 2001;27:101–6.
67. Major A, Brazzini B, Campolmi P et al. Nd:YAG 1064 nm laser in the treatment of facial and leg telangiectasias. J Eur Acad Dermatol Venereol 2001; 15:559–65.
68. Trelles MA, Allones I, Levy JL et al. Combined nonablative skin rejuvenation with the 595- and 1450-nm lasers. Dermatol Surg 2004; 30:1292–8.
69. Paithankar DY, Clifford JM, Saleh BA et al. Subsurface skin renewal by treatment with a 1450-nm laser in combination with dynamic cooling. J Biomed Optics 2003; 8:545–51.
70. Leffell DJ. Clinical efficacy of devices for nonablative photorejuvenation. Arch Dermatol 2002; 138:1503–8.
71. Kopera D, Smolle J, Kaddu S, Kerl H. Nonablative laser treatment of wrinkles: meeting the objective? Assessment by 25 dermatologists. Br J Dermatol 2004; 150:936–9.
72. Ross EV, Domankevitz Y, Skrobal M, Anderson RR. Effects of CO_2 laser pulse duration in ablation and residual thermal damage: implications for skin resurfacing. Lasers Surg Med 1996; 19:123–9.
73. Walsh JT, Jr, Flotte TJ, Deutsch TF. Er:YAG laser ablation of tissue: effect of pulse duration and tissue type on thermal damage. Lasers Surg Med 1989; 9:314–26.
74. Smith KJ, Skelton HG, Graham JS et al. Depth of morphologic skin damage and viability after one, two, and three passes of a high-energy, short-pulse CO_2 laser (Tru-Pulse) in pig skin. J Am Acad Dermatol 1997; 37:204–10.
75. Majaron B, Verkruysse W, Kelly KM, Nelson JS. Er:YAG laser skin resurfacing using repetitive long-pulse exposure and cryogen spray cooling: II. Theoretical analysis. Lasers Surg Med. 2001; 28:131–38.
76. Koch RJ. Radiofrequency nonablative tissue tightening. Facial Plastic Surg Clin N Am 2004; 12:339–46.
77. Sadick NS, Makino Y. Selective electro-thermolysis in aesthetic medicine: a review. Lasers Surg Med 2004; 34: 91–7.
78. Zelickson BD, Kist D, Bernstein E et al. Histological and ultrastructural evaluation of the effects of a radiofrequency-based nonablative dermal remodeling device: a pilot study. Arch Dermatol 2004; 140:204–9.

79. Bjerring P, Zachariae H, Sogaard H. The flashlamp-pumped dye laser and dermabrasion in psoriasis – further studies on the reversed Kobner phenomenon. Acta Dermatol Venereol 1997; 77:59–61.
80. Hern S, Allen MH, Sousa AR et al. Immunohistochemical evaluation of psoriatic plaques following selective photothermolysis of the superficial capillaries. Br J Dermatol 2001; 145:45–53.
81. Zelickson BD, Mehregan DA, Wendelschfer-Crabb G et al. Clinical and histologic evaluation of psoriatic plaques treated with a flashlamp pulsed dye laser. J Am Acad Dermatol 1996; 35:64–8.
82. Alora MB, Anderson RR, Quinn TR, Taylor CR. CO_2 laser resurfacing of psoriatic plaques: a pilot study. Lasers Surg Med 1998; 22:165–70.
83. Taylor CR, Racette AL. A 308-nm excimer laser for the treatment of scalp psoriasis. Lasers Surg Med 2004; 34:136–40.
84. Cather JC, Abramovits W. Investigational therapies for psoriasis. J Am Acad Dermatol 2003; 49(2):133–138.
85. Ibbotson SH. Topical 5-aminolaevulinic acid photodynamic therapy for the treatment of skin conditions other than non-melanoma skin cancer. Br J Dermatol 2002; 146:178–88.
86. Szeimies RM, Landthaler M, Karrer S. Non-oncologic indications for ALA-PDT. J Dermatol Treat 2002; 13:13–18.
87. Hartmann A, Brocker EB, Becker JC. Hypopigmentary skin disorders: current treatment options and future directions. Drugs 2004; 64:89–107.
88. Walsh J. Pulsed laser angioplasty: a paradigm for tissue ablation. In: Welch AJ, van Gemert MJ, eds. Optical–thermal response of laser-irradiated tissue. New York: Plenum; 1995:925.
89. Friedman PM, Jih MH, Skover GR et al. Treatment of atrophic facial acne scars with the 1064-nm Q-switched Nd:YAG laser: six-month follow-up study. Arch Dermatol 2004; 140:1337–41.
90. Fulchiero GJ, Jr., Parham-Vetter PC, Obagi S. Subcision and 1320-nm Nd:YAG nonablative laser resurfacing for the treatment of acne scars: a simultaneous split-face single patient trial. Dermatol Surg 2004; 30:1356–59.
91. Hirsch RJ, Dayan SH. Nonablative resurfacing. Facial Plastic Surg 2004; 20:57–61.
92. Bowes LE, Alster TS. Treatment of facial scarring and ulceration resulting from acne excoriee with 585-nm pulsed dye laser irradiation and cognitive psychotherapy. Dermatol Surg 2004; 30:934–8.
93. Elman M, Lebzelter J. Light therapy in the treatment of acne vulgaris. Dermatol Surg 2004; 30:139–46.
94. Hongcharu W, Taylor CR, Chang Y et al. Topical ALA-photodynamic therapy for the treatment of acne vulgaris. J Invest Dermatol 2000; 115:183–92.
95. Kang W, Lee E, Choi GS. Treatment of Ota's nevus by Q-switched alexandrite laser: therapeutic outcome in relation to clinical and histopathological findings. Eur J Dermatol 1999; 9:639–43.
96. Taylor CR, Anderson RR. Ineffective treatment of refractory melasma and postinflammatory hyperpigmentation by Q-switched ruby laser. J Dermatol Surg Oncol 1994; 20: 592–7.
97. Chan HH, Kono T. The use of lasers and intense pulsed light sources for the treatment of pigmentary lesions. Skin Ther [Letter]. 2004; 9:5–7.
98. Negishi K, Kushikata N, Tezuka Y et al. Study of the incidence and nature of 'very subtle epidermal melasma' in relation to intense pulsed light treatment. Dermatolog Surg 2004; 30:881–6.
99. Koster PH, van der Horst CM, van Gemert MJ, van der Wal AC. Histologic evaluation of skin damage after overlapping and nonoverlapping flashlamp pumped pulsed dye laser pulses: A study on normal human skin as a model for port wine stains. Lasers Surg Med 2001; 28:176–81.
100. Fournier N, Brisot D, Mordon S. Treatment of leg telangiectasias with a 1064-nm Nd YAG laser in multipulse mode emission and contact cooling (abstract poster book ICO 865). World Congress Dermatol 2002.
101. Fournier N, Brisot D, Mordon S. Treatment of leg telangiectases with a 532 nm KTP laser in multipulse mode. Dermatol Surg 2002; 28:564–71.
102. Ross EV, Ladin Z, Kreindel M, Dierickx C. Theoretical considerations in laser hair removal. Dermatol Clin 1999; 17:333–55, viii.
103. Svaasand LO, Nelson JS. On the physics of laser-induced selective photothermolysis of hair follicles: Influence of wavelength, pulse duration, and epidermal cooling. J Biomed Optics 2004; 9:353–61.
104. Dover JS, Margolis RJ, Polla LL et al. Pigmented guinea pig skin irradiated with Q-switched ruby laser pulses. Morphologic and histologic findings. Arch Dermatol 1989; 125:43–9.
105. Bouzari N, Tabatabai H, Abbasi Z et al. Laser hair removal: comparison of long-pulsed Nd:YAG, long-pulsed alexandrite, and long-pulsed diode lasers. Dermatol Surg 2004; 30:498–502.
106. Goh CL. Comparative study on a single treatment response to long pulse Nd:YAG lasers and intense pulse light therapy for hair removal on skin type IV to VI – are longer wavelengths lasers preferred over shorter wavelengths lights for assisted hair removal. J Dermatol Treat 2003; 14:243–7.
107. Goldberg DJ, Silapunt S. Hair removal using a long-pulsed Nd:YAG laser: comparison at fluences of 50, 80, and 100 J/cm. Dermatol Surg 2001; 27:434–6.
108. Goldberg DJ, Silapunt S. Histologic evaluation of a millisecond Nd:YAG laser for hair removal. Lasers Surg Med 2001; 28:159–61.
109. Gold MH, Bell MW, Foster TD, Street S. One-year follow-up using an intense pulsed light source for long-term hair removal. J Cut Laser Ther 1999; 1:167–71.
110. Zhao Z, Fairchild P. Dependence of light transmission through human skin on incident beam diameter at different wavelengths. Proc Soc Photo-instrument Eng 1998; 2681: 468–77.
111. Greppi I. Diode laser hair removal of the black patient. Lasers Surg Med 2001; 28:150–5.
112. Anderson RR. Shedding some light on tattoos? Photochem Photobiol 2004; 80:155–6.
113. Taylor CR, Gange RW, Dover JS et al. Treatment of tattoos by Q-switched ruby laser. A dose–response study. Arch Dermatol 1990; 126:893–9.
114. Taylor CR, Anderson RR, Gange RW et al. Light and electron microscopic analysis of tattoos treated by Q-switched ruby laser. J Invest Dermatol 1991; 97:131–6.
115. Ross V, Naseef G, Lin G et al. Comparison of responses of tattoos to picosecond and nanosecond Q-switched neodymium: YAG lasers. Arch Dermatol 1998; 134:167–71.
116. Chen H, Digbold G. Chemical generation of acoustic waves. A giant photoacoustic effect. Science 1995; 270:963–6.
117. Anderson RR, Geronemus R, Kilmer SL et al. Cosmetic tattoo ink darkening. A complication of Q-switched and pulsed-laser treatment. Arch Dermatol 1993; 129:1010–14.
118. Ross EV, Yashar S, Michaud N et al. Tattoo darkening and nonresponse after laser treatment: a possible role for titanium dioxide. Arch Dermatol 2001; 137:33–7.

119. Haedersdal M, Bech-Thomsen N, Wulf HC. Skin reflectance-guided laser selections for treatment of decorative tattoos. Arch Dermatol 1996; 132:403–7. [erratum appears in Arch Dermatol. 1996; 132(7):818. Note: Hodersdal M (corrected to Haedersdal M)].
120. Zelickson BD, Mehregan DA, Zarrin AA et al. Clinical, histologic, and ultrastructural evaluation of tattoos treated with three laser systems. Lasers Surg Med 1994; 15:364–72.
121. Aguilar G, Majaron B, Karapetian E et al. Experimental study of cryogen spray properties for application in dermatologic laser surgery. IEEE Trans Biomed Eng 2003; 50:863–9.
122. Choi B, Pearce JA, Welch AJ. Modelling infrared temperature measurements: implications for laser irradiation and cryogen cooling studies. Phys Med Biol 2000; 45:541–57.
123. Zenzie HH, Altshuler GB, Smirnov MZ, Anderson RR. Evaluation of cooling methods for laser dermatology. Lasers Surg Med 2000; 26:130–44.
124. Paithankar D, Ross E. Comparison of cryogen spray and surface contact cooling through heat transfer modeling: LaserExpress 2000; 1(2):1–14. Online. Available at http://www.lasernews.net
125. Hohenleutner U, Walther T, Wenig M et al. Leg telangiectasia treatment with a 1.5 ms pulsed dye laser, ice cube cooling of the skin and 595 vs 600 nm: preliminary results. Lasers Surg Med 1998; 23:72–8.
126. Greve B, Hammes S, Raulin C. The effect of cold air cooling on 585 nm pulsed dye laser treatment of port-wine stains. Dermatol Surg 2001; 27:633–6.
127. Chan HH, Lam LK, Wong DS, Wei WI. Role of skin cooling in improving patient tolerability of Q-switched alexandrite (QS Alex) laser in nevus of Ota treatment. Lasers Surg Med 2003; 32:148–51.
128. Raulin C, Greve B, Hammes S. Cold air in laser therapy: first experiences with a new cooling system. Lasers Surg Med 2000; 27:404–10.
129. Huang PS, Chang CJ. Cryogen spray cooling in conjunction with pulse dye laser treatment of port wine stains of the head and neck. Chang Gung Med J 2001; 24:469–75.
130. Weiss RA, Sadick NS. Epidermal cooling crystal collar device for improved results and reduced side effects on leg telangiectasias using intense pulsed light. Dermatol Surg 1015; 26:1015–18.
131. Tunnell JW, Nelson JS, Torres JH, Anvari B. Epidermal protection with cryogen spray cooling during high fluence pulsed dye laser irradiation: an ex vivo study. Lasers Surg Med 2000; 27:373–83.
132. Chang CW, Reinisch L, Biesman BS. Analysis of epidermal protection using cold air versus chilled sapphire window with water or gel during 810 nm diode laser application. Lasers Surg Med 2003; 32:129–36.
133. Muccini J, O'Donnell F, Fuller T, Reinisch L. Laser treatment of solar elastosis with epithelial preservation. Lasers Surg Med 1998; 23:121–7.
134. Manstein D, Herron GS, Sink RK et al. Fractional photothermolysis: a new concept for cutaneous remodeling using microscopic patterns of thermal injury. Lasers Surg Med 2004; 34:426–38.
135. Ross EV, Grossman MC, Duke D, Grevelink JM. Long-term results after CO_2 laser skin resurfacing: a comparison of scanned and pulsed systems. J Am Acad Dermatol 1997; 37:709–18.
136. Svaasand LO, Aguilar G, Viator JA et al. Increase of dermal blood volume fraction reduces the threshold for laser-induced purpura: implications for port wine stain laser treatment. Lasers Surg Med 2004; 34:182–8.
137. Choi B, Tsu L, Chen E et al. Determination of chemical agent optical clearing potential using in vitro human skin. Lasers Surg Med 2005; 36:72–5.
138. Dolotov LE, Sinichkin YP, Tuchin VV et al. Design and evaluation of a novel portable erythema-melanin-meter. Lasers Surg Med 2004; 34:127–35.
139. Anderson RR. Polarized light examination and photography of the skin. Arch Dermatol 1991; 127:1000–5.
140. Pitsillides CM, Joe EK, Wei X et al. Selective cell targeting with light-absorbing microparticles and nanoparticles. Biophys J 2003; 84:4023–32.
141. Reinisch L. Scatter-limited phototherapy: a model for laser treatment of skin. Lasers Surg Med 2002; 30:381–8.
142. Berns MW. A possible two-photon effect in vitro using a focused laser beam. Biophys J 1976; 16:973–7.
143. Black JF, Barton JK. Chemical and structural changes in blood undergoing laser photocoagulation. Photochem Photobiol 2004; 80:89–97.
144. Prahl SA. Skin optics summary. Online. Available: http://www.omlc.ogi.edu/news/jan98/skinoptics.html [1999].

Chapter 2

Laser Treatment of Cutaneous Vascular Lesions

Mitchel P. Goldman

Laser treatment of cutaneous vascular lesions began with Dr Leon Goldman in 1963 at the Children's Hospital Research Foundation in Cincinnati, Ohio, with the treatment of port-wine stain (PWS) and cavernous hemangioma using ruby, neodymium:yttrium-aluminum-garnet (Nd:YAG), and argon lasers. His initial report of 45 patients treated with these three lasers appeared in 1968 and stimulated great interest in this new treatment modality.[1] Beginning in 1970, early pioneering work in argon laser surgery was accomplished at the Palo Alto Medical Clinic by Apfelberg, Maser, and Lash[2] for treatment of cutaneous vascular lesions. By 1984 the argon laser was generally accepted as the treatment of choice for PWS.[3] Indeed, before the development of the argon laser, no effective form of treatment could be recommended to patients.

The next major advance was the development of the flashlamp pumped pulse dye laser (PDL) in the mid-1980s to treat PWS. This laser was developed to encompass the theory of selective photothermolysis. This theory states that a specific laser wavelength and energy be delivered to vaporize a specific target. The target was oxygenated hemoglobin in the red blood cell in the blood vessel of the PWS. The most important factor was to keep the thermal damage within the blood vessel's 20–50-μm diameter through the use of a pulsed laser output of 350 μsec, which has been expanded to 450 μsec then 1500 μsec and now up to 40 ms. The original wavelength chosen was 577 nm, which soon changed to 585 nm and then 595 nm to allow both deeper penetration as well as more efficient use of the excitation dye between the flashlamps of the laser. Finally, techniques providing epidermal cooling and copper vapor lasers emitting a wavelength of 577 nm were also developed to target oxygenated hemoglobin. The use of a scanning hand-piece for use with non-pulsed lasers was used to keep the laser energy within the thermal relaxation time of the blood vessel.

The latest advance was the development of the intense pulsed light (IPL) devise in 1993. This therapeutic modality did not use a single wavelength of light, but a broad spectrum of visible light where the lower portion was cut off to limit the wavelength to various band-widths between 515 nm and 1000 nm. The output was pulsed in single, double or triple pulses of 1.5–20 ms with delays between the pulses to allow for epidermal cooling. IPL technology, which at first was stated by the 'experts' as being both dangerous and ineffective is now adopted by every laser manufacturer and laser surgeon and is the single most popular technology for the treatment of vascular lesions word-wide. This chapter reviews current laser and IPL technologies in the treatment of vascular lesions. Other chapters specifically discuss the treatment of leg veins, pigmented lesions, photorejuvenation and light activation of photosensitizers: photodynamic therapy.

Selective Photothermolysis

Importance of Pulse Duration

To limit thermal damage to the intended target, the pulse duration must be shorter than the thermal relaxation time of the target tissue (Tables 2.1 and 2.2). The thermal relaxation time of tissue is defined as the time necessary for target tissue to cool down by 50% through transfer of its heat to surrounding tissue through thermal diffusion. If a targeted tissue can be heated sufficiently to affect it irreversibly before its surrounding tissue is damaged by thermal diffusion, selective photocoagulation occurs.[4,5]

Box 2.1 *Classification of Vascular Malformations*

Capillary Malformation (CM)
Port-wine stain
  Sturge–Weber syndrome
Telangiectasia

Lymphatic Malformation (LM)
Localized
Diffuse

Venous Malformation (VM)
Localized
Diffuse

Arterial Malformation (AM)
Bonnet–Dechaume–Blanc syndrome
Cobb syndrome

Complex-Combined Malformation
Capillary-lymphatic malformation (CLM)
  Circumscribed
  Angiokeratomas
Regional
  Klippel–Trenaunay syndrome (CLM, VM)
  Parkes–Weber syndrome (CLM, VM, AM)
Diffuse
  Maffucci syndrome (LM, VM, enchondromas)
  Solomon syndrome (CM, VM, intracranial AM, epidermal nevi, osseous defects, tumors)
  Riley–Smith syndrome (LM, VM, macrocephaly, pseudopapilledema)
  Bannayan syndrome (AM, LM, VM, macrocephaly, lipomas)
  Proteus syndrome (CM, VM, macrodactyly, hemihypertrophy, lipomas, pigmented nevi, scoliosis)

Modified from Mulliken JB The classification of vascular birthmarks. In: Tan OT, ed. Management and treatment of benign cutaneous lesions. Philadelphia: Lea & Febiger; 1992.

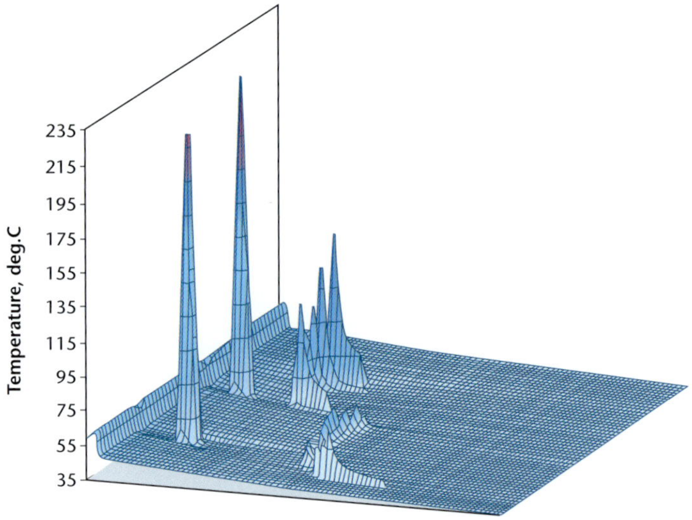

Figure 2.1 Temperature distribution achieved during treatment of four different-size vessels with PDL. Two 0.05-mm-diameter vessels are located at 0.4-mm and 0.5-mm depths. A large 1-mm-diameter vessel is located at a depth of 1.1 mm; a medium-sized 0.4-mm-diameter vessel is located at a depth of 0.6 mm. Treatment conditions: 585-nm wavelength, 6-mm-diameter spot size, 10-J/cm^2 fluence. (Reprinted with permission from Goldman MP, Eckhouse S et al: Dermatologic Surgery: Official Publication for American Society for Dermatologic Surgery 22:323, 1996. With permission from Blackwell Publishing Ltd.)

Table 2.1 *Approximate Thermal Relaxation Time (Tr) for Vessels of Different Diameters*

Diameter (μm)	Tr (ms)
10	0.048
20	0.19
50	1.2
100	4.8
200	19.0
300	42.6

Data from Anderson RR, Parrish JA. Lasers Surg Med 1981; 121:217.

Table 2.2 *Thermal Relaxation Time (Tr) of Laser Targets*

Target	Diameter (μm, approx)	Tr
Epidermis	60	2 ms
Basal layer	20	400 μs
Melanosome	1	0.2 μs
Erythrocyte	5	5 μs

For vascular lesions, the exposure time should be long enough to conduct heat from the red blood cell (RBC)-filled lumen to the entire blood vessel wall. The thermal relaxation time of vessels 10 to 50 μm in diameter is 0.1 to 10 ms, averaging 1.2 ms.[4,5] However, pulse durations less than 20 μs result in vessel rupture and hemorrhage secondary to RBC explosion.[6] This will lead to hemosiderin pigmentation. Therefore, with single laser pulses, the therapeutic window is small. This argues for the development of a wider single pulse or a multipulsed laser that is able to transfer absorbed heat to the endothelium without causing its rupture (Figs 2.1 and 2.2).

Extension of the pulse duration of the PDL from 0.45 ms to over 1.5 ms limits purpura without decreasing efficacy. The immediate purpuric threshold increases from 6.2 to 8, 10.4, and 13.8 J/cm^2 with an increase in the pulse duration from 0.5 to 2.0, 20 and 40 ms.[7] Even though a decrease in purpura can be obtained by extending the pulse duration to 10 ms, patients are still erythematous for 3–4 days and posttreatment edema is present to a similar extent.[7]

Importance of Wavelength

The theory of selective photothermolysis is the basis for the development of the PDL with a wavelength of 577, 585 or 595 nm to increase penetration into the dermis without loss of vascular specificity.[8] Although blood

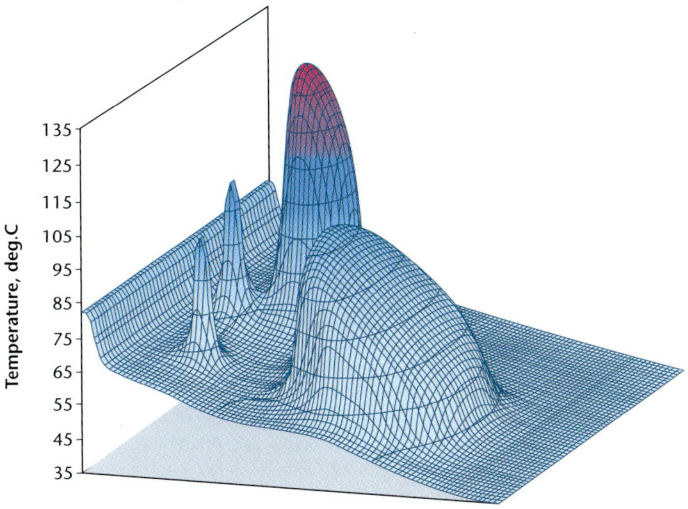

Figure 2.2 Temperature distribution achieved during treatment of four different-size vessels with IPL. Two 0.05-mm-diameter vessels are located at 0.4- and 0.5-mm depths. A large 1-mm-diameter vessel is located at a depth of 1.1 mm; a medium-sized 0.4-mm-diameter vessel is located at a depth of 0.6 mm. Treatment conditions: 590-nm cutoff filter, double pulse of 5 and 10 ms, 150-ms delay between pulses, irradiance of 55 J/cm^2. (Reprinted with permission from Goldman MP, Eckhouse S et al: Dermatologic Surgery: Official Publication for American Society for Dermatologic Surgery 22:323, 1996. Blackwell Publishing Ltd.)

absorbs 585-nm light about one-half as efficiently as it absorbs 577-nm light,[9] 585-nm light will coagulate larger vessels better than 577-nm light at a given depth because of deeper penetration of laser energy. In addition, deeper vessels absorb laser energy at longer wavelengths.[10]

The tissue depth to which a given fluence will coagulate the target vessel depends largely on the blood volume of vessels above the target vessels. Superficial vessels containing blood will absorb laser light before it reaches deeper target vessels. This explains why multiple treatments are necessary for complete PWS resolution.

Because blood also has an absorption peak at 532 nm, the frequency doubled Nd:YAG laser is also effective in treating superficial vascular lesions. However, to obtain a degree of selectivity over the high melanin absorption at 532 nm and to penetrate to clinically useful depths, cooling the overlying epidermis is important.

Effect of Epidermal Cooling

Cooling the epidermis has been shown to increase the depth of penetration of effective thermocoagulation.[11,12] Addition of the pretreatment epidermal cooling allows treatment to occur at higher energy fluences (9–10 J/cm^2 versus 6–7 J/cm^2 without cooling) without increasing the incidence of scarring or pigmentary changes.

The Beckman Laser Institute developed the concept of delivering a cryogen spurt of tetrafluorethane (boiling point –26.2°C) just before laser impact. They term this 'dynamic cooling'. The Candela Laser Corporation and CoolTouch Corporation have proprietary rights to this technology. Skin surface temperature is reduced by as much as 40°C with a 20- to 80-ms cryogen spurt after PDL exposure. The skin surface usually cools to about –30°C, whereas the temperature of the epidermal basal layer will not drop below 0°C.[13] This allows for higher fluences to be given without adverse epidermal effects. The result of epidermal cooling and higher laser fluences increases efficacy, allows deeper laser penetration, and minimizes treatment pain.[14,15]

One potential problem is the effect on the cryogen spray on laser light. One study on 594 and 785-nm light demonstrated a 3% decrease in light transmission after a 30-ms pulse and a 30-ms delay before the laser pulse.[16]

Other methods for cooling the epidermis are air cooling, contact cooling through a quartz or sapphire crystal or topical cold gel or ice. The cold air cooling devise commonly used, SmartCool or Cryo 5 (Zimmer Elektromedizin, Ulm, Germany) generates a continual air current of 500–1000 L/min at a minimal temperature of –30°C. The level of airflow can be regulated. At a cooling level of 6 (1–6 scale), a temperature of –15°C has been measured at the skin surface after 8 seconds of cooling.[17] In addition, the air transport system can be modified with an adapter so that the stream of cold air hits the skin exactly at the laser impact site. A study on 166 patients treated with a variety of lasers for hair removal, tattoo removal and the treatment of vascular abnormalities were treated with air cooling or ice pack cooling or chilled tip cooling; 86% of patients felt that the cold air cooling was better than other cooling methods.[18] The analgesic effect was better in 37% of patients than ice gel. There was also a reduction in erythema and purpura of 70% and 83% respectively.

However, contact cooling has certain advantages in comparison to air cooling. As a physician you can use the contact cooling handpiece to compress the skin up to a certain degree. By doing this, the amount of blood in the vein to be coagulated can be adjusted and optimized. This procedure can reduce pain and result in good coagulation. In this connection it is important to have a handpiece that provides parallel cooling through a cooled sapphire window as well as long post cooling through an integrated cooled metal piece. The handpiece of the long-pulsed Nd:YAG laser MYDON from WaveLight is the only device that features not only these options but also has a removable cooled sapphire window. The advantage of this possibility is remarkable when it comes to treating fine vessels where you need optimal vision at the treatment area. Additionally, it also avoids the blood disappearing completely by the pressure of the contact cooling when treating these very small veins.

The effect of epidermal cooling to enhance clinical efficacy has been shared by other therapeutic modalities, particularly the IPL and long-pulsed Nd:YAG systems described later in this chapter and hair removal lasers and IPLs.

Lasers Commonly Used to Treat Vascular Lesions

Flashlamp-pumped Pulsed Dye Lasers

Tan et al's successful treatment of children with PWSs established the safety and efficacy of the PDL.[19] Garden

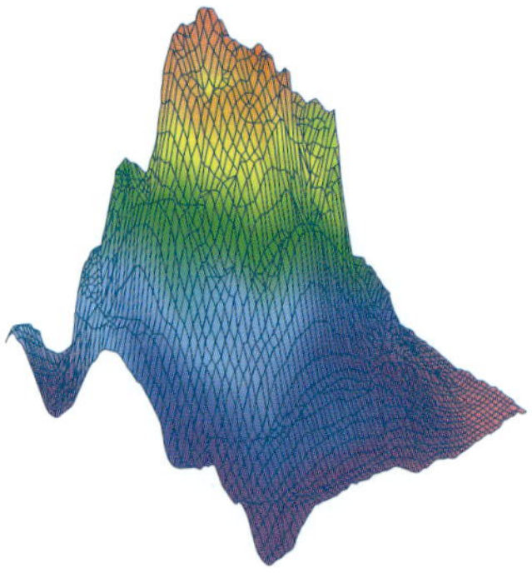

Figure 2.3 Beam profile of Candela SPTL-1 from laser head. It exhibits Gaussian-like distribution of energy with some irregularities. (Reprinted from Jackson BA, Arndt KA, Dover JS. Journal of the American Academy of Dermatology 34:1000, 1996, with permission from the American Academy of Dermatology.)

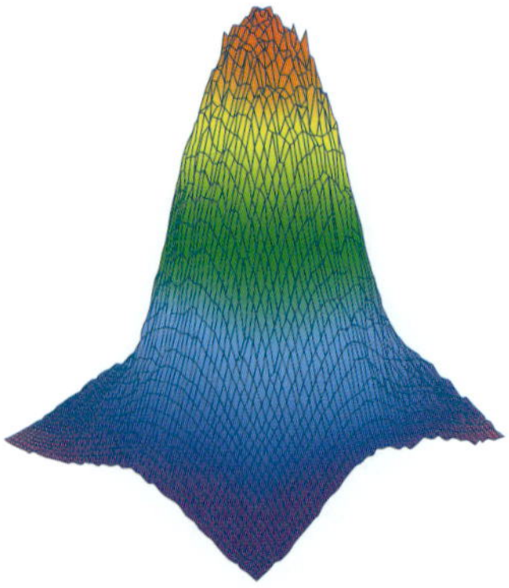

Figure 2.4 Cynosure PhotoGenica V laser from laser head. Like the Candela SPTL-1 (see Fig. 2.3), it exhibits Gaussian energy distribution with irregularities. (Reprinted from Jackson BA, Arndt KA, Dover JS. Journal of the American Academy of Dermatology 34:1000, 1996, with permission from the American Academy of Dermatology.)

and others[20–22] further refined the treatment parameters and expanded the use to lesions in adults. This clinical efficacy has been confirmed by other authors,[23–29] and the use has been expanded to include the early treatment of capillary hemangiomas as well as many different cutaneous lesions that have a vascular component.[30–32]

Three manufacturers produce this type of laser. Candela Corporation (Wayland, MA) manufactures the SPTL line of machines, which originally emitted a wavelength of 585 nm and now can emit wavelengths of 590, 595, and 600 nm. The original pulse duration was 450 μs and now can be increased to 40,000 μs. The beam profile can be circular at 3, 5, 7, 10 and 12 mm in diameter or elliptic at 2 × 7 mm. Maximal energy fluences of 10 or 20 J/cm^2 are available. The Candela machine uses cryogen spray cooling. Another PDL is the PhotoGenica V with a 585 nm wavelength and the Photogenica V-Star with a 595 nm wavelength and similar spot sizes and power as the Candela machine manufactured by Cynosure, Inc. (Chelmsford, MA). Currently produced Candela systems, according to their website, include the Vbeam (6 J output, 595-nm, 0.45- to 40-ms, with 5-, 7-, 10-, 3 × 10-mm handpieces) and Cbeam (6 J output, 585-nm, 0.45-ms, 5-, 7-, 10-mm handpieces). Cynosure currently produces the PhotoGenica V-Star (8 J output, 585- or 595-nm, 0.5- to 40-ms, with 7-, 10-, 12-mm and elliptical handpieces and PhotoGenica V (4 J output, 585-nm, 0.45-ms, with 7- and 10-mm handpieces). Currently, no manufacturer produces a multi-wavelength dye laser. Both the Candela Sclerolaser and the Cynosure VLS multi-wavelength systems have been discontinued, although they may be available on the used market. The Cynosure PDL uses cold air cooling. The third company is DEKA (Florence, Italy), which produces the Dermobeam at 595 nm with similar spot sizes and pulse durations as the other PDL. DEKA uses an integrated cooling system.

The PDL beam profiles may be different between laser companies. With the Candela PDL a 10% to 20% overlapping spot provides for an even distribution of energy fluence. This is because of the Gaussian distribution of beam output. An 18% overlap has been found to cover the largest surface area with the least overlap.[33] In contrast, the Cynosure PDL has a 'top hat' distribution of energy fluence (Figs 2.3 and 2.4).[34] In addition, when the 5-mm-diameter spot size of the two lasers were tested, the Candela laser spot size was up to 35% larger than 5 mm while the Cynosure laser was up to 8% smaller. Therefore it is prudent to check the diameter of the spot with burn paper before switching from one PDL machine to another.

Neodymium:Yttrium-Aluminum-Garnet (Nd:YAG) Laser

Doubling the frequency and halving the wavelength to 532 nm has made the 1064 nm Nd:YAG laser more potentially useful in the management of vascular lesions. This laser is produced by Continuum (CB Diode/532), and other laser companies. The 532-nm wavelength is at one of the hemoglobin peaks for 50-μm superficial blood vessels. This allows some selectivity in treating vascular lesions. However, its shorter wavelength does not allow deep penetration. A preliminary study using the Con-Bio Laser (Continuum) at fluences ranging from 1 to 6 J/cm^2 (maximum 10 ns, 150 mJ) in mice and rabbit ear veins showed a depth of coagulation of 0.73 ± 0.44 mm and hemorrhage of 0.68 ± 0.41 mm. In addition, edema (blistering) was observed at all fluences tested with mild subcutaneous fibrosis and epidermal hypertrophy. Therefore this laser can produce vascular injury, but because of its interaction with epidermal melanin, it is relatively nonselective.

Potassium Titanyl Phosphate (KTP) Laser

LaserScope (San Jose, CA) has developed a modulated KTP laser that uses an arc lamp running at a constant current pulsed to a much higher current than the lamp can tolerate under current operation. This produces an average power up to 160 W packaged into a single pulse that can be adjusted to pulse durations of 1 to 100 ms at pulse rates that are adjustable from one to ten pulses per second. Ten watts of power are available, with peak power of up to 60 W for pulse widths of 1 to 50 ms. The fluence is delivered through a bare fiber 1–5 mm in diameter, which can be connected to various scanning delivery systems.

The KTP lasers are used in three modes when treating vascular lesions. In one mode the laser is used with the Dermastat (LaserScope), which applies a spot size to the skin varying in size from 0.1 to 2.0 mm in diameter. The maximum average laser power is 5 W, and the pulse duration can be varied in the range of 0.1 to 1.0 s. The 1-mm spot size at 5 W with a pulse duration of 0.2 s generates a fluence of 127 J/cm^2 on the skin. Higher fluences can be selected by using longer pulse durations or smaller spot sizes. These high energies may not be appropriate for treating PWS in children or pink superficial lesions.

Intense Pulsed Noncoherent Light

The PhotoDerm VL is the original intense pulsed light source emitting a continuous light spectrum with most of its energy fluence between 515 and 1000 nm. Xenon-filled flashlamps are the primary light source with the lamps powered by a capacitor bank. The lamps are cooled by water which surrounds the lamps and helps in cutting down longer infra-red emissions. The intense pulse light source produces incoherent light whose spectrum can be cut off through the use of colored filters. Filters in standard use are 515, 550, 560, 570, 595, 610, 645, 695 and 755 nm. These filters block out the shorter wavelengths, allowing the energy fluence to be concentrated up to 1000 nm with resulting deeper penetration of the high-intensity pulsed light (Fig. 2.5). Different manufacturers use different absorbing filters to cut-off the lower wavelengths. Palomar uses a fluorescent filter to shift the wavelengths to the right preserving the 800–950-nm band (this is said by the company to help with dermal heating).

The pulse durations of the Lumenis IPLs can be adjusted from 2 to 25 ms/pulse given as a single, double, or triple pulse with delays between pulses of 2 to 100 ms. The total energy fluence emitted can range from 3 to 90 J/cm^2. Other IPL devises do not have this degree of variability. Most systems have only one or two pulse durations that are directly correlated with the energy fluence, so that if a higher fluence is needed, the pulse duration is longer. The Palomar Palmalite/Prolite features advanced pulse-forming. The target tissue experiences the pulse burst as continuous. The first third of the pulse train with higher power is said to heat up the target tissue with the lower power last third of the pulse train maintaining the target tissue temperature.

The fluence is delivered through a quartz or sapphire light guide with a spot size/surface area of 8 × 15 to 15 × 35 mm (Figs 2.6–2.8). This spot size can be further minimized by covering the surface area with any opaque covering, such as white paper. All settings are computer controlled to deliver the desired energy to a flashlamp. The exact wavelength spectral output is proprietary.

The ability to pulse the intense light rapidly within the thermal relaxation time of the target vessel allows an accumulation of heat to occur within the target vessel with dissipation of heat within the epidermis (Figs 2.9 and 2.10). The use of a cool gel on the skin surface and/or a cooled crystal that touches the epidermis provides epidermal protection to heat generated by the light output (Fig. 2.11). The ability of the epidermis to cool more quickly than the target vessel is a function of the vessel size. When one combines the longer wavelength, longer pulse duration, larger spot size, and ability to deliver multiple pulses within the thermal relaxation time of the target vessel, treatment efficacy is enhanced. Multiple sequential pulsing is a proprietary technology of Lumenis. All other IPL devises use variations of increasing fluence with pulse duration and various methods of epidermal cooling to selectively heat blood vessels.

The BBL™ intense pulsed light is available as a module for the ScitonProfile platform or as a stand-alone system (Sciton, Sunnyvale, CA). BBL has the widest single pulse width of presently available IPLs and can also deliver double or triple pulses. An integrated thermo-electric cooled sapphire crystal cools the treatment area and can control skin temperature to within 1°C during an entire

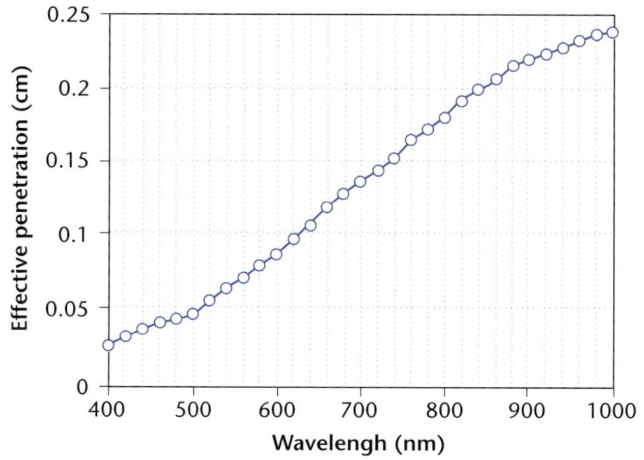

Figure 2.5 Light penetration into tissue. (Courtesy ESC Medical, Inc.)

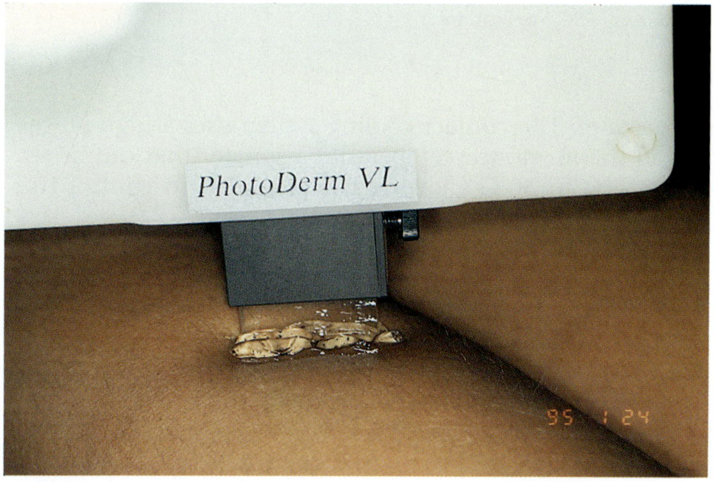

Figure 2.6 Application of intense pulsed light (IPL) treatment head to the skin. Pulsed light passes through quartz crystal light guide and layer of clear coupling gel before going into skin.

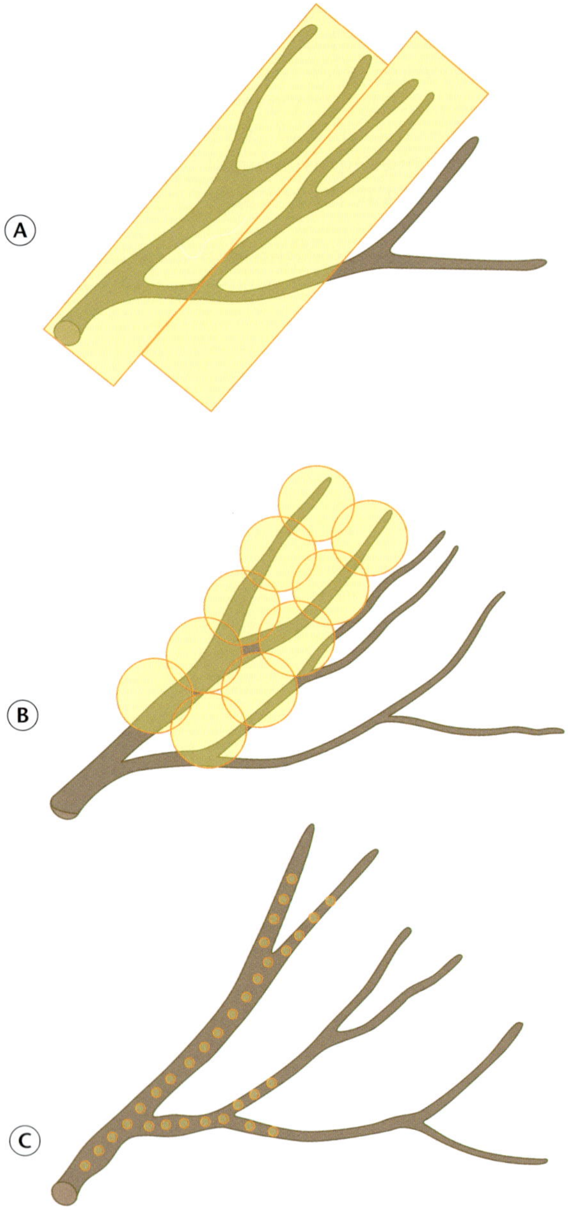

Figure 2.7 (A) Footprint of the intense pulsed light. (B) Footprint of 5-mm-diameter pulsed dye laser (PDL). (C) Footprint of typical CVL. (Courtesy ESC Medical, Inc.)

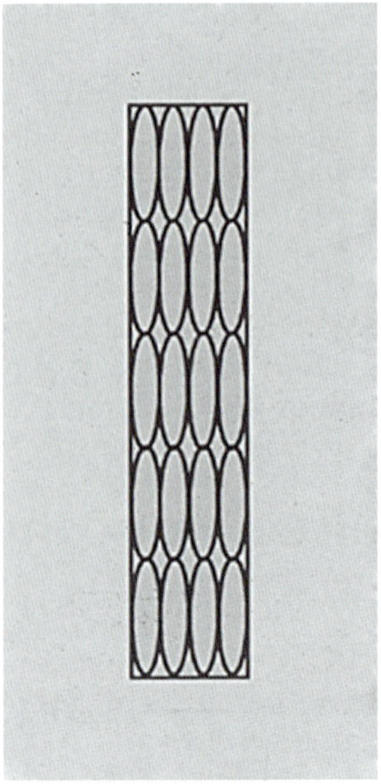

Figure 2.8 Footprint of elliptic pulsed dye laser (PDL) compared with intense pulsed light (IPL) footprint. (Courtesy ESC Medical, Inc.)

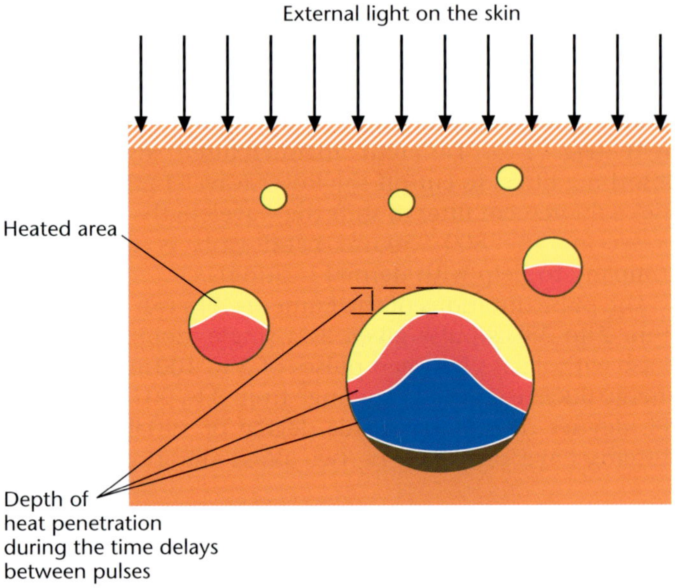

Figure 2.9 Diagram of effect of repetitive pulses of intense pulsed light on 2-mm vessel, 1 mm below epidermis. (Courtesy ESC Medical, Inc.)

procedure. The contact cooling system uses a high-power quad thermoelectric temperature regulator that can be set from 0°C to 30°C allowing the physician to control the level of epidermal cooling.

The vascular network leading to facial flushing, redness and fine telangiectasia is very near the surface as is dyspigmentation. Surface cooling systems may affect the response of the superficial vascular targets and surface pigmentation to the IPL. With the proper temperature control BBL is able to treat vascular conditions and pigmented lesions with only 50% of the fluence of many other systems leading to greater comfort, safety, and consistency. For deeper targets the high power of the quad-thermoelectric system can provide deep regulated cooling for maximum patient comfort.

BBL uses an advanced dual-lamp configuration. The lifetime of lamps decreases rapidly as they are driven to higher energies. Using dual lamps results in each lamp supplying half of the energy for a lifetime that is an order of magnitude greater than that of a typical single-lamp system. As a result, BBL comes with a standard 300,000-shot warranty. BBL has the following filters: 420 nm, 515 nm, 560 nm, 590 nm, 640 nm, 695 nm, and 755 nm.

Table 2.3 details the present variety of vascular-specific lasers available.

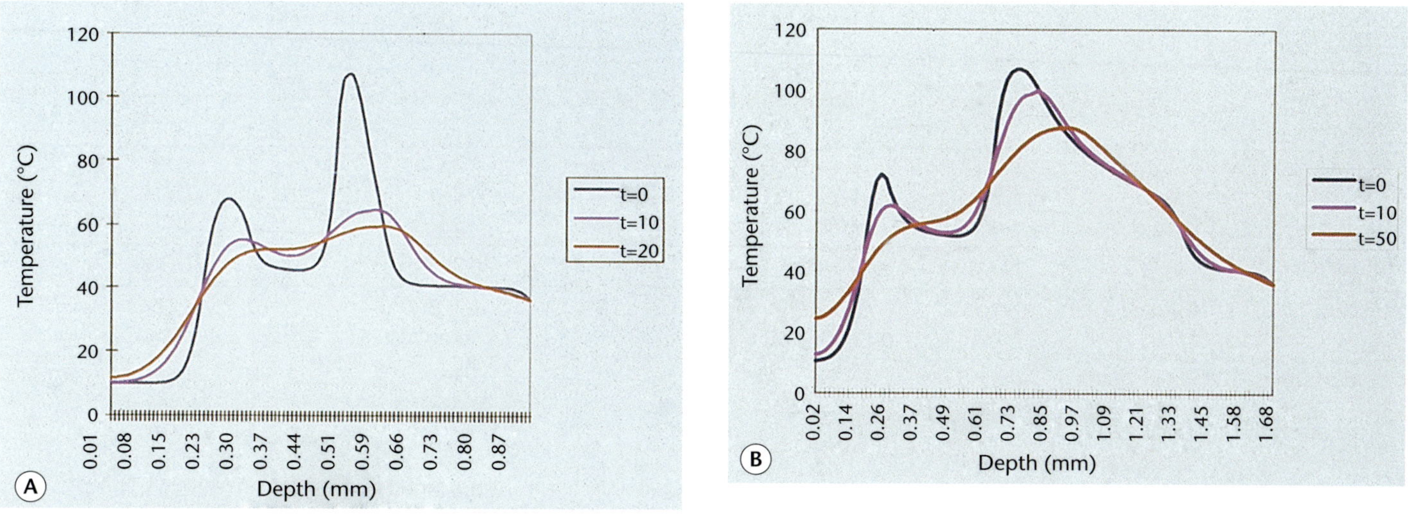

Figure 2.10 (A) Vessel size is 0.2 mm in diameter. Double pulse with 550-nm cut-off filter is used with energy of 35 J/cm^2 given in 2.4-ms pulses. (B) Vessel size is 1 mm in diameter. Double pulse is given with 590-nm cutoff filter and energy of 40 J/cm^2 given in 2.4- and 4.0-ms pulses. (Courtesy ESC Medical, Inc.)

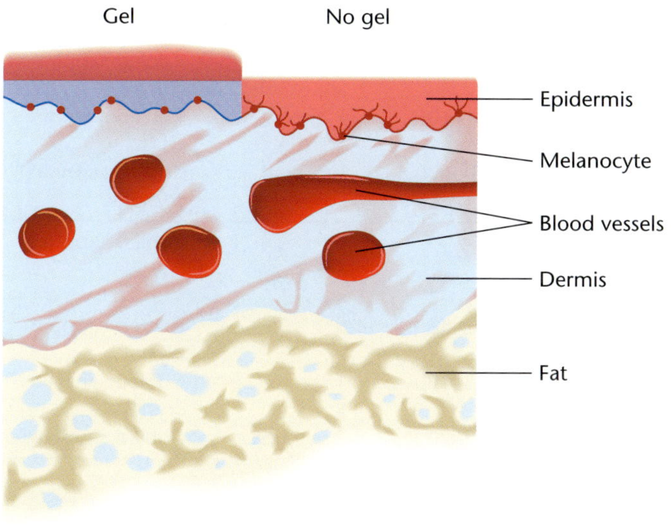

Figure 2.11 Application of cool gel to skin minimizes thermal damage and allows thermocoagulation to occur in vessel. Without gel, skin is thermally damaged before the underlying vessel is thermocoagulated.

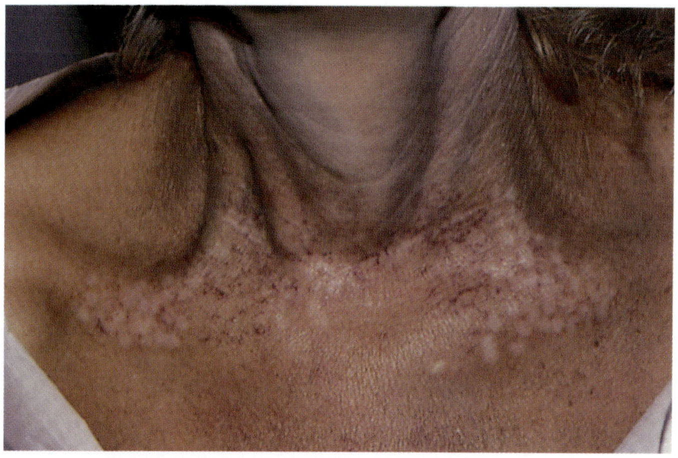

Figure 2.12 A 48-year-old woman 20 years after radiation therapy for thyroid tumor with development of telangiectasia. Clinical appearance 6 months after treatment with pulsed dye laser at 7 J/cm^2. Hypopigmented macules took approximately 18 months for complete resolution.

Adverse Effects of Vascular Lasers

Hypopigmentation can occur in treated areas in dark-skinned patients and was found in 3.2% of patients in one study, who were Hispanic or Middle Eastern treated with the PDL.[35] Persistent hypopigmentation is more common on the neck, legs, and chest (Fig. 2.12). Persistent hyperpigmentation may also occur with premature sun exposure on facial areas and after treatment of vascular lesions on the leg. This is especially common and appears as 'skipped' areas of normal skin on a background of sun-damaged skin. (Fig. 2.13) Fortunately, most hypopigmented areas resolve spontaneously within 6–12 months. Treating these areas with an Eximer laser or Relume narrow band UVB light source (Relume, Lumenis, Santa Clara, CA) can speed repigmentation.

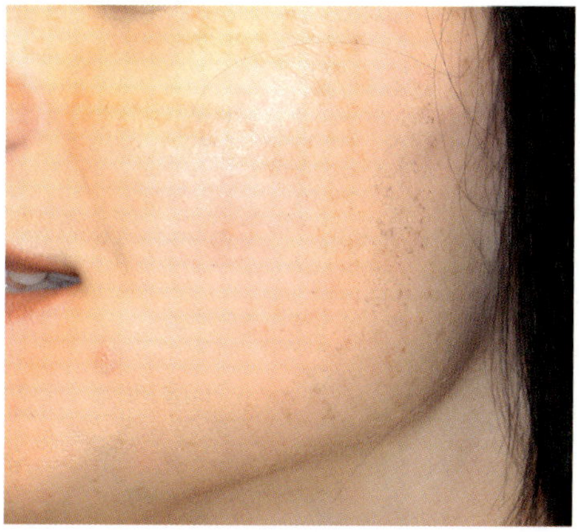

Figure 2.13 Patient treated with the intense pulsed light. Each impulse is spaced too far apart and areas of 'skipped' treated skin are apparent.

Table 2.3 *Vascular Specific Lasers and Intense Pulsed Light*

Supplier	Product name	Device type	Wavelength (nm)	Energy (Joules)	Pulse duration (ms)	Spot diameter (mm)	Cooling
American BioCare	OmniLight FPL	Fluorescent pulsed light	480, 515, 535, 550, 580–1200	Up to 90	Up to 500		External continuous
Candela	Vbeam	Pulsed dye	595	25	0.45–40	5, 7, 10, 12	DCD
	Cbeam	Pulsed dye	585	8–16	0.45	5, 7, 10	DCD
	Gentle YAG	Nd:YAG	1064	Up to 600	0.25–300		DCD
CoolTouch	Varia	Nd:YAG	1064	Up to 500	0.3–500	2–10	DCD
Cutera	Vantage	Nd:YAG	1064	Up to 300	0.1–300	3, 5, 7, 10	Copper contact
	XEO	Pulsed light	600–850	5–20	?Automatic		None
Cynosure/Deka	PhotoGenicaV	Pulsed dye	585	20	0.45	3, 5, 7, 10	Cold air
	PhotoGenica V-Star	Pulsed dye	585–595	40	0.5–40	5, 7, 10, 12	Cold air
	SmartEpill II	Nd:YAG	1064	1–200	Up to 100	2, 3, 5, 7, 10	Cold air
	Acclaim 7000	Nd:YAG	1064	300	0.4–300	2, 3, 5, 7, 10	Cold air
	PhotoLight	Pulsed light	400–1200	3–30	5–50	46 × 18; 46 × 10	None
DermaMed USA	Quadra Q4	Pulsed light	510–1200	10–20	60–200		None
Laserscope	Lyra	Nd:YAG	1064	5–900	20–100	1–5 cont. adjustable	Cooled sapphire crystal
	Aura	KTP	532	1–240	1–50	1–5 cont. adjustable	Cooled sapphire crystal
	Gemini	KTP	532	Up to 100	1–100	1–5 cont. adjustable	Cooled sapphire crystal
		Nd:YAG	1064	Up to 990	10–100	1–5 cont. adjustable	Cooled sapphire crystal
Lumenis	Quantum	Pulsed light	515–1200				Cooled sapphire crystal
	Vasculite Elite	Pulsed light	515–1200	3–90	1–75	35 × 8	
		Nd:YAG	1064	70–150	2–48	6	Cooled sapphire crystal
	Lumenis One	Pulsed light	515–1200	10–40	3–100	15 × 35, 8 × 15	Cooled sapphire crystal
		Nd:YAG	1064	10–225	2–20	2 × 4,6,9	Cooled sapphire
Med-Surge	Quantel Viridis	Diode	532	Up to 110	15–150		
	Prolitell	Pulsed light	550–900	10–50		10 × 20, 20 × 25	None
Orion Lasers	Harmony	Fluorescent pulsed light	540–950	5–20	10, 12, 15	40 × 16	None
		Nd:YAG	1064	35–145	40–60	6 mm	None
		Nd:YAG	1064	35–450	10	2 mm	None
Palomar	MediLux	Pulsed light	470–1400	Up to 45	10–100	12 × 12	None
	EsteLux	Pulsed light	470–1400	Up to 45	10–100	12 × 12	None
	StarLux	Pulsed light/Nd:YAG	550–670/870–1400/1064	Up to 700	0.5–500		
Sciton	Profile	Nd:YAG	1064	4–400	0.1–200		Contact sapphire
	Profile BBL	Pulsed light	400–1400	Up to 30	Up to 200	30 × 30, 13 × 15	
Syneron	Aurora SR	Pulsed light /RF	580–980	10–30/2–25 RF	Up to 200	12 × 25	Contact sapphire
	Polaris	Diode/RF	900	Up to 50/Up to 100 RF		8 × 12 5 × 8	Contact sapphire Contact sapphire
	Galaxy	Diode	580–980	Up to 140/Up to 100RF	Up to 200		
WaveLight	Mydon	Nd:YAG	1064	10–450	0.5–90	1.5, 3, 5	Contact or air cooling

Although rare, hypertrophic scarring has been reported with high laser fluences and when treating lesions on the neck, arms, or shoulder with any vascular specific laser.[35–37] Another report described 'isolated, superficial, depressed scars' in 2 of 35 children treated, reportedly in areas traumatized within 24 hours after PDL treatment.[19] Two of 92 adults with facial telangiectasia developed dermal atrophy with normal skin texture on the nose, nasolabial folds, and malar regions that lasted at least 6 months. These areas were treated with a 1-mm spot diameter PDL at a fluence of 7 J/cm^2.[38] Laser fluence, lesion location, and posttreatment care are important factors that may contribute to the risk of scarring.

Port-wine Stain (Capillary Malformation)

Port-wine stains (PWSs) occur in 0.3% to 0.5% of newborns[39,40] and represent a congenital malformation of the superficial dermal capillaries. They should not be confused with the common pink patches known as 'nevus flammeus neonatorum', 'angel's kiss', 'stork bite', or 'salmon patch'. These 'stains' fade within the first year of life in 50% of patients. A midline PWS-appearing lesion may represent a capillary malformation that clears quickly with one or two treatments and thus is not typical of the more ectatic and venular PWS (Fig. 2.14). These midline lesions may represent a maturation delay in autonomic innervation because up to 60% of lesions resolve spontaneously.[41]

Most PWSs are superficial, with a mean vessel depth of 0.46 mm.[42] The lesion is first present as a relatively sharply marginated pink patch, most often involving the head and neck in 90% of patients, especially in the areas of the first and second trigeminal nerves.[39,40]

Videomicroscopy has demonstrated two patterns of vascular abnormality: type 1 consists of tortuous, superficial, dilated capillary loops (blobs); type 2 consists of dilated ectatic vessels in the superficial horizontal vascular plexus (rings)[43] (Figs 2.15 and 2.16). Patients with type 1 vascularity have a better response to PDL treatment because type 2 PWS lesions are more deeply situated and consist of freely anastomosing dilated vessels of the superficial horizontal vascular plexus. Videomicroscopy may allow the physician to choose the most appropriate laser or pulsed light source for treatment of PWS.

Adverse Medical Effects

In addition to their abnormal cosmetic appearance, PWSs may be associated with medical problems, the most common and serious being glaucoma and less common and serious being inflammation. Glaucoma occurs in approximately 45% of patients with a PWS involving both the ophthalmic (V_1) and maxillary (V_2) divisions of

A

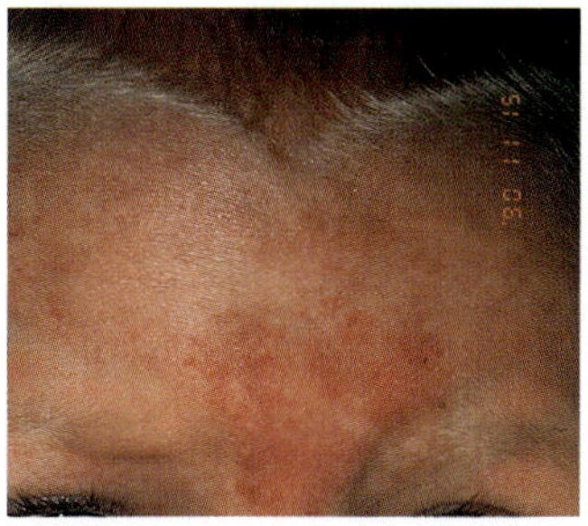

B

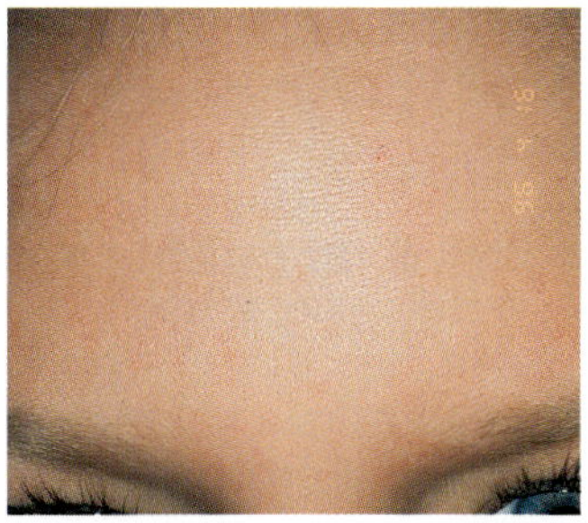

Figure 2.14 (A) Four-month-old girl with urticaria pigmentosa and midline port-wine stain before treatment. (B) 6½ years after single treatment with pulsed dye laser at 5.5 J/cm^2 using 5-mm-diameter spot size, lesions show 100% clearance without adverse sequelae and no evidence of recurrence.

A

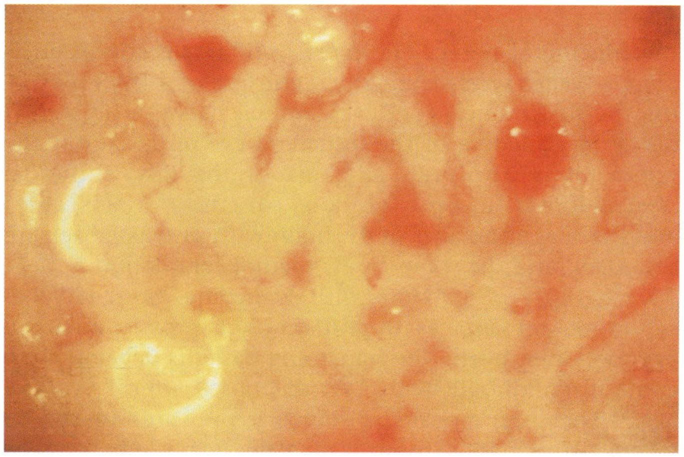

B

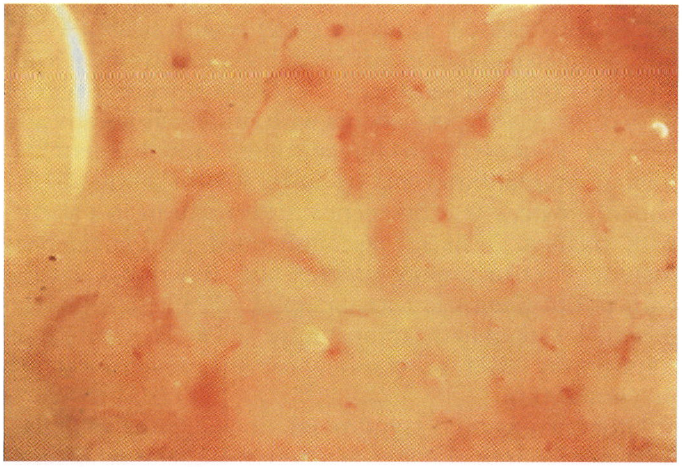

Figure 2.15 (A) Results of transcutaneous videomicroscopy of patient with port-wine stain (PWS) showing type 1 blob abnormalities (×200). (B) Results of transcutaneous videomicroscopy of patient with PWS showing type 2 ring abnormalities. Note the small, fine capillary dots that are capillary loops in normal dermal papillae. Dilated vessels of horizontal plexus lie in a deeper plane (×200). (Reprinted from Arch Dermatol 133:921, 1997. Copyright © 1997 American Medical Association. All rights reserved.)

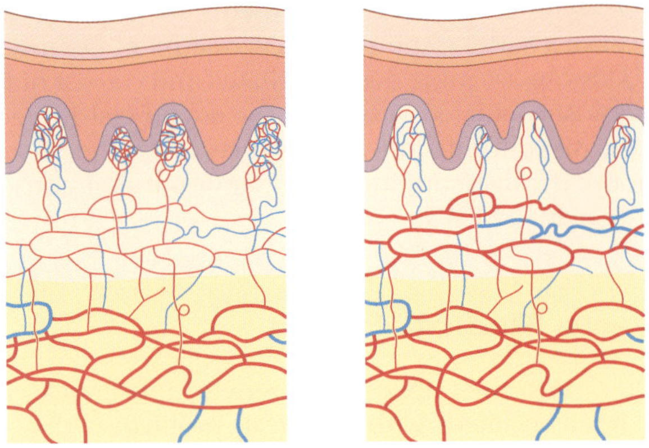

Figure 2.16 Diagrammatic representations of vascular abnormalities found with videomicroscopy. (Left) Tortuous, dilated papillary tip vessels. (Right) Dilated vessels of superficial horizontal vascular plexus. Note that type 1 abnormality (left) presents a superficial target with limited blood supply. Type 2 abnormality (right) is more deeply situated, and vessels anastomose freely. (Reprinted from Arch Dermatol 133:921, 1997. Copyright © 1997 American Medical Association. All rights reserved.)

the trigeminal nerve. The most well-known condition is Sturge–Weber syndrome, which consists of a PWS involving the first branch of the trigeminal nerve, a high incidence of glaucoma of the ipsilateral eye (especially if the upper lid is involved), angioma of the lids, choroidal hemangiomas (in up to 40% of patients),[44] calcification and vascular anomalies of the brain with associated seizure disorders, and, in some cases, mental retardation.[45–47] In 70% to 80% of patients with glaucoma, Sturge–Weber syndrome presents as buphthalmos, a grossly enlarged eye soon after birth. The remaining patients develop glaucoma in childhood, with 44% diagnosed after 4 years of age.[48] Therefore repeated intraocular pressures should be taken every 3 to 4 months if glaucoma is not present initially.

The extent of the PWS does not usually correlate with neurologic disease.[49] However patients with bilateral PWS have a greater likelihood of neurologic involvement with an earlier onset of seizures.[46,50] Epileptic seizures occur in 72% of Sturge–Weber patients with unilateral lesions and 93% of patients with bihemispheric involvement.[44,46] Mental retardation occurs in up to 30% of Sturge–Weber patients, with a 92% incidence of retardation in patients with bilateral lesions.[46] Recommended neurologic tests include electroencephalography and functional testing with positron emission tomography (PET), single-photon emission computed tomography (SPECT), computed tomography (CT) of cranium, or magnetic resonance imaging (MRI).[51]

Other congenital syndromes include the Klippel–Trenaunay and Klippel–Trenaunay–Weber syndromes (PWS with associated varicose vein and hypertrophy of skeletal tissue[52] with or without arteriovenous malformations [AVMs], respectively) and Cobb syndrome (PWS with underlying AVM of the spinal cord).[53] A PWS may be associated with an underlying venous malformation or occasionally an arterial malformation or AVM,[54] so the existence of these associated lesions should not cause confusion in diagnosis.

Various support groups are available for children with congenital vascular abnormalities and their families. The Sturge–Weber Foundation (PO Box 460931, Aurora, CO 80046, USA) publishes an excellent booklet for children that clearly explains the syndrome as well as multiple treatment options. The Klippel–Trenaunay Support Group (4610 Wooddale Ave, Edina, MN 55424, USA) publishes a useful quarterly newsletter and holds support group and educational meetings for the public. The National Congenital Port-Wine Stain Foundation (125 E. 63rd St, New York, NY 10021, USA) also provides information and support to patients and families of children with PWSs; www.birthmarks.com is an excellent website for patient information. Patients and parents should be encouraged to use these resources.

PWSs can also present with an inflammatory component consisting of scaling, excoriations, oozing, and crusting, resembling a dermatitis.[55] PWS with this secondary inflammation has been reported in lesions on the nuchal and occipital areas. Treatment with topical steroids helps decrease the inflammation, but the PDL is curative after one treatment.

The natural history of a PWS is that the vessels become progressively ectatic over time.[42,56] This results in gradual darkening, thickening, and development of nodularity (Fig. 2.17). One study found that two-thirds of patients develop hypertrophy and nodularity by age 46, with a mean age of 37 years for hypertrophy.[57] Rarely, spontaneous improvement may occur,[58] possibly during the first 3 years of life.

Giant proliferative hemangiomas may also arise in PWSs and can develop without any prior history of trauma.[59]

Psychologic Impact

In addition to lesion characteristics that may cause bleeding and produce physical deformity, a PWS carries a definite risk for lasting detrimental effects on a child's psychologic, social, interpersonal, and cognitive development.[60–62] The exact age when psychosocial development is affected is speculative. A psychiatric study of 19 children 3 to 5 years old with face, head, or neck hemangiomas found no association with major problems in psychosocial development.[63,64] However, early treatment improves the responsiveness, decreases the number of treatments, and reduces the likelihood of permanent adverse sequelae.[19,26–28,64] Therefore we recommend that treatment be started at the earliest possible age.

A common misperception regarding PWS in adults is that if one has reached adulthood without psychologic damage from a cosmetic deformity, one does not require treatment. Former Soviet president Mikail Gorbachev is an example of successful 'coping' with a cosmetic handicap. (Interestingly, the Soviet news agency, Tass, airbrushed out Gorbachev's PWS from published photographs until *perestroika*.) However, such presumptions are often incorrect.

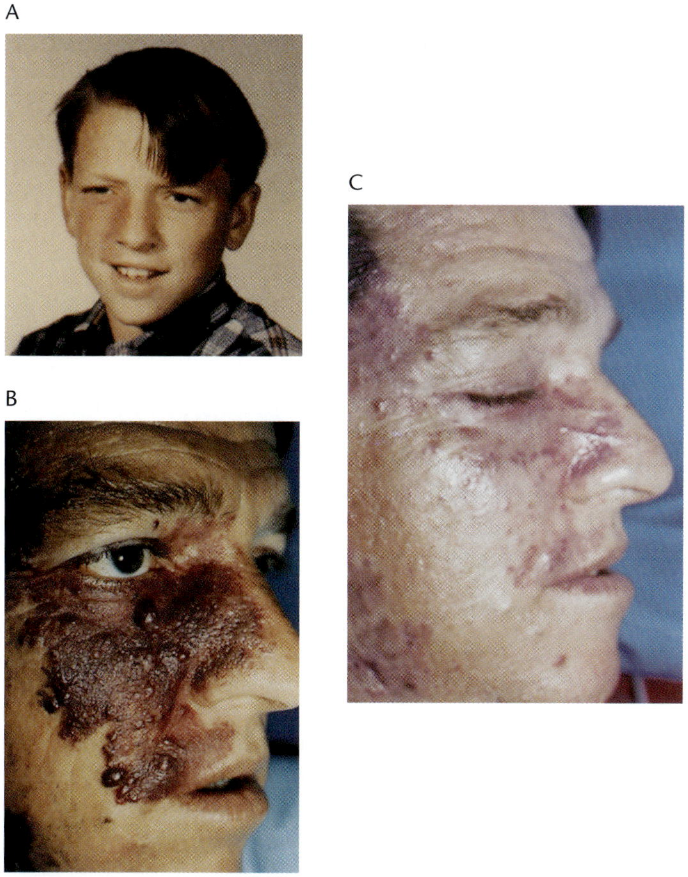

Figure 2.17 Progressive nodularity of port-wine stain (PWS) is noted with aging. (A) Patient, age 15, has light-pink PWS on right cheek. (B) Patient, age 35, has marked nodularity and darkening of PWS. (C) Clinical appearance after 12 separate treatments with pulsed dye laser at average fluence of 7.0 to 7.5 J/cm^2. Each treatment averaged 600 5-mm impacts. (Courtesy of Gerald Goldberg, MD.)

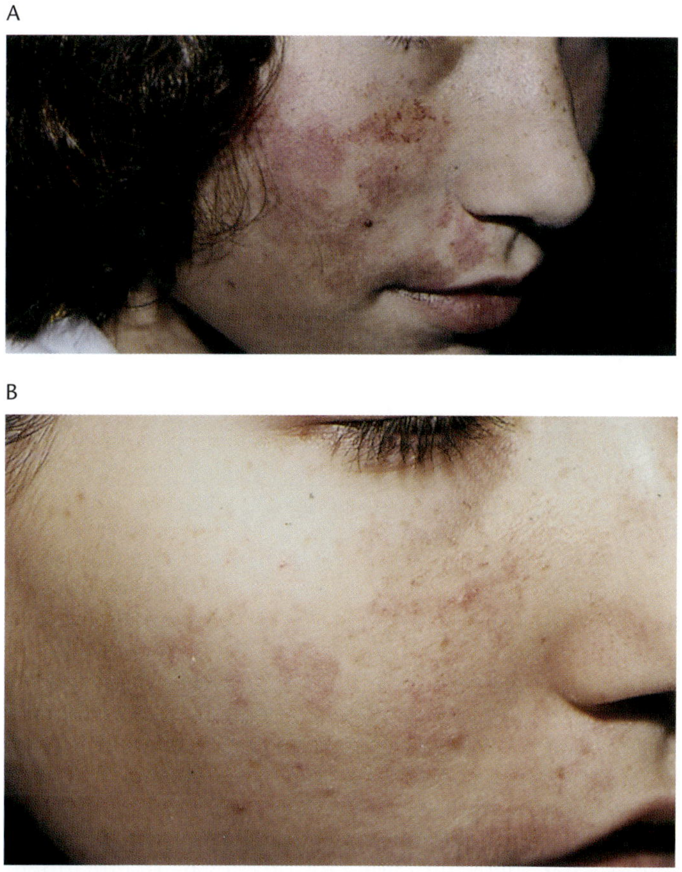

Figure 2.18 (A) Twelve-year-old girl with congenital port-wine stain on her right cheek. (B) After third treatment with pulsed dye laser. First treatment used a fluence of 7.25 J/cm^2 with 213 5-mm pulses, second treatment 7.5 J/cm^2 with 109 5-mm pulses, and third treatment 7.5 J/cm^2 with 40 5-mm pulses. Patient and parents noted 90% resolution of entire lesion. (From Goldman MP, Fitzpatrick RE, Ruiz-Esparza J. J Pediatr 1993; 122:71.)

More often, the misperception of treatment complications along with cost considerations are the primary reasons for avoiding treatment. These misconceptions are often used by insurance companies to deny coverage and save money. Unfortunately, cosmetic considerations are not the only reasons PWS should be treated in adults. Hypertrophy, hemorrhage, and infection are the medical reasons for treatment.

Adult PWS can also have an adverse impact on social relationships. A questionnaire given to 186 patients who sought treatment for their PWS found that 29% thought the PWS was disadvantageous in forming interpersonal relationships with members of the opposite sex.[65] Half rated their PWS as unattractive, although only 33% thought that other people perceived their PWS to be moderately to very unattractive. The true incidence of psychologic problems from PWS may be higher or lower because this study was obviously skewed to patients who were actively seeking treatment. Nevertheless, the survey does show that a significant number of adults with PWS would benefit psychologically from treatment.

Psychologic difficulties in interactions with others occur as often in adults as in children. An experiment during the 1989 annual meeting of the American Academy of Dermatology dramatically demonstrates this point. A model had a PWS painted on her face and then feigned an illness that led to unconsciousness on a public bus. Not one passenger came to her aid. When the same model feigned the same illness on a bus without the facial PWS, all those present eagerly came to her aid. Pena Clementina Masclarelli,[66] a senior occupational therapist who also has an extensive PWS, wrote a poignant chapter about her interactions with others that should be required reading for all physicians.

Multiple studies have demonstrated an improvement in psychological health after successful treatment of PWS.[63,67,68] We have noted a change in personal perceptions dramatically in our treated patients. A 12-year-old girl first sought treatment in our practice for a PWS on the right cheek. Initially, although of above-average intelligence, she was introverted and interacted sparingly with her classmates. After three treatment sessions, resulting in 75% clearance, she began dating, joined the school band, and excelled academically (Fig. 2.18). These are the obser-

Table 2.4 *Childhood Port-wine Stains: Treatment Response by Age*

No. patients	No. lesions	Average range	Average age	Average treatments	Average improvement (%)	Median improvement (%)	95% Improvement No. lesions	95% Improvement Average treatments
Age 0–4 years								
21	25	2 weeks to 4 years	2.15 years	3.4	70	75	5 (20%)	3.8
Age 4.5–14 years								
22	24	6–14 years	10.3 years	4.0	68	75	3 (12.5%)	6.5
Total 0–14 years								
43	49	2 weeks to 14 years	6.2 years	3.7	69	75	8 (16.3%)	4.8

From Goldman MP, Fitzpatrick RE, Ruiz-Esparza J. J Pediatr 1993; 122:71.

vations so gratifying to the physician and medical staff involved in laser treatment.

Despite the psychologic and medical complications of PWS, insurance coverage in the US for laser treatment of PWS varies from state to state. A study by McClean and Hanke[69] of insurance reimbursement in 18 States found that determination for approval of treatment was made on a case-by-case basis, with the majority requiring preauthorization. The percentage of requests approved for coverage varied from 50% to 100% without apparent reason. Some insurance carriers would only approve treatment if functional impairment existed and some only if the patient was less than 1 year of age. Only Minnesota has a law requiring all health insurance to cover the elimination or maximum feasible treatment of PWS.

Treatment

Many therapeutic methods have been attempted to treat PWSs. These include surgery (excision, grafts, flaps, dermabrasion),[45,70,71] radium implants,[72] X-ray therapy,[45] cryosurgery,[73] electrocautery,[21] sclerotherapy,[64] tattooing,[74,75] and cosmetic camouflage.[76] These methods all have limited and unpredictable results as well as potentially serious complications.[64] In addition to currently recommended laser treatments, the CO_2 laser,[77–80] Nd:YAG laser,[81] copper vapor laser (CVL),[82,83] and argon laser[56,84–87] have previously been used to treat PWS in children. As previously discussed, cosmetic results with these lasers have been poor in children, with the risk of scarring unacceptably high.

Childhood Port-wine Stains

The PDL was specifically designed to treat the small vessels found in childhood PWSs.[19,21] The first published reports noted complete clearing of pink-to-red macular PWSs in 35 children less than 14 years old (mean age 7 years 2 months) with an average of 6.5 treatments.[19] Subsequent clinical studies demonstrated notable efficacy and defined more reasonable expectations. Reyes and Geronemus[26] successfully treated 73 patients between age 3 months and 14 years. The overall average lightening after one treatment was 53%, and the percentage of lightening increased with subsequent treatments. More than 75% lightening was achieved with an average of 2.5 treatments in 33 patients.

Morelli and Weston[88] advocate beginning treatment as early as 7 to 14 days of age so that three treatments can be done before the infant reaches 6 months of age. They noted a 50% resolution with this protocol by the third treatment. In their population of 132 patients, complete clearance was obtained in 25% of PWSs when treatment was begun before 18 months of age (average 7.8 treatment sessions) versus 7% to 10% having total clearance when treatment was begun between ages $1\frac{1}{2}$ and 18 years (average 7.0 treatment sessions). A follow-up evaluation of this patient population confirmed the authors' initial observations with 83 children: 32% of children who began treatment before 1 year of age had complete clearing of their PWS compared with 18% of children treated after 1 year of age.[89] In this later study, 32% of patients with PWS less than 20 cm^2 in size completely cleared compared with an 8% complete clearance rate in patients with larger PWSs.

Our studies on the treatment of 43 children between ages 2 weeks and 14 years with 49 lesions of capillary malformation confirm these results.[28] Lesions treated in children under age 4 had greater overall improvement with less treatment sessions compared with those in children over age $4\frac{1}{2}$ years (Table 2.4). In general, improvement and clearance were gradual and required 5 to 10 treatments. However, very superficial lesions cleared more quickly, with four lesions reaching a level of 95% clearing in one or two treatments (Table 2.5).

Table 2.5 *Childhood Port-wine Stains: Response Per Number of Treatments*

No. treatments	No. lesions	Improvement of nonclear lesion						
		Average treatment energy (J)	Mean (%)	Median (%)	No. lesions			
					>95% clear	Percent	Mean (%)	Median (%)
1	10	6.73	51	50	1	10	46	40
2	12	6.96	70.4	72	3	25	61	50
3	5	6.55	62	60	0	0	62	60
4	4	6.86	70	70	0	0	70	70
5	10	7.05	77.5	80	2	20	72.5	77
6–11	8	6.50	85	90	3	37.5	78	80

From Goldman MP, Fitzpatrick RE, Ruiz-Esparza J. J Pediatr 1993; 122:71.

An additional study of 12 children 6 to 30 weeks of age confirmed that treatment of infants only a few weeks old can be undertaken safely and with an accelerated response: 45% demonstrated 75% or more lightening of their lesions after a mean of 3.8 treatments.[64] Alster and Wilson[90] reported an 87% clearance rate in patients less than 2 years of age, 78% clearance in patients ages 3 to 8, and 73% clearance rate in patients 16 years and older. All these studies demonstrate a better treatment outcome with younger patients.

Only one study of 23 facial PWS lesions in patients up to age 17 showed no difference among different ages in the average number of treatments to obtain maximum lesion lightening.[91] However, this study only evaluated four lesions in children less than 1 year of age and eight lesions in those 1 to 7 years of age.

Although treatment is efficacious and most laser surgeons recommend treatment at the earliest sign of a lesion, photothermolysis of blood vessels does result in the release of free Hb into the circulation. Hemoglobinemia may theoretically lead to renal impairment in a young patient. Therefore a study of 15 patients under age 5 treated with the PDL tested serum haptoglobin and urine hemosiderin postoperatively.[92] Even though patients had a treatment region more than 3% of total body surface area and received more than 1500 5-mm-diameter pulses in some cases, the authors found no evidence of urine hemoglobin and reported normal levels of serum haptoglobin levels.

Therefore the advantages of early treatment are: (1) quicker resolution requiring fewer treatments; (2) fewer laser pulses because of smaller size (children triple in size from birth to age 2 and further double in size from ages 2 to 8); and (3) less need for anesthesia.

Unfortunately, pediatricians and family practitioners are reluctant to refer their patients for treatment. This is most likely a result of too few reports in all but the most recent pediatric literature and thus lack of knowledge. Second, older physicians may remember the failures of the argon laser in treating these lesions and equate all laser treatment with the argon laser. Third, treatment is usually painful to the child.

In our experience, treatment is considerably eased with topical anesthetic creams, cooling the epidermis with cryogen spray or ice, or conscious sedation administered by a pediatric anesthesiologist, but necessary only in children 8 years old or younger. Fortunately, earliest childhood memories usually occur after 2 or 3 years of age.[93] Thus treatments given before this time should not have long-term psychologic effects. We have been treating infants with the PDL since 1985 and have yet to observe adverse psychologic effects in our patients with continuing long-term follow-up. Some of our initial patients, treated in the first few months of life with continued treatment at 4- to 6-month intervals, are now 8 to 10 years old and continue to receive treatment without apparent psychologic trauma.

For children less than age 12 years, we recommend laser fluences that generate slight purpura. We like to use a large spot size (10–12 mm in diameter for PDL or the large footprint of the IPL) to minimize skipped areas. The initial treatment session usually results in an average improvement of approximately 50%. Each subsequent treatment provides an additional increment of approximately 10% improvement. After six treatments, 40% of our patients completely clear, and those who are not clear have an average improvement of approximately 80% (Fig. 2.19). We have not had patients with scarring or persistent pigmentary changes despite rare episodes of vesiculation and crusting after treatment. Skin type (I–III) also does not appear to influence the ultimate treatment outcome, but darker skin requires more treatment sessions to achieve the same degree of clearing as in PWSs of fair-skinned patients as we recommend lower fluences and a higher degree of epidermal cooling. Lesions on distal limbs respond with less fading than lesions elsewhere, such as on the neck and torso (Table 2.6). The diminished response of PWS on the limbs has been reported by others.[94,95]

Fortunately, treatment of PWS in childhood and infancy not only has been very efficacious with the PDL, but also

A

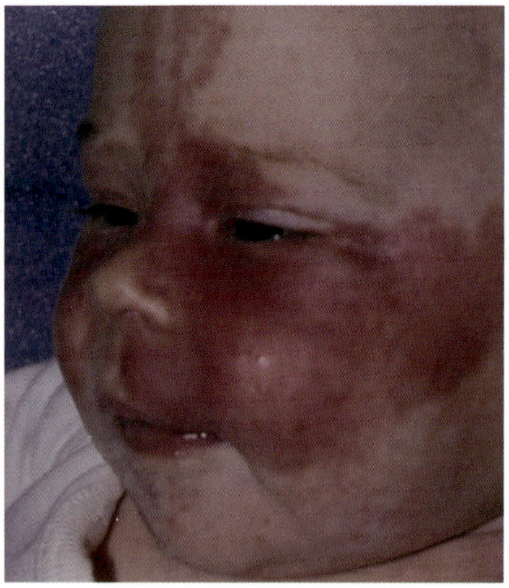

B

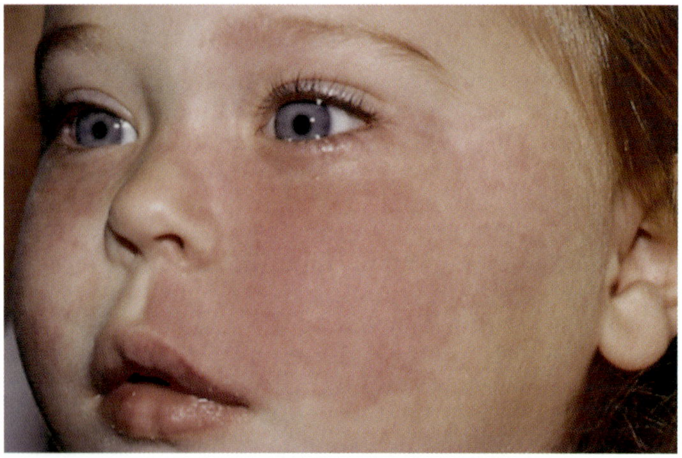

Figure 2.19 (A) Initial appearance of extensive port-wine stain (PWS) on a 10-week-old girl. Evaluation by pediatric neurologist was entirely within normal limits. (B) The same patient 4 months after her fourth treatment with the pulsed dye laser. First and second treatments were performed at an energy of $6\,J/cm^2$ and third and fourth treatments at $6.25\,J/cm^2$. Total of 400 pulses were given to the entire PWS during each treatment visit. Parents and physician noted almost 90% resolution of PWS. (From Goldman MP, Fitzpatrick RE, Ruiz-Esparza J. J Pediatr 1993; 122:71.)

has proved to be safe. Swelling and erythema are frequently present immediately after treatment, especially around the eyes, but resolve within 24 to 48 hours. Hyperpigmentation of the treated site occurs in 25% to 30% of patients but is temporary and resolves over 2 to 3 months. Hypopigmentation occurs infrequently and resolves spontaneously over 3 to 6 months. Cutaneous depressions or atrophic scars have occurred in isolated laser impact sites and have been associated with excessive delivery of energy, excessive spot overlap, or posttreatment trauma to the site. Almost all reported cases have resolved spontaneously within 1 year.[21,26,28]

Adult Port-wine Stains

The treatment of PWS in adults has been as equally gratifying as our experience in children (Figs 2.20 and 2.21). The PDL is used in the same manner as with children except that fluences are usually increased depending on the lesion's color and thickness. A 7- to 12-mm-diameter spot size is preferred because of its deeper penetration. We recommend beginning with a fluence of 5.0 to $5.5\,J/cm^2$ with a 7-mm-diameter spot size and increasing by $0.5\,J/cm^2$ with each subsequent treatment at 3- to 4-month intervals.

A mathematical model as well as clinical experience predict a 10% clearance of the PWS with each of the first five or six treatments. Additional treatments result in a decreased therapeutic response so that 20 treatments are required to produce a 90% clearing.[96]

The IPL can also be used in a number of different settings to effect vascular-specific thermocoagulation of PWS. Multiple studies have demonstrated an enhanced efficacy of clearing in comparison to the PDL. This holds true even for Asian patients.[97–101]

Different settings are used with each treatment, which can be given at monthly intervals. We usually increase the fluence with each subsequent treatment as well as the pulse duration, cutoff filter, and number of simultaneous pulses (Fig. 2.22). The following settings are effective for initial and subsequent treatments (these settings apply for the Lumenis vasculite system; parameters will vary with other IPL systems):

Table 2.6 *Childhood Port-wine Stains: Treatment Response by Location*

Location				>95% clear		
	No. lesions	Average no. treatments	Average improvement (%)	No. lesions	Percent	Average no. treatments
Face	33	3.5	65	4	12	4.0
Neck	4	5.3	90	2	50	4.5
Torso	6	3.0	85	3	50	3.0
Hand and arm	6	3.7	63	0	–	0

From Goldman MP, Fitzpatrick RE, Ruiz-Esparza J. J Pediatr 1993; 122:71.

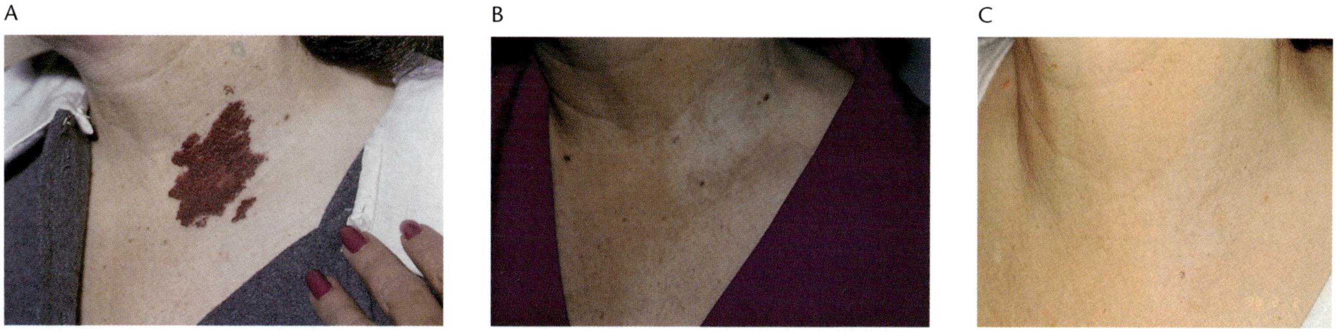

Figure 2.20 Port-wine stain on left anterior chest of 44-year-old woman. (A) Before treatment. (B) Near 100% resolution after six treatments. Each treatment used a fluence of 7.25 J/cm^2 with PDL. First treatment used 136 5-mm impacts, second treatment 175 5-mm impacts, third treatment 117 5-mm impacts, fourth treatment 87 5-mm impacts, fifth treatment 77 5-mm impacts, and sixth treatment 37 5-mm impacts. Fig. 2.20A and B: Reprinted from Fitzpatrick RE: American Journal of Cosmetic Surgery 9:107, 1992. With permission from American Academy of Cosmetic Surgery. (C) Continued clearance 12 years after original treatment clearance.

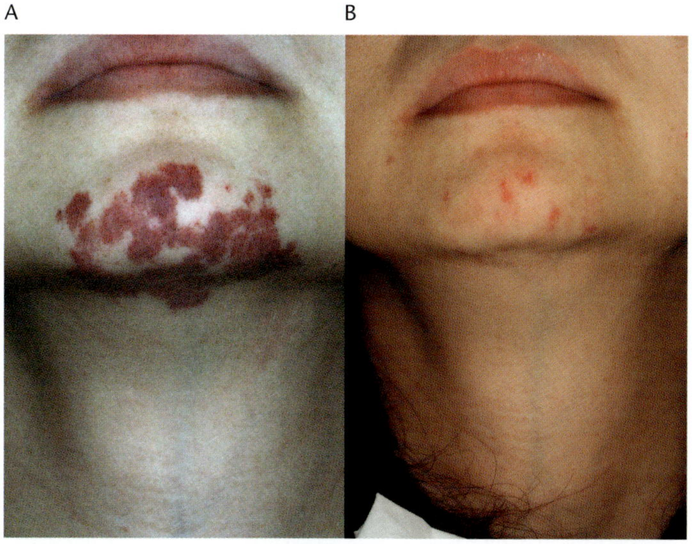

Figure 2.21 This 34-year-old patient had a port-wine stain of her chin (A). She underwent a series of five pulsed dye laser treatments with approximately 2 months between sessions. Treatment parameters were the following: 585-nm wavelength; 7- to 10-mm spot size; 8–12 J/cm^2; cryogen spray cooling spurt duration of 30–50 ms with a 30–50-ms delay. The patient achieved an excellent result (B). (Courtesy Kristen Kelley, MD.)

- 515-nm or 550-nm cutoff filter, single pulse at 2 to 5 ms with 20 to 25 J/cm^2
- 550-nm cutoff filter, double-pulsed at 2.4 ms with 10-ms delay, 4.0 ms with 35 to 42 J/cm^2
- 570-nm cutoff filter, double-pulsed at 3.0 ms with 20-ms delay, 6 ms with 40 to 45 J/cm^2
- 590-nm cutoff filter, triple-pulsed at 3 ms with 30-ms delay, 4.5 ms with 30-ms delay, 7 ms with 30-ms delay at 50 to 60 J/cm^2

As with other lesions, patients with more darkly pigmented skin are treated with higher cutoff filters to circumvent melanin absorption and longer delay times between double and triple pulses because epidermal heat is higher in these patients. Ice-cold coupling gel and/or cold contact crystals are used.

One advantage when using the IPL is the minimization of purpura after treatment (Fig. 2.23). Other advantages are described later.

Complications and Adverse Sequelae

Complications and adverse sequelae when treating vascular lesions with the PDL, IPL or any vascular specific laser as described previously are rare. Adverse sequelae are usually temporary and limited to purpura and epidermal crusting. Purpura is more common with the PDL.

The most common long-term adverse sequelae are pigmentary changes. Because melanin competes as an absorber with Hb in patients with Fitzpatrick type III skin or greater, hypopigmentation (especially in patients with tanned skin) is not uncommon. Alternatively, postinflammatory melanocytic hyperpigmentation may occur. At times this may appear as a 'checkerboard' pigmentation (Fig. 2.24). When this occurs, additional treatments are usually necessary to even out the skin color. Oftentimes, switching to the IPL, which with its larger spot size evens out the dyspigmentation in addition to the nontreated areas (discussed later). In addition, the use of depigmenting agents such as hydroxyquinone, alpha-hydroxy acids, azelaic acid, and kojic acid alone or in combination with retinoic acid both before and after treatment is helpful. Fortunately, permanent scars or pigmentary changes are very rare.

More serious potential adverse events include atrophic and hypertrophic scarring and keloid formation. The formation of keloids may be enhanced when the patient is also taking isotretinoin. Multiple case reports of the development of keloid formation in patients receiving isotretinoin have been reported with argon laser and dermabrasion treatment.[102,103] A single case report of this occurrence with PDL treatment of a neck PWS has appeared in the literature.[104] Although the mechanism for enhancing scarring is speculative and the length of time

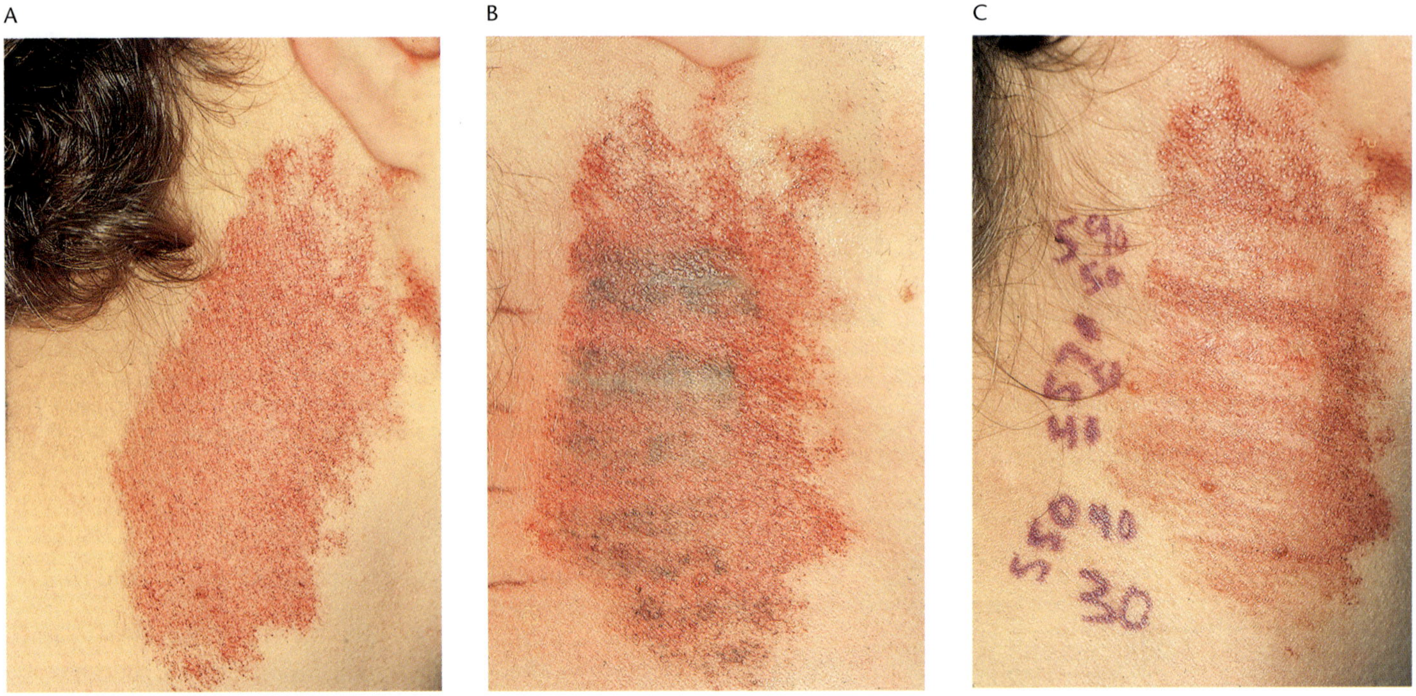

Figure 2.22 (A) Port-wine stain on 24-year-old male before treatment. (B) Immediately after treatment with PhotoDerm VL. Note purpuric response to treated areas (C) One month after treatment. Note resolution at various treatment parameters, all given in single pulses. (Top to bottom) 590-nm cutoff filter at 50 J/cm^2, 570-nm cutoff filter at 40 J/cm^2, 550-nm cutoff filter at 30 J/cm^2.

from cessation of treatment to 'safety' is unknown, it would seem prudent to avoid laser treatment within 1 to 2 years of isotretinoin use.

Numerous retrospective studies have detailed adverse sequelae. A study of 133 patients (89 females, 44 males) with PWS who had been treated with the PDL over a 2-year period showed good or excellent results in 84% of the PWSs.[27] The average number of treatments increased from 1.7 to 2.3 to 3.5 as the clinical results improved from slight to good to excellent, accordingly. After a treatment session, discoloration and purpura were seen in all patients, crusting in 51.9%, and scaling or peeling in 19.6%. Three patients reported swelling, and two reported blisters. Many patients reported crusting only after their first treatment and not with subsequent treatments. The average duration of these immediate skin changes was reported to be 7 to 14 days. Long-term skin changes with PDL therapy included hyperpigmentation in six patients, hypopigmentation in five, and isolated punctate depressions in two. Pigmentation changes in patients who had completed therapy lasted an average of 6 months. Atrophic surface changes noted in two patients involved small areas of excoriation. No hypertrophic scarring was noted. This apparent scarring was transient in nature, and both episodes resolved completely within 12 months. No significant differences in adverse sequelae were apparent between original lesions that were flat or raised.

An additional study of 500 patients treated with the PDL found an incidence of atrophic scarring of less than 0.1%. Hyperpigmentation was seen in 1% of patients and transient hypopigmentation in 2.6%. Patients with atrophic scarring were treated in the early stages of the PDL development, when problems with the dosage meter were common.

A study of 701 patients who received 3,877 full treatments with the PDL using a 5- or 7-mm-diameter spot and fluences of 5.5 to 9.5 J/cm^2 with the Candela and the Cynosure systems reported severe blistering in 1.08%, severe crusting in 0.13%, hypopigmentation in 0.26%, hyperpigmentation in 1.7%, atrophic scarring in 0.7%, and hypertrophic scarring in 0.13% of treatments.[105] Seven patients developed atrophic scarring despite uneventful test area treatments. Thirty percent of patients with scarring had clinical resolution over 6 to 12 months. Hypertrophic scarring also occurred after an uneventful test and four or five uneventful treatments. Hypertrophic scarring showed no resolution in these patients.

Complaints of discomfort from treatment were rated as moderate in 49.1% of patients, which is higher than previously reported.[21] However, pain in adults was not a limiting factor in treatment. Although patients, in retrospect, have rated treatment pain as moderate, treatment was not discontinued because of pain in any patient.

Variable Treatment Response by Lesion Location and Size

In addition to an obvious decrease in responsiveness to treatment on the extremities compared with the face (see the next section), PWSs responded differently even within the same anatomic location. The centrofacial regions

A

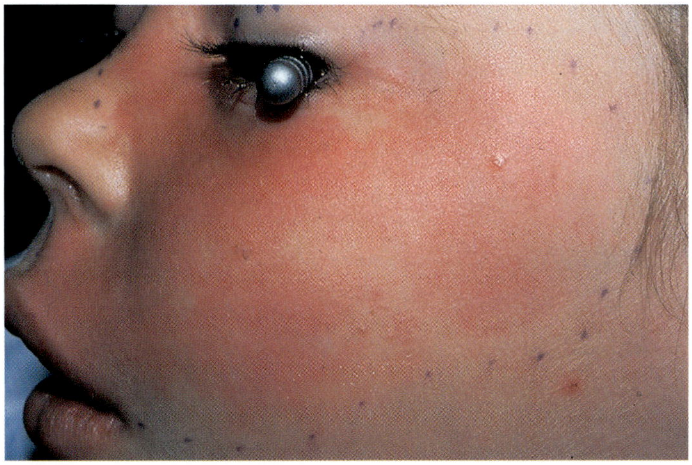

B

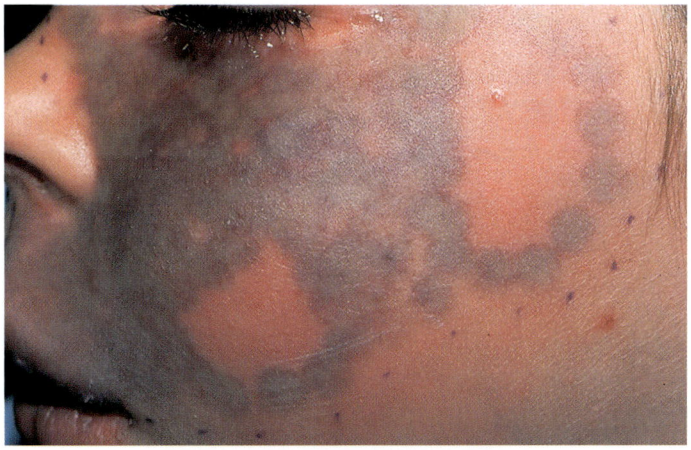

C

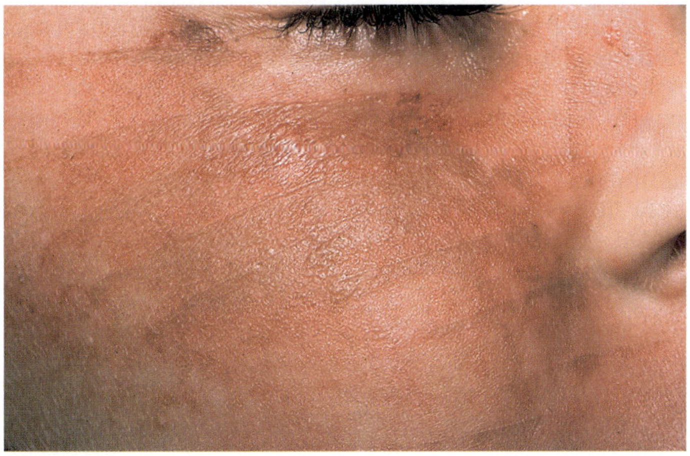

Figure 2.23 (A) Port-wine stain (PWS) on the cheek of 4-year-old girl immediately before treatment. (B) Purpuric response immediately after treatment with PDL at 7.0 J/cm^2 delivered through 7-mm-diameter spot size. (C) Opposite cheek with identical PWS immediately after treatment with PhotoDerm VL with 570-nm cutoff filter at 40 J/cm^2 given as a single 8-ms-duration pulse. Note diminished purpuric response.

A

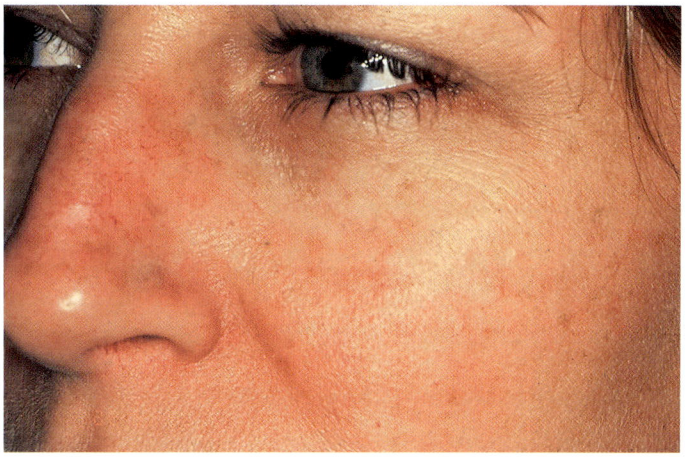

B

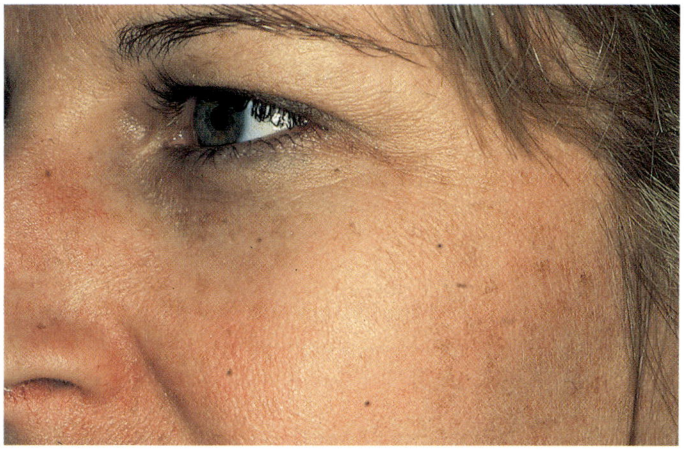

Figure 2.24 (A) Facial telangiectasia in 32-year-old woman 3 years after one treatment with the PDL at 7.0 J/cm^2 with 5-mm-diameter spot. Note hypopigmented circles and persistent telangiectasia. (B) Ten months after three treatments with PhotoDerm VL. First treatment was with 570-nm cutoff filter at 37 J/cm^2 given as a double pulse of 2.4 and 2.4 ms with a delay time of 10 ms. Second and third treatments given 4 weeks apart, 4 weeks later through a 550-nm cutoff filter at 40 J/cm^2 given as a 2.4- and 4.0-ms double pulse with a 10-ms delay. Note complete resolution of the telangiectasia and hypopigmented circles.

(medial aspect of the cheek, upper cutaneous lip, nose) respond less favorably than the periorbital, forehead, temple, lateral cheek, neck, and chin areas.[91,106] Evaluation by dermatomal distribution revealed that V_2 lightened on average 74%, whereas combined dermatomes V_1 and V_3 lightened on average 82% when treated with the PDL at 585 nm, 5-mm-diameter spot size, and 5.75 to 8.5 J/cm^2 in an average of four treatments. V_2 lesions also require more treatments to reach maximal clearance than V_1 or V_3 lesions (Fig. 2.25). Lesions in the V_3 dermatome have been found to have more superficially ecstatic blood vessels, whereas lesions in V2 dermatome and on distal extremities have more deeply placed vessels.[107]

Lesion size may be an independent factor determining lesion response. A study of 74 adult PWSs on various loca-

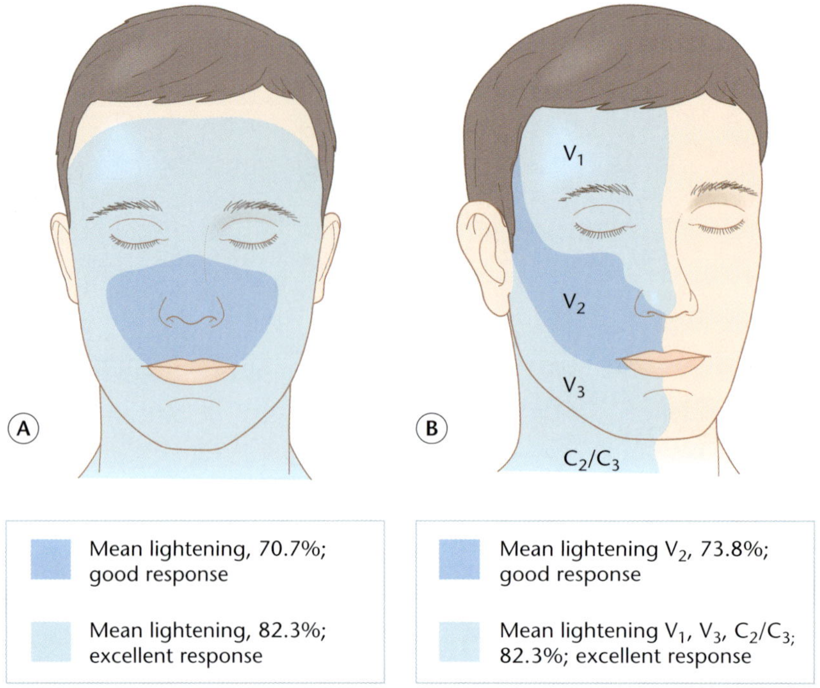

Figure 2.25 (A) Anatomic subdivision of therapeutic response of port-wine stain (PWS) to pulsed dye laser (PDL) treatment. (B) Dermatomal distribution of therapeutic response of PWS to LPDL treatment. (Reprinted from Arch Dermatol 129:182, 1993. Copyright © 1993 American Medical Association. All rights reserved.)

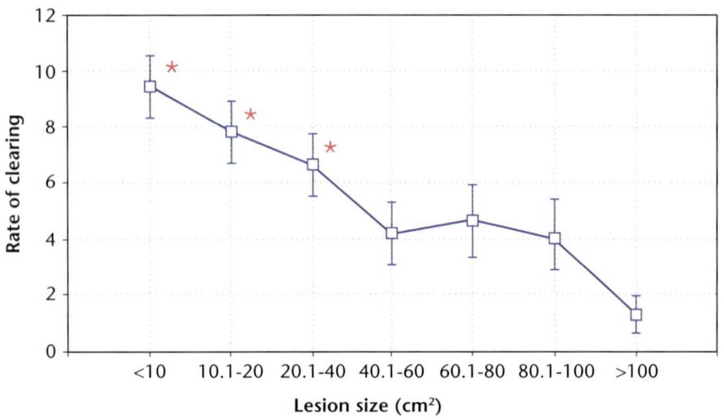

Figure 2.26 Facial PWS lesion size affects rate of clearing after PDL treatment in adults. Data are represented as mean ± standard error of mean for each lesion-size category. Asterisk (*) designates significant difference ($p < 0.05$) in rate of clearing versus size category of greater than 100 cm^2. (From Yohn JJ, Huff JC, Aeling JL et al. Reprinted with permission from Cutis. 1997; 59:267–270. © 1997, Quadrant Healthcom Inc.)

tions found that all lesions responded, with 25% to 90% lightening.[108] However, only 36.5% achieved 50% clearing despite 4 to 19 treatments, depending on the size of the lesion. No lesions had greater than 75% clearance despite 6 to 15 treatments when their size was greater than 60 cm^2, and no lesions had greater than 50% clearance despite a mean of 17 treatments when their size was larger than 100 cm^2 (Fig. 2.26).

PDL Treatment of Extremity Lesions

The poor response of lesions located on the distal extremities has been seen in our practice and reported by others. In one review, 7 of 10 patients with PWS on the extremities responded only slightly or poorly.[94] This finding might reflect an artifact of fewer treatments because the average number of treatments was 2.6 (Fig. 2.27). In contrast, those lesions on the face and neck that responded slightly or poorly had an average of only 1.1 treatments. Twenty-seven patients with lower limb PWS treated with the PDL at fluences up to a maximum of 8.5 J/cm^2 also had a poor response.[95] In this population, only one patient had greater than 95% clearance, despite these patients having an average of 9.4 treatments. Overall, 26% of these patients had no response, 22% had a poor response, 33% had less than 50% lightening, 15% had 50% to 75% lightening, and only one had greater than 95% clearance after seven treatments. In addition, 18% of patients developed hyperpigmentation, which lasted for an undisclosed period.

The effect of decreased response to treatment with lesions located in extremities was also noted by Orten et al,[91] who found only 33% lightening despite a mean of approximately six treatments, compared with 80% to 90% lightening of PWS lesions in fewer or similar number of treatments in other locations. Lanigan[109] also reported poor response to treatment in 23 patients with lower limb PWS. Ten patients had no discernible lightening after one treatment at 7.75 J/cm^2. Seventeen patients with a median of seven treatments at a median fluence of

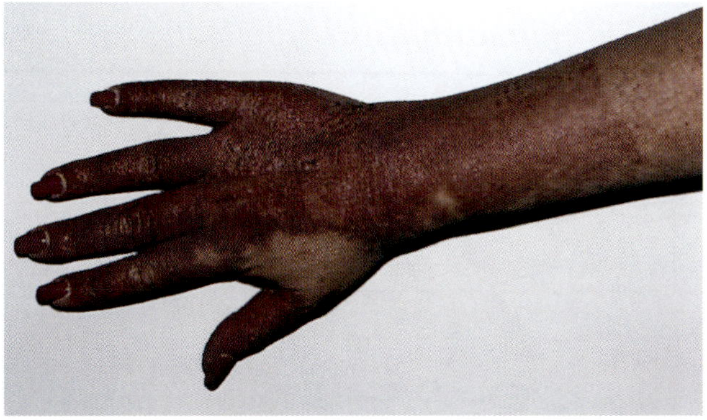

Figure 2.27 Port-wine stain on entire right hand, arm, and chest of 38-year-old woman. Photograph was taken 2 years after treatment of hand and arm. Right dorsal hand has been treated three times with the pulsed dye laser at fluences ranging between 7 and 7.5 J/cm^2. Area from wrist to elbow has been treated once at an energy of 7 J/cm^2. Area of demarcation from midforearm to lateral aspect of photograph was treated a second time with a fluence of 7.5 J/cm^2. Note significant improvement in proximal forearm without noticeable improvement (by comparison) of distal forearm, dorsal hand, or fingers.

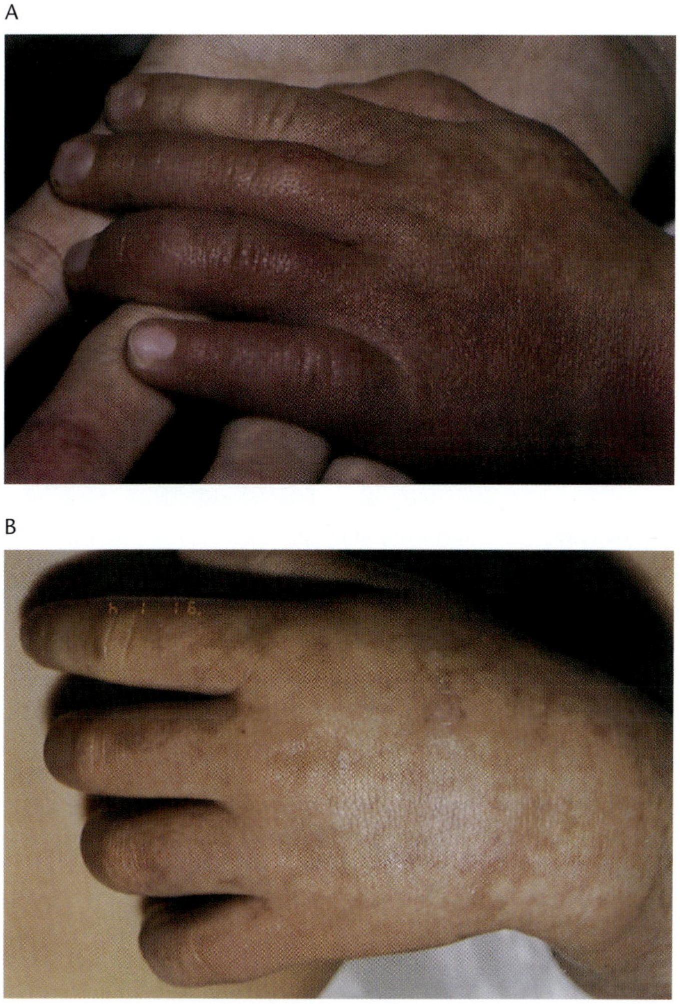

Figure 2.28 Extensive port-wine stain (PWS) of left hand, forearm, and chest of 18-month-old boy. (A) Before treatment. (B) Six months after two treatments to dorsal hand with pulsed dye laser using a fluence of 6.75 J/cm^2. Total of 80 5mm impacts were given during each treatment session. Note significant resolution of PWS.

7.25 J/cm^2 showed median lightening of 40%. Of those responding, only three patients had lightening of 70% or greater after six, ten, and five treatments. However, some authors have reported a similar treatment efficacy despite lesion location with a similar average number of treatments.[90]

The reason PWSs on the distal limbs respond slowly is unknown but may be related to gravitational or deoxygenation effects on circulation. Distal vessels have a thicker wall, which may require increased thermal effects for irreversible damage (see p. 50). Because distal areas respond more poorly than more proximal areas, early treatment of extremity lesions, before ambulation, may be beneficial. We have found this to be true in the small number of patients we have treated at an early age with distal limb PWS (Figs 2.28 and 2.29).

As previously mentioned, even treating extremity lesions with high-energy fluences has been unsuccessful. Near-complete resolution in only two treatments has been reported when fluences of 9 J/cm^2 are used. However, this degree of laser energy poses a risk of pigmentary and nonspecific epidermal changes.[88] Epidermal cooling may allow these necessary higher fluences to be used.

Treatment Protocol

The treatment protocol involves first performing a test of several different energy densities to determine efficacy. Immediately after impact, a dark purple discoloration occurs. Conversely, if the site does not discolor, too low an energy fluence may have been chosen. If edema, blistering, or blackening of the impact site occurs, too high an energy density may have been chosen. Generally, three or four energy fluences are tested and evaluated at approximately 6 weeks (Fig. 2.29). The most effective one is then chosen for treatment. If none of the test sites shows improvement, a second series of test energies is chosen. With experience, the test period may be eliminated and the treatment energy chosen by evaluation of the laser's immediate effects.

Treatment of the entire lesion or a portion of the lesion may be accomplished by covering the treatment area with laser or IPL impacts that overlap 10%. Overlapping can minimize a mottled 'egg crate' or 'foot-print' appearance. However, as previously described, the degree of overlapping is determined by the type of PDL used, with the Cynosure PDL better used without any overlapping, except with a 'fuzzy spot'. Overlapping may also be achieved with the Candela PDL by use of the so-called fuzzy spot.[110] With this treatment modification, the laser handpiece is moved away from the skin beyond the laser's focal point, resulting in a

A B

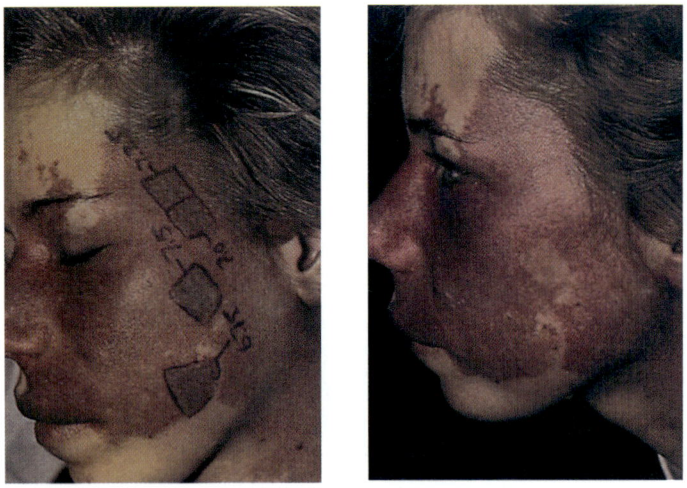

Figure 2.29 (A) Immediately after application of test doses with pulsed dye laser at laser energies specified. (B) Four months after test doses. Note significant clearing in all areas, with maximum clearing at fluences of 7.0 and 7.25 J/cm^2. Patch treated at 7.5 J/cm^2 shows light-brown hyperpigmentation. Treatment will therefore proceed at an energy of 7.0 J/cm^2.

A

B

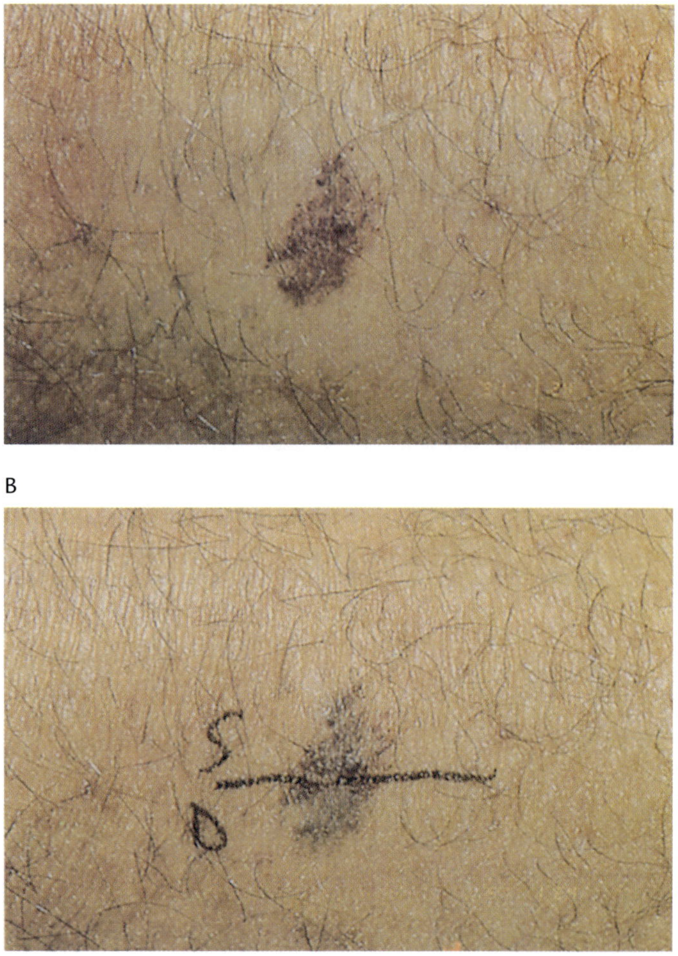

Figure 2.30 Congenital port-wine stain on thigh of 66-year-old man. (A) Before treatment. (B) Immediately after treatment with pulsed dye laser at 7 J/cm^2. S, area treated with single pulse; D, area treated with double pulse. Double-pulse area has darker pigmentation.

larger, defocused impact spot. This has a lower energy density than that indicated for the focused spot and also a more indistinct or 'fuzzy' border that blurs the edges of clearing from a single treatment. Re-treatments are generally done at 1½- to 4-month intervals.

The use of overlapping pulses should be undertaken with caution, however, because biopsies of PWSs treated with single impact and consecutive double-impact therapy reveal an additive thermal effect resulting in nonspecific thermal damage to the superficial dermis and epidermis (Figs 2.30 and 2.31). This double-pulsing technique does promote greater resolution of nodular, thicker, and darker lesions but results in loss of specificity.

The reason for multiple treatments is the layered nature of ectatic vessels of a PWS. Modeling studies using the histologically correct layered vessel demonstrate that the more superficial vessels receive most of the delivered energy. The deeper vessels receive less energy and are therefore not thermocoagulated because of mutual shadowing of the superficial vessels[111] (Fig. 2.32).

Other Factors in Treatment Response

In addition to size and location of the PWS (lesions on extremities), other factors may be important in predicting responsiveness to treatment. PWSs that are dark red or purple may be less responsive to laser treatment. The relative difficulty in treating these lesions results from the presence of deeper, larger vessels that are beyond the laser's penetration depth[19,21] or that are too large to be photocoagulated completely within treatment parameters of the PDL.[10] (As discussed previously, the thermal relaxation time of target vessels is related to their diameter, with the effective wavelength related to their depth.) However, purple lesions are not completely or always unresponsive to treatment. We found that although purple lesions are graded most often as excellent responders (52%), they also are the leading group of poorly responsive lesions (21%).[27] This paradox may occur because two distinct populations of purple lesions exist: macular and nodular. Exophytic nodular lesions respond well, whereas purple and macular lesions respond poorly because of deeper and larger dermal vessels.

Paradoxically, lesions that respond poorly may appear clinically similar to good responders. In these lesions, biopsy demonstrates vessel walls that are thicker despite a vessel diameter that is smaller than 0.056 to 0.102 mm.[112,113] Such lesions are usually on the trunk or extremities. Alternatively, lesions with deeper vessels respond poorly, because the PDL at 585 nm and 6 to 8 J/cm^2 has been found to coagulate the entire vessel wall only to a maximum depth of 0.65 mm (mean 0.37 mm), even in vessels not shielded by more superficial vessels.[114] Superficial PWS vessels up to 0.15 mm in diameter were found

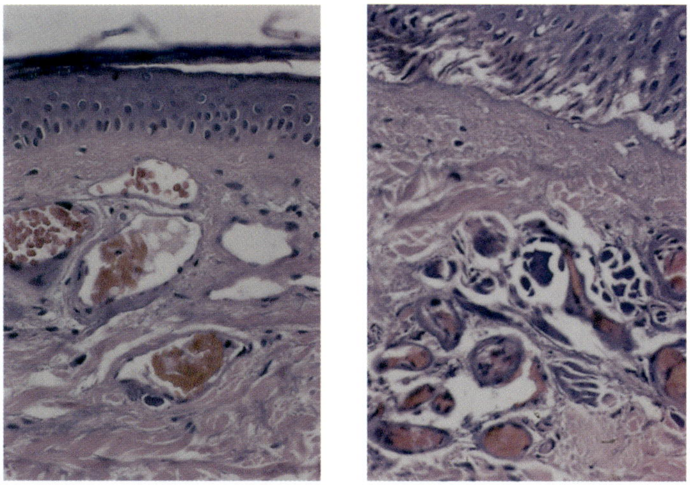

Figure 2.31 (A) Biopsy specimen immediately after single pulse as described in Figure 2.47A. Note coagulation of superficial dermal ectatic blood vessels without any change in overlying epidermis or perivascular tissue (hematoxylin–eosin; ×40). (B) Biopsy specimen immediately after double-pulse technique as described in Figure 2–47B. Note nonspecific thermal damage to overlying epidermis and perivascular tissue. Ectatic blood vessels in superficial papillary dermis are thrombosed with evidence of perivascular collagen homogenization (hematoxylin–eosin ×40).

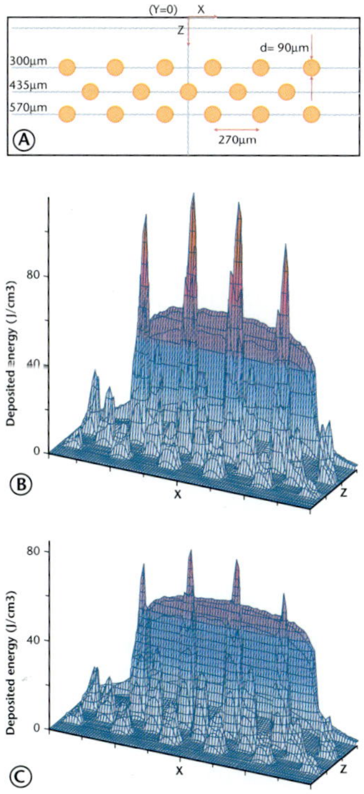

Figure 2.32 (A) Geometry with 17 multiple straight vessels in three layers at different depths z of 300, 435, and 570 μm, and lateral spacing between vessels' centers of 270 μm. Energy deposition in multi-blood-vessel geometry for (B) wavelength 577 nm, and (C) wavelength 585 nm. Laser beam diameter is 1 mm. Upper vessels receive most of the energy. Deeper vessels receive less energy by decreasing light fluence with depth and also by mutual shadowing of vessels. (Fig. 2.32A, B and C. Lucassen GW, Verkruysse W, Keijzer M et al: Lasers in Surgery and Medicine 18:345, © 1996. Reprinted with permission of Wiley-Liss, Inc., a subsidiary of John Wiley & Sons, Inc.)

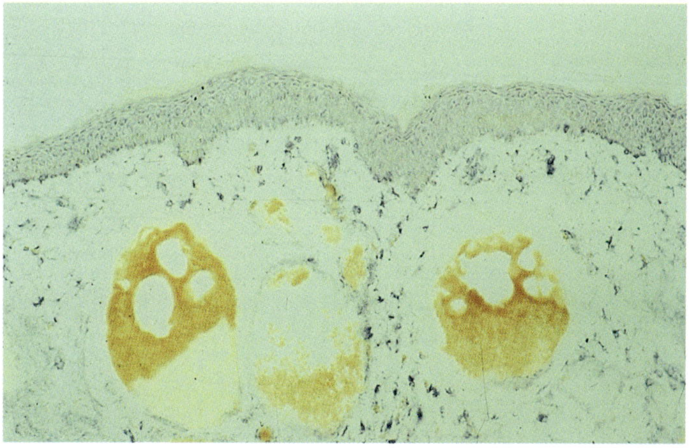

Figure 2.33 Biopsy of port-wine stain on the face of a 43-year-old female. Lesion is violaceous and thick immediately after treatment with pulsed dye laser at 6.5 J/cm^2. There is complete coagulation of red blood cells (RBCs) and vessel wall in a 150-μm vessel (right) and no damage to the lower third of RBCs and vessel wall in a larger vessel. Note the 'steam bubble' formation in upper half of vessels and perivascular dermal coagulation zone. (Reprinted from Hohenleutner U, Hilbert M, Wlotzke U et al: Journal of Investigative Dermatology 104:798, 1995. With permission from Blackwell Publishing Ltd.)

histologically to coagulate completely without nonspecific damage to epidermal or perivascular tissues (Table 2.7 and Fig. 2.33).

Therefore both vessel size and vessel depth in addition to vascular wall thickness are important determinants in predicting treatment efficacy. Vessel size has an important effect because the entire vessel (not just the superficial portion) must be thermocoagulated. This assumes that for vessel coagulation, heating the center of the vessel is necessary for thermal radiation to the entire vessel wall. This requires both an adequate wavelength (for depth of penetration) and an adequate pulse duration (thermal relaxation).

Finally, Waner[115] has proposed that autonomic innervation is an important determinant of treatment efficacy. In a study of 118 PWSs in 102 patients, recurrence of the PWS depended on the time lapsed since the completion of treatment. Although only 3% of patients showed evidence of recurrence at 1 year, 20% and 40% showed evidence for recurrence at 1 to 2 and 2 to 3 years after treatment, respectively. Cutaneous venules of the PWS vasculature are innervated by sympathetic postganglionic neurons as well as sensory neurons.[116–118] The apparent underlying cause of a venular malformation is an absolute or relative deficiency of autonomic innervation of the cutaneous vascular plexus. Smaller and Rosen[116] demonstrated a deficit in the number of perivascular nerves in PWS. Kane et al[119] also found a decrease in autonomic innervation in six patients with poorly response PWS despite 5 to 21 treatments with the PDL at fluences up to 10 J/cm^2.

Therefore Waner[115] postulates and we concur that even though effective treatment decreases the number of ectatic vessels significantly, the remaining milieu allows for a continuing course of progressive ectasia. Recurrence of com-

Table 2.7 *Treatment of Port-wine Stains with Flashlamp-pumped Pulsed Dye Laser (PDL, 6.5 J/cm²): Lightening Per Vessel Size and Depth*

Measurement (μm; mean ± SD)	Poor lightening (*n* = 8)	Moderate lightening (*n* = 12)	Good lightening (*n* = 22)
Diameter	19 ± 7	38 ± 17	38 ± 19
Depth	280 ± 46	315 ± 89	202 ± 56
Wall thickness	5.3 ± 1.8	5.4 ± 2.1	4.5 ± 1.7

From Fiskerstrand EJ, Svaasand LO, Kopstad et al. J Invest Dermatol 1996; 107:671.

pletely resolved capillary malformations, however, has not been observed by the authors.

Multiple Treatments

Improvement and clearance are gradual and usually require 5 to 10 treatments, although some lesions may not fully clear despite more than 20 separate treatments. It is sometimes difficult to determine when a lesion has reached a point of maximum improvement, but treatments should be continued as long as each results in an increment of improvement. We have found the point of diminishing return to occur about the seventh treatment. Finally, areas within a PWS that fail to respond to treatment should be closely examined because we and others have reported the development of basal cell carcinoma within a PWS.[119]

A retrospective photographic analysis was performed on 69 patients who failed to achieve greater than 75% lesional lightening in nine treatment sessions with the PDL at typical treatment parameters.[120] Retreatment at similar parameters with a 5-mm-diameter spot size and fluences of 5.75 to 8.0 J/cm² resulted in continued improvement in these patients. An additional 25% to 100% lightening was achieved in these patients treated up to 25 separate times. Extensive surface area involvement and limb lesions were the slowest to respond.

As mentioned previously, the dominant vessel size in childhood PWS is 10 to 50 μm in diameter. The average thermal relaxation time of PWS vessels is estimated at 1.2 ms.[4] As the child grows to adulthood, progressive ectasia results in larger and deeper vessels up to 300 μm in diameter with a thermal relaxation time of approximately 10 ms. It is reasonable to assume that these larger vessels would be more common in the darker, thicker lesions of adults. Although the PDL has been shown to be very effective in the treatment of adult PWS,[22,23,25,27] larger vessels in these lesions are not ideally suited for the specific parameters of this laser. Therefore other laser or pulsed light sources or photodynamic therapy may be useful.

Treatment of 'Resistant' Lesions

Multiple methods are available for treating PWS lesions that fail to respond to the PDL. The first is to switch to the IPL as previously discussed. To enhance the therapeutic effects of the PDL one can use cryogen spray with higher fluences, increase the spot size of the PDL, change from a 595 to a 585 dye, increase the pulse duration from 0.45 ms to 1.5–20 ms, and perform multiple passes at the same session with variable pulse durations.

The primary purpose of cryogen cooling is to allow higher fluences to be used without damage to the epidermis. Higher fluences will produce higher temperatures within the dermal ecstatic vessels. Studies have found that the use of cooling with higher fluences enhances the resolution of PWS.[121–123]

Performing multiple passes with 0.45-ms and 1.5-ms pulse durations has been reported to accelerate resolution of PWS.[124] However, this has not been uniformly confirmed by our group and others.[125]

Increasing the pulse duration from 0.45 ms to 1.5 or even 2.0 ms has been reported to result in further clearing of 'resistant' PWS.[126,127]

Changing from a 585-nm dye to a 595-nm dye has resulting in enhanced clearing in some PWS. It appears that pink or red PWS do best with 585 nm whereas blue or dark red PWS do better with 595-nm dyes.[127–131] This is due to the shift of absorption to higher wavelengths with production of methemoglobin, which is formed by a photoinduced oxidation of hemoglobin with laser treatment.[132]

Finally, other maneuvers, such as increasing the diameter of the blood vessels by using a proximal tourniquet has also enhanced absorption with a 585-nm, 1.5-ms PDL.[133]

Recurrence of Port-wine Stains

The use of the PDL in treating PWS has been widely practiced for almost 20 years. Recently, we and others have begun to evaluate our patients treated in the early years for signs of persistent or recurrent lesions. Although we have not seen a significant number of patients returning to our practice with progressing lesions, other physicians have reported recurrence after completion of treatment (see Fig. 2.17). Orten et al[91] have evaluated a small number of patients who were 2, 3, and 4 years posttreatment. They have reported recurrence (darkening of the lesion) in 5 of 24 patients at 2 years, 4 of 10 patients at 3 years, and 2 of 4 patients at 4 years posttreatment. The most obvious patient, an adult female whose PWS was on the midlateral cheek, had near-complete clearance of the PWS only to have almost total recurrence after 42 months. Whether these recurrent lesions would respond more favorably to alternative treatment modalities (e.g. IPL) or respond equally as well to additional treatment is unknown. Recurrence of PWS in a subset of patients may support a 'neuronal' theory of PWS evolution.

Raulin et al[134] reported complete resolution of a facial PWS in a 35-year-old male that did not respond to a single treatment with the PDL at 6.5 J/cm². They used a 550-nm cutoff filter with single and double pulses of 25 J/cm² 3 ms in duration. Treatments were given every 8 weeks until clearance occurred after the fourth treatment.

Treatment with Other Lasers

Carbon Dioxide Laser

In our opinion, nodular lesions are best treated with the UltraPulse CO_2 ($UPCO_2$) laser (see Chapter 6) or the IPL. With the $UPCO_2$ laser the lesion can be sculpted to reestablish a normal facial contour in addition to thermocoagulating the ectatic blood vessels. The advantages of the $UPCO_2$ laser are its precise hemostasis and avoidance of nonspecific thermal damage (Fig. 2.34). After normal contours are obtained, the PDL or IPL can be used to lighten the remaining erythema.

Potassium Titanyl Phosphate Laser

The 532-nm Starpulse KTP laser (LaserScope) has been used in conjunction with a scanner to treat adults with PWS. Best clearing of the test sites was obtained with 3- or 5-ms pulses at 15 or 20 J/cm². Posttreatment purpura developed at all effective treatment sites. No scarring or ulceration occurred. Histology showed that selective vessel closure was achieved without hemorrhage. Perivascular collagen damage was always present at the effective treatment sites. These findings show that a 532-nm laser pulsed in the 1- to 30-ms domain is capable of inducing selective vessel closure.[135]

532 nm Nd:YAG Long-pulse Laser

By extending the pulse duration to within the thermal relaxation time of the vessel treated, purpura is avoided without loss of efficacy (see earlier). This laser has been effective in treating PWSs that have sometimes proved to be recalcitrant to treatment with other laser modalities[136] (Fig. 2.35). Our experience in using this modality, both with and without epidermal cooling, has been variable but positive. The 532 nm laser is less effective in Asian patients with a higher risk of complications.[137] A dual pulsed 532 and 1064 nm laser (Dualis KTP+, Fotana d.d., Ljubljana, Slovenia) has been found in a pilot study on 10 patients to be effective in treating PWS. Cryogen spray cooling as well as topical anesthesia is necessary but atrophic scars still occurred.[138]

1064 nm Nd:YAG Long-pulse Laser

Most recently, this longer wavelength laser has been used in the treatment of PWS. It is thought that the deeper penetration of the 1064 nm wavelength would allow further improvement especially in blue PWS. Although effective, this laser has a relatively high incidence of hypertrophic and atrophic scarring due to the high energies needed

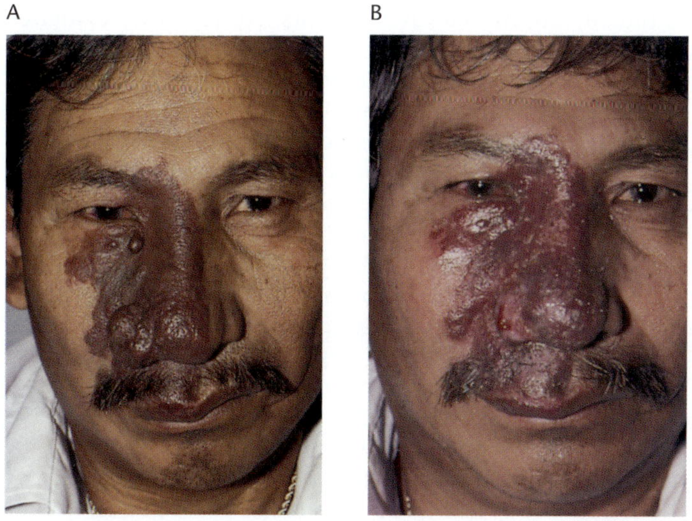

Figure 2.34 (A) Congenital port-wine stain with large hypertrophic mass on right lateral distal nose and nodules on right inner canthus present in 47-year-old Hispanic man. Over last 20 years, lesion has grown progressively darker in appearance as well as developing nodular hypertrophies. (B) Three weeks after treatment with Coherent Ultra Pulse CO_2 Laser (Coherent Laser Corp., Palo Alto, CA) at 250 mJ, pulse width of 794 ms at 20 W, 80 pulses per second, in continuous-wave mode with 2-mm spot.

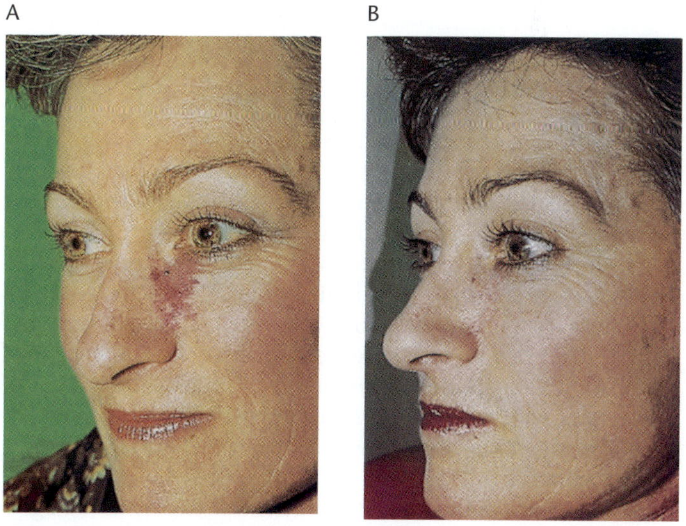

Figure 2.35 Port-wine stain on left upper cheek of female patient treated under general anesthesia with copper bromide laser (CBL); actual treatment required about 15 minutes. (A) Before treatment. (B) After treatment with exposure time of 7 ms, 2.5 W, and spot size of 0.7 to 1.0 mm (4.5 J/cm²), with 10 ms (6.5 J/cm²) for darker areas. (Courtesy Sue McCoy, MD.)

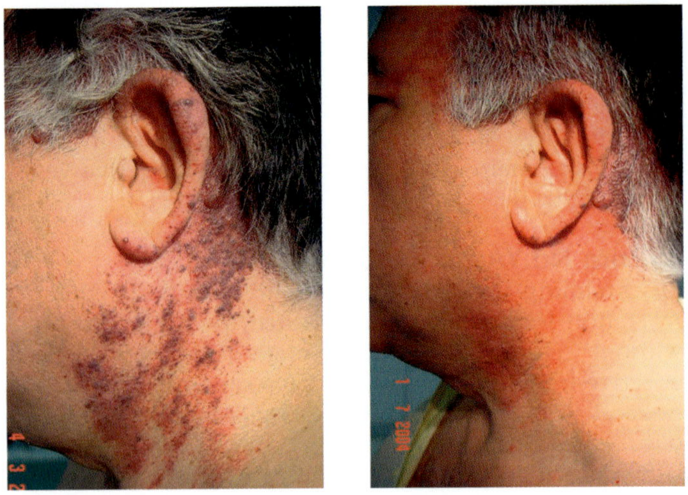

Figure 2.36 Long-standing PWS before and 1 month after 4-monthly treatments with a long-pulse Nd:YAG laser using a 7-mm-diameter handpiece with a fluence of 60–65 J/cm^2 at 10–15 ms pulse duration. (Courtesy of Don Groot, MD.)

to thermocoagulate red blood cells at this wavelength. Although patients prefer the lack of significant purpura with the 1064 nm laser, scarring has been noted to occur even with epidermal cooling after establishing a minimal purpuric laser fluence.[139] This may be related to the different absorption characteristics of the vessels of a PWS in different locations within the same lesion. At this time, this laser modality is only recommended for thick, blue lesions recalcitrant to other treatment modalities (see Fig. 2.36).

Hemangioma

The treatment of hemangiomas remains a challenge. Part of the problem in evaluating published reports and in designing rational therapeutic plans resides in the confusion in terminology that still exists.

Hemangiomas are benign vascular tumors composed of proliferative, plump, endothelial cells. They can occur in skin, mucous membranes, and other soft tissues. A hemangioma often begins as a field transformation, frequently in multiple sites simultaneously or over a large area of skin.[140] The tumor may begin in subcutaneous tissue or muscle or may infiltrate the skin densely without elevating it, giving an appearance similar to that of a PWS.[141] However, whether superficial, deep, or mixed, the lesion is thought to have the same histologic and biologic behavior pattern throughout.[140] Hemangioma typically present with both a superficial component and a deep cutaneous component as well as a subcutaneous proliferation of ectatic vessels.

The term 'cavernous' is confusing. At times this term is used to refer to the deep dermal component of a hemangioma. Other times it is used to (mis)label a noninvoluting 'cavernous hemangioma', which in reality is a venous malformation with spongy architecture.[141] A venous malformation may be difficult to differentiate clinically from a deep hemangioma. Failure to evacuate blood with compression occurs in hemangiomas, not in venous malformations, and this is a useful maneuver to differentiate the two conditions.

Natural History

Hemangiomas are the most common tumor of infancy; 60% occur on the head and neck, 25% on the trunk, and 15% on the extremities.[142] Eighty percent of hemangiomas are present as a single, well-circumscribed lesion 0.5 to 5.0 cm in diameter, and the remainder occur as multiple cutaneous and visceral lesions.[141] The lesions are generally absent at birth, but a localized area of pallor or macular erythema or telangiectasia may be present. The majority of hemangiomas (70%–90%) appear during the first month of life, and by age 12 months the incidence is reported to be in the 10% to 12% range.[39,143,144]

Hemangiomas present at birth result from in utero growth. They are difficult to diagnose with routine ultrasonic evaluation, even when associated with Kasabach–Merritt syndrome. They tend not to grow after birth and usually regress by 14 months, leaving atrophic, redundant, or scarred skin.[145]

When lesions have distinct borders, homogeneous color, no overlying telangiectasia they are usually a capillary malformation. When the borders are indistinct and the lesions are variably colored with visible overlying telangiectasia they are true hemangiomas.

Congenital hemangiomas of eccrine glands have also been reported.[146] These rare lesions usually appear at birth as bluish, slightly elevated tumors. None shows evidence of hyperhidrosis, and all resolve spontaneously. Diagnosis is made on histologic examination of dilated capillary-like vessels located around sweat glands.

The female/male ratio for hemangiomas is estimated to be 3 : 1.[142,147] Caucasian infants have been reported to have an increased incidence over other racial groups.[119,143,144] The clinical appearance is related to the depth of the proliferating lesion. Superficial lesions are raised and bright red (Fig. 2.37). Deeper dermal lesions appear as bluish subcutaneous nodules. The overlying skin may have a fine network of telangiectasia (Fig. 2.38). With regression, superficial lesions leave a flaccid, pedunculated, waxy, yellow-colored skin (Fig. 2.39). Deep lesions usually leave a smooth skin surface with overlying telangiectasia. A mottled grayish mantle spreads towards the periphery of the lesion and is less tense to palpation. Parents note that deep lesions do not swell as much as superficial lesions when the child cries.

The hallmark of hemangiomas is a rapid proliferative phase. Immunohistochemical cellular markers that indicate proliferation include type IV collagenase, vascular endothelial growth factor, basic fibroblast growth factor, and other endothelial markers (CD31 and von Willebrand

A

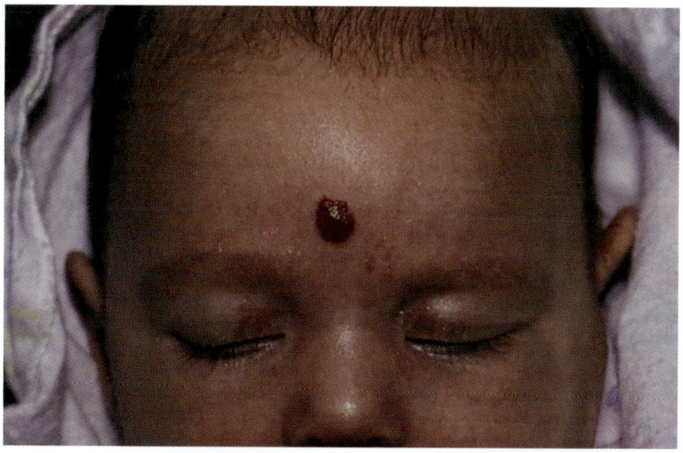

B

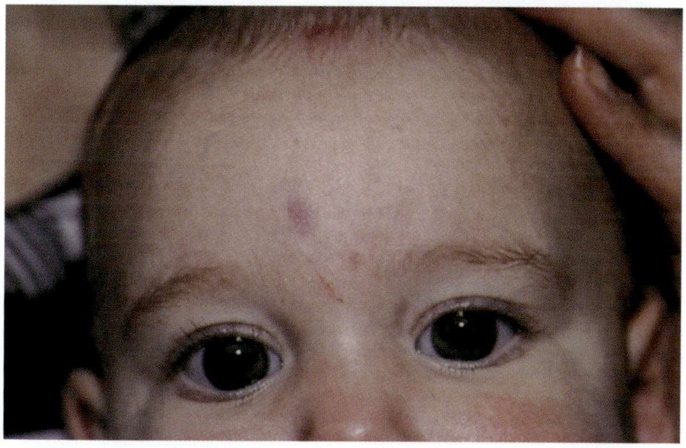

Figure 2.37 Hemangioma on forehead of infant appeared at 2 weeks of age and gradually enlarged. (A) Appearance at 9 weeks of age. (B) Clinical appearance 4 months after initial laser treatment and 1 month after fifth treatment with PDL at a fluence of 7 J/cm^2. Treatments were given at 3-week intervals. Although some persistence of the lesion is seen clinically as a faint pink macule, parents elected to discontinue treatment. (Reprinted from Fitzpatrick RE: American Journal of Cosmetic Surgery 9:107, 1992. With permission from American Academy of Cosmetic Surgery.)

A

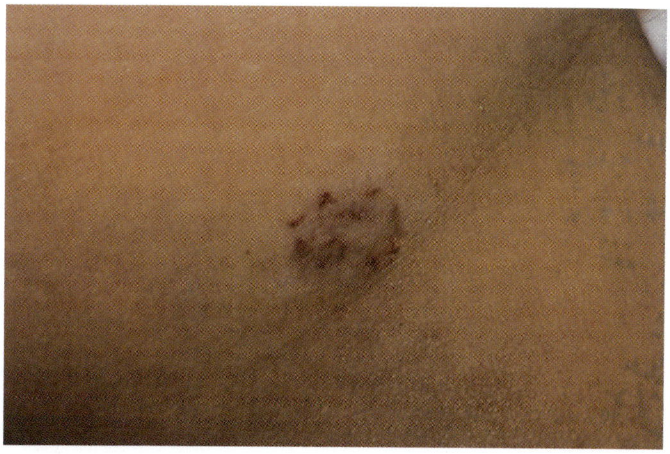

B

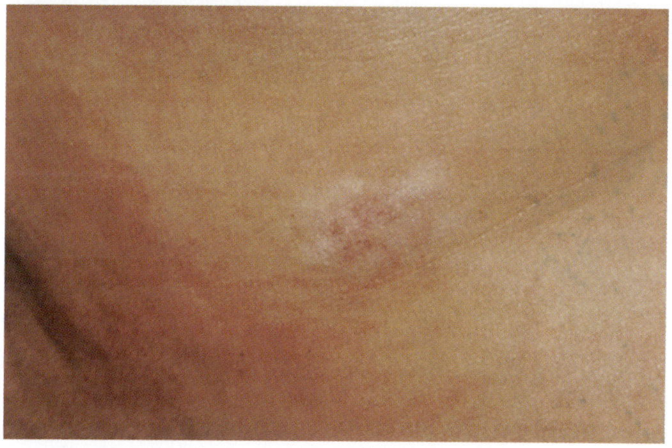

Figure 2.38 (A) Clinical appearance of deep hemangioma with overlying telangiectasias on lateral trunk of 3-month-old girl. (B) After five treatments with PDL at a fluence of 7 J/cm^2. Note complete resolution of hemangioma with only very faint persistence of overlying telangiectatic component. Hypopigmented area was present before any treatment commenced.

factor).[148] Growth is particularly rapid during the first 6 months of life but may continue until 12 months of age. Gradual spontaneous involution begins between the sixth and tenth month.[39,149,150] These stages are not distinct, because proliferation continues while involution slowly begins to dominate. The first sign of regression is a change in color from crimson to dull purple. Clinical studies indicate that involution proceeds on the same time schedule for both deep and superficial hemangiomas.[142,147] Lesions located on the nose and lips are thought to involute more slowly.[147]

Adult hemangiomas are composed of mature, capillary-sized vessels approximately 100 μm in diameter, resembling dermal venules with virtually no endothelial growth.[151] Basement membrane thickness ranges from 0.6 to 14 μm because of multiple superimposed layers of basal lamina. At times an ingrowth of dermal collagen fibers is seen in the vessel wall. Pericytic cells are also immersed in the basement membrane, further thickening the vessel wall. Therefore, although response to laser treatment occurs, it may not be as dramatic as in thinner-walled hemangiomas of infancy.

Studies of the natural history of hemangiomas reveal that complete resolution occurs in 50% of children by age 5 and in 70% by age 7, with continued improvement in the remaining children until ages 10 to 12.[39,40,143,150–152] However, 15% to 25% of lesions do not completely involute, and lesions that do not show significant signs of regression by age 6 to 8 years are not likely to regress completely.[152,153] Rate and extent of resolution are unrelated to lesion size[147] (Fig. 2.40).

Complications and Adverse Sequelae

Complications from the proliferative phase include ulceration (5% to 11% of patients) and infection, which is more

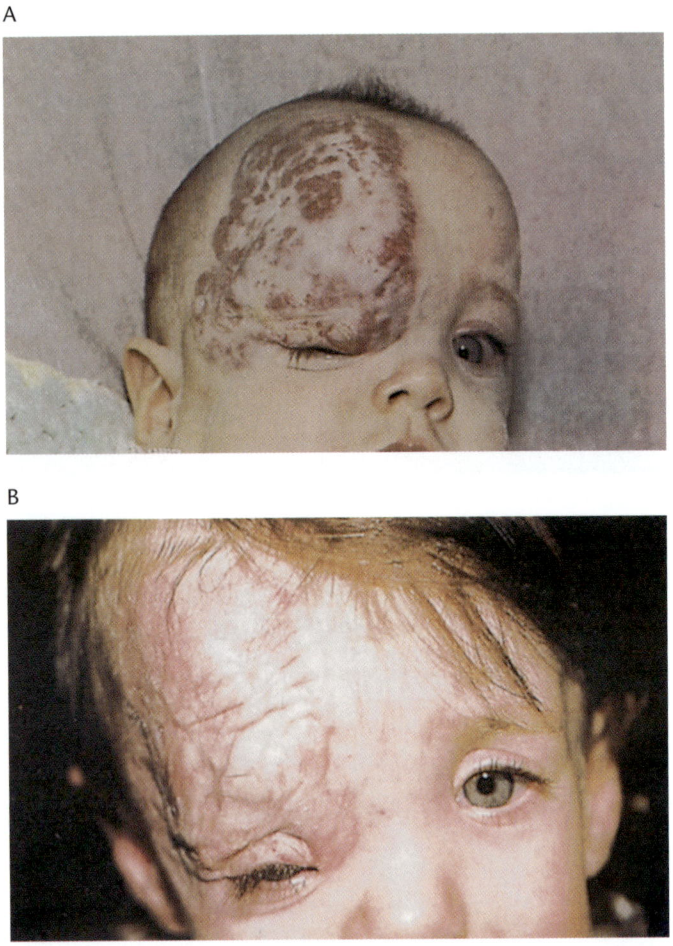

Figure 2.39 Extensive hemangioma on right forehead and upper eyelid of 9-month-old girl. (A) Clinical appearance before any therapy. (B) Clinical appearance 7 months after systemic prednisolone therapy per protocol described in this text, plus six separate treatments with PDL at a fluence of 7 J/cm^2. CT scan demonstrated no intracranial connection with hemangioma. Severe orbital dystopia will be corrected when her bones are more fully developed at age 6. In addition, periorbital atrophy and loss of subcutaneous tissue in area of hemangioma will be corrected with surgical excision after bony correction has been achieved. (Reprinted from Fitzpatrick RE: American Journal of Cosmetic Surgery 9:107, 1992. With permission from the American Academy of Cosmetic Surgery.)

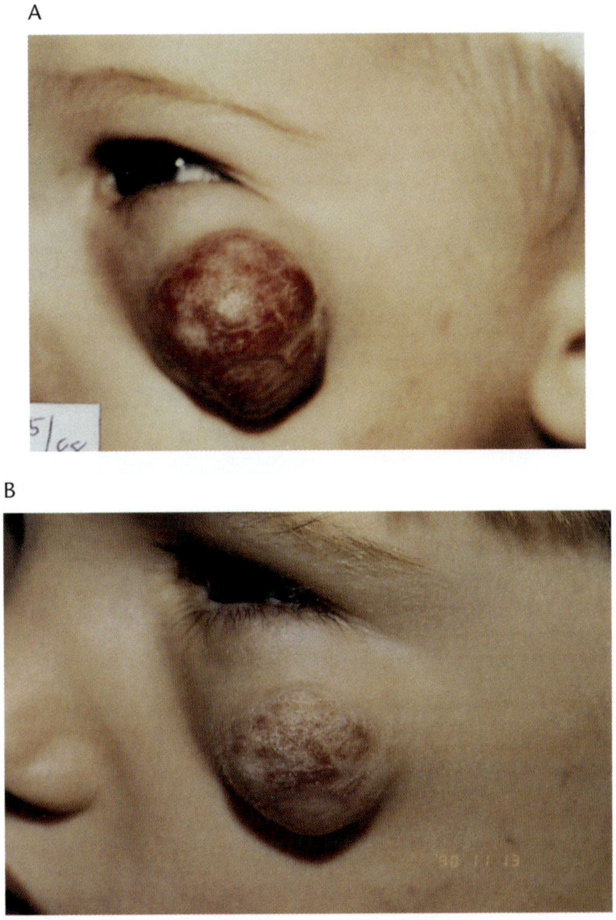

Figure 2.40 (A) Hemangioma on left cheek of 15-month-old child. Lesion arose at 3 weeks of age and increased in size over first year before beginning a short resolution. Patient was treated with oral prednisolone at 6 weeks of age until 6 months of age without noticeable effect on size of hemangioma. (B) Appearance at 3 years of age. Note redundant skin with some superficial atrophic scarring and persistent superficial telangiectasia.

common on the lip and genitoanal areas, where abrasion is common[149,154] (Fig. 2.41). Bleeding from trauma is an annoying and relatively common problem that usually responds to pressure. At times, superficial ulcerations appearing on buttock, sacral, or lip skin in infants can precede the development of hemangiomas by a few weeks. The reason for this evolution in some infants is unknown.[155]

A retrospective analysis of 60 pediatric patients showed that in the 37% of ulcerations that were treated with the PDL, 50% showed definite improvement, 18% showed no response and 5% showed worsening. Other forms of treatment included surgical excision (3%), interferon (8%), systemic antibiotics (43%) and systemic corticosteroids (37%).[156]

Skeletal distortion is rare but may occur from a mass effect on underlying bone. Lesions of the nasal tip often distort underlying cartilage (Fig. 2.42). Deviation of facial bones or orbital enlargement may occur.[157]

Lesions of the upper eyelid may obstruct the visual axis, causing deprivation amblyopia with failure to develop binocular vision.[158] Interruption of vision in infancy for as briefly as 1 to 2 weeks can cause permanent damage, with longer periods of obstruction being more harmful. Upper eyelid lesions may also distort the growing cornea by direct pressure producing refractive errors (strabismic amblyopia).[159] Large hemangiomas of the lower eyelid may result in similar problems, but even the smallest hemangioma within the upper eyelid can cause visual disturbances.[160] Therefore all children with hemangiomas involving either the upper or the lower eyelid should be referred to an ophthalmologist promptly, even if vision appears normal.

Other functional problems may occur because of the sheer bulkiness of lesions in critical locations causing obstruction. Lesions of the nose may interfere with breath-

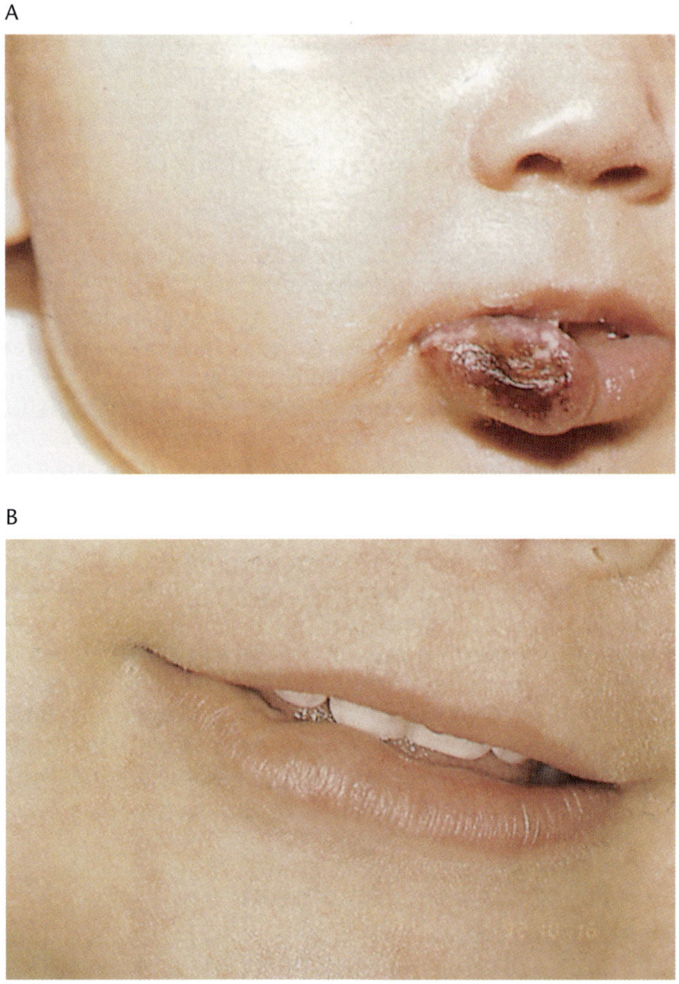

Figure 2.41 (A) Three-month-old girl with hemangioma on right lower lip that was flat and pink at birth and slowly enlarged during first 2 months before rapid enlargement over last 4 weeks, at which point it interfered with eating and was bleeding. (B) Clinical response 2 years later and 1 year after last treatment with PDL. Total of nine laser treatments were given at 4- to 6-week intervals with a fluence of 7 J/cm^2. Within 2 weeks of first laser treatment, definite improvement with rapid resolution of lesion was seen, as well as near-immediate resolution of pain associated with eating. Slight depression appears in midportion of lower lip underlying previous hemangioma. However, there is no distortion of the vermilion border. (Reprinted from Fitzpatrick RE: American Journal of Cosmetic Surgery 9:107, 1992. With permission from American Academy of Cosmetic Surgery.)

ing. Lesions in the subglottic airway may obstruct the larynx, causing life-threatening asphyxiation.[161] Lesions may obstruct the external auditory canal and cause a mild to moderate hearing loss. Lesions in the anogenital area may cause obstruction, pressure, or tenderness when ulcerated and inflamed.

Medical complications include the Kasabach–Merritt syndrome[162]: generalized bleeding from profound thrombocytopenia associated with a large hemangioma or extensive hemangiomatosis. Congestive heart failure is a potentially lethal complication in an infant with multiple cutaneous and visceral hemangiomas.[163]

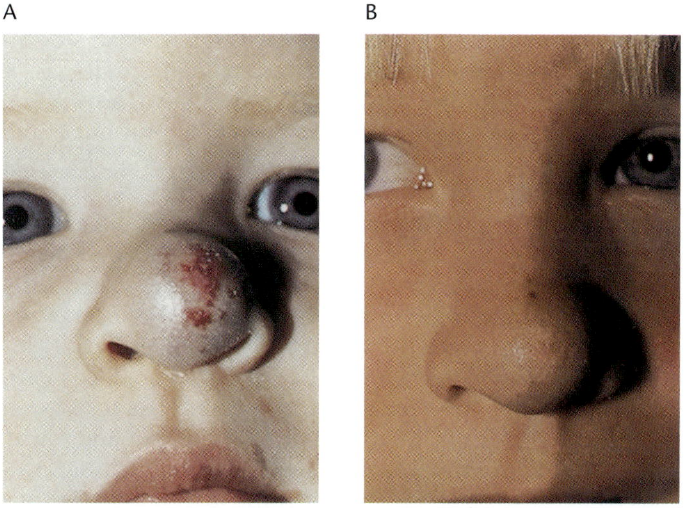

Figure 2.42 (A) Five-month-old boy with 1.5-cm hemangioma on tip of nose and overlying 4 × 8-mm strawberry-red mark in center of lesion, which is very fluctuant. Hemangioma was present at birth and is continuing to enlarge. (B) Approximately 3 years later, after four treatments with pulsed dye laser at a fluence beginning initially at 6.75, then 7.5, 8.0, and 8.5 J/cm^2. In addition to laser treatment, patient received intralesional injection of triamcinolone, with a total of 10 mg given over five injections Although nose has assumed normal appearance, it is still slightly boggy and increases in size with hot weather and when patient cries. (Reprinted from Fitzpatrick RE: American Journal of Cosmetic Surgery 9:107, 1992. With permission from American Academy of Cosmetic Surgery.)

Extensive facial hemangiomas may also be associated with cardiac and abdominal anomalies. Associated anomalies can be right-sided aortic arch coarctation, a supraumbilical midabdominal raphe defect, associated laryngeal and duodenal hemangiomas, and posterior brain fossa abnormalities such as Dandy–Walker malformations.[164–168] The constellation of findings consisting of large facial hemangiomas, posterior fossa malformations, arterial anomalies, coarctation of the aorta and cardiac defects, and eye abnormalities has been given the acronym PHACE syndrome.[168] This syndrome represents a spectrum of malformations of varying degrees of severity caused by a common morphogenetic event or events in utero.[167,169]

The facial hemangiomas seen in the PHACE syndrome are usually plaque like in quality and cover at least one dermatome; 88% occur in females. Infants who have large facial hemangiomas should be evaluated with head circumference measurements and neurologic studies, including brain imaging with cranial ultrasound and MRI scans. These patients also appear at risk for developing airway abnormalities and should be evaluated closely for cardiac defects as well.

Sacral hemangiomas have also been associated with several anomalies, including imperforate anus, genitourinary abnormalities (absent or hypoplastic kidney, abnormal genitalia), and tethered spinal cord without neurologic dysfunction.[170,171]

In a study of 175 cases of severe superficial hemangiomas, defined as lesions involving large surface areas, symptomatic visceral hemangiomas were present in 11.4% and associated malformations in 6.9%.[172] The authors found that MRI was the best imaging modality to detect the deep growth. Hemangiomas give signals that are different from lymphatic or arteriovenous malformations. It may also indicate the rapidity of blood flow movement. Color-flow duplex ultrasonography was helpful but could not accurately distinguish a hemangioma from an AVM because both may have a high-flow pattern.

As described later, many hemangiomas resolve spontaneously without any form of treatment. However, even when resolution is complete, the skin that remains after involution exhibits mild atrophy, has a wrinkled texture with a few telangiectatic vessels, or is paler than the surrounding skin.[141] Resolution that is considered cosmetically acceptable has been said to occur in 70% to 82% of patients.[154] However, in an analysis of 298 hemangiomas, 80% that had not involuted by age 6 left a significant residual cosmetic deformity.[173] In addition, 38% of those lesions that had completely resolved by age 6 left a significant residual deformity. Scarring after ulceration generally leaves a white, flat area of fibrosis. When the hemangioma has been large, there is often redundant skin and a residual subcutaneous fibrofatty tissue mass.[141] Therefore, our opinion, supported by the clinical studies detailed next, is to treat lesions at the first available opportunity.

In addition to medical complications, including persistent scarring, the psychologic consequences are real. A child develops a sense of self-awareness between 18 and 24 months of age. This awareness may be transmitted to psychosocial developmental disorders. Parental guilt, anger, and disappointment as well as over protectiveness are common. These feelings may affect the dynamics of the entire family. A study consisting of interviews of the parents of 25 children aged 6 months to 8 years with facial hemangiomas at least 1 cm in diameter reported negative social stigmatization in the majority of families.[174] For 32% of parents this interfered with outings. Common feelings that the parents expressed were grief, loss, isolation and guilt. For the children, social sensitivity occurred after age 4. This study underscores a family's need for more than just medical management of an infant's hemangiomas.

Traditional Treatment

Treatment of hemangiomas has been oriented toward waiting for natural regression to occur since Lister's article in 1938 outlined a predictable course for these lesions.[152] However, contemporaries of Lister recognized the effectiveness of early treatment before and during the proliferative stage of growth.[175] Therapeutic intervention historically has been reserved for lesions causing recurrent bleeding, ulceration, infection, or serious distortion of facial features and lesions that interfere with normal physiologic functions, such as breathing, hearing, eating, vision, and bladder and bowel function. Despite these therapeutic guidelines, there is tremendous pressure on anguished, concerned parents observing an enlarging hemangioma on their child, particularly when it is a facial lesion of any size. Because of this, there have been many ill-advised attempts at treatment that have resulted in excessive scarring.[176]

Surgical intervention,[177] X-ray therapy,[72,176,178] sclerotherapy,[176,179] diathermy,[180] CO_2 snow cryotherapy,[181] and electrocautery[182] have all been attempted, resulting in significant scarring. A basal cell carcinoma (BCC) presenting 58 years after thorium X applications to a birthmark when the patient was 3 years old has been reported.[183] Thorium X, a rich source of alpha radiation, was frequently used for treating hemangiomas until the 1960s.[184,185] BCC developing after thorium X treatment of hemangiomas has also been reported.[186] Angiosarcomas have also occurred after radiation treatment of hemangiomas, with a review of the literature uncovering 11 such cases.[187] The prognosis is poor, with a 10% 5-year survival rate.

Thus these prior methods of treatment, because of unacceptable side effects and lack of efficacy, have been replaced with laser therapy as a destructive and antiproliferative modality and with other antiproliferative medical treatments. As discussed later, some patients require multiple forms of therapy.

When the pathogenesis of these lesions is considered, an antiangiogenic agent that would prevent proliferation and induce involution of the entire lesion is the most logical therapeutic approach.[188] At present, the only treatment of this type is the use of systemic steroids with or without interferon-alpha.

Systemic and Intralesional Corticosteroids

If a hemangioma is steroid responsive (30%–60% of cases),[188,172] the result is often immediate and dramatic.[176] A treatment schedule of 2 to 3 mg/kg/day of prednisone, rapidly tapered, when the tumor has reduced in size, is given for a cycle of 4 to 6 weeks, followed by a rest period. Complications have been few.[188] In patients who fail to respond, however, increasing the dose of prednisone to 4 to 5 mg/kg/day may trigger growth of the lesion.[172] Loss of appetite and diminished growth rate have been observed but resolve quickly when steroids are discontinued. However, because the proliferative activity of the tumor continues for 6 to 12 months, the need for prolonged steroid suppression persists, with rebound growth of the hemangioma occurring when treatment is discontinued. This often results in an escalating steroid dosage or abandonment of this regimen because of concern regarding potential steroid side effects.

A second steroid schedule has been used throughout the entire proliferative phase of the hemangioma. Prednisolone is given in a dosage of 3 to 5 mg/kg/day for 2 to 4 weeks until control of growth of the hemangioma is achieved. An alternate-day schedule is then instituted by doubling the dose on the 'on' day and eliminating the alternate-day dosage gradually over 2 weeks. Prednisolone is then tapered every 2 weeks by 5 mg if the hemangioma does not enlarge.[189] This treatment schedule is maintained for 6 to 10 months. In 43 infants treated, only one infant had transient side effects. However, it is advisable to use

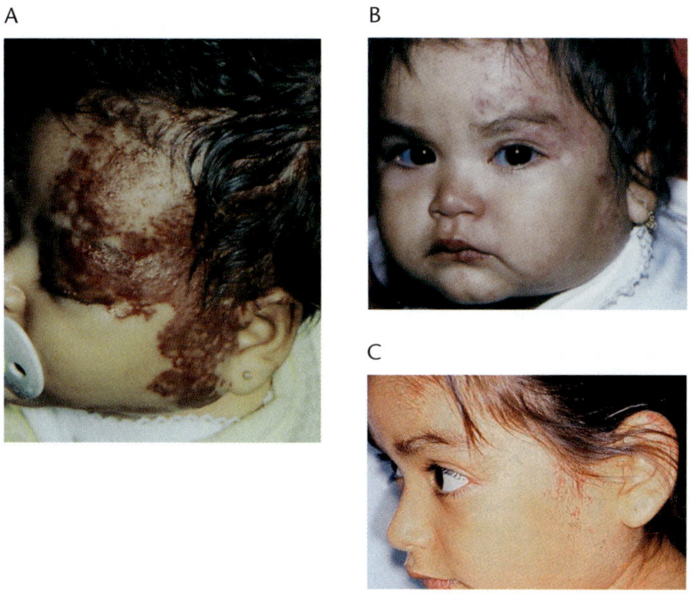

Figure 2.43 (A) Large hemangioma over right side of face of 4-week-old girl. This lesion began as a red macule 5 mm in diameter, first noted over right cheek 2 days after birth. Hemangioma spread rapidly over left forehead, cheek, neck, and eyelid over only 2 to 3 days. Patient was initially treated with pulsed dye laser (PDL) alone at a fluence of 7.25 J/cm^2. However, when seen 2 weeks later, although there was definite improvement in laser-treated site, hemangioma was continuing to enlarge rapidly, involving entire orbit and right parotid and neck area. Subcutaneous masses were present, and prednisolone was begun at a dosage of 4.5 mg/kg/day. Laser treatment was continued at a fluence of 7.5 J/cm^2 at 2-week intervals. Almost immediately after institution of oral prednisolone, hemangioma stopped growing and began a resolution phase. Prednisolone dosage was tapered 2 weeks after institution. When it was discontinued totally on pediatrician's advice 6 weeks later, hemangioma again began to enlarge. We therefore restarted prednisolone therapy, increasing it to a dosage of 5 mg/kg/day to initiate resolution of hemangioma. During this time, lesion was continually treated at 2- to 3-week intervals with PDL at fluences ranging from 7.0 to 7.5 J/cm^2. Interestingly, on alternate-day prednisolone therapy, patient's parents noticed hemangioma increasing in size during the day off therapy, with it regressing in size during the day on prednisolone therapy. Prednisolone therapy was tapered over 2 years before being discontinued. (B) Patient, now 11 months old, has marked resolution of hemangioma. At this point she is continuing to have prednisolone therapy and has had total of nine treatments with PDL, with last treatment 4 months previous to this photograph. (C) Patient is now 7 years old without recurrence. (Reprinted from Fitzpatrick RE: American Journal of Cosmetic Surgery 9:107, 1992. With permission from American Academy of Cosmetic Surgery.)

the lowest effective dose of steroid for the shortest period until the hemangioma enters the regression phase (Fig. 2.43).

Adverse effects of systemic corticosteroids include immunosuppression, osteoporosis, hypertension, cushingoid features, hypothalamic–pituitary–adrenal (HPA) axis suppression, impaired glucose tolerance, growth suppression and ocular complications. One study of 22 patients with hemangiomas treated with an average corticosteroid dose of 2.23 mg/kg/day for an average of 28.1 weeks found irritability, fussiness or insomnia in 73%, hypertension in 45% and HPA suppression in 87%.[190] This review emphasizes the need for close monitoring of patients who require systemic steroids.

Intralesional steroids have been used successfully in the treatment of periorbital hemangiomas.[191,192] Soft tissue atrophy is common but seems to be temporary.[191] Intralesional steroid injection carries a risk of hemorrhage or hematoma in the retrobulbar space, which is a threat to vision.[167] It may cause occlusion of the central retinal artery and damage to the optic nerve.[193] When the hemangioma extends posterior into the orbital cone, systemic steroids should be considered.[176]

A study of 70 children with 74 hemangiomas treated with intralesional corticosteroids showed more than 75% reduction in volume in 58% of patients, 50% to 75% improvement in 22%, 25% to 50% improvement in 12%, and less than 25% improvement in 8%.[194] No patient had regrowth after treatment with a mean follow-up of 14 months. The authors used doses of 10 to 120 mg per injection of triamcinolone and betamethasone acetate (1.5–18 mg/injection) given in a total volume of 0.5 to 6.0 mL, depending on the hemangioma's size. Side effects included temporary cushingoid facies and hypopigmentation, each in two patients. No apparent correlation existed between response and lesion location, size, patient gender, or age.

Enjolras and Mulliken[195] advise giving 3 to 5 mg/kg/procedure (either intralesional or systemic) of triamcinolone with or without cortisone acetate. They believe that intralesional and systemic corticosteroids have a similar response rate. They advise caution when injecting hemangiomas of the upper eyelid because particles in the steroid suspension can potentially occlude retinal or choroidal microvessels or the central retinal artery.

Interferon

Interferon is the second-line drug for treating severe, large hemangiomas. Interferon-alpha$_{2a}$ (IFN-α2a) is a potent, fairly well-tolerated cytokine that requires liver and hematologic monitoring during therapy. Long-term treatment carries the risk of thyroid dysfunction and neurologic complications. Interferon is known to inhibit angiogenesis, probably through inhibition of vascular smooth muscle cells and capillary endothelial cells.[196]

In a study of 20 patients with vision-threatening hemangiomas resistant to corticosteroids, 18 patients had more than 50% regression after an average of 8 months of treatment.[197]

Combination Therapy

At times, especially when treating large or extensive hemangiomas and conditions such as diffuse neonatal hemangiomatosis, multiple modalities may be required. In these patients, systemic prednisone with or without interferon, embolization of hemangiomas, surgical debulking and excision of the dermal component, and PDL treatment to superficial lesions may all be used[198] (Fig. 2.44). Although one might believe that the laser is cosmetic, its use in these patients prevents cutaneous hemorrhage and facilitates routine skin care.

A

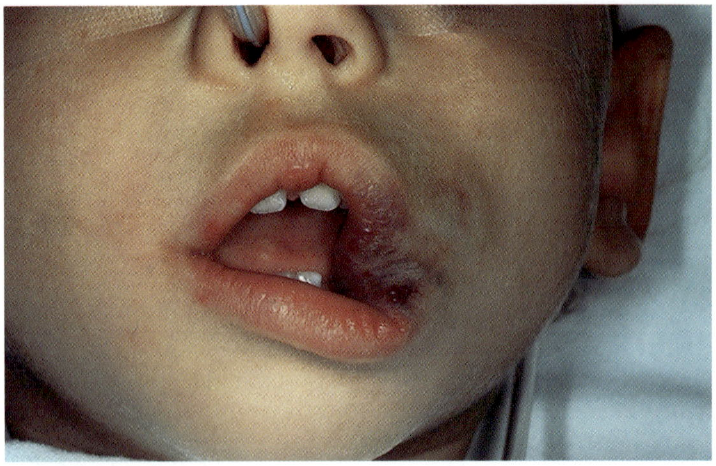

B

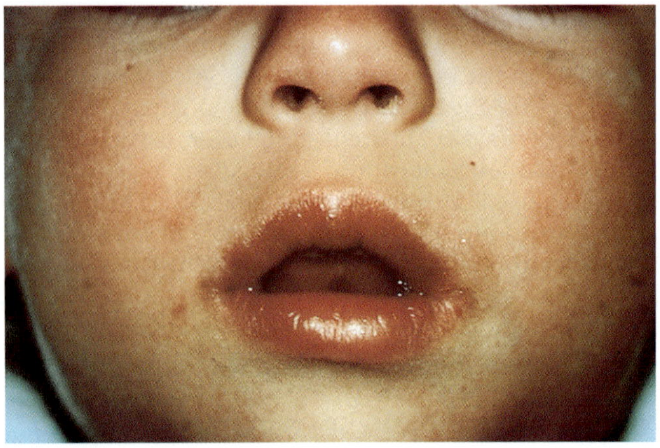

Figure 2.44 (A) Venous malformation involving lip and mucosa before treatment. (B) After therapy with Nd:YAG laser delivered as two separate treatments 6 weeks apart. Laser was used with 600-μm filter in noncontact mode and energy fluence of 30W delivered in 0.2-s pulses to shrink malformation. This was followed 6 weeks later by surgical resection. This photograph is clinical appearance 6 months after surgery. (Courtesy Milton Waner, MD.)

Early therapeutic intervention with laser photocoagulation of the vessels of a hemangioma when it is in a thin, flat stage or on initial presentation as localized telangiectasia is advocated to minimize enlargement of the tumor, ulceration, bleeding, and obstruction of vital organs.[30,32] This may be effective theoretically if the laser is capable of reaching all the vessels present. However, the notion that superficial photocoagulation will initiate regression of the entire hemangioma, including adjacent untreated tumor, does not appear to be true. Our experience, along with that of several colleagues, is that the deep portion of hemangiomas beyond the depth of laser penetration continues to proliferate despite involution of the superficial components treated by laser.[28,30,32]

Laser Treatment

The necessary requirements for any laser or pulsed light source to thermocoagulate effectively the ectatic vessel of a hemangioma are its depth of penetration, energy fluence, and pulse duration. Lasers with short wavelengths (<585 nm) can only deliver sufficient energy required for thermocoagulation to a depth less than 1 mm. Pulse durations necessary range from 0.5 to 10 ms, depending on the size of the ectatic vessels. Energy fluences should be greater than 6 J/cm^2. With these parameters, many different pulsed-light modalities have demonstrated efficacy.

Argon Laser

The argon laser[199–201] has been used effectively to treat hemangiomas. The potential benefit of the argon laser is limited by its depth of penetration into the dermis (<1 mm) and its tendency to cause hypertrophic scarring through nonspecific thermal injury, as reported in children with PWS.[25] However, with PWSs thicker than 1 mm, nonspecific thermal injury may be advantageous with a physician experienced in the laser's use. In addition, one physician noted atrophic, hypopigmented scarring in three of five cases of hemangioma treated with the argon laser.[202]

Nd:YAG Laser

The Nd:YAG laser at 1064 nm can penetrate deeply into tissue (2–8 mm) but produces widespread tissue injury because of its nonspecific absorption. This tends to result in scar formation. The Nd:YAG laser has been successful in shrinking large symptomatic lesions through nonspecific thermal injury,[203] but the risk of scarring, which always occurs to some extent,[204] must be weighed against potential benefits.

Some physicians believe the Nd:YAG laser should be limited to treating mucous membrane lesions (e.g., oral mucosa). Treatment technique also makes a difference. Treatment using 3- to 4-mm-diameter spots with 6- to 8-mm untreated lesion between spots has been advocated as a method to decrease scarring while still effectively debulking a lesion.

In 160 patients treated with the Nd:YAG laser at energy fluences of 400 to 1600 J/cm^2 in a continuous manner with pulses of 0.5 s, 13% had excellent results, 55% had a reduction in hemangioma size by more than 50%, 35% had a reduction in lesion size by less than 50%, and 2% had negligible results.[205] Ten percent of patients had scarring from superficial necrosis. The incidence of textural or pigmentary changes to the overlying skin was not reported. The authors noted an advantage of surgical resection of bulky tumors after thermocoagulation was obtained with the Nd:YAG laser.

Dr Berlien in Germany has successfully used the Nd:YAG laser to coagulate tissue, with its fluence being transferred to the bulk of the tumor through a 600-μm bare fiber at 8 to 10 W on a continuous mode until tumor coagulation occurs. The fiber is introduced through an 18-gauge Teflon cannula, and the skin is monitored with a thermal probe and cooled to minimize thermal injury to the epidermis. The fiber is slowly extracted at a rate approximating 0.5 mm/s, and monthly treatments are given to allow resorption of coagulated tissue. Postoperative edema and some pain occur for about 6 hours. A study of 100 pediatric patients treated over 3 years with intralesional 532 nm KTP and 1064 nm Nd:YAG laser in continuous mode for one to four treatments showed a 90% reduction in size in 446 patients and 50–90% reduction in 56 patients of the hemangiomas with no difference between the two lasers used.[206] Surgical resection was required in 76 patients. Thus, the intralesional laser decreased the size of the lesion to permit a smaller, more cosmetic resection of the lesion.

Use of the sapphire-tip contact probe with the Nd:YAG laser allows excision of vascular lesions with control of bleeding and offers another therapeutic approach in debulking the lesion.[207,208] However, a retrospective analysis of 11 patients treated with this technique demonstrated only three 'aesthetically acceptable' results despite four separate treatments.[209] In contrast, Afpelberg[210] has reported total removal without complications or side effects in 16 patients treated in this manner. The difference in treatment results may be related to preoperative preparation of the patient with intralesional corticosteroids or waiting until the lesion is in a stable or regressive stage before proceeding with surgical correction.

Cryogen spray cooling of the epidermis overlying hemangiomas may protect the epidermis and papillary dermis while achieving deep tissue photocoagulation during Nd:YAG laser irradiation.[211] A preliminary study on the highly vascularized chicken comb demonstrated 6.1-mm-deep photocoagulation while preserving epidermal integrity. To be effective, however, surface temperature monitoring must occur simultaneously with laser treatment and cooling to prevent epidermal damage. Therefore this technique may allow treatment of thick hemangiomas with a deep component.

One study detailing the treatment of 61 deep vascular malformations with a contact cooling 1064 nm Nd:YAG laser showed that 50% of treated lesions demonstrated 55% or greater resolution after a single treatment session with 35% having less than 50% improvement and 20% having 100% resolution.[212] Unfortunately, many of the lesions presented in this paper did not have specified treatment parameters.

532 nm Potassium Titanyl Phosphate (KTP) and Nd:YAG Laser

The KTP laser used through an intralesional 0.6-mm-diameter bare fiber has been found to shrink hemangiomas.[213] With this technique the fiber is passed through a 20-gauge needle positioned in the center of the hemangioma. Laser energy is then delivered at 15 J until shrinkage is seen or the overlying skin begins to feel warm to the touch. However, this is inaccurate and potentially dangerous because once the overlying skin is warm, excessive nonspecific damage has probably occurred. In a series of 12 patients 1 month to $3^1/_2$ years of age, 92% had a greater than 50% reduction in the hemangioma size at 3 months, with 8% maintaining this reduction at 6 months. To achieve these results, 50% required two treatments and 8% three treatments; 33% of hemangiomas ulcerated after therapy. Thus this aggressive form of treatment is best reserved for large, voluminous hemangiomas that have functional significance (e.g. airway obstruction, visual change).

The 532 nm Nd:YAG laser can be used on the skin to treat superficial hemangiomas. A retrospective study of 50 infants with 62 superficial hemangiomas found that complete regression occurred in 41% of lesions with PDL treatment versus 30% with the 532 nm Nd:YAG laser.[214] The 532 nm Nd:YAG laser was used at 20 J/cm^2 with a 50-ms pulse through a 5-mm-diameter spot. The PDL was a 0.45-ms, 585 nm laser with a 7-mm spot size.

Carbon Dioxide Laser

The CO_2 laser is also useful as a scalpel to excise and debulk vascular tissue with minimal blood loss. It has been used to excise laryngeal lesions causing airway obstruction,[30,161] oral hemangiomas,[215–217] and facial lesions.[218] Because this treatment modality has also been associated with a higher rate of scarring, it is not recommended for cutaneous lesions and is most efficacious in treating internal and mucosal hemangiomas.[30] In our practice the UPCO_2 laser has been used to resurface scarred hemangiomas and tighten those with redundant and stretched tissue with excellent results (Fig. 2.45).

Pulse Dye Laser

Although initially developed to treat vessels present in PWS, the similar vessel diameter and depth in hemangiomas explains the PDL's clinical efficacy. The depth of penetration of 585 nm is 0.6 to 1.2 mm, which limits its efficacy to relatively superficial lesions. Its safety and specificity are the reasons for its appeal. Early studies have demonstrated efficacy in hastening resolution of lesions beyond the proliferative phase,[28,32] as well as slowing or arresting proliferative growth.[28,30,32] The PDL is best utilized and most effective in eradicating lesions in a macular stage before proliferation.[30,32]

The PDL will not affect hemangioma vasculature below 1.5 mm, because proliferation of deeply situated hemangioma vessels proceeds despite involution of superficial laser-treated areas.[10,32,188]

Of 50 patients (mean age 13 months) treated with the PDL an average of 3.8 times, 53% had significant improvement in color without an appreciable reduction in lesion bulk.[219] Four of seven patients with flat lesions completely cleared after two treatments, with the remaining three patients achieving satisfactory results requiring no further treatment. Eight flat, ulcerated hemangiomas healed completely with PDL treatment after one to three treatments. Ten patients with slightly raised lesions required a mean of 5.2 treatments to achieve clearance in four and a good degree of flattening and improvement in the remaining six patients. Red raised lesions with a

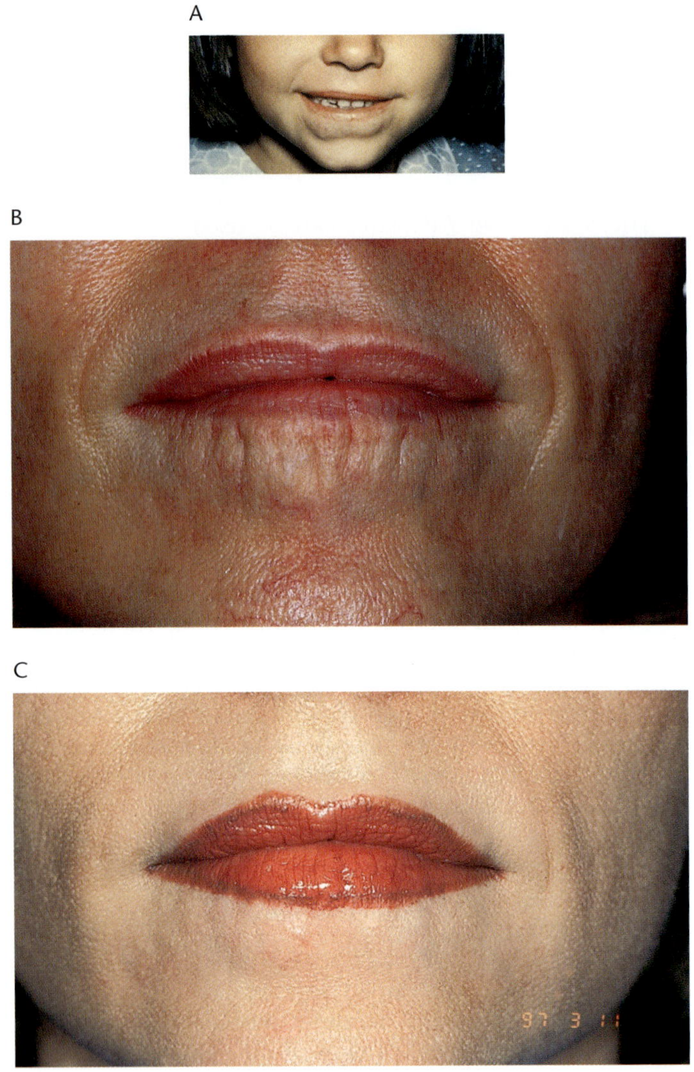

Figure 2.45 (A) Appearance of hemangioma in 5-year-old girl. (B) Clinical appearance 30 years later. Note flaccid, wrinkled skin. (C) Six months after resurfacing with Coherent Ultra Pulse CO_2 Laser. Three passes were given at 500 mJ through 3-mm collimated spot size handpiece.

significant subcutaneous component showed elimination of the red coloration and any ulcerations without change in lesion bulk.

Morelli and Weston[220] reported their 2-year experience in treating 55 lesions. Five patients with hemangiomas less than 3 cm^3 treated once or twice with the PDL in the proliferative phase had a good response with arrest of lesion growth. An additional five patients with large lesions greater than 20 cm^3 had an excellent response and resolution of lesions in those who continued treatment. Twenty patients with superficial and deep lesions had resolution of the superficial component only. Purely nodular older lesions resisted treatment. Ulcerated painful hemangiomas, when treated, heal and become painless, providing the best indication for treatment. Morelli et al[221] reported a total of 37 infants with ulcerated hemangiomas treated with the PDL between 2 and 40 weeks of age. All ulcerations healed with one to three treatments at 2- to 4-week intervals at fluences of 6.0 to 6.5 J/cm^2. Almost 70% healed within 2 weeks after a single laser treatment.

Garden et al[222] have reported that the best results occur when the hemangioma is elevated 3 mm or less and advise treatment in the first weeks of life. They studied 33 hemangiomas in 24 patients 2 weeks to 7 months of age in whom a 93.9% lightening occurred in the superficial lesions in 4.1 treatment sessions. Seven lesions 4 mm or more in thickness lightened 83.7% in seven treatment sessions. They found that compressing the hemangioma with a glass slide to bring the deeper vascular component closer to the surface did not increase efficacy.

A report on treating 68 infants with 100 hemangiomas within 12 weeks of their development further confirms PDL efficacy.[223] Seventy-three lesions required a single treatment and 27 up to five treatments; 23% of lesions showed complete remission, 55% showed partial remission, and 14% stopped growing. Only 8% of lesions continued to grow despite treatment. This efficacy occurred with virtually no serious adverse sequelae.

Proliferative hemangiomas causing functional impairment in seven patients 8 to 24 weeks of age showed significant reduction in size, normalization of color, and resolution of superficial ulceration.[224] Lesions were treated at fluences of 7.0 to 9.25 J/cm^2 at 4- to 8-week intervals (two to six times) until the hemangioma completely regressed or stopped regressing further. As reported in the previous studies, all patients with ulceration responded to treatment. Four of seven patients had complete resolution of the hemangioma. No adverse events or complications were noted.

Our experience is similar to that of most reports.[225] The following is a summary of our experience with a total of 34 infants and children. We used the PDL at fluences of 6.25 to 8.0 J/cm^2 at 2- to 3-week intervals with spots overlapping 10% to 15% to produce an endpoint of homogenous darkening of the entire lesion until one of the following circumstances: resolution occurred, the treatment was judged to be ineffective, or the parents discontinued treatment for unrelated reasons. Treatment was offered to all parents of children with hemangiomas after explanation of the natural resolution history of the lesions and the potential benefits and risks of laser therapy and steroid therapy. Some patients had medical reasons for treatment (visual obstruction, interference with feeding or breathing, or lesional bleeding), but treatment was also offered to patients with lesions that caused concern because of proliferative activity, tissue distortion, or cosmetic disfigurement.

Seventeen hemangiomas had only a superficial component, with 13 of these less than 1 cm in diameter, averaging 7 mm. The lesions appeared as a red macule initially, at an average age of 15 days. The lesions typically began to proliferate, causing parental concern. The average age at first treatment was 5.5 months. The most common reason for the delay in treatment was difficulty in finding an appropriate treatment center. The average patient received 3.6 treatments over 3.3 months. The average fluence used was 6.8 J/cm^2. Nine patients (53%) cleared completely.

Table 2.8 *Superficial Capillary Hemangiomas: PDL Treatment*

No. lesions	Diameter >1 cm	Average age lesion appeared	Average age first treatment	Average no. treatments	Average time of treatment	Average treatment fluence	Complete clearing	Average improvement if not clear
17	13	15 days	5.5 months	3.6	3.35 months	6.8 J/cm^2	9 (53%)	67%

Table 2.9 *Mixed Superficial/Deep Capillary Hemangioma: Early PDL Treatment*

No. lesions	Diameter >1 cm	Average age lesion appeared	Average age first treatment	Average no. treatments	Average time of treatment	Average treatment fluence	Adjunctive steroid therapy	Average improvement	
								Superficial	Deep
8	8	6 days	4.5 months	4.5	7.4 months	6.8 J/cm^2	4 (50%)	96%	73%

Table 2.10 *Mixed Superficial/Deep Capillary Hemangioma: Late PDL Treatment*

No. lesions	Diameter >1 cm	Average age lesion appeared	Average age first treatment	Average no. treatments	Average time of treatment	Average treatment fluence	Adjunctive steroid therapy	Average improvement	
								Superficial	Deep
9	8	40 days	41 mo	3.5	7.2 mo	6.9 J/cm^2	2 (22%)	62%	32%

Those lesions not clearing had an average improvement of 67% (Table 2.8).

Seventeen infants had hemangiomas classified as mixed, with both a superficial and a deep component. All these lesions were large, some encompassing the entire side of the face. Eight lesions were treated relatively early, during the proliferative phase, and nine lesions were treated later, during the involution-dominant phase (Table 2.9).

Those hemangiomas treated early had appeared at an earlier age (average age 6 days). Treatment was initiated at an average age of 4.5 months and continued for an average 7.4 months, during which time 4.5 treatments were administered, using an average fluence of 6.8 J/cm^2. Four patients (50%) received adjunctive therapy with steroids during this period, two receiving systemic prednisolone and two receiving intralesional steroids. Interestingly, in these four patients, treatment with steroids abruptly halted the proliferation of the deep component and resulted in shrinking this deep portion, but it had no visible effect on the superficial component. Likewise, the PDL treatment abruptly halted proliferation and resulted in clearance of the superficial component without apparent effect on the deep component, which continued to proliferate unless steroids were used. Treatment resulted in near-complete (96%) clearing of the superficial component in all patients and an average improvement of 73% in the deep component (Table 2.9).

Lesions treated later in their course appeared at an average age of 40 days but were not treated until an average age of 41 months. These nine lesions received an average of 3.5 treatments, using an average fluence of 7.2 J/cm^2 and a treatment interval averaging 9 weeks. Two patients received intralesional steroids in an attempt to shrink the persistent deep component of the lesion. These nine patients achieved a much more modest degree of improvement than the other eight patients treated early, with the superficial component improving an average 62% and the deep component only 32% (Table 2.10).

Most authors report cessation of the proliferative phase as a consequence of treatment with the PDL.[30,31,222] Controversy has surrounded the question of whether early treatment can prevent the proliferative phase and especially whether it may have an effect on the deep component that the PDL cannot reach.[226] Indeed, the case reported by Glassberg et al[30] showed deep proliferation despite cutaneous involution during PDL therapy. Mulliken[176] reported his experience of the same phenomenon. This was our experience as well: four patients with superficial and deep components showed response of only the superficial component to treatment with the PD laser, while the deep component continued to proliferate. Interestingly, the opposite was true as well; only the deep component was responsive to steroid therapy, the superficial component being unaffected. Glassberg et al[30] also have mentioned this point.

The cases reported by Glassberg et al,[30] Sherwood and Tan,[31] and us well illustrate that the PDL can rapidly and dramatically halt the proliferative superficial component.

In two of these three series, the hemangiomas were very extensive and were responsive throughout the superficial component. Because the depth of penetration is limited, a series of treatments is usually necessary gradually to reach deeper layers of vessels. We recommend a treatment schedule of every 2 to 3 weeks for three to six treatments, using a fluence of 5 to 7 J/cm^2 for most lesions. Lesions with only a superficial component are very responsive to treatment because 90% will completely involute (see Fig. 2.37). Those with a deep component and a superficial component may require intralesional steroid therapy for the deep component and laser therapy for the superficial component (see Figs 2.42 and 2.43). Widespread and deep lesions may require laser therapy and systemic steroids to arrest the growth of the deep component. Treatment at the earliest opportunity is critical in determining success in these cases.

Kauvar[227] presented the 1.5-ms pulsed, 595 nm PDL in the treatment of ten hemangiomas. Two superficial lesions cleared in two or three treatments, and eight lesions with both a superficial and a deep component cleared in two to four treatments. In the latter group, the superficial component cleared completely, but with only a 10% to 50% reduction in the deep component. Kauvar recommends the following parameters:

- infants: 7-mm-diameter spot, 7 J/cm^2
- adults: 7-mm-diameter spot, 8 J/cm^2
- hypertrophic lesions: 7-mm-diameter spot, 9 J/cm^2.

A total of 165 children with 225 separate hemangiomas treated with the PDL with a mean of two treatments were separated out as superficial or mixed hemangiomas.[228] Flat cutaneous hemangiomas had an excellent response in 32% and good results in 52%. Of the mixed hemangiomas, 39% had a response of the superficial component with continued proliferation in 61% and no change in the dermal component. The authors concluded that early treatment is only effective for superficial lesions and did not prevent progression of deep or mixed lesions. The drawback of this study was that the investigators used an old PDL at 585 nm, 300-ms pulse and a 5-mm spot beam without epidermal cooling allowing for only 5–7 J/cm^2 to be delivered. One would suspect that the use of a 595 nm PDL with a 7- to 10-mm-diameter spot and epidermal cooling would allow deeper therapeutic effects to be obtained.

The largest study on the treatment of childhood hemangiomas evaluated 548 children with 692 hemangiomas who were treated with the PDL.[229] After 1 to 12 treatments (mean 2.5) further growth was stopped in 96.6% of all hemangiomas; 13.8% achieved a complete remission with a significant regression in another 14.9%. Small and superficial hemangiomas responded best to treatment. As with previous studies, the drawback of this study was the use of a first-generation PDL with a pulse duration of 0.45 ms and a spot size of 5 to 7 mm. A mean fluence of 8.4 J/cm^2 was used. Adverse effects even with this high fluence were rare with 7% developing temporary pigmentary changes and 4% developing small atrophic scars. The age at the start of treatment was not important in this study (Fig 2.46).

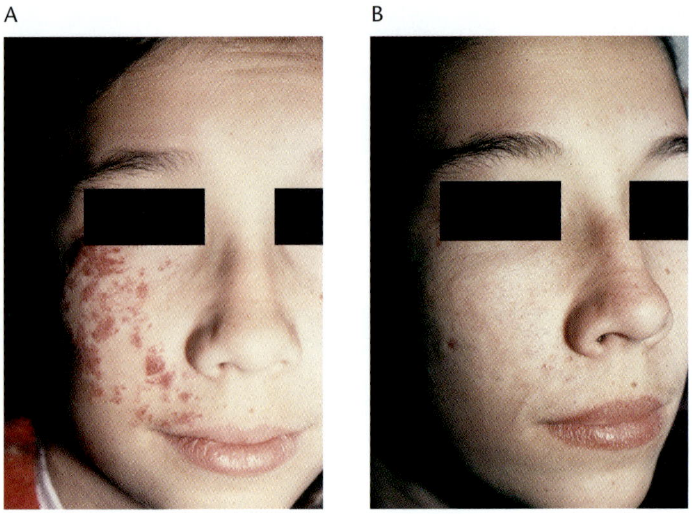

Figure 2.46 (A) Fifteen-year-old girl with facial hemangioma. (B) Appearance after 6 treatments with the PDL. (Courtesy Gerald Goldberg, MD.)

Intense Pulsed-light Treatment

In addition to monochromatic light, noncoherent light has also been found to be effective in treating hemangiomas when used within an adequate wavelength range and with proper fluence and pulse duration. We have used the IPL with a cutoff filter at 550, 570, or 590 nm to treat multiple hemangiomas with excellent results (Fig. 2.47). We have used this light source to treat evolving as well as long-established tumors. One 66-year-old patient developed a hemangioma after trauma 15 years before treatment. One treatment with a 570-nm cutoff filter at 80 J/cm^2 given as a double pulse of 9 and 13 ms separated by a 50-ms delay resulted in 100% resolution. The lesion immediately became purpuric, then crusted before completely involuting (Fig. 2.48).

Foster and Gold[230] reported 90% involution of a 7.5 × 4-cm ulcerated cavernous hemangioma on the abdomen of an 11-week-old black infant. They used a 550-nm cutoff filter at a fluence of 38 J/cm^2 in a triple-pulse mode (T_1 3 ms, T_2 2 ms, T_3 1.7 ms) with a 10-ms delay between pulses. Two additional treatments at 2-week intervals with a 570-nm cutoff filter at fluences of 30 and 38 J/cm^2 using a triple pulse (T_1 4 ms, T_2 3 ms, T_3 2 ms) with a 20-ms delay between pulses resulted in maximal resolution with minimal hypopigmentation.

Surgical Treatment

Surgical therapy should be considered for certain lesions. Hemangiomas of the vermilion border, mucous membranes, and nasal tip are very slow to involute and may seriously interfere with a child's self-esteem. In these cases, excision before entering school may be considered.[176] Microsurgical techniques with hemostatic lasers have been successful at debulking lesions and coagulating vessels to allow for easier surgical excision.[231] The use of tissue

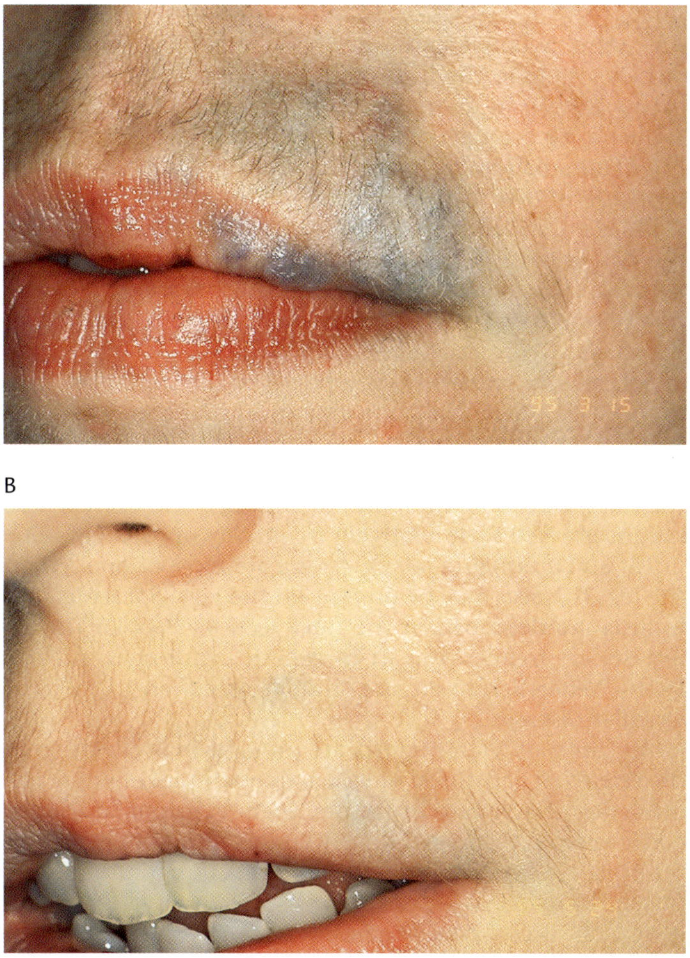

Figure 2.47 (A) Persistent hemangioma/venous malformation despite four treatments with argon laser (0.5-s pulses at 2W) and one treatment with the PDL (8 J/cm^2 with 5-mm-diameter spot size). (B) After three treatments with Photoderm VL with 590-nm cutoff filter, double pulse of 4.2 and 7.7 ms with 300-ms delay between pulses at 65, 71, and 69 J/cm^2, respectively.

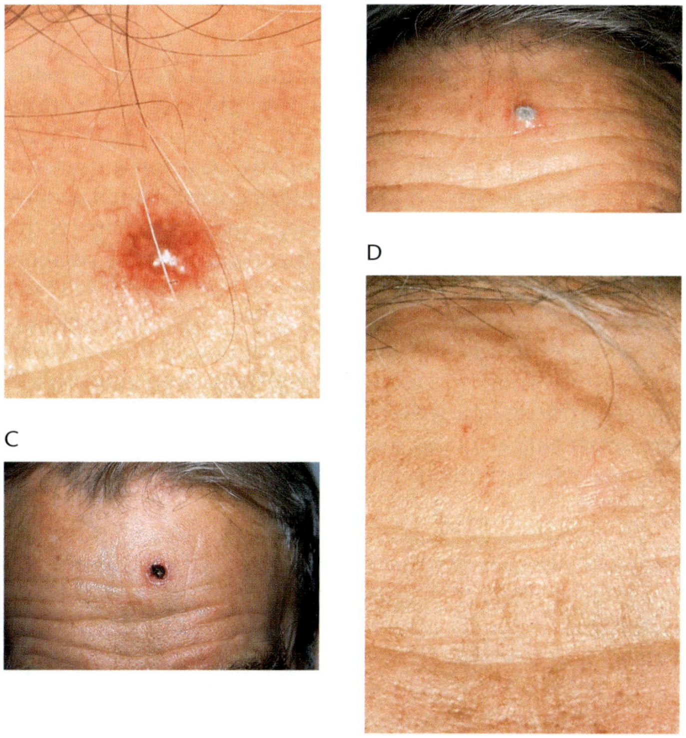

Figure 2.48 (A) This 66-year-old male had a 15-year history of hemangioma on forehead before treatment. (B) Immediately after treatment with PhotoDerm VL (see text). (C) Nine days after treatment an eschar developed, which healed without scarring 3 months later. (D) Complete resolution 4 weeks later.

expansion further improves excision cosmesis.[232] Facial or neck hemangiomas that have incompletely resolved with sagging skin or excessive fibrofatty residuum may be excised.[233]

Ideally, a team approach should be used in treating extensive hemangiomas. Multiple specialties, including but not limited to vascular surgeons, radiologists, dermatologists, plastic surgeons, and pediatricians, may combine their expertise to optimize patient care. Apfelberg et al[207,234] have reported the use of the Nd:YAG laser with sapphire tip in conjunction with intralesional steroids and also in a team approach using superselective embolization before resection.

Summary Recommendations

Mulliken[140] correctly calls for a biologic approach to the treatment of hemangiomas of infancy. He points out that the only antiangiogenic agents currently available are corticosteroids and that they may afford dramatic benefit without significant risks as one might expect. When this therapeutic approach is considered in light of the recent information available regarding laser responsiveness of the superficial component, we conclude that the PDL should be used at the earliest sign of a capillary hemangioma and certainly as soon as active proliferation begins. In conjunction with this treatment, intralesional or systemic steroids should be given to halt the proliferation of the deep component when that portion proceeds despite laser therapy. The risks of therapy have been demonstrated to be minimal.

Extensive hemangiomas that have not responded to other treatments have reduced with IPL treatment.[235]

The recommendations of the American Academy of Dermatology's Guidelines of Care Committee for treatment of hemangiomas are summarized as follows[236]:

1. Prevent or reverse life-threatening or function-threatening complications.
2. Prevent permanent disfigurement left by residual skin changes.
3. Minimize psychosocial stress.
4. Avoid scarring procedures.
5. Prevent or treat ulcerative lesions to minimize scarring, infection, and pain.

Pyogenic Granuloma

Pyogenic granuloma (PG) is an acquired vascular lesion, a true neoplasm distinct from granulation tissue, usually solitary, 0.5 to 2.0 cm in diameter, bright red, and pedunculated.[237–239] The surface is soft, bleeding easily with trauma. It may become ulcerated and develop a granulomatous surface with a brown or black crust. Lesions usually appear suddenly and may enlarge rapidly. There is no history of preceding trauma or infection in most patients (75%),[240] although this typically is assumed.[241] These lesions also frequently occur as a superimposed growth on the surface of a PWS.[158] Repeated episodes of bleeding and unresponsiveness to electrocautery have been reported in up to 50% of patients.[240] This may be secondary to the extension of vascular proliferation deep into the dermis, often with a unique lobular arrangement of capillaries.[242]

The argon laser,[243] as well as the CO_2 laser,[244] has been shown to be effective in treating PGs. The PG is photocoagulated until the entire lesion blanches and turns a dusty gray color. Treatments are repeated at 3- to 4-week intervals as needed.

PG lesions have been unpredictably responsive to the PDL.[78] They have been shown to respond,[38,241,245,246] but in most cases lesions are too thick for the laser to penetrate throughout the lesion in one treatment. Tan and Kurban[245] use a glass slide to compress the superficial ectatic vessels and use the laser through the glass to treat the deeper component of this lesion. This maneuver presumably allows treatment of deep vessels, after which the slide is removed and the treatment is repeated to coagulate more superficially located vessels. When effective by itself, the PDL must be used with multiple, 100% overlapping pulses to turn the lesion deep purple. As previously demonstrated, this technique produces nonselective photo-thermolysis and is therefore no different than CW argon, copper vapor, or 577-nm dye lasers.

A study of 18 patients with PG treated with the PDL demonstrated both symptomatic and clinical clearing in 16 patients with excellent cosmetic results.[247] Seven of the lesions had been previously treated with electrosurgery or excision. The authors flattened the lesions with a glass slide and used fluences of 6.5 to 9.0 J/cm^2 in an overlapping manner to cover the lesion completely. Treatments were repeated up to four times to achieve success. Treatment outcomes were excellent, but two postoperative photos showed textural changes that resembled a scar, although this was not noted by the authors.

We have not been able to achieve uniform success in treating PG lesions with or without the diascopy maneuver with the PDL. In addition, multiple treatments are impractical because of the ease with which lesions are traumatized between sessions. We therefore recommend shave excision of the lesion's papular component if a histologic specimen is necessary or CO_2 vaporization of the lesion followed by PDL therapy to the remaining flat macular lesion if necessary.

Telangiectasia

The term 'telangiectasia' refers to superficial cutaneous vessels visible to the human eye.[248] These vessels measure 0.1 to 1.0 mm in diameter and represent a dilated venule, capillary, or arteriole. Telangiectasia that are arteriolar in origin are small in diameter, bright red in color, and do not protrude above the skin surface. Those that arise from venules are wider, blue in color, and often protrude above the skin surface. Telangiectasia arising at the capillary loop are often initially fine, red lesions but become larger and purple or blue with time because of venous backflow from increasing hydrostatic pressure.[249]

Telangiectasia have been subdivided into four classifications based on clinical appearance: (1) simple or linear, (2) arborizing, (3) spider, and (4) papular[250] (Fig. 2.49). Red linear and arborizing telangiectasia are very common on the face, especially the nose, midcheeks, and chin. These lesions are also seen relatively frequently on the legs. Blue linear and arborizing telangiectasia are most often seen on the legs but also may be present on the face. Spider telangiectasia are described in the next section. Papular telangiectasia are frequently part of genetic syndromes, such as Osler–Weber–Rendu disease, and also are seen in collagen vascular diseases.

All forms of telangiectasia are thought to occur through the release or activation of vasoactive substances under the influence of a variety of factors, such as anoxia, estrogen, corticosteroids (topical or systemic), various chemicals, multiple types of bacterial or viral infection, and multiple physical factors, with resultant capillary or venular neogenesis.[249] Box 2.2 lists the associated diseases and causes of telangiectasia.

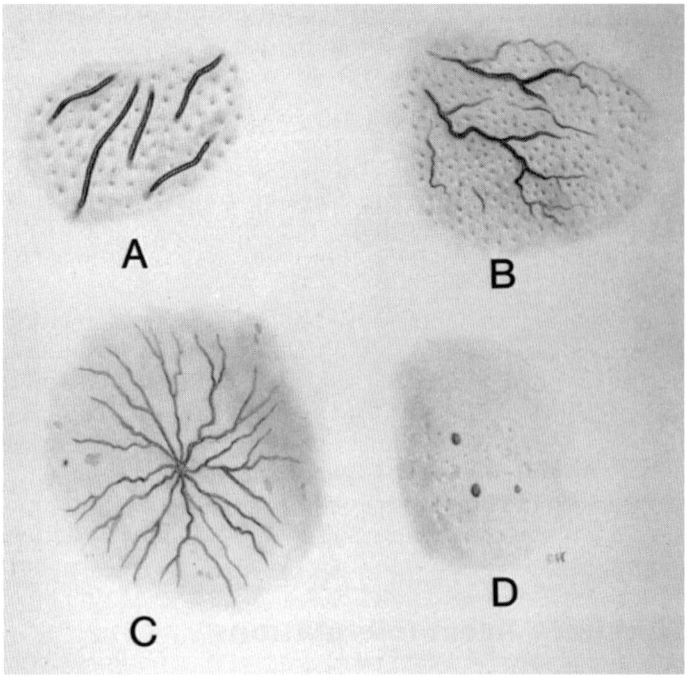

Figure 2.49 Four types of telangiectasia. (A) simple; (B) arborized; (C) spider; and (D) popular. (Modified from Goldman MP, Bennett RG. J Am Acad Dermatol 1987; 17:167.)

Box 2.2 *Causes of Cutaneous Telangiectasia*

Genetic
Vascular nevi
- Nevus flammeus
- Nevus araneus

Congenital neuroangiopathies
- Ataxia telangiectasia
- Sturge–Weber syndrome
- Maffucci syndrome
- Klippel–Trenaunay–Weber syndrome

Congenital poikiloderma (Rothmund–Thomson syndrome)
Bloom syndrome
Cockayne syndrome
Hereditary hemorrhagic telangiectasia (Osler–Weber–Rendu disease)
Essential progressive telangiectasia
Generalized essential telangiectasia
- Familial (autosomal dominant)
- Acquired (hormonal or infectious stimulation)

Unilateral nevoid telangiectatic syndrome
Diffuse neonatal hemangiomatosis
Hereditary benign telangiectasia

Acquired disease with secondary cutaneous component: Collagen vascular diseases
Lupus erythematosus (especially periungual)
Dermatomyositis
Progressive systemic sclerosis (especially periungual, and with the *c*alcinosis, *R*aynaud, *e*sophageal dysmotility, *s*clerodactyly, and *t*elangiectasia [CREST] syndrome)
Cryoglobulinemia

Other
- Telangiectasia macularis eruptiva perstans (mastocytosis)
- Carcinoma telangiectasia (metastatic tumors)

Component of a primary cutaneous disease
Rosacea
Varicose veins
Basal cell carcinoma
Merkel cell tumor
Necrobiosis lipoidica diabeticorum
Poikiloderma vasculare atrophicans
Capillaritis (purpura annularis telangiectodes)
Xeroderma pigmentosum
Pseudoxanthoma elasticum
Degos disease
Superficial epithelium with sebaceous differentiation

Hormonal
Pregnancy
Corticoid induced
- Cushing syndrome/disease
- Iatrogenic (from systemic, topical, or intralesional use)
- Estrogen therapy (usually with high dose)

Physical damage
Actinic dermatitis
Radiodermatitis
Postsurgical, especially in suture lines under tension and after rhinoplasty
Physical trauma

Modified from Goldman MP, Bennett RG Treatment of telangiectasia: a review. Journal of the American Academy of Dermatology 1987; 17:167.

Telangiectasia of the face are most often seen in patients with fair complexion (Fitzpatrick types I and II skin). These lesions are especially common on the nasal alae, nose, and midcheeks and are probably caused by persistent arteriolar vasodilatation resulting from vessel wall weakness. The vessels dilate further when damage to the surrounding connective and elastic tissue occurs from factors such as chronic sun exposure or use of topical steroids. These lesions have a definite familial or genetic component. Rosacea may be an accompanying condition.

Telangiectasia: Clinical Variants

Linear Facial Telangiectasia

These telangiectasia often carry an unjustified social stigma implying alcoholism. Thus patients are understandably distressed by this otherwise benign condition. Treatment of large vessels on the nasal ala or nasal alar groove is difficult and often leads to noticeable scarring when conventional methods are used. We have found the PDL to be a powerful and effective tool in the treatment of these lesions, virtually without the risk of scarring or other permanent skin changes.

Carbon Dioxide Laser

The CO_2 laser has been used for treatment of facial telangiectasia.[231] Because tissue destruction is nonselective with this laser, occurring by vaporization of water within cells, the skin surface and dermis overlying the telangiectasia are destroyed as well as the vessel. Because of this nonselective action, the CO_2 laser has no advantage over electrosurgery in the treatment of telangiectasia.

Argon Laser

The argon laser has often been used for treatment of facial telangiectasia. Treatment parameters have varied, with laser powers of 0.8 to 2.9 W; exposure times of 50 ms, 0.2 s, and 0.3 s; and continuous output with spot sizes of 0.1 and 1 mm. Although the success rate has been reported to be good to excellent in 65% to 99% of patients treated,[2,252] pitted and depressed scars, hypopigmentation, hyperpigmentation, and recurrence of veins have been noted.[3,253] One area of particular concern is the nasal alae and nasolabial creases, where depressed scarring is relatively common, although resolution gradually occurs over time.[3]

Adverse healing may occur with the argon laser because of nonspecific thermal damage to perivascular tissue and the overlying epidermis. This is caused by competition for absorption of laser fluence from epidermal melanin and extensive radial diffusion and dissipation of heat from the target blood vessels.[254] Both these factors result in relatively nonspecific thermal destruction. To minimize these effects, a small beam size (100 µm) has been advocated to trace vessels precisely,[83,255,256] and a low power or pulsing with a 50-ms shutter has been recommended.[255,257,258] As mentioned previously, these parameters must be monitored closely, because the successful treatment of vascular lesions with the argon laser requires experience and artful expertise. As described previously, the use of a very small beam (100 µm) greatly increases the scattering of laser photons within the dermis and limits treatment to the most superficial of dermal vessels. With these parameters, many physicians find the argon laser effective in treating facial telangiectasia, with only minimal risk of adverse healing. This application is its most successful use.

To limit heat diffusion with the argon laser, robotized scanning laser handpieces have been used (see earlier section on treatment of PWS in adults). The use of this device has been reported to be successful in the treatment of facial and leg telangiectasia when the telangiectasia occur in densely interlacing mats.[259] This technique is effective and greatly reduces the risk of adverse response, but it is not well suited for individual or widespread isolated telangiectasia.

Argon-Pumped Tunable Dye Laser

The argon-pumped tunable dye laser (ATDL) is a CW laser, although mechanically shuttered pulses as short as 20 ms are achievable. Beam size may be varied from 50 µm to 6.0 mm. Yellow light (577–595 nm) is usually chosen for treatment of vascular lesions. The tracing technique using a 100-µm beam with this laser has been used extensively and advocated by Scheibner and Wheeland[255] as a technique that produces good to excellent results with minimal risk in a variety of cutaneous vascular lesions,[83,256] including facial telangiectasia.[260] The proper endpoint of treatment is disappearance of the vessel, not blanching, blistering, or charring of the overlying skin. Because the tracing hand motion cannot be accurately quantified, treatment parameters are difficult to teach except by direct monitoring. In addition, this technique is more tedious and time-consuming than the PDL, even when one becomes a skilled operator. Multiple treatments are usually required, with hypopigmentation rarely occurring.[261] The laser also may be used with a robotized scanning device if large areas of matted telangiectasia are to be treated.[259,262] However, multiple treatments are required, including spot vessel tracing to eliminate the hexagonal appearance.

A prospective, side-by-side comparison of the ATDL with the PDL in 14 patients found better efficacy with the PDL.[263] The ATDL used was a modified ophthalmic laser at 585 nm, focused to a 0.1-mm circular spot with a power of 0.7 to 0.8 W at a pulse duration of 0.1 s (Coherent Medical, now Lumenis). Treatment times were about three times longer for the ATDL than the PDL. The PDL was more painful than the ATDL. Swelling and erythema was similar between the two lasers, but hyperpigmentation was greater with the ATDL. Excellent clearance occurred with the LPDL in 78% of patients compared with 28% with the ATDL.

Copper Vapor/Copper Bromide Laser

The CVL or CBL operates at two specific wavelengths, 578 nm (yellow) and 511 nm (green), and delivers a 'quasi-continuous wave' composed of pulsed laser light energy in 20-ns pulses at a frequency of 15,000 pulses per second. This train of pulses interacts with tissue in the same manner as a continuous beam because of the accumulation of heat with the large number of pulses delivered. Because of resulting thermal diffusion, it may be necessary to gate the pulse electronically with 20- to 50-ms secondary pulses or to use a scanning device.

The ability to pulse the CVL between 20 and 50 ms allows this laser to work within the thermal relaxation time of many telangiectasia (Fig. 2.50). When the laser is used

A

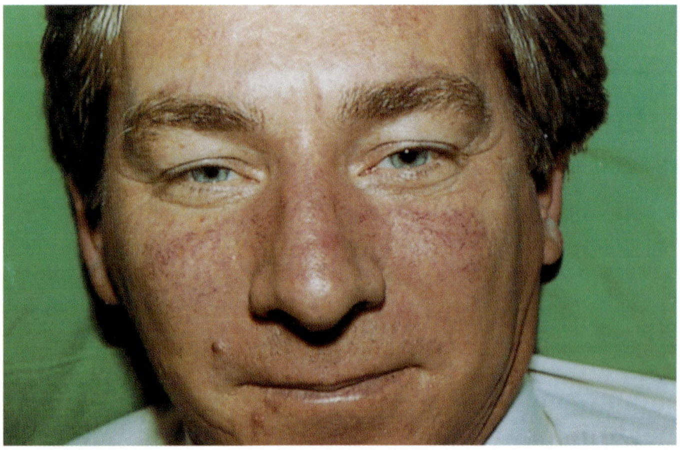

B

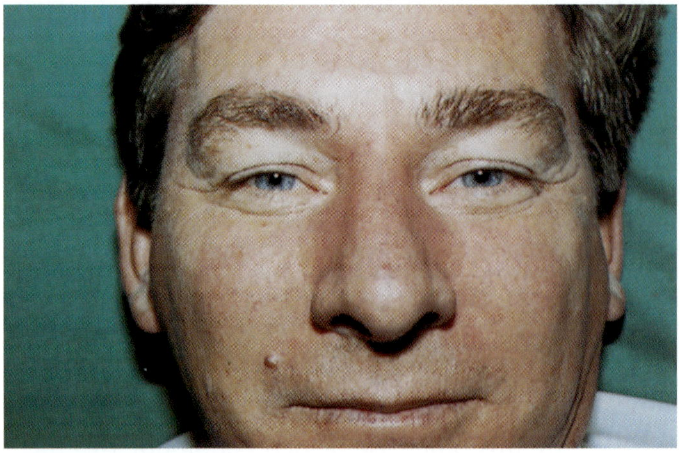

Figure 2.50 This man with telangiectasias was treated for about 20 minutes on two occasions with a copper bromide laser. (A) Before treatment. (B) After treatment. First treatment was at 2.2 W and 0.7 mm spot size, with 20-ms pulses (11.4 J/cm^2) for smaller vessels and 30-ms pulses (17.1 J/cm^2) for larger vessels. Second treatment 2 months later was at 2 W with 20-ms pulses for all remaining vessels (10.4 J/cm^2). (Courtesy Sue McCoy, MD.)

with these refinements, it is somewhat safer and more effective than the argon laser for treatment of facial telangiectasia and has the advantage of leaving only very minor superficial crusts overlying treated vessels, in contrast to the very visible, dark purpuric impact spots of the PDL.[264] A comparison of the CVL with the PDL in 10 adults with facial telangiectasia resistant to electrosurgical therapy demonstrated no difference in efficacy or adverse sequelae.[265] However, Dinehart et al[188] report a 10% incidence of transient hyperpigmentation. Whether this represents melanin or hemosiderin is unknown.

Of 33 patients with facial telangiectasia treated with the CVL, 69% had good to excellent results and 19% had poor results.[266] Treatment occurred with a 1-mm-diameter spot size at pulse durations of 50 to 200 ms at energy densities from 8 to 32 J/cm² or continuous until vessel blanching occurred. Best results were seen on the cheeks, with poor results on the nose or nasolabial folds. Atrophic scarring was reported on nasal lesions (7 of 33 patients), and edema lasting 1 to 3 days occurred on the cheeks and lower eyelids.

Thibault[267] reported the results of a patient questionnaire of 180 patients treated with the CVL with or without sclerotherapy for facial telangiectasia. He used a CVL (VisErase 3 w, Visiray Pty Ltd., Hornsby, NSW, Australia) with a 200-μm fiber delivering a spot size of 150 to 400 μm. A clinical endpoint of vessel blanching was used, which required a power of 600 to 700 mW impinging on the vessel for less than 1 s delivered continuously. Patients developed blistering 24 to 48 hours after treatment, with crusting lasting 7 to 17 days. Edema usually lasted 3 days. Almost half of patients treated with the CVL alone developed hypopigmentation. Good results were seen in 47% of vessels treated with the CVL alone, and these patients were satisfied with treatment, versus 86% of patients who had combination treatment with CVL and sclerotherapy being satisfied with treatment.

Waner et al[268] compared the CVL with the PDL in 12 patients with facial telangiectasia. Treatment times and patient satisfaction were equivalent. Postoperative swelling and prolonged healing occurred with the PDL. The CVL used was the Vasculase (Metalaser), with a spot size of 150 μm at a power of 0.35 to 0.55 W chopped at 0.2-s intervals. Waner concludes that both lasers have equal efficacy, with most patients preferring the CVL.

McCoy[269] has reported her results in treating 570 patients with facial telangiectasia. Similar results were reported in another study of 23 patients evaluated in a blinded manner.[270] In both studies, greater than 75% clearance was achieved in 70% of patients, 50% to 75% clearance in 17%, and less than 50% clearance in 13%. Vessels on the cheeks cleared much better than nasal telangiectasia, which only had an excellent response in 26% of patients. Vessels less than 100 μm or greater than 300 μm did not respond as well as vessels 100 to 300 μm in diameter. McCoy used the CBL at 578 nm only (Norseld CuB D-10, Adelaide, South Australia) in a train of 30-ns pulses at 16 kHz. The average power through the 600-μm fiber was 2 W. The fiber was used in a slightly defocused mode to produce a 0.9-mm-diameter spot. Although the chopped pulse duration varied from 7 to 60 ms, the treatment endpoint was vessel spasm without epidermal blanching. About 45% of patients required one treatment, and 35% of patients required two treatments. The remaining 20% of patients received three to five treatments. Treatment sessions ranged from 5 to 60 minutes, with the average treatment requiring 16.7 minutes. Moderate erythema occurred in most patients and lasted 2 to 3 hours. Swelling and crusting were rare. There were no reports of scarring or hyperpigmentation.

McCoy et al[270] postulate that the reduced effectiveness in treating vessels less than 100 μm results from the thermal relaxation time being much less than the delivered pulse durations. The reduced effectiveness in vessels greater than 300 μm results from absorption of laser fluence in the superficial portion of the vessel with 'protection' to the deeper endothelium. McCoy recommends using sclerotherapy for vessels greater than 300 μm in diameter.

When used with the modulating influence of a secondary shuttered pulse or scanning device, the risk of adverse response is further minimized without significant change in clinical effectiveness. In a comparison of 144 patients treated with the point-by-point technique and 105 patients treated by the Hexascan, French investigators determined that the incidence of hypertrophic scarring was less than 1% in the Hexascan group versus 7% in the point-by-point group. Treatment time was also reduced to 20% of the point-by-point time. Patients treated by Hexascan also experienced less pain, and local anesthesia was rarely required.[271] The balance between these two results (vessel obliteration and adverse healing) must be weighed and the treatment technique altered to be consistent with the goals of treatment.

532 nm KTP Laser

The Starpulse KTP laser (LaserScope) operates at 532 nm and emits a train of 1-ms Q-switched pulses at 25 kHz. What distinguishes this system from other frequency-doubled Nd:YAG lasers is that the arc lamp is modulated and can provide pulse durations ranging from 1 to 50 ms. This produces very-high-energy pulses that can be projected onto the skin in spots ranging in diameter from 0.25 to 4.0 mm while still maintaining fluences within the 5 to 10 J/cm² therapeutic range. The combination of high-energy pulses and ability to adjust pulse duration to match the thermal relaxation time of blood vessels allows modulated KTP lasers to remove vascular lesions with less purpura than the PDL (Figs 2.51 and 2.52). One study demonstrated a 75–100% improvement in 94% of patients using 16–22.5 J/cm² through a 500- to 700-μm spot with pulse durations of 15–30 ms. Telangiectasia were treated with complete vessel blanching or visible intravascular coagulation.[272]

A comparison study of the KTP laser (Starpulse) with the PDL found less swelling, pain, bruising, and redness with the KTP laser.[273] The Starpulse was used with a 2-mm-diameter spot size, 17 J/cm², 10 ms. The PDL was used with a 3-mm-diameter spot size at 6.8 J. No significant difference in efficacy was found between the two lasers.

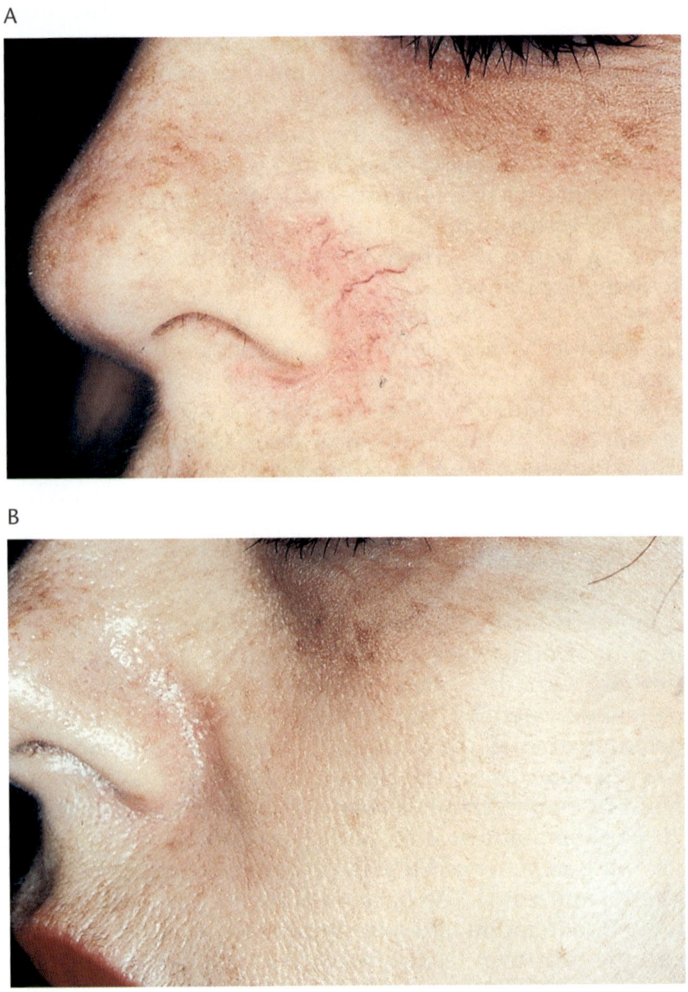

Figure 2.51 (A) Perinasal telangiectasia before treatment. (B) Two weeks after treatment with Orion potassium titanyl phosphorus (KTP) at 5 W, tracing vessels once with 250-μm spot Dermastat with 10-ms exposure duration, 5 pulses per second (pps). (Courtesy Burton E Silver, MD.)

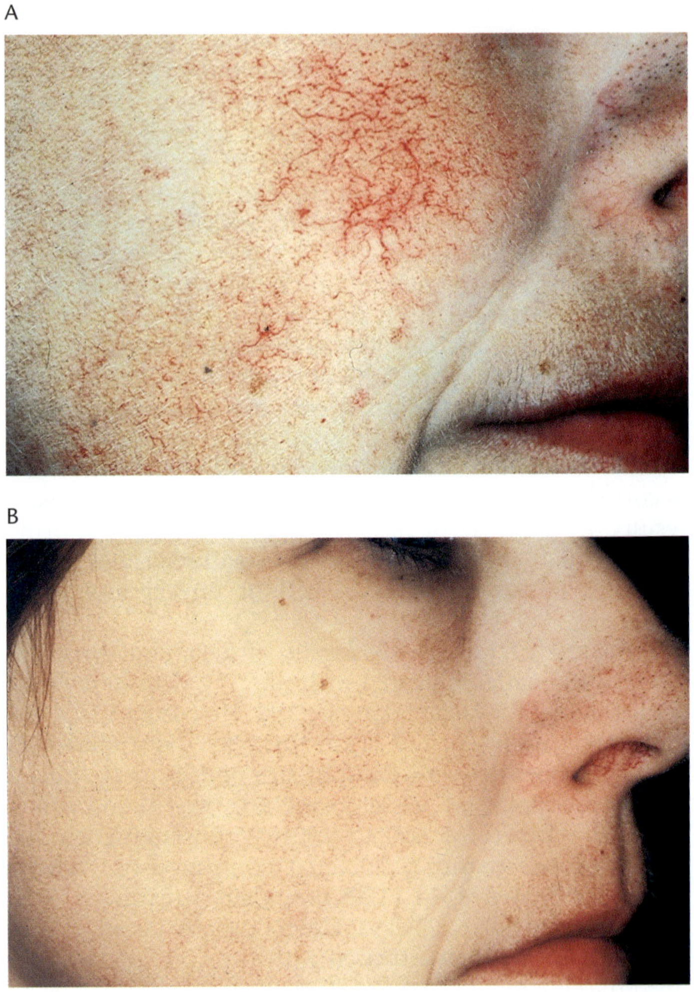

Figure 2.52 (A) Facial telangiectasia before treatment. (B) Three months after treatment with Orion KTP at 40 W, 4-mm Dermastat with 20-ms exposure duration, 1 pps. (Courtesy Burton E Silver, MD.)

Q-switched Nd:YAG laser, 532 nm

Even without consideration for the thermal relaxation time of vascular lesions, the 532-nm laser has been shown to be effective in clearing facial telangiectasia. Ten patients treated with the Nd:YAG laser at 532 nm in the Q-switched mode with 5-ns pulses at 1 to 2 and 3 to 4 J/cm^2 demonstrated clearance.[274] Excellent results occurred in 30% of patients treated at 1 to 2 J/cm^2 versus 70% of patients having excellent results when treated at 3 to 4 J/cm^2. However, at 3 to 4 J/cm^2, purpura occurred in all patients, with hyperpigmentation developing in 20% at 30 days and 10% at 60 days. The effectiveness and pigmentation were probably caused by the explosive effects to the absorption of the laser energy in a very short time (5 ns) with rupture of the vessel and release of hemosiderin.

Long-pulse Nd:YAG laser, 532 nm

By extending the pulse duration to within the thermal relaxation time of the vessel treated, purpura is avoided without loss of efficacy (see earlier discussion) (Fig. 2.53). This laser has been effective in treating facial telangiectasia that have sometimes proved to be recalcitrant to treatment with other laser modalities[260] (Fig. 2.54). Our experience in using this modality both with and without epidermal cooling has been variable but positive.

An evaluation of four different 532nm Nd:YAG lasers showed improvement with all four lasers without significantly different adverse effects. One was a Q-switched laser with a train of 5–10 ms pulses producing a pulse duration of 10–400 ms; a second machine used a quasi-continuous train of pulses delivering pulse durations of 10–25 ms; a third system was a diode-pumped system delivering 1–100 ms pulses and the fourth laser delivered 2–10 ms pulses.[275]

To decrease pain associated with the use of 532 nm lasers, cold clear gel has been demonstrated under a cooled sapphire window to decrease pain and erythema. Cooling the skin did not decrease efficacy.[276]

Pulse Dye Laser

The clinical treatment technique involves delivering a train of pulses overlapping 10% to 20%, tracing the vessels

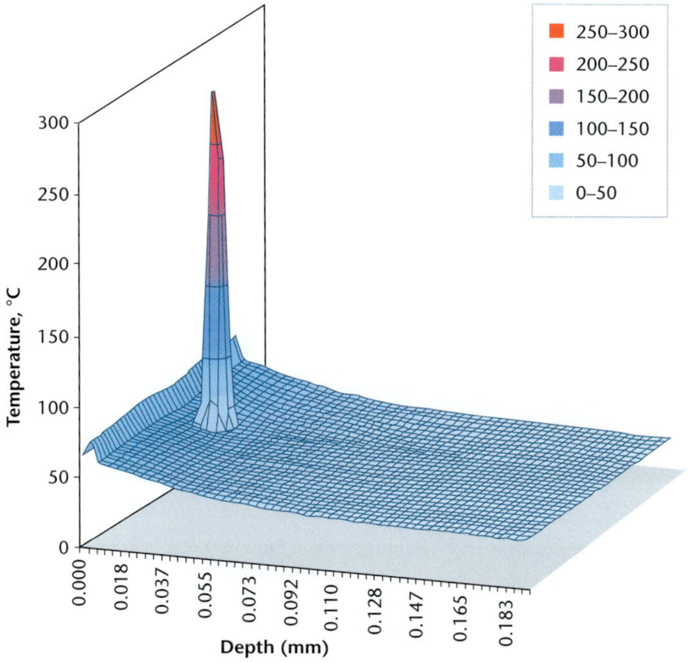

Figure 2.53 Temperature distribution achieved in treating 0.1-mm-diameter, 0.2-mm deep vessel with 532-nm laser with 2-ms pulse duration, 5-mm-diameter spot size, 15 J/cm^2 with epidermal cooling to 4°C. (Courtesy ESC Medical, Inc.)

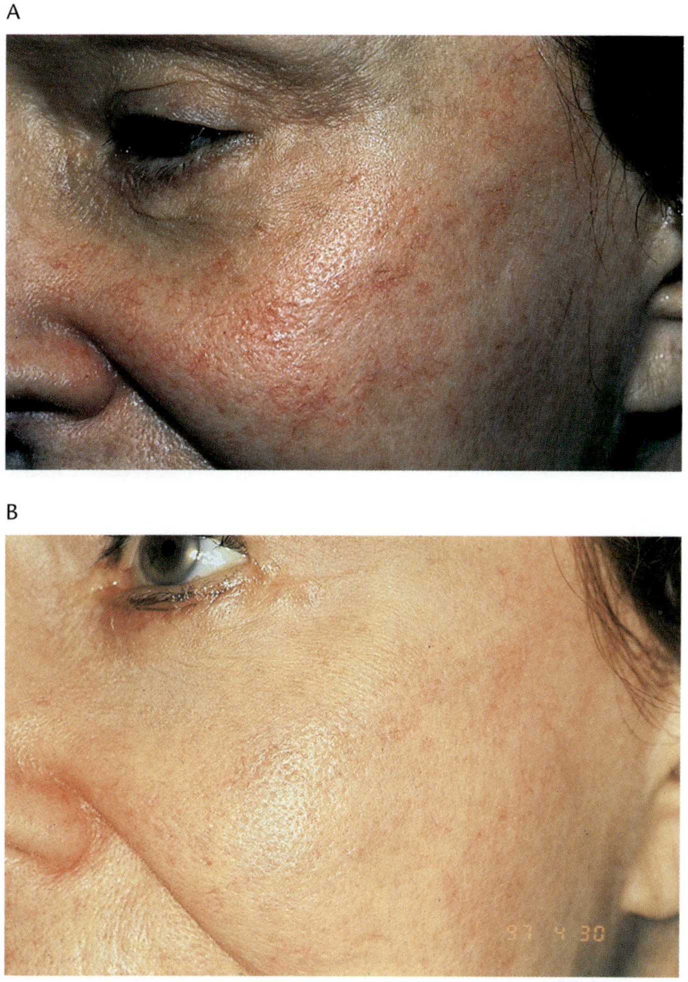

Figure 2.54 (A) Facial telangiectasia on cheek of 60-year-old woman before treatment. (B) Two months after single treatment with Versapulse, 532 nm at 10-ms pulse duration, 3-mm-diameter spot size, 10 J/cm^2 with epidermal cooling to 4°C.

to be treated with a 3-, 5-, 7- or 10-mm delivery spot, and treating an area of interlacing telangiectasia with overlapping spots to cover the involved area. Delivery energies range from 5 to 8 J/cm^2 with a 0.45-ms pulse and higher with longer duration pulses as described below and are adjusted according to lesion response and location. Disruption of blood flow occurs with resultant purpura which varies with pulse duration and fluence but without excessive swelling or crusting. Treatments of telangiectasia are generally done without the use of test spots, although these may be used if the patient or physician is unsure and wants to observe response in a small area. If test spots are used, the entire length of the vessel must be treated to eliminate the vessel (Fig. 2.55).

One study reports a 77% response rate to PDL treatment of adult facial linear telangiectasia.[38] Although vessel diameter was not measured, larger blue vessels were less responsive than smaller red vessels. The poorer response to treatment of these larger vessels may result from: (1) the thermal relaxation time in larger-diameter telangiectasia being longer than the pulse duration of the laser; and (2) the deoxygenated Hb absorbing at a lower wavelength of the laser (545 nm.)

Our published series shows 97.5% of 182 patients achieving good to excellent results (14% good, 83.5% excellent), indicating resolution of more than 50% of the treated lesions in one or two treatments[277] (Figs 2.56 and 2.57). In 152 of these patients, more than 75% of their telangiectasia was removed. Scarring did not occur in any patient, and skin texture remained unchanged. As expected, all patients experienced a transient bluish purple discoloration at the treatment site that resolved spontaneously in 10 to 14 days. This discoloration was well tolerated by our patient population, who were informed in advance of its occurrence. They could therefore modify their social and business schedules accordingly. Typically, makeup foundation was used to camouflage the purpura approximately 5 days after treatment. A small number of patients experienced other transient skin changes at the treatment site. Even though no anesthesia was used, patients experienced only mild to moderate discomfort in 93% of the cases. Most patients (62%) underwent only one treatment, although further improvement and a better response were seen in patients with more than one treatment. The largest percentage of patients had an excellent response with fluences above 7 J/cm^2 (93% versus 78%). There was a noticeable trend toward increasing effectiveness with increasing fluence. Our experience is that vessels larger than 0.2 mm in diameter require multiple treatments. Vessels larger than 0.4 mm in diameter are responsive to PDL treatment when the pulse duration is 20–40 ms.

A method for using the PDL without purpura formation consists of giving two to three pulses over the telangiecta-

A

B

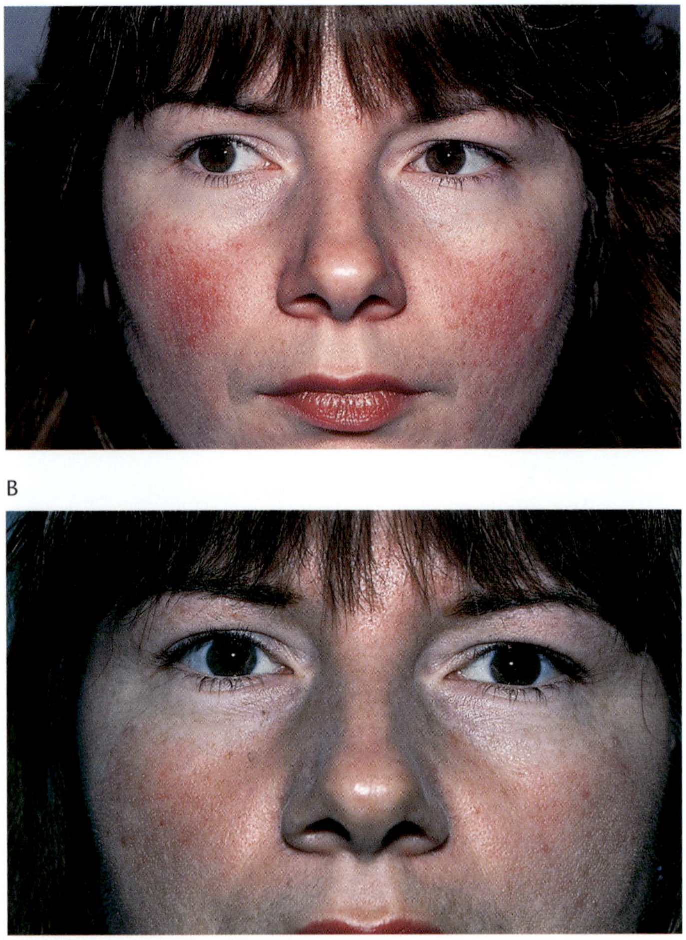

Figure 2.55 (A) Facial rosacea and telangiectasia in 32-year-old woman before treatment. (B) Three years after single treatment with PDL at 7 J/cm^2 delivered through 5-mm-diameter spot.

A

B

C

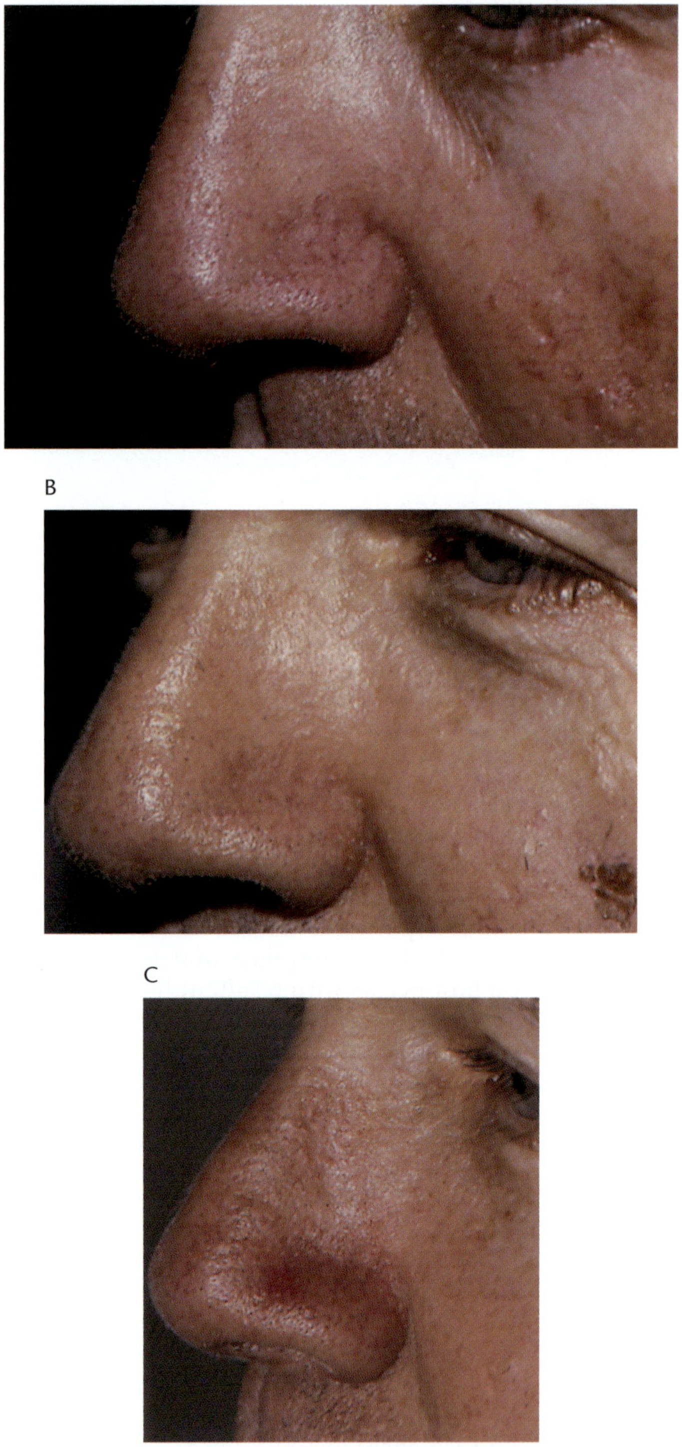

Figure 2.56 (A), Bright-red linear telangiectasia 0.1 mm in diameter over nasal alar crease in 46-year-old man. (B) Three months after PDL treatment at 7 J/cm^2. Note complete resolution of nasal alar telangiectasia. (C) One year after laser treatment. Note persistent resolution of nasal telangiectasia.

sia at lower fluences (pulse stacking). Typically, with a 595nm PDL, a 10-mm-diameter spot size is used at 4–5 J/cm^2. Multiple pulses even with short pulse durations (0.45 ms) allow a gradual increase in intravascular temperature to effect selective photothermolysis without vessel rupture. The only drawback is that multiple treatments are required. One study demonstrated a good effect using the above-mentioned parameters with a 1.5-ms pulse. Patients required 7.4 ± 2.3 weekly treatments for vessel resolution to occur. A second study compared the PDL used at purpura-free parameters (595 nm, 10-ms pulse, 10-mm spot size dynamic cooling with a 30-ms spray and 20-ms delay at 7.5 J/cm^2) as a single pulse on one side of the face with three or four pulses on the other side. Although side effects were similar with both single and stacked pulses, vessel clearance was 74.3% in the pulse stacked side and 58.5% in the single pulse side.[278]

Another method of achieving purpura-free resolution of telangiectasia with the PDL is to increase the pulse duration. One study used a 7-mm-diameter spot at 10-ms pulse duration with a dynamic cooling device delivering a 30-ms spray with a 20-ms delay. One pass was used at a fluence 1 J/cm^2 lower than a purpuric fluence, typically 9 J/cm^2. This study divided the face so that one side was treated with purpura-free settings and the other side with purpuric settings. The study demonstrated that in 82% of the patients, the purpuric side had better resolution.[279]

A

B

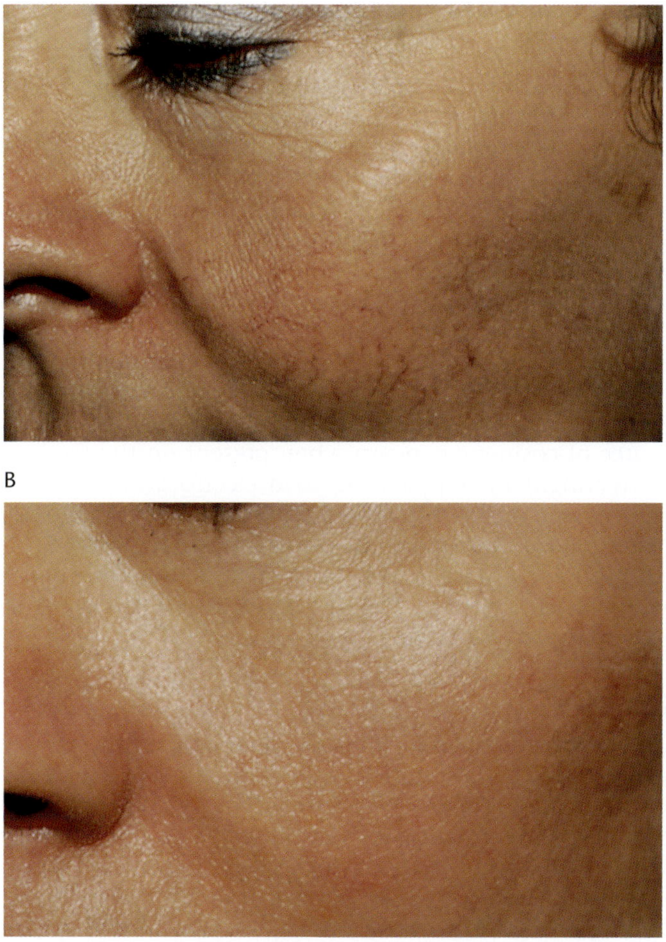

Figure 2.57 (A) Extensive telangiectasia bilaterally on cheeks of 56-year-old woman. (B) Six months after one treatment with pulsed dye laser at 7.25 J/cm^2. Total of 40 5-mm impact pulses were given to entire left cheek.

940 nm Diode-Pumped Laser

This laser (Medilas D SkinPulse; Dornier MedizinLaser GmbH, Germering, Germany) has been reported to be effective at clearing 1- to 3-mm-diameter periocular vessels in 86% of patients when used at 141 J/cm^2, 20-ms pulse through a 3-mm-diameter spot size.[280]

1064 nm Long Pulse Nd:YAG Laser

In an effort to treat deeper, larger and bluer vessels, a longer wavelength system has been developed. Using this wavelength requires fluences over ten times that used with 532 nm to 595 nm lasers since the absorption of Hb and HbO_2 at 1064 nm is ten times less. These higher fluences necessitate epidermal cooling. One laser uses dynamic cryogen cooling to achieve epidermal protection. A study using the CoolTouch laser (New Star Lasers, Rosemont, CA) found greater than 75% improvement in 97% of treated sites with a 125–150 J/cm^2 fluence through a 6-mm-diameter spot and 25-ms pulse duration for small diameter vessels and 75- to 100-ms pulse durations for reticular veins (Fig. 2.58). All treated reticular veins including periorbital and temporal veins resolved 100%. One or two passes were required to achieve vessel spasm or coagulation.[281]

A

B

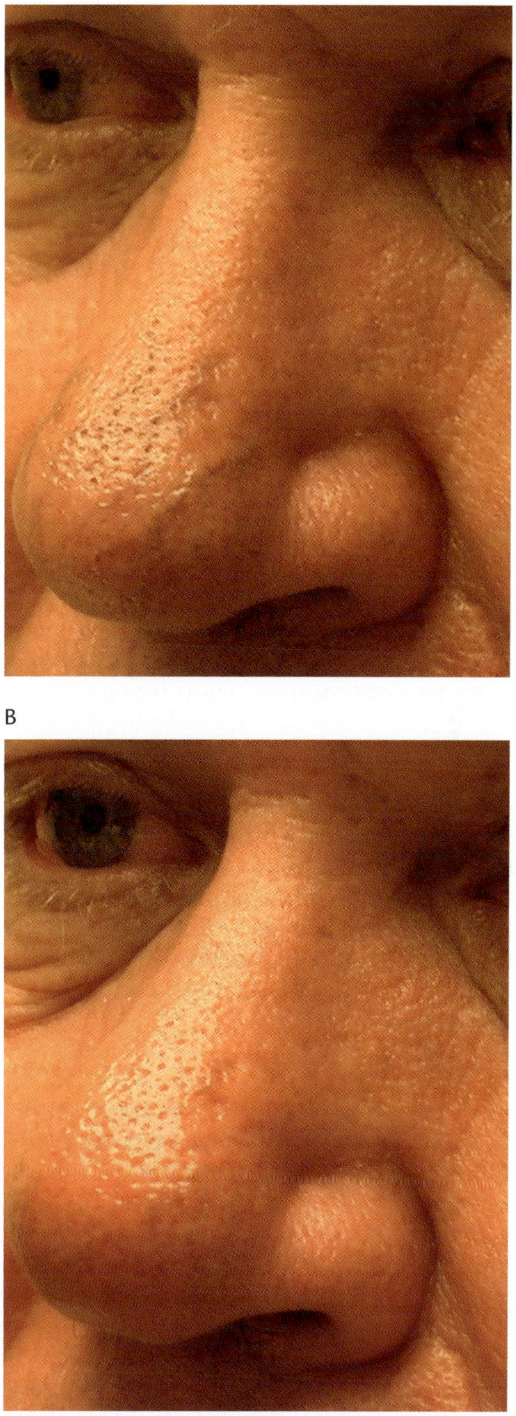

Figure 2.58 (A) Nasal telangiectasia 1–2 mm in diameter. (B) Complete resolution after 1 treatment with the LP 1064nm CoolTouch Varia. A 3.5-mm-diameter spot size was used at 200 J/cm^2 with a 25-ms pulse duration and 25 ms of cryogen cooling given immediately after the laser pulse. A total of 22 laser pulses were given.

Another long-pulse 1064 nm laser using precooling through a copper contact probe demonstrated moderate to significant vessel improvement in 80% of patients.[282] This laser (CoolGlide Excell, Cutera, Burlingame, CA) is used at 120–170 J/cm^2 with a 3-mm-diameter spot size and 5–

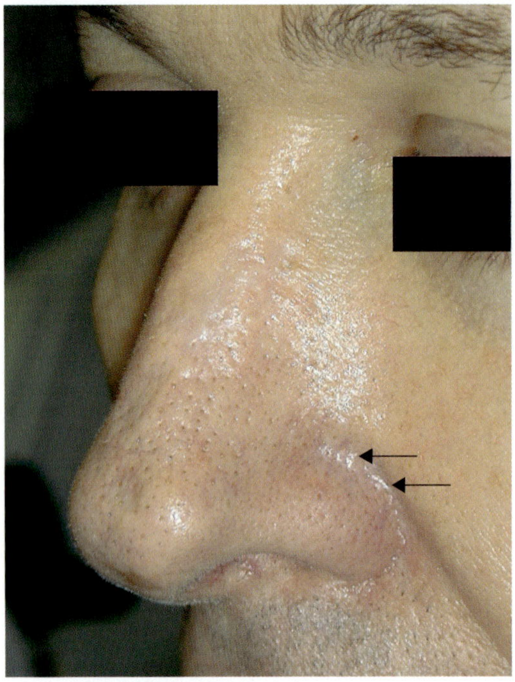

Figure 2.59 Multiple depressed 3mm scars at the point of treatment with the CoolGlide (now Cutera) 1064-nm long pulse laser (see arrows).

40-ms pulses until vessel blanching or coagulation occurs. These patients received two treatments 4 weeks apart to achieve therapeutic efficacy. Cutaneous blistering and scarring with 2- to 3-mm depressions and/or hypopigmentation was reported in this study and is not uncommonly seen by this author with the use of this laser (Fig. 2.59). It is presumed that pre- and postcontact cooling can be insufficient in some patients.

Intense Pulsed Light

This high-energy pulsed light source described previously is very effective in treating facial telangiectasia. Advantages are the almost complete lack of purpura and adverse sequelae. Energy fluences of 25 to 45 J/cm^2 are required for vessel ablation given as a double pulse of 2.4 to 6.0 ms each with a 10–30-ms delay between pulses. A 550 nm, 560 nm or 570 nm cutoff filter works best. Lesions usually clear in one treatment in 90% of patients.[283] Lesions are treated with one or two pulses until initial vessel spasm or slight purpura occurs (Figs 2.60 and 2.61). The only potential side effects are slight purpura, which lasts 2 to 4 days, or epidermal desquamation when treatment is performed on tanned or type III or IV skin. Epidermal desquamation in pigmented patients can be avoided by changing the filter to a longer wavelength or increasing the delay time between double or triple pulses (see Chapter 8).

A dual-mode filtering IPL (Ellipse Flex, Danish Dermatologic Development, Hoersholm, Denmark) that restricts the filtered light to between 555 and 950 nm (median wavelength of 705 nm) has been show to provide more than 50% reduction in facial telangiectasia in 79% of patients after one to four treatments; 37.5% of patients had greater than 75% improvement.[284] The decreased efficacy with this IPL may be due to the lower fluence used (13 and 22 J/cm^2) and single pulse durations of 10, 15 or 30 ms.

Spider Telangiectasia

Spider telangiectasia represents telangiectasia with a central feeding arteriole. They typically appear in preschool and school-age children. The peak incidence appears to be between ages 7 and 10,[285] and as many as 40% of girls and 32% of boys less than 15 years old have at least one lesion.[286,287] The incidence in healthy adults is about 15%.[288] The difference between these stated incidences implies that 50% to 75% of childhood lesions regress. However, this is not easily observable because most lesions seem to persist without change and become a source of cosmetic concern when present on the face.

Treatment in the past included electrocautery and the argon laser. Both modalities have the disadvantages of being painful and prone to causing punctate scarring. In addition, recurrence is common if treatment is done lightly to avoid scarring. The PDL has proved to be a very effective treatment for these benign lesions.[289,290]

Pulse Dye Laser

Geronemus[289] reported 100% success without any adverse sequelae in 12 children treated with the PDL for facial spider telangiectasia. We retrospectively evaluated the response to treatment with the PDL in 23 children with 55 spider telangiectasia.[290] Lesions were treated at energy fluences of 6.5 to 7.5 J/cm^2 (mean 6.9 J/cm^2). One or two pulses were given to the central punctum of the 'spider', with additional pulses with a 10% overlap given to the radiating 'arms' of the lesion if the lesion was greater than 5 mm in diameter. Local anesthesia was not used. Seventy percent of lesions resolved completely with one treatment. Twelve lesions required a second treatment for complete resolution. The remaining five lesions not treated a second time had an average clearance of 78% (Fig. 2.62). The three patients with five lesions who did not have a second treatment were either satisfied with the degree of resolution from their first treatment or were unavailable for further treatment.

Spider telangiectasia respond equally as well in adults, with 93% of patients having total resolution with one treatment between 6.5 and 7.0 J/cm^2[238] (Fig. 2.63).

With the PDL, lesions become purpuric immediately after laser treatment. Purpura resolves within 7 to 10 days. We have not seen permanent pigmentary changes or scarring. Although adverse effects from treating spider telangiectasia are extremely rare, one case of granuloma telangiectaticum (pyogenic granuloma) after argon laser therapy has been reported.[291] This complication occurred 3 months after the central vessel was treated at 5 W, 50 ms, with a 0.5-mm-diameter spot size. The authors speculated that laser trauma, in addition to the lack of complete destruction of the spider telangiectasia endothelium, led to a focal capillary proliferation. This effect has also been reported with laser treatment of PWS, with development of 'hemangiomas' within the treated areas.

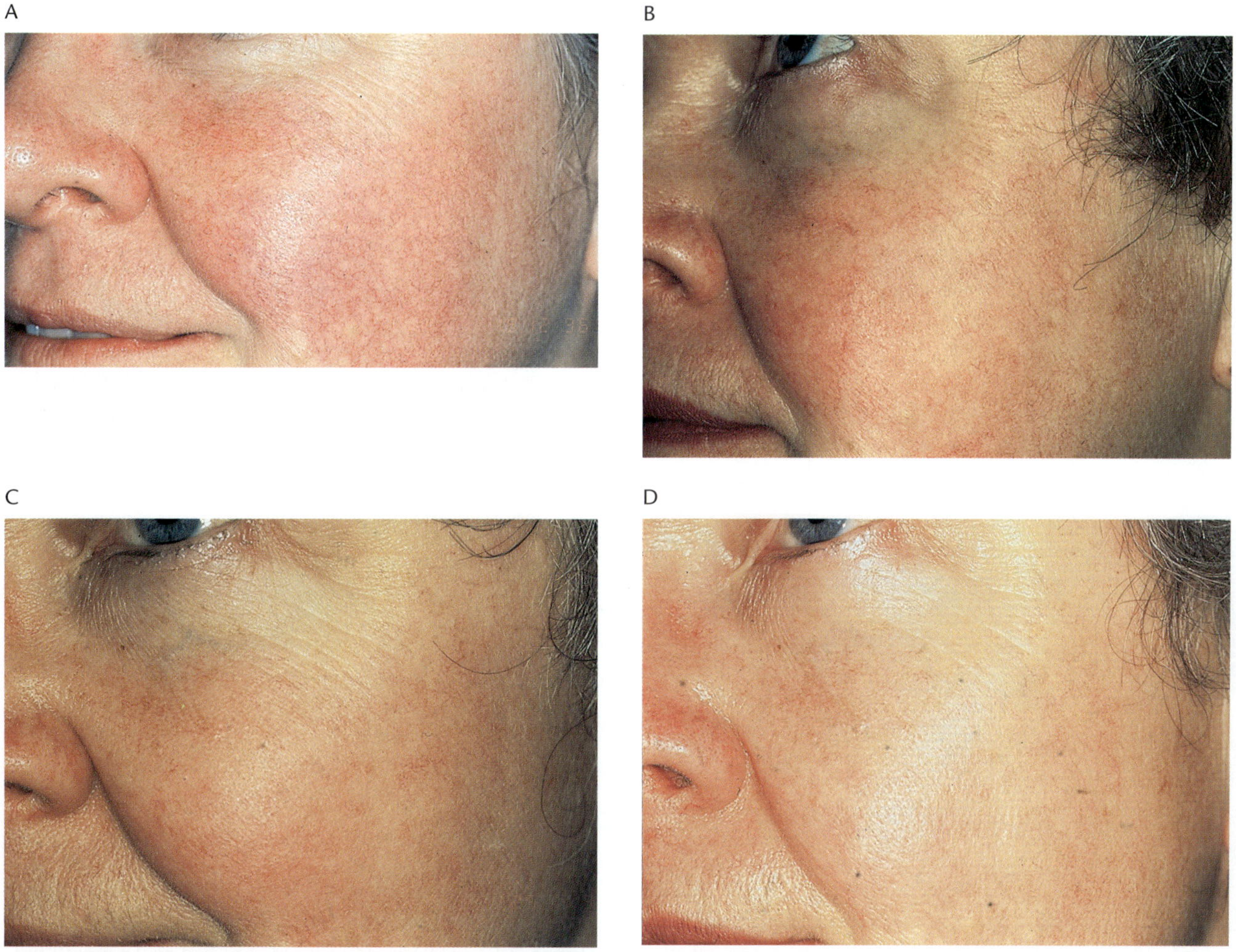

Figure 2.60 (A) Extensive facial telangiectasia on 55-year-old woman after automobile airbag impacted her face. (B) Eight weeks after treatment with PhotoDerm VL, 550-nm cutoff filter, 40 J/cm^2, double pulse of 2.4 and 4.0 ms with 10-ms delay. Note 50% improvement. (C) Four weeks after second PhotoDerm VL treatment with 570-nm cutoff filter, 44 J/cm^2 delivered in two pulses of 2.4 and 4.0 ms with 10-ms delay. (D) Complete resolution 8 weeks after third and fourth treatments, with parameters similar to those in (C).

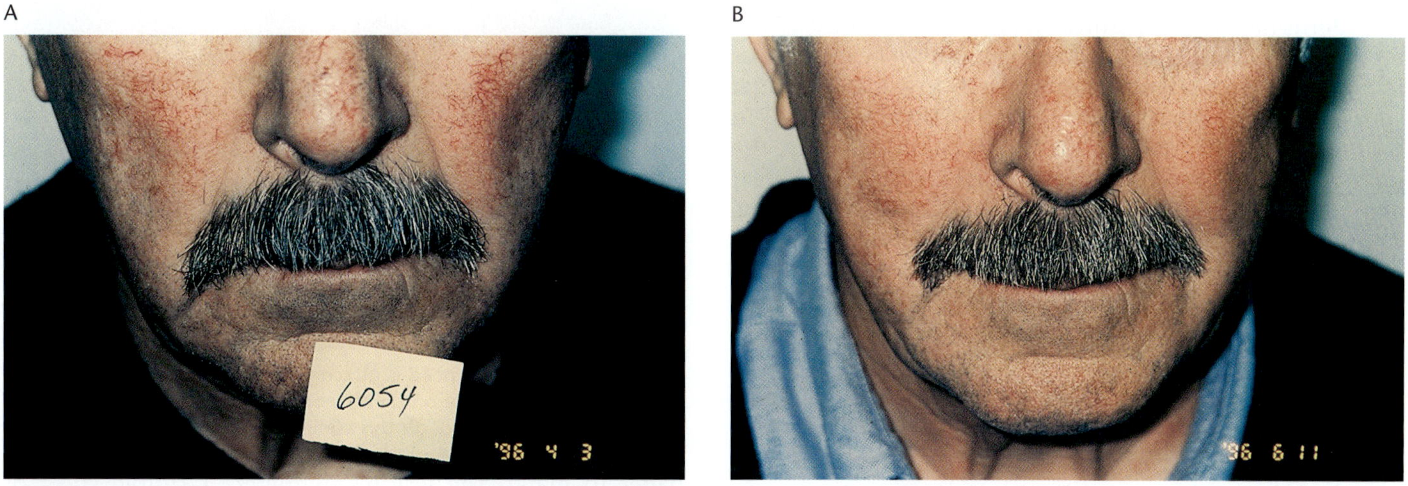

Figure 2.61 (A) Facial telangiectasia before treatment. (B) After two treatments with PhotoDerm VL with 570- or 550-nm cutoff filters, 37 J/cm^2 given as double pulse of 3 and 4 ms with 10-ms delay between pulses. (Courtesy Beverly Kemsley, MD, Calgary, Canada.)

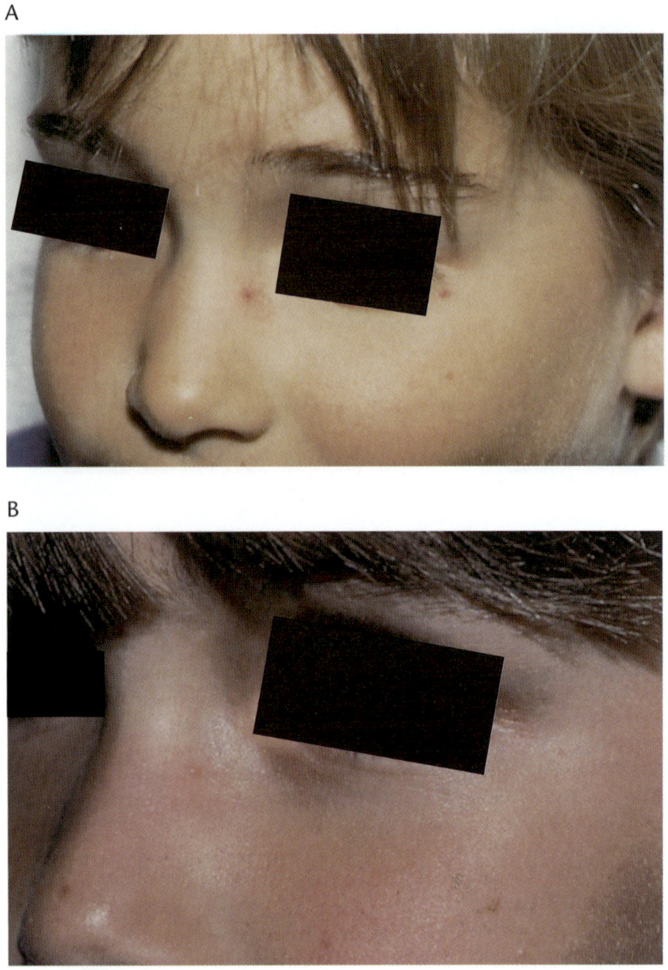

Figure 2.62 (A) Two spider telangiectasia on left inner canthal area and outer canthal area of 10-year-old girl for 6 months. (B) Four weeks after single treatment with PDL at 7 J/cm^2. Note complete resolution of telangiectasia without any evidence of cutaneous changes. (Reprinted from Fitzpatrick RE: American Journal of Cosmetic Surgery 9:107, 1992. With permission from American Academy of Cosmetic Surgery.)

532 nm KTP or Nd:YAG Laser

An additional nearly painless treatment modality is the long-pulse 532 nm laser. Parameters found to be efficacious in treating spider telangiectasia are a 3- to 4-mm-diameter spot with an energy fluence of 12 to 14 J/cm^2 delivered in a 10-ms pulse. The treatment is almost painless because the laser beam is delivered through a double-chambered clear quartz crystal cooled in its center to 4°C with water (Fig. 2.64). The quartz cooling device is placed over the lesion on the skin surface, and the laser fluence is delivered one to three times until the lesion blanches. This laser has an efficacy of almost 100% for this treatment in our practice.

The KTP laser (Orion/Aura, Laserscope, Palo Alto, CA) has been found to be effective when used with a 1- to 2-mm diameter spot size, at 13–10 J/cm^2 respectively with a 5–8 ms pulse duration.

Intense Pulsed Light

The IPL has also been useful in treating these lesions. Because one needs only to treat the lesion, we use a hole punch or scissors to cut out an open area in a sheet of white paper to match the lesion's diameter. A simple sheet of white paper, cardboard, or self-sticking label is sufficient to block out the light delivered through the quartz or sapphire light guide. Fluences of 35 to 40 J/cm^2 delivered in a double pulse of 2.4 and 4.0 ms with a 10-ms delay through

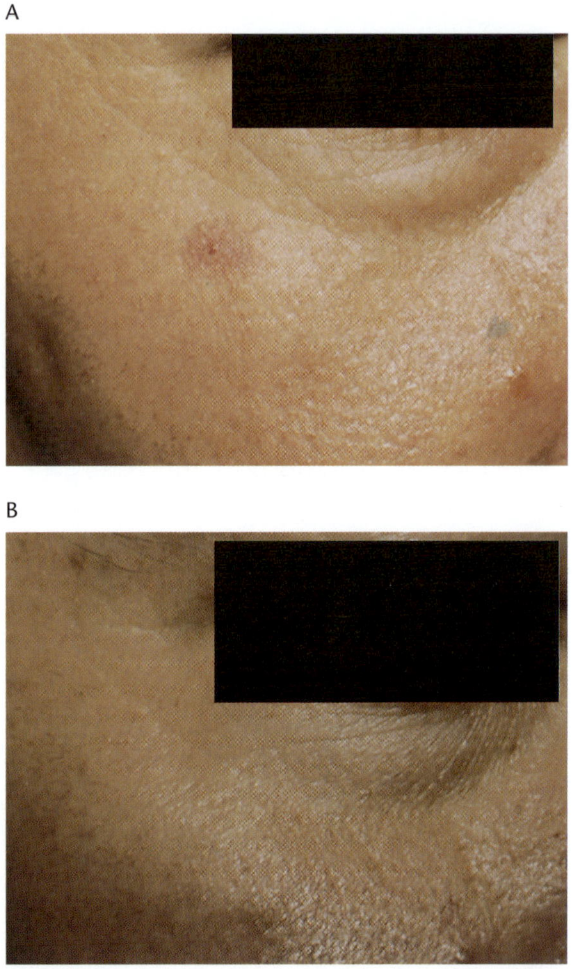

Figure 2.63 (A) This 44-year-old man had an 18-month history of enlarging spider telangiectasia on right cheek. (B) Six months after single treatment with PDL at 7 J/cm^2. A total of six 5-mm pulses were given, with complete resolution of telangiectasia.

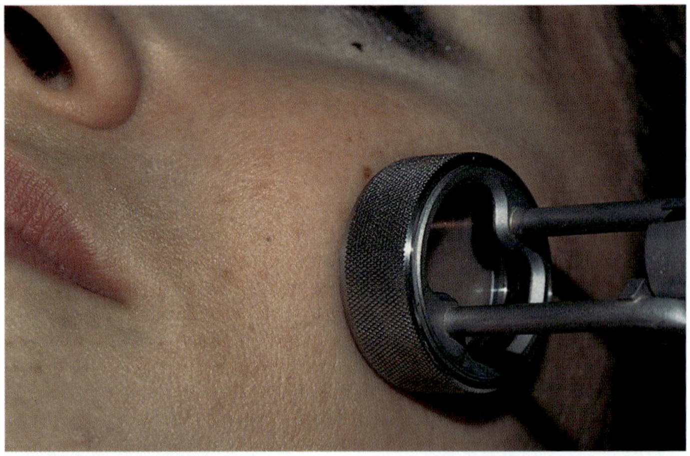

Figure 2.64 Cooling head is attached to handpiece of Versapulse 532-nm laser and placed on skin over target vascular lesion. Laser energy is then given through this cooling device.

A

B

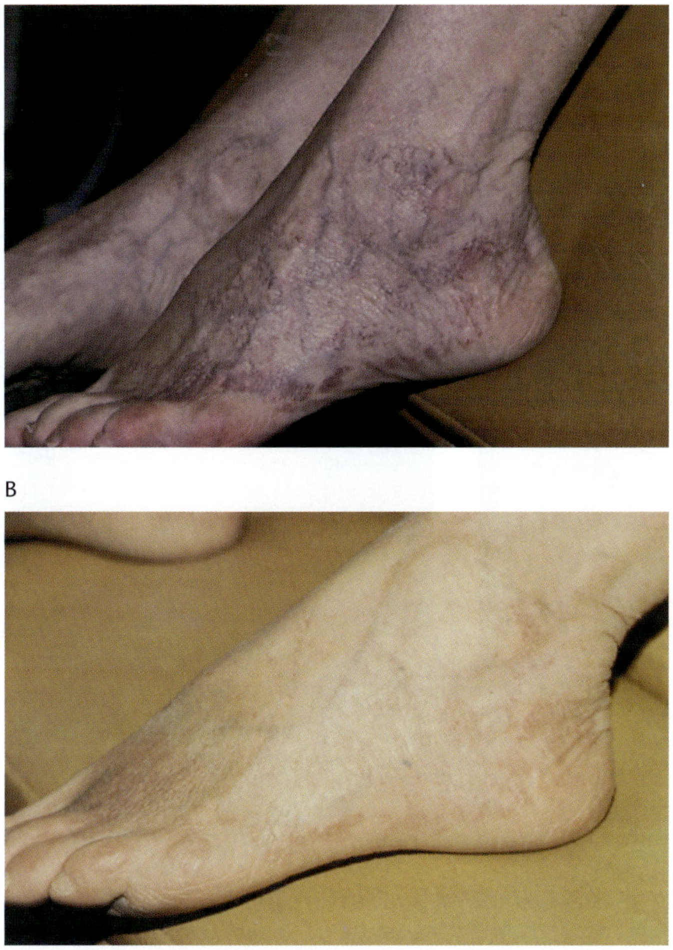

Figure 2.65 Extensive vascular ectasia on both feet of 54-year-old woman. (A) Before treatment. (B) Six months after initial treatment and 3 months after second treatment with PDL at 7.25 J/cm^2 using 84 and 115 pulses, respectively. (From Goldman MP. Sclerotherapy: treatment of varicose and telangiectatic leg veins, 2nd edn. St Louis: CV Mosby; 1995.)

a 550-nm cutoff filter usually gives near 100% efficacy with almost no pain. Even small children and male adults tolerate the treatment without complaint. Lesions are rarely purpuric and usually without adverse sequelae, making this modality a treatment of choice.

Generalized Essential Telangiectasia

This telangiectasia generally occurs on the legs but may also involve other cutaneous surfaces. Various treatments have been proposed, with variable efficacy.[249] Tan and Kurban[245] reported successful treatment with the PDL at fluences of 6 J/cm^2. We also treated four patients with the PDL at fluences ranging from 6.0 to 7.5 J/cm^2. Two patients responded with total resolution, but two patients had almost no improvement in their appearance (Fig. 2.65). Therefore we believe that intrinsic factors in these patients may preclude predictable results. We recommend performing a patch test for such patients.

IPL treatment has also been found to be effective (Fig. 2.66).[292]

Rosacea

Rosacea is essentially a cutaneous vascular disorder. It is best thought of not as a disease but as a typology of a cluster of patients with a characteristic combination of cutaneous stigmata consisting of telangiectasia, papules, pustules, and rhinophyma.[293] A comprehensive review of the literature finds that of the 18 histologic studies on rosacea, 14 showed an increase in Demodex mites.[294] It is hypothesized that these mites may play a role in the inflammation of rosacea.[295] Studies have demonstrated thermal destruction of these mites after IPL therapy, which may contribute to the therapeutic effects of IPL.[295,296] Telangiectasia represents the later phase of vascularization and probably results from a reduction in mechanical integrity of the upper dermal connective tissue, allowing a passive dilatation of capillaries. Inflammation and associated angiogenesis may contribute to the telangiectasia. Interestingly, facial temperature is higher in rosacea and this has been associated with a difference in the nature and behavior of skin bacteria, particularly coagulase-negative staphylococci.[297] Therefore, the elimination of excessive blood vessels may not only decrease the erythematous appearance of rosacea but also modify the bacterial flora further decreasing the cutaneous erythema.

Pulse Dye Laser

Rosacea-associated telangiectasia and erythema respond well to treatment with the PDL. We have reported good to excellent results in 24 of 27 patients (89%).[298,299] In addition to the cosmetic improvement resulting from elimination of the vascular component of this disorder, PDL treatment also appears to alter the pathophysiology of this condition because a decrease in papule and pustule activity occurs in up to 59% of patients (Fig. 2.67). After PDL treatment, patients who responded to treatment with elimination of the vascular component required less or no topical or systemic antibiotic therapy to maintain disease resolution.[299] Anecdotal reports from Tan and Kurban[245] confirm our more formal evaluations. An additional study of 12 patients with rosacea treated with the PDL to one cheek with the other as a control at purpuric settings of 5-mm diameter, 5.5–6.5 J/cm^2, 0.45-ms pulse without cooling also demonstrated a 75% reduction in telangiectasia is 11 of 12 patients and a decrease in erythema of 50% after three treatments.[300]

The efficacy of the first-generation PDL was reproduced in a study of a 6 ms PDL at 595 nm with fluence between 7 and 9 J/cm^2 and cryogen spray cooling.[301] Here, two of 12 patients had over 75% improvement with one treatment. Another two had 50–75% improvement; five had 25–50% improvement. These parameters did not produce significant purpura.

A questionnaire rating of Dermatology Life Quality Index and symptoms of flushing, burning, itching, dryness, swelling and skin sensitivity was performed on 16 patients treated with a PDL for their rosacea.[302] PDL parameters of treatment were 10 J/cm^2, 7-mm-diameter spot, 1.5-ms pulse duration with cryogen skin cooling

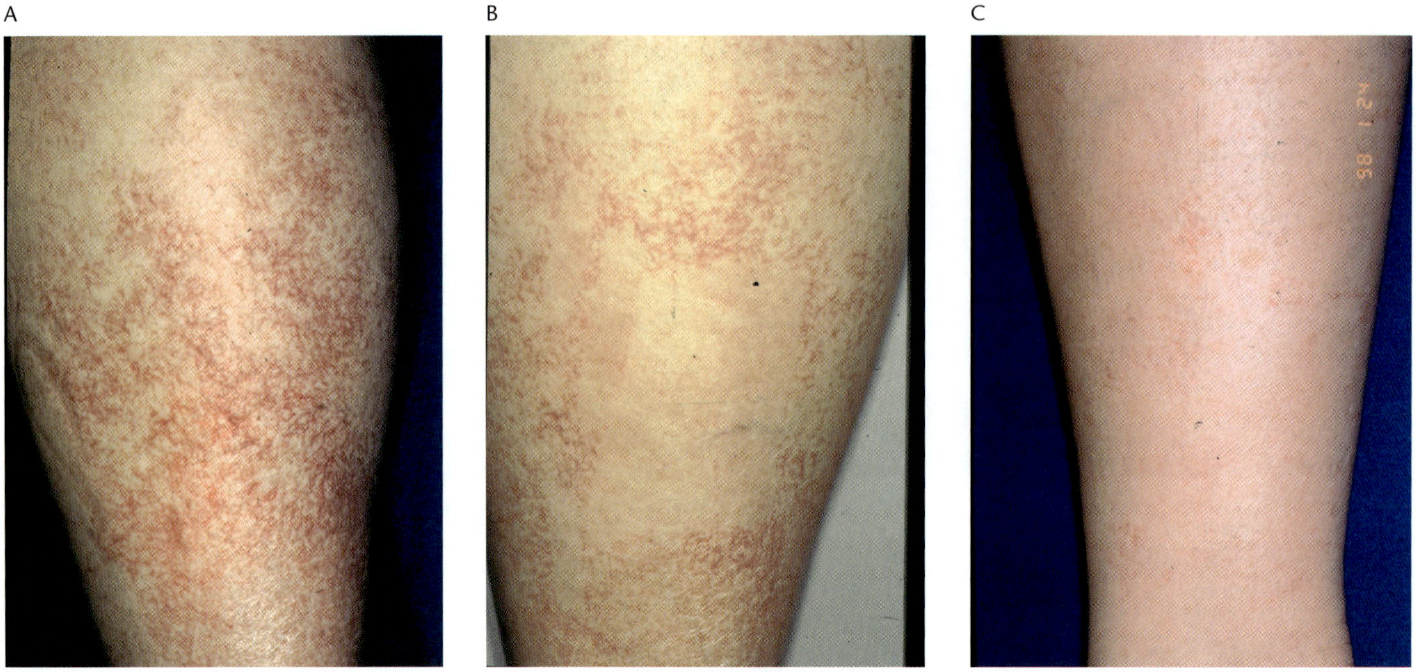

Figure 2.66 (A) Essential telangiectasia before treatment in a 38-year-old women. (B) After one treatment with the Lumenis Vasculite IPL at 32 J/cm^2 with a 570 cut-off filter and a double pulse of 2.4 and 4.0 ms with a 10-ms delay. (Reprodued with permission from Goldman MP, Bergan JB: Sclerotherapy treatment of varicose and telangiectatic leg veins, 3rd Ed. Mosby, 52 Louis, 2001.)

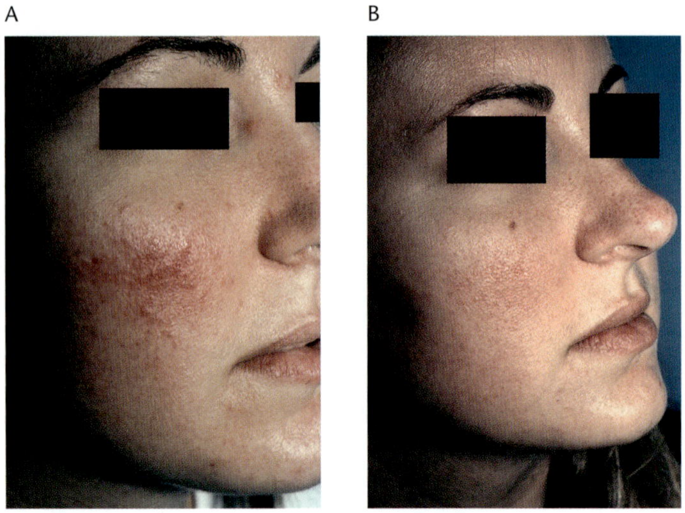

Figure 2.67 (A) 24-year-old women with rosacea on the cheeks. (B) One month after the second of two treatments with the PDL.

of 40–50-ms spray after a 20-ms delay. Two treatments were performed. The Dermatology Quality of Life Index improved in each patient from an average score of 7.8 before treatment to 3 after the first treatment and 1.9 after the second treatment (75.6%). Symptoms of burning, flushing, stinging and itching improved by at least 57% after treatment. Therefore, a cosmetic improvement is not the only benefit of laser treatment of rosacea.

The improvement in symptoms was reproduced in another study of 32 patients with rosacea treated with the first-generation 0.45-ms, 5-mm-diameter PDL with purpura lasting 5–14 days.[303] These patients all had a positive lactic acid (Stinger) test indicating skin sensitivity. 24 of the 32 patients became stinger negative after one PDL treatment. Seven patients had less symptoms and only one patient was unchanged. Superficial nerve fiber density and number of substance P immunoreactive nerve fibers were decreased.

In assessing the overall success and potential risk of each laser used in the treatment of facial telangiectasia with rosacea, we believe that the PDL provides effective and relatively risk-free results. However, purpura resulting after treatment is an inconvenience that must be recognized in advance in scheduling treatment. In addition, one study of ten patients showed that only 50% had less papulopustular lesions after an average of 2.4 treatments with parameters of the PDL previously described above.[304] However, even in this 'negative' paper, two of the ten treated patients had excellent results when evaluated 5 years after treatment.

532 nm KTP Laser

A study of 47 patients treated with the KTP 532 nm laser with variable-sized handpieces depending on the type of telangiectasia showed good results.[305] Matted telangiectasia were treated with a 4-mm-diameter spot and 20-ms pulse width at an average energy of 0.7 W. Vessels 0.1 to 0.3 mm in diameter were treated with a 0.25-mm-diameter spot size and 20-ms pulse width at an average energy of 0.12 W. Vessels greater than 0.3 mm in diameter were treated with a 1-mm-diameter spot and 10-ms pulse width at an average energy of 0.2 W. Vessels were treated by tracing them with the laser until they disappeared. This required one to several tracings. Of the 47 patients, 38% had more than 70% resolution of their telangiectasia, and 32% required a second treatment to achieve the same result. The only adverse effect consisted of linear crusting along the path of the telangiectasia.

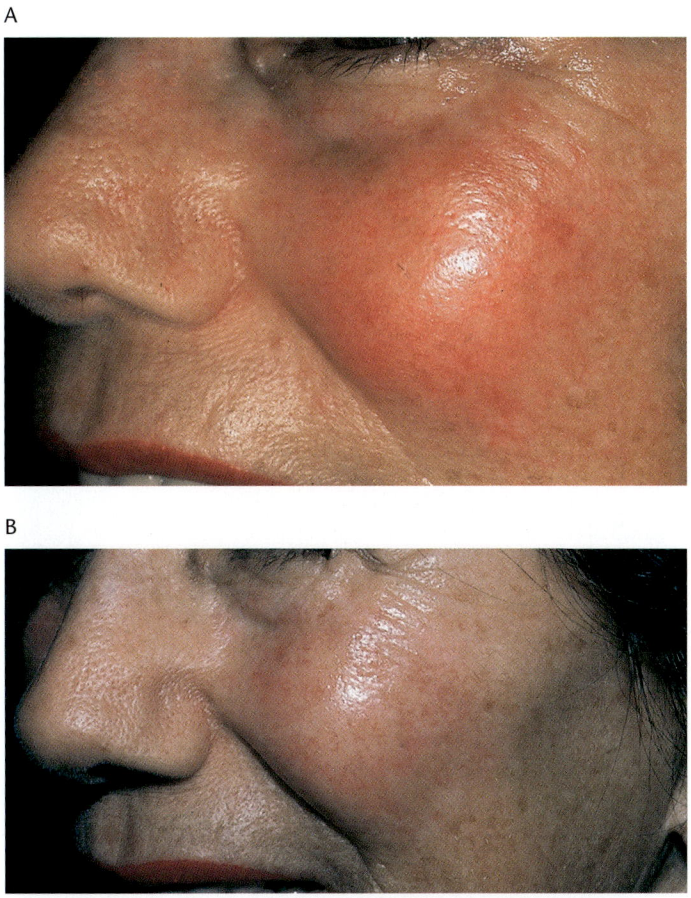

Figure 2.68 (A) Erythematous cheeks of 66-year-old woman before treatment. (B) After three treatments with PhotoDerm VL using 570-nm cutoff filter and 12-ms pulse at 52 J/cm^2; followed 4 weeks later by 590-nm cutoff filter and 12-ms pulse at 55 J/cm^2; then followed 4 weeks later by 550-nm cutoff filter at 44 J/cm^2 given as double pulse of 4.2 and 7.7 ms with 20-ms delay.

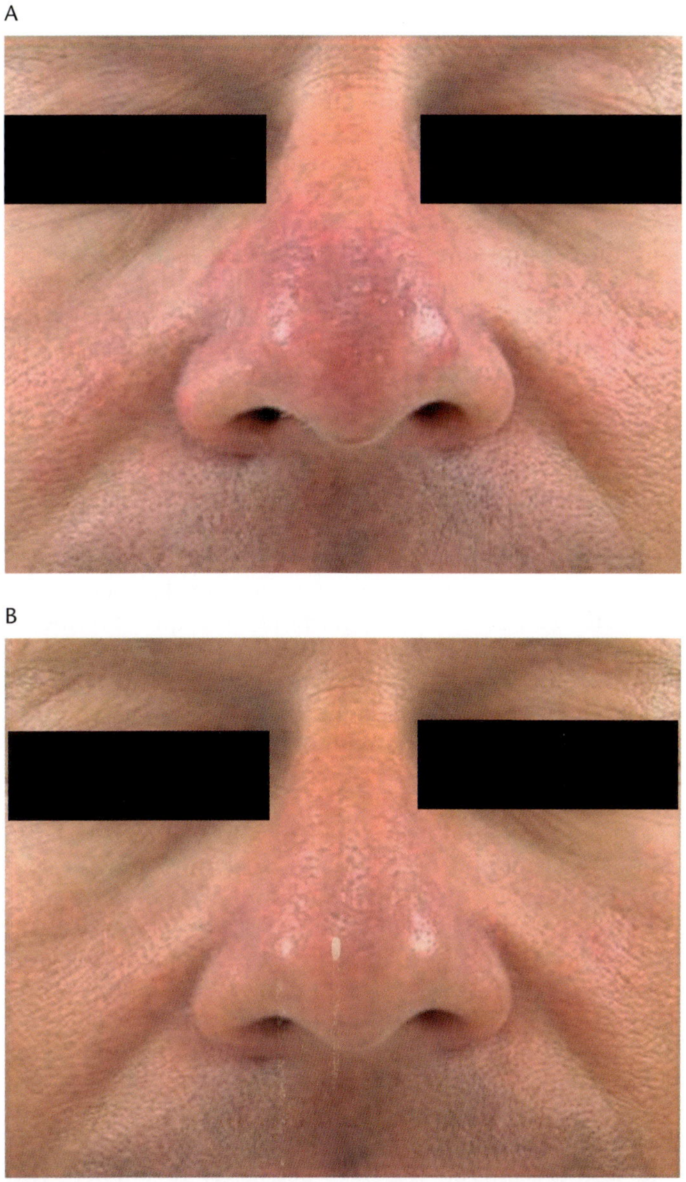

Figure 2.69 (A) Diffusely red telangiectatic nose of 58-year-old male. (B) After one treatment with Lumenis 1 intense pulsed light using 560-nm cutoff filter at 20 J/cm^2 given as double pulse of 3, 5 and 3.5 ms with a 10-ms delay.

Intense Pulsed Light

The IPL has also been found to be effective in treating rosacea. As described previously, this light source has the advantage of relatively quick vessel elimination without significant purpura or crusting (Figs 2.68 and 2.69). Scanning Doppler evaluation demonstrated a 30% decrease in blood flow after five IPL treatments.[306] In addition, a 21% decrease in erythema intensity as well as a 29% decrease in the actual size of the cheek with telangiectasia was noted in this study of four patients. A larger study of 60 patients were treated with the IPL with pulse durations of 4.3 to 6.5 ms and energy density of 25–35 J/cm^2.[307] A mean clearance of 77.8% was achieved and maintained for a follow-up period averaging 51.6 months. An additional study of 32 consecutive patients treated with an average of 3.6 IPL treatments similar to the above-mentioned parameters showed that 83% of patients had reduced redness, 75% experienced reduced flushing and 64% noted fewer acne breakouts.[308]

Treatment Recommendations

We treat the entire facial area affected by the erythematous rosacea. Short pulses appear to be most effective. We typically use a 550 or 560 cutoff filter with a double pulse of 2.4 ms and 4.0 ms with a 10-ms delay and an energy density of 30 J/cm^2 (26 J/cm^2 with the QuantumSR) and 3.0 ms and 3.0 ms at 18 J/cm^2 with the Lumenis One). Patients are retreated every 3–4 weeks until clear. We have found that most patients clear in two or three treatments. A certain percentage of patients (20%) do not respond to the IPL and need to be treated with the PDL. Most of our patients need to return for retreatment every year or so.

Poikiloderma of Civatte

Poikiloderma of Civatte is a variant of telangiectasia involving the neck and upper chest and occurring from accumulated ultraviolet exposure and associated photosensitization of various chemicals, most notably fragrances.[309] Poikiloderma consists of a combination of telangiectasia, irregular pigmentation, and atrophic changes of the skin. Histologic changes on biopsy confirm this clinical combination. These changes are best treated by addressing the telangiectatic and pigmentary components simultaneously.

In the past, poikiloderma treatment focused on the telangiectatic component and solely on various laser modalities. Fair efficacy was reported, but treatments were lengthy because of the large surface areas involved and multiple sessions required. The argon laser is only partially successful and frequently results in areas of hypopigmentation with a low incidence of scarring. The 532 nm KTP laser has also been reported to be successful in a one patient case report.[310]

Pulse Dye Laser

The PDL, as reported by Tan and Kuran,[245] Wheeland and Applebaum,[311] and us, has good efficacy at fluences of 6 to 7 J/cm^2 with a 5-mm-diameter spot size. Our recommended fluence at a 7-mm-diameter is 5 to 6 J/cm^2. Problems with the PDL include extensive purpura, multiple treatments because of large surface area, and mottled response with circular imprints (Figure 2.70). In addition, by mainly targeting the vascular component, these treatments often do little to change the hyperpigmentation. Scarring has also been reported when the PDL was used at fluences greater than 6 J/cm^2.[312]

We recommend that if the PDL is used to treat poikiloderma of Civatte, it be used with a 10-mm-diameter spot size, 0.45- to 0.5-ms pulse duration if pigmentation is prominent and 1.5- to 2-ms pulse duration if erythema is prominent. Fluence should be just strong enough to give a minimal purpuric response and epidermal cooling should be performed. Patients must be told that three to five treatments will be necessary and that the treated area may appear to be polka-dotted until all treatments are given.

A

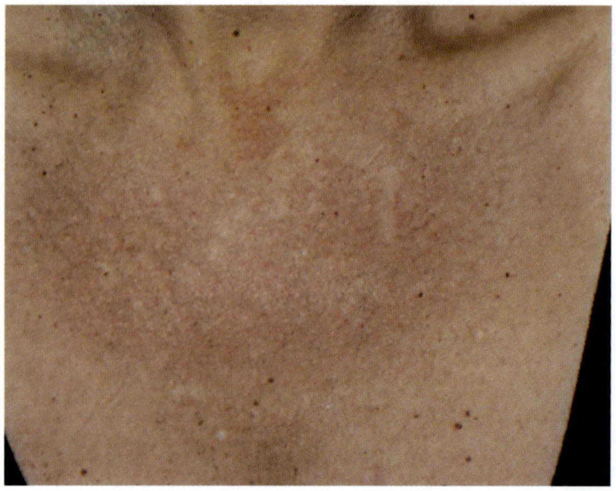

B

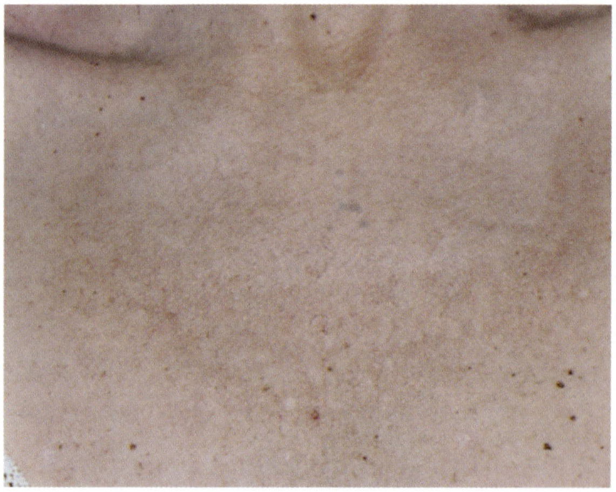

Figure 2.70 (A) Extensive poikilodermic changes from sun damage on central chest of 36-year-old woman. (B) After three treatments with FLPDL at a fluence of 7 J/cm^2 during each treatment session. Between 200 and 300 5-mm impact pulses were given at each session. Note excellent clearing of poikilodermic changes. Somewhat mottled pigmentation remains between laser impact sites and on peripheral aspect of poikiloderma.

Intense Pulsed Light

Our results using an IPL have been very favorable. With this pulsed light system, the target is both vascular and epidermal and dermal melanin. Multiple wavelengths are used, usually with a 515-nm filter first. This filter is used with a single pulse of 3 ms at a fluence of 22 to 25 J/cm^2. These treatment parameters are effective in removing epidermal melanin and very superficial telangiectasia. A second or third treatment spaced at least 4 weeks apart is usually necessary and typically uses a 550-nm cutoff filter with a double pulse of 2.4 and 4 ms with a 10-ms delay. This is helpful in treating slightly larger or deeper telangiectasia. A total fluence from 35 to 42 J/cm^2 is usually necessary to achieve an optimal clinical result. With these parameters, few or no side effects have been noted in our patients (Fig. 2.71). This experience has been detailed in a study in which 66 patients with typical changes of poikiloderma of Civatte on the neck were treated with IPL at various settings every 4 weeks until desired improvement occurred. A 50%–75% improvement in the extent of telangiectasias and hyperpigmentation comprising poikiloderma was observed in an average of 2.8 treatments. Incidence of hypopigmentation was 5%.[313,314] A second expanded study of 135 patients randomly selected with typical changes of poikiloderma of Civatte on the neck and/or upper chest were treated one to five times every 4 weeks with the IPL. Clearance of over 75% of telangiectasias and hyperpigmentation comprising poikiloderma was observed. Incidence of side effects was 5% including pigment changes. In many cases, improved skin texture was noted both by physician and patient (Figs 2.71 and 2.72).[315,316]

Approximately 75% improvement occurs after one treatment. Side effects include transitory erythema from 24 to 72 hours. Purpura occurs only 10% of the time and only with some pulses in variable locations. This purpura is different from that seen with the PDL in that it is intravascular and resolution occurs within 3 to 5 days. A slight stinging pain during treatment is easily tolerated for up to 60 pulses per session. No anesthesia is required, and the entire neck and chest area can be treated during one treatment session. Patients must be informed that ‘foot-prints’ representing the shape of the contact crystal may be

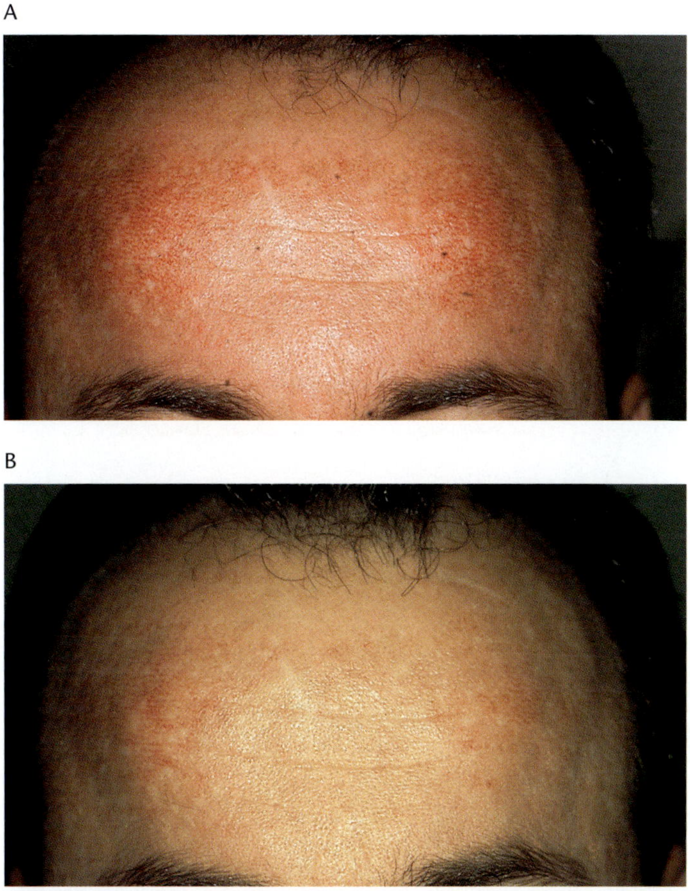

Figure 2.71 (A) Poikiloderma of Civatte in 44-year-old male before treatment. (B) One month after a second treatment with IPL using a 550-nm cutoff filter at 40 J/cm^2 given as a double pulse of 2.4 and 4.0 msec separated by a 10 msec delay.

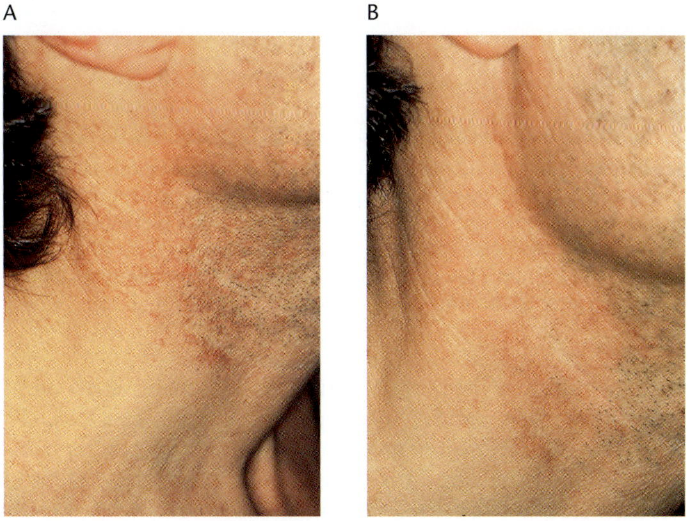

Figure 2.72 (A) Poikiloderma of Civatte in 52-year-old male before treatment. (B) Six months after third treatment with PhotoDerm VL using 550-nm cutoff filter at 37 to 40.5 and 43.5 J/cm^2 given over three treatments as a double pulse of 2.4 and 2.4 ms with 10-ms delay between pulses.

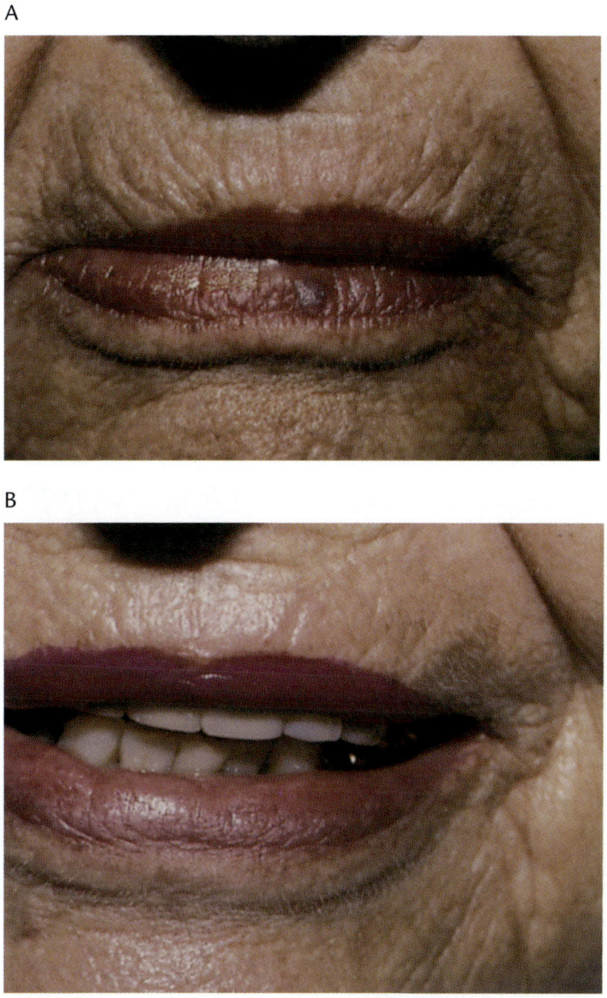

Figure 2.73 (A) Progressively enlarging venous lake on lower lip of a 78-year-old women for 2 years. (B) Three months after single treatment with PDL at 7.5J/cm^2 with a total of four 4-mm impacts.

present after the first and even second treatment and is a normal response.

Venous Lake

Venous lakes are dilated 'lake-like' venules in the upper dermis typically seen on the lips or ears of elderly patients. These lesions are dark-blue to purple, soft, raised nodules, usually 2 to 10 mm in diameter.[317] Patients generally request treatment because of concern over possible medical consequences and recurrent bleeding with trauma or for cosmetic improvement.

Treatment of venous lakes of the lips and ears has been effective with the argon laser, requiring from one to four treatment sessions.[318,319] Use of laser spot size less than 1 mm in diameter may promote excessive bleeding.[320] Lesions less than 5 mm in diameter almost always heal without scarring, whereas those larger than 5 mm healed with scarring in 21% of patients treated in one study.[321] Treatment of venous lakes with electrocautery has been unsatisfactory.[322] The PDL has been reported to be successful in treating venous lake lesions (Fig. 2.73).[245,269]

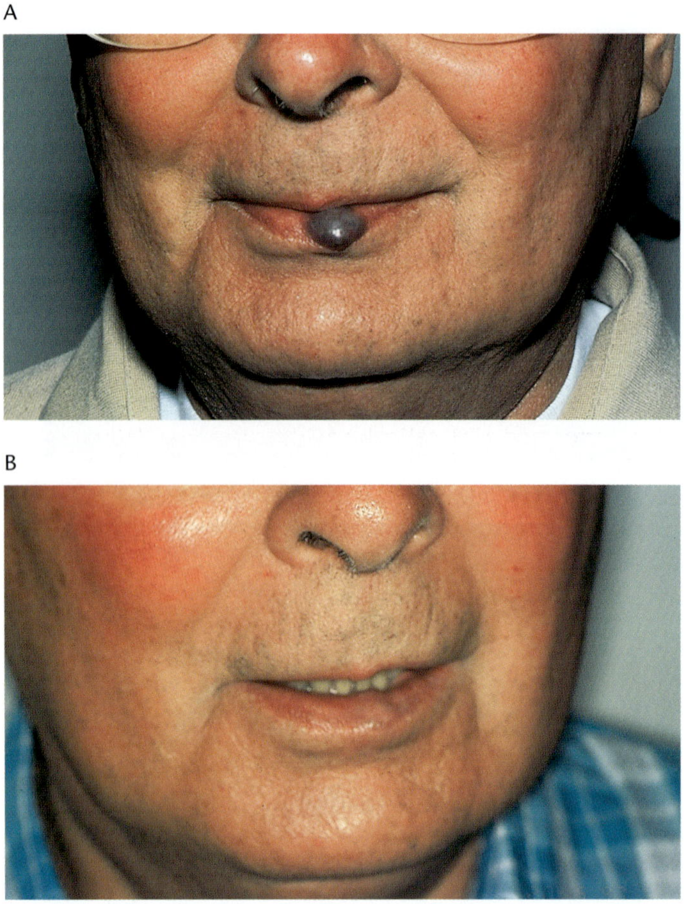

Figure 2.74 (A) Venous lake present for more than 20 years on the lower lip. (B) Four weeks after second treatment with intense pulsed light at 590-nm cutoff filter, 38J/cm^2 given as a double pulse of 3 ms and 2 ms with a 10-ms delay.

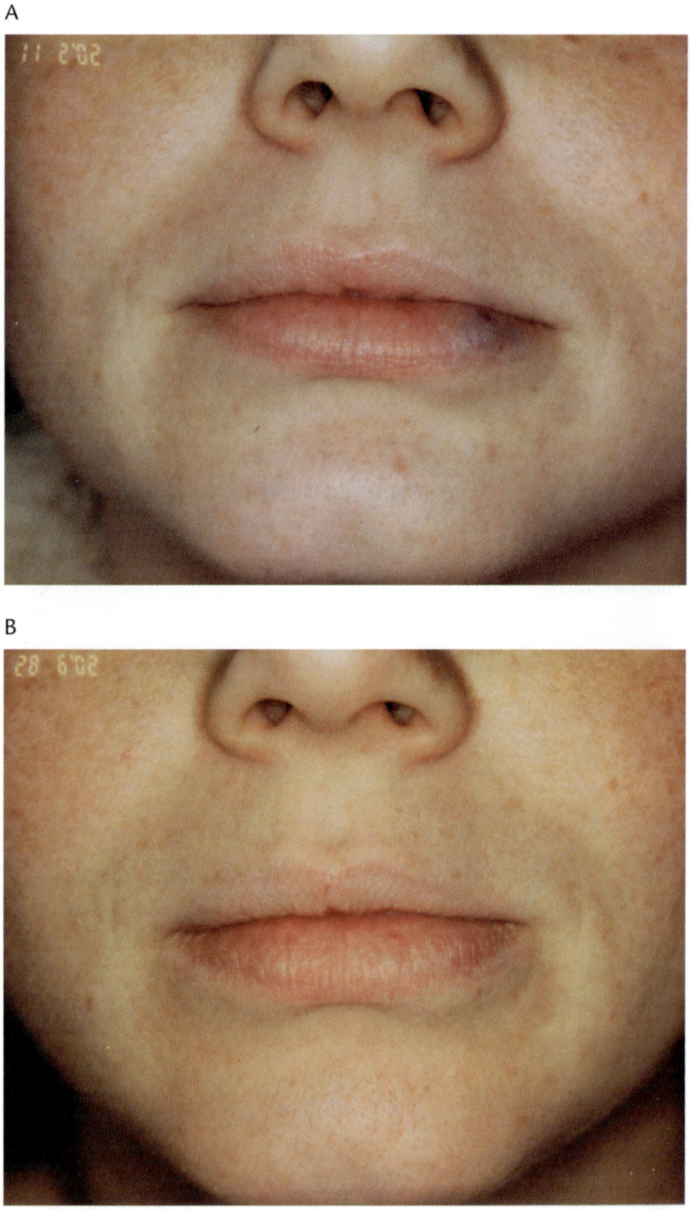

Figure 2.75 (A) A 32-year-old woman who had a venous lake on the lower lip for 18 years and requested removal for cosmetic reasons. One treatment was given with a long-pulse Nd:YAG laser with a 7-mm diameter spot size, a pulse duration of 45 ms and a fluence of 120 J/cm^2. Six pulses were given. (B) Complete resolution 4 months after treatment. (Courtesy of Don Groot, MD.)

When using the PDL, selective photothermolysis is not the goal. Multiple pulses over the same area with or without diascopy are usually required for efficacy. This has resulted in epidermal and perivascular thermal damage as previously described. A tunable dye laser at 577 nm used with diascopy in a continuous wave at 1 W also gives excellent cosmetic results.[323]

The IPL has also been found to be effective in resolving venous lakes in one or two treatments. Treatment parameters are similar to those used for treating hemangiomas (Fig. 2.74). The long-pulse Nd:YAG is also suitable for treating this vascular lesion. Figure 2.75A shows a 32-year-old woman who had had a venous lake on the lower lip for 18 years and requested removal for cosmetic reasons. One treatment was given with a long-pulse Nd:YAG laser with a 7-mm-diameter spot size, a pulse duration of 45 ms and a fluence of 120 J/cm^2; six pulses were given. Figure 2.75B shows complete resolution 4 months after treatment.

Verruca Vulgaris

Verrucae represent benign tumors of epidermal cells induced by the human papillomavirus (HPV). They occur in about 10% of adults and children.[324] Verrucae develop from epidermal hyperproliferation in response to viral genome incorporation into epidermal cellular DNA. To maintain a proliferative growth, neovascularization is stimulated. This is reflected histologically in prominent, dilated blood vessels in dermal papillae.[325] Theoretically, vaporization and coagulation of the new capillaries should halt viral replication and promote verrucae resolution. To produce vascular coagulation, the CVL has been reported to treat genital warts effectively.[326]

Nemeth and Reyes[326] postulated that using epidermal melanin as the 'surrogate' target produces epidermal-dermal separation with removal of the wart. In a population of resistant warts, only 12 of 137 patients failed to respond to treatment with a CVL. However, one-third of patients developed recurrent lesions at the 6-month follow-up.

In an effort to coagulate deeper vessels, using a laser with a longer wavelength should be effective. Therefore we have used the PDL to treat common verrucae. Lesions are treated at a fluence of 7.0 to 7.5 J/cm^2 with single pulses to flat warts and two to four pulses to hypertrophic verrucae. Paring down the warts is recommended but not to the point of bleeding, which would cause the laser light to be absorbed by surface blood. Lesions are treated until they appear gray. They then become black after 24 hours. Patients are retreated every 1 to 2 weeks until resolution. We combined a limited series of patients with those of Webster et al[327] at Jefferson Medical College and found that flat warts were most responsive to treatment, with 71% resolving completely in an average of 2.4 treatments. Palmar and plantar warts had a 65% total resolution response in 2.3 treatments, and periungual warts only cleared completely in 33% of patients despite an average of 3.3 treatments. Some warts cleared after one treatment, and some required several treatments. There was no significant difference in the number of treatments or fluence used. Very few warts failed to show some response to treatment, with smaller warts responding more quickly than larger warts. None of our patients developed postprocedural debility.

Tan et al[328] treated 39 patients with verrucae recalcitrant to multiple treatment modalities with the PDL after paring the warts at fluences ranging from 6.25 to 7.5 J/cm^2. As with our patients, excellent resolution occurred, warts totally clearing in 72% of patients after an average of 1.68 treatments. The more rapid response was most likely related to enhanced efficacy by allowing deeper vascular coagulation through paring the surface of the verrucae. Only one of the patients had a recurrence in the 5- to 6-month follow-up period. The authors examined 15 patients histologically and found marked agglutination of RBCs accompanied by vessel wall necrosis. Necrotic keratinocytes surrounded these vessels.

Kauvar et al[329] have reported the highest efficacy with PDL treatment: 93% overall efficacy in treating 142 patients with 703 verrucae that had been recalcitrant to previous treatment with various modalities, including liquid nitrogen and CO_2 laser vaporization. Warts were pared and hemostasis obtained with aluminum chloride 3 weeks before treatment. When warts cleared, they did so in an average of 2.5 treatments (range 2–5). In addition to an enhanced therapeutic response from therapy, 60% of patients reported adverse effects that were minimal enough to prevent a change in their daily activities, and 70% thought PDL treatment was less painful than liquid nitrogen cryosurgery. Interestingly, the study found no difference in efficacy among 7, 8, 9, or 10 J/cm^2 fluences, as well as no apparent difference between two to five pulses and six to ten pulses. The authors concluded that each wart should receive two or three pulses at a fluence of 6 to 7 J/cm^2 at 3-week intervals.

An additional study of 156 warts in 32 individuals treated with the PDL at 8 J/cm^2 showed resolution of 68% of recalcitrant warts and 47% of never-treated warts with an average of 1.78 treatments.[330] Recalcitrant warts had a higher clearance rate because they were usually treated up to three times, whereas never-treated were usually only treated once or twice. These patients generally preferred PDL treatment to cryosurgery, with only 2 of 32 patients having residual pain lasting 1.5 days to 1.5 weeks.

Increasing the fluence of the PDL to 8.1 to 8.4 J/cm^2 has increased clearance. Of 97 verrucae treated at this higher fluence, 70% had 100% clearance.[331]

A prospective randomized study of PDL vs. conventional treatment on 40 adults with 194 warts showed a 70% response with conventional and 66% response with PDL treatment. Conventional treatment was LN_2 with 2, 15 second freeze thaw time. PDL treatment was with a 5-mm-diameter spot, 9–9.5 J/cm^2 given in two pulses. Both groups also performed 17% salicylic acid treatments daily to their warts. A mean number of two treatments was necessary in both groups to achieve clearance. There appeared to be a slight advantage of the PDL in the treatment of recalcitrant lesions.

Unfortunately, not all studies report the same degree of significant efficacy with PDL therapy.[332] A study of 27 patients with 79 recalcitrant palmoplantar, digital, periungual, and body lesion warts found that 36% of the patients had complete resolution of their warts and 59% partially responded. Of the total number of warts treated, only 21% completely resolved.[333] Of those warts that cleared, 40% recurred within 4 months with a mean follow-up of 7 months. Exact treatment parameters and techniques were not noted in this abstract, but this study from a major laser center casts doubt on the absolute efficacy of PDL treatment.

Reasons for the difference in therapeutic response is unknown. Because of a wart's tendency toward spontaneous resolution, however, a blinded controlled study of PDL versus sham laser is necessary. Nevertheless, the efficacy of this treatment, in addition to its ease and lack of scarring, is encouraging. In addition to the proposed mechanism of vascular coagulation for wart destruction, direct thermal effects from treatment may be significant.

Nonlaser-induced hyperthermia has been demonstrated to result in regression of warts in a high percentage of patients.[334] The mechanism of action for heat may be related to direct epidermal protein coagulation or coagulation of nutritive blood vessels or to the subsequent inflammatory response to thermal injury. Other lasers have been used to produce local hyperthermia, and the term 'laserthermia' has been used specifically with Nd:YAG laser therapy.[335,336] As with PDL treatment, Nd:YAG laserthermia has advantages over CO_2 laser treatment because the skin remains intact and bleeding usually does not occur. Thirty-one patients with recalcitrant warts (previous unsuccessful cryosurgery, keratolytic treatment, antimitotic therapy, and excision alone or in combination) were treated with the Nd:YAG at 10 W with 8-mm-diameter spot size and irradiation time of 20 s. These parameters resulted in heating of wart tissue to 40°C for 30 s. Patients were treated up to three times at 3-week intervals. At 9-month follow-up, 77% of patients cleared completely without scarring or recurrence.[337] Local anesthesia was not necessary because patients felt only a slight burning sensation during and after treatment.

The frequency doubled Nd:YAG laser has also been found to be effective in the treatment of flat warts.[338] This laser was used with a 3-mm-diameter spot size at 2.5 J/cm^2 with multiple 10 ns pulses. Lesions were treated until whitening occurred and all lesions turned into eschars after a few days. In the seven patients treated, hyperpigmentation developed but all lesions resolved without adverse effects.

Finally, the treatment of warts in sensitive areas such as the anogenital region is less traumatic with the PDL than with conventional techniques.[339]

Technique: PDL

The warts are first paired down just before bleeding occurs. If bleeding occurs it must first be stopped with pressure. The PDL is used with a 5-mm-diameter spot size. A 2-ms pulse, at 9 J/cm^2 is given with slight epidermal cooling (air cooling at 2). Two to four pulses are given until the lesion turns grey. Treatments are repeated every 2 weeks.

Technique: IPL

Another system that incorporates both vascular specificity and thermal effects is the IPL. As previously described, this system produces deep vascular coagulation and thermal effects. We have achieved excellent success with this modality.

With the IPL, the wart is exposed through a hole-punch in a white index card. The IPL crystal is then placed on the wart which is exposed through the hole-punch. IPL energy does not penetrate through the white index card and the treatment is not painful. With the IPL a 550-, 560-, or 570-nm filter is used, with a double pulse of 2.4 ms and 4.0 ms or 3.0 ms and 3.0 ms (with the Lumenis One) with a 10-ms delay between the pulses, 45 J/cm^2 (30 J/cm^2 with the Lumenis One) is used; one to three pulses are given until the wart turns gray.

Acknowledgment

This chapter is extensively updated from: Goldman MP, Fitzpatrick RE: 'Laser Treatment of Cutaneous Vascular Lesions' in Cutaneous Laser Surgery: The Art and Science of Selective Photothermolysis 2nd Ed. Goldman MP, Fitzpatrick RE (eds) Mosby, St. Louis, 1999.

References

1. Solomon H et al. Histopathology of the laser treatment of port-wine lesions. J Invest Dermatol 1968; 50:141.
2. Apfelberg DB, Maser MR, Lash H. Argon laser management of cutaneous vascular deformities: a preliminary report. West J Med 1976; 124:99.
3. Dolsky RL. Argon laser skin surgery. Surg Clin North Am 64:861, 1984.
4. Anderson RR, Parrish JA. Microvasculature can be selectively damaged using dye lasers: a basic theory and experimental evidence in human skin. Lasers Surg Med 1981; 1:263.
5. Anderson RR, Parrish JA. Selective photothermolysis: precise microsurgery by selective absorption of pulsed radiation. Science 1983; 220:524.
6. Garden JM, Tan OT, Kerschmann R et al. Effect of dye laser pulse duration on selective cutaneous vascular injury. J Invest Dermatol 1986; 87:653.
7. Tanghetti E, Sierra RA, Sherr EA, Mirkov M. Evaluation of pulse-duration on purpuric threshold using extended pulse pulsed dye laser (Cynosure V-Star). Lasers Surg Med 2002; 31:363–366.
8. Tan OT, Murray S, Kurban A. Action spectrum of vascular specific injury using pulsed irradiation. J Invest Dermatol 1989; 92:868.
9. van Gemert MCJ et al. Can physical modeling lead to an optimal laser treatment strategy for port-wine stains? In Wolbarsht ML, ed. Laser applications in medicine and biology, vol 5. New York: Plenum; 1991.
10. Pickering TW, van Gemert MJC. 585 nm for the laser treatment of port-wine stains: a possible mechanism. Lasers Surg Med 1991; 11:616 (letter).
11. Gilchrist BA, Rosen S, Noe JM. Chilling port-wine stains improves the response to argon laser therapy. Plast Reconstr Surg 1982; 69:278.
12. Dreno B, Patrice T, Litoux P et al. The benefit of chilling in argon laser treatment of port-wine stains. Plast Resconstr Surg 1985; 75:42.
13. Pope K, Kask G. Epidermal temperature evaluation during dynamic spray cooling, contact cooling, and ice. Presented at the 20th Annual meeting of the ASLMS, Reno, Nevada, April 2000.
14. Nelson JS, Milner TE, Anvari B et al. Dynamic epidermal cooling during pulsed laser treatment of port-wine stain. Arch Dermatol 1995; 131:695.
15. Nelson JS, Milner TE, Anvari B. Dynamic epidermal cooking in conjunction with laser-induced photothermolysis of port-wine stain blood vessels. Lasers Surg Med 1996; 19;224.
16. Edris A, Choi B, Aguilar G, Nelson JS. Measurements of laser light attenuation following cryogen spray cooling spurt termination. Laser Surg Med 2003; 32:143–7.
17. Greve B, Hammes S, Raulin C. The effect of cold air cooling on 585 nm pulsed dye laser treatment of port-wine stains. Dermatol Surg 2001; 27:633–636.
18. Raulin C, Hammes S. Cold air in laser therapy: First experiences with a new cooling system. Lasers Surg Med 2000; 27:404–10.
19. Tan OT, Sherwood K, Gilchrest BA. Treatment of children with port-wine stains using the flashlamp-pulsed tunable dye laser. N Engl J Med 1989; 320:416.
20. Garden JM, Tan OT, Parrish JA. The pulsed dye laser: its use at 577 nm wavelength. J Dermatol Surg Oncol 1987; 13:134.
21. Garden JM, Polla LL, Tan OT. The treatment of port-wine stains by the pulsed dye laser. Analysis of pulse duration and long-term therapy. Arch Dermatol 1988; 124:889.
22. Garden JM et al. The pulsed dye laser for the treatment of port-wine stains. J Dermatol Surg Oncol 1986; 12:757.
23. Glassberg E et al. The flashlamp-pumped 577 nm pulsed tunable dye laser: clinical efficacy and in vitro studies. J Dermatol Surg Oncol 1988; 14:1200.
24. Rios WR. Flashlamp-excited dye laser: treatment of vascular cutaneous lesions. Facial Plast Surg 1989; 6:167.
25. Morelli JG, Tan OT, Garden J. Tunable dye laser (577 nm) treatment of port-wine stains. Lasers Surg Med 1986; 6:94.
26. Reyes BA, Geronemus R. Treatment of port-wine stains during childhood with the flashlamp-pumped pulsed dye laser. J Am Acad Dermatol 1990; 23:1142.
27. Ruiz-Esparza J, Goldman MP, Fitzpatrick RE, Lowe NJ, Behr KL. Flashlamp-pumped dye laser for port-wine stains. Lasers Surg Med 1993; 19(11):1000–3.

28. Goldman MP, Fitzpatrick RE, Ruiz-Esparza J. Treatment of port-wine stains (capillary malformation) with the flash-lamp-pumped pulsed dye laser. J Pediatr 1993; 122:71.
29. Glassberg E et al. The flashlamp-pumped 577 nm pulsed tunable dye laser: clinical efficacy and in vitro studies. J Dermatol Surg Oncol 1988; 14:1200.
30. Glassberg E et al. Capillary hemangiomas. Case study of a novel laser treatment and a review of therapeutic options. J Dermatol Surg Oncol 1989; 15:1214.
31. Sherwood KA, Tan OT. Treatment of a capillary hemangioma with the flashlamp-pumped dye laser. J Am Acad Dermatol 1990; 22:136.
32. Ashinoff R, Geronemus RG. Capillary hemangiomas and treatment with the flashlamp-pumped pulsed dye laser. Arch Dermatol 1991; 127:202.
33. Dinehart SM, Flock S, Waner M. Beam profile of the flash-lamp-pumped pulsed dye laser: support for overlap of exposure spots. Lasers Surg Med 1980; 15:277.
34. Jackson BA, Arndt KA, Dover JS. Are all 585 nm pulsed dye lasers equivalent? J Am Acad Dermatol 1996; 34:1000.
35. Archauer BM, Vander Kam VM, Padilla III JF. Clinical experience with the tunable pulsed-dye laser (585 nm) in the treatment of capillary vascular malformations. Plast Reconstr Surg 1993; 92:1233.
36. Glassberg E et al. The flashlamp-pumped 577 nm pulsed tunable dye laser: clinical efficacy and in vitro studies. J Dermatol Surg Oncol 1988; 14:1200.
37. Swinehart JM. Hypertrophic scarring resulting from flash-lamp-pumped pulsed dye laser surgery. J Am Acad Dermatol 1991; 25:845.
38. Gonzalez E, Gange RW, Momtaz K. Treatment of telangiectases and other benign vascular lesions with the 577 nm pulsed dye laser. J Am Acad Dermatol 1992; 27:220.
39. Jacobs AH, Walton RG. The incidence of birthmarks in the neonate. Pediatrics 1976; 58:218.
40. Pratt AG. Birthmarks in infants. Arch Dermatol 1953; 67:302.
41. Warner M. Personal communication, 1996.
42. Barsky SH et al. The nature and evolution of port-wine stains: a computer-assisted study. J Invest Dermatol 1980; 74:154.
43. Motley RJ, Lanigan SW, Katugampola GA. Videomicroscopy predicts outcome in treatment of port-wine stains. Arch Dermatol 1997; 133:921.
44. Susan JO et al. The 'tomato catsup' fundus in Sturge–Weber syndrome. Arch Ophthalmol 1974; 92:69.
45. Mulliken JB. Capillary (port-wine) and other telangiectatic stains. In: Mulliken JB, Young AE, eds. Vascular birthmarks, hemangiomas, and malformations. Philadelphia: WB Saunders; 1988.
46. Bebin EM, Gomez MR. Prognosis in Sturge–Weber disease: comparison of unihemispheric and bihemispheric involvement. J Child Neurol 1988; 3:181.
47. Paller AS. The Sturge–Weber syndrome. Pediatr Dermatol 1987; 4:300.
48. Iwach AG et al. Analysis of surgical and medical management of glaucoma in Sturge–Weber syndrome. Ophthalmology 1990; 97:904.
49. Uram M, Zubillaga C. The cutaneous manifestations of Sturge–Weber syndrome. J Clin Neurol Ophthalmol 1982; 2:245.
50. Tallman B, Tan OT, Morelli JG et al. Location of port-wine stains and the likelihood of ophthalmic and/or central nervous system complications. Pediatrics 1991; 87:323.
51. Roach ES. Congenital cutaneovascular syndromes. In: Vinkin PV, Bruyn GW, Klawans HL, eds. Handbook of clinical neurology: vascular diseases, vol 2. Amsterdam: Elsevier; 1989.
52. Stern R. Syndromes associated with port-wine stains. In: Arndt K, Noe J, eds. Cutaneous laser therapy: principles and methods. New York: Wiley & Sons; 1983.
53. Jessen RT, Thompson S, Smith EB. Cobb syndrome. Arch Dermatol 1977; 113:1587.
54. Mulliken JB. Classification of vascular birthmarks. In: Mulliken JB, Young AG, eds. Vascular birthmarks, hemangiomas and malformations. Philadelphia: WB Saunders; 1988.
55. Tay Y-K, Morelli J, Weston WL. Inflammatory nuchal-occipital port-wine stains. J Am Acad Dermatol 1996; 35:811.
56. Noe JM et al. Port-wine stains and the response to argon laser therapy: successful treatment and the predictive role of color, age, and biopsy. Plast Reconstr Surg 1980; 65:130.
57. Geronemus RG, Ashinoff R. The medical necessity of evaluation and treatment of port-wine stains. J Dermatol Surg Oncol 1991; 17:76.
58. Wilson BB, Brewer PC, Cooper PH. Spontaneous improvement of port-wine stain. Cutis 1995; 55:93.
59. Holloway KB, Ramos-Caro FA, Brownlee RE Jr et al. Giant proliferative hemangiomas arising in a port-wine stain. J Am Acad Dermatol 1994; 31:675.
60. Wagner KD, Wagner RF. The necessity for treatment of childhood port-wine stains. Cutis 1990; 45:317.
61. Malm M, Calberg M. Port-wine stain: a surgical and psychological problem. Ann Plast Surg 1988; 20:512.
62. Lanigan SW, Cotterill JA. Psychological disabilities amongst patients with port-wine stains. Br J Dermatol 1989; 121:209.
63. Hansen K, Kreiter CD, Rosenbaum M, Whitaker DC, Arpey CJ. Long-term psychological impact and perceived efficacy of pulsed-dye laser therapy for patients with port-wine stains. Dermatol Surg 2003; 29:49–55
64. Ashinoff R, Geronemus RG. Flashlamp-pumped pulsed dye laser for port-wine stains in infancy: earlier versus later treatment. J Am Acad Dermatol 1991; 24:467.
65. Tan E, Vinciullo C. Pulsed dye laser treatment of port-wine stains. Dermatol Surg 1996; 22:119.
66. Masclarelli PC. Living with a port-wine birthmark. In: Tan OT, ed. Management and treatment of benign cutaneous vascular lesions. Philadelphia: Lea & Febiger; 1992.
67. Troilius A, Wrangsjo B, Ljungren B. Patients with port-wine stains and their psychosocial reactions after photothermolytic treatment. Dermatol Surg 2000; 26:190–196.
68. Kurwa HA, Mills CM, Langian SW. Improvement in the psychological impact of a port wine stain after successful pulsed dye laser therapy. J Dermal Ther 1999; 10:277–282
69. McClean K, Hanke CW. The medical necessity for treatment of port-wine stains. Dermatol Surg 1997; 23:663.
70. Clodius I. Excision and grafting of extensive facial haemangiomas. Br J Plast Surg 1977; 30:185.
71. Clodius I. Surgery for the extensive facial port-wine stain? Aesthetic Plast Surg 1985; 9:61.
72. Wilson GM, Kilpatrick R, Eckert H. Thyroid neoplasms following irradiation. Br Med J 1958; 2:929.
73. Hidano A, Ogihara Y. Cryotherapy with solid carbon dioxide in the treatment of nevus flammeus. J Dermatol Surg Oncol 1977; 3:213.
74. Conway H, Montroy RE. Permanent camouflage of capillary hemangiomas of the face by interdermal injection of insoluble pigments (tattooing): indications for surgery. NY State J Med 1965; 65:876.

75. Thomson HG, Wright A. Surgical tattooing of the port-wine stain: operative technique, results and critique. Plast Reconstr Surg 1971; 48:113.
76. Cosman B. Clinical experience in the laser therapy of port-wine stains. Lasers Surg Med 1980; 1:133.
77. Bailin PL. Treatment of port-wine stains with the CO_2 laser: early results. In: Arndt KA, Noe JM, Rosen S, eds. Cutaneous laser therapy: principles and methods. Chichester, UK: Wiley & Sons; 1983.
78. Buecker JW, Ratz JL, Richfield DF. Histology of port-wine stains treated with carbon dioxide laser. J Am Acad Dermatol 1984; 10:1014.
79. Ratz JL, Bailin PL, Levine HL. CO_2 laser treatment for port-wine stains: a preliminary report. J Dermatol Surg Oncol 1982; 8:1039.
80. Lanigan SW, Cotterill JA. The treatment of port-wine stains with the carbon dioxide laser. Br J Dermatol 1990; 123:229.
81. Landthaler M, Haina D, Brunner R. Neodymium-YAG laser therapy for vascular lesions. J Am Acad Dermatol 1986; 14: 107.
82. Walker EP, Butler PH, Pickering JW. Histology of port-wine stains after copper vapor laser treatment. Br J Dermatol 1989; 121:217.
83. Scheibner A, Applebaum J, Wheeland RG. Treatment of port-wine hemangiomas in children. Lasers Surg Med (Suppl) 1989; 1:42.
84. Dixon J, Huether S, Rotering R. Hypertrophic scarring in argon laser treatment of port-wine stains. Plast Reconstr Surg 1984; 73:771.
85. Hobby LW. Argon laser treatment of superficial vascular lesions in children. Lasers Surg Med 1986; 6:16.
86. Brauner GJ, Schliftman A. Laser surgery for children. J Dermatol Surg Oncol 1987; 13:178.
87. Brauner G, Schliftman A, Cosman B. Evaluation of argon laser surgery in children under 13 years of age. Plast Reconstr Surg 1991; 87:37.
88. Morelli JG, Weston WL. Pulsed dye laser treatment of port-wine stains in children. In: Tan OT, ed. Management and treatment of benign cutaneous vascular lesions, Philadelphia: Lea & Febiger; 1992.
89. Morelli JG, Weston WL, Huff JV et al. Initial lesion size as a predictive factor in determining the response of port-wine stains in children treated with the pulsed dye laser. Arch Pediatr Adolesc Med 1995; 149:1142.
90. Alster TS, Wilson F. Treatment of port-wine stains with the flashlamp-pumped dye laser: extended clinical experience in children and adults. Ann Plast Surg 1994; 32:474.
91. Orten SS, Waner M, Flock S et al. Port-wine stains: an assessment of 5 years of treatment. Arch Otolaryngol Head Neck Surg 1996; 122;1174.
92. Eppley BL, Sadove M. Systemic effects of photothermolysis of large port-wine stains in infants and children. Plast Reconstr Surg 1994; 93:1150.
93. Pao D. Personal communication, 1994.
94. Levine VJ, Geronemus RG. Adverse effects associated with the 577- and 585-nm pulsed dye laser in the treatment of cutaneous vascular lesions: a study of 500 patients. J Am Acad Dermatol 1995; 32:613.
95. Lanigan SW. Port-wine stains on the lower limb: response to pulsed dye laser therapy. Clin Exp Dermatol 1996; 21:88.
96. Koster PHL, Horsr CMAM van der, Bossuyt PMM, Gemert MJC van. Prediction of portwine stain clearance and required number of flashlamp pumped pulsed dye laser treatments. Lasers Surg Med 2001; 29:151–155.
97. Raulin C, Schroeter C, Weiss RA, Keiner M, Werner S. Treatment of port-wine stains with a noncoherent pulsed light source. Arch Dermatol 1999; 135:679–683.
98. Cliff S, Misch K. Treatment of mature port wine stains with the photoderm VL. J Cutan Laser Ther 1999; 1:101–104.
99. Bjerring P, Christiansen K, Troilius A. Intense pulsed light source for the treatment of dye laser resistant port-wine stains. J Cosmetic Laser Ther 2003; 5:7–13.
100. Hellbrugge G, Stockmeier M, Henschel R, Drosner M. Port wince stains: comparison of intense pulsed light with pulsed dye laser. Lasers Surg Med 2004; S16:14.
101. Ho WS, Ying SY, Chan PC, Chan HH. Treatment of portwine stains with intense pulsed light: a prospective study. Dermatol Surg 2004; 30:887–891.
102. Zachariea H. Delayed wound healing and keloid formation following argon laser treatment or dermabrasion during isotretinoin treatment. Br J Dermatol 1988; 118:703.
103. Rubenstein R, Roenigk HH, Stegman S et al. Atypical keloids after dermabrasion of patients taking tretinoin. J Am Acad Dermatol 1986; 15:280.
104. Bernestein LJ, Geronemus RG. Keloid formation with the 585-nm pulsed dye laser during isotretinoin treatment. Arch Dermatol 1997; 133:111.
105. Seukeran DC, Collins P, Sheehan-Dare RA. Adverse reactions following pulsed tunable dye laser treatment of port-wine stains in 701 patients. Br J Dermatol 1997; 136:725.
106. Renfro L, Geronemus RG. Anatomical differences of port-wine stains in response to treatment with the pulse dye laser. Arch Dermatol 1993; 129:182.
107. Eubanks LE, McBurney EI. Videomicroscopy of port-wine stains: correlation of location and depth of lesion. J Am Acad Deramtol 2001; 44:948–51.
108. Yohn JJ, Huff JC, Aeling JL et al. Lesion size is a factor for determining the rate of port-wine stain clearing following pulsed dye laser treatment in adults. Cutis 1997; 59: 267.
109. Lanigan SW. Poor response of port wine stains on lower limb to pulsed tunable dye laser therapy. Lasers Surg Med 1995; Suppl 7:58.
110. Taylor MB. Flashlamp laser treatment of port-wine stain hemangiomas and other vascular lesions using a defocused 'fuzzy spot'. Lasers Surg Med 1991; Suppl 3:68.
111. Lucassen GW, Verkruysse W, Keijzer M et al. Light distributions in port-wine stain model containing multiple cylindrical and curved blood vessels. Lasers Surg Med 1996; 18: 345.
112. Fiskerstrand EJ, Dalaker M, Norvang LT. Laser treatment of port-wine stains: a study comparing therapeutic outcome with morphologic characteristics of the lesions. Acta Derm Venerol (Stockh) 1995; 75:92.
113. Fiskerstrand EJ, Svaasand LO, Kopstad G et al. Photothermally induced vessel-wall necrosis after pulsed dye laser treatment: lack of response in portwine stains with small sized or deeply located vessels. J Invest Dermatol 1996; 107:671.
114. Hohenleutner U, Hilbert M, Wlotzke U et al. Epidermal damage and limited coagulation depth with the flashlamp-pumped pulsed dye laser: a histochemical study. J Invest Dermatol 1995; 104:798.
115. Orten SS, Waner M, Flock S, Roberson PK, Kincannon J. Port-wine stains: an assessment of 5 years of treatment. Arch Otolaryngol Head Neck Surg 1996; 122(11):1174–9.
116. Smaller RB, Rosen S. Port-wine stains: a disease of altered neural modulation of blood vessels. Arch Dermatol 1986; 122:177.

117. Rydh M, Malm M, Jernbeck J et al. Ectatic blood vessels in port-wine stains lack innervation: possible role in pathogenesis. Plast Reconstr Surg 1991; 87:419.
118. Kauvar AN, Geronemus RG. Repetitive pulse dye laser treatments improve persistent port-wine stains. Dermatol Surg 1995; 21:515.
119. Kane KS, Smoller BR, Fitzpatrick RE et al. Pulsed dye laser-resistant port-wine stains. Arch Dermatol 1996; 132:839.
120. Lo JS, Sgouros GN, Laohs FE et al. Basal cell carcinoma within a nevus flammeus: report of a case. Int J Dermatol 1991; 30:723.
121. Chang C-J, Nelson JS. Cryogen spray cooling and higher fluence pulsed dye laser treatment improve port-wine stain clearance while minimizing epidermal damage. Dermatol Surg 1999;25:767–772.
122. Geronemus RG. High-fluence modified pulsed dye laser photocoagulation with dynamic cooling of port-wine stains in infancy. Arch Dermatol 2000; 136:942–943.
123. Kelly KM, Nanda VS, Nelson JS. Treatment of port-wine stain birthmarks using the 1.5-msec pulsed dye laser at high fluences in conjunction with cryogen spray cooling. Dermatol Surg 2002; 28:309–313.
124. Bencini PL. The multilayer technique: a new and fast approach for flashlamp-pumped pulsed (FLPP) dye laser treatment of port-wine stains (preliminary report). Dermatol Surg 1999; 25;786–789.
125. Lorenz S, Brunnberg S, Landthaler M, Hohenleutner U. Regading the multilayer technique for treatment of PWS. Dermatol Surg 2001; 27:90.
126. Bernstein EF. Treatment of a resistant port-wine stain with the 1.5-msec pulse duration, tunable, pulsed dye laser. Dermatol Surg 2000; 26:1007–1009.
127. Greve B, Raulin C. Prospective study of port wine stain treatment with dye laser: Comparison of two wavelengths (585 nm vs. 595 nm) and two pulse durations (0.5 milliseconds vs. 20 milliseconds). Lasers Surg Med 2004; 34:168–173.
128. Laube S, Taibjee S, Lanigan S. Treatment of resistant port wine stains with the V Beam® pulsed dye laser. Lasers Surg Med 2003; 33:282–287.
129. Scherer K, Lorenz S, Wimmershoff M, Landthaler M, Hohenleutner U. Both the flashlamp-pumped dye laser and the long-pulsed tunable dye laser can improve results in port-wine stain therapy. Br J Dermatol 2001; 145:79–84.
130. Kimel S, Svaasand LO, Hammer-Wilson MJ, Nelson JS. Influence of wavelength on response to laser photothermolysis of blood vessels: implications for port wine stain therapy. Lasers Surg Med 2003; 33:288–295.
131. Chang C-J, Kelly KM, van Gemert MJC, Nelson JS. Comparing the effectiveness of 585-nm vs. 595-nm wavelength pulsed dye laser treatment of port wine stains in conjunction with cryogen spray cooling. Lasers Surg Med 2002; 31:352–358.
132. Randeberg LL, Bonesronning JH, Dalaker M, Nelson JS. Methemoglobin formation during laser induced photothermolysis of vascular skin lesions. Lasers Surg Med 2004; 34:414–419.
133. Svaasand LO, Aguilar G, Viator JA, Randeberg LL, Kimel S, Nelson JS. Increase of dermal blood volume fraction reduces the threshold for laser-induced purpura: Implications for port wine stain laser treatment. Lasers Surg Med 2004; 34:182–188.
134. Raulin C, Hellwig S, Schonermark MP. Treatment of a nonresponding port-wine stain with a new pulsed light source (Photoderm VL). Lasers Surg Med 1997; 21:203.
135. Dierickx CC, Farinelli WA, Flotte T et al. Effect of long-pulsed 532 nm ND-YAG laser on port-wine stains (PWS). Lasers Surg Med 1996; Suppl 8:188.
136. Woo WK, Jasim ZF, Handley JM. Evaluating the efficacy of treatment of resistant port-wine stains with variable-pulse 595-nm pulsed dye and 532-nm Nd:YAG lasers. Dermatol Surg 2004; 30:158–162.
137. Chan H, Chan E, Kono T, Ying SY, Wai-Sun H. The use of variable pulse width frequency doubled Nd:YAG 532 nm laser in the treatment of port-wine stain in Chinese patients. Dermatol Surg 2000; 26:657–661.
138. Ahcan U, Zorman P, Recek D, Ralca S, Mararon B. Port wine stain treatment with a dual-wavelength Nd:YAG and cryogen spray cooling: a pilot study. Lasers Surg Med 2004; 34:164–167.
139. Yang MU, Yaroslavsky AN, Farinelli WA, Flotte TJ, Rius-Dias F, Tsao SS, Anderson RR. Long-pulsed Nd:YAG laser treatment of portwine stains. J Am Acad Dermatol 2005; 52:480–490.
140. Mulliken JB. A plea for a biologic approach to hemangiomas of infancy. Arch Dermatol 1991; 127:243 (editorial).
141. Mulliken JB. Diagnosis and natural history of hemangiomas. In: Mulliken JB, Young AE, eds. Vascular birthmarks, hemangiomas and malformations. Philadelphia: WB Saunders; 1988.
142. Finn MC, Glowacki J, Mulliken JB. Congenital vascular lesions: clinical application of a new classification. J Pediatr Surg 1983; 18:894.
143. Jacobs AH. Strawberry hemangiomas: the natural history of the untreated lesion. Calif Med 1957; 86:8.
144. Holmdahl K. Cutaneous hemangiomas in premature and mature infants. Acta Paediatr 1955; 44:370.
145. Boon LM, Enjolras O, Mulliken JB. Congenital hemangioma: evidence of accelerated involution. J Pediatr 1996; 128:329.
146. Rositto A, Ranalletta M, Drut R. Congenital hemangioma of eccrine sweat glands. Pediatr Dermatol 1993; 10:341.
147. Bowers RE, Graham EA, Tomlinson KM. The natural history of the strawberry nevus. Arch Dermatol 1960; 82:667.
148. Takahashi K, Mulliken JB, Kozakewich HPW et al. Cellular markers that distinguish the phases of hemangioma during infancy and childhood. J Clin Invest 1994; 93:2357.
149. Margileth AM, Museles M. Cavernous hemangiomas in children: diagnosis and conservative management. JAMA 1965; 194:523.
150. Bivings L. Spontaneous regression of angiomas in children: twenty-two years' observation covering 236 cases. J Pediatr 1954; 45:643.
151. Tuder RM, Young R, Karasek M et al. Adult cutaneous hemangiomas are composed of new replicating endothelial cells. J Invest Dermatol 1987; 89:594.
152. Lister WA. The natural history of strawberry naevi. Lancet 1938; 1:1429.
153. Baker ER, Manders E, Whitney CW. Growth of cavernous hemangioma with puberty. Clin Pediatr 1985; 24:596.
154. Moroz B. The course of haemangiomas in children. I: Ryan TJ, Cherry GW, eds. Vascular birthmarks: pathogenesis and management. New York: Oxford University Press; 1987.
155. Liang MG, Frieden IJ. Perineal and lip ulcerations as the presenting manifestation of hemangioma of infancy. Pediatrics 1997; 99:256.
156. Kim HJ, Colombo M, Frieden IJ. Ulcerated hemangiomas: clinical characteristics and response to therapy. J Am Acad Dermatol 2001; 44:962–72.
157. Williams HB. Facial bone changes with vascular tumors in children. Plast Reconstr Surg 1979; 63:309.

158. Thomson G, Stigmar G et al. Hemangiomas of the eyelid: visual complications and prophylactic concepts. Plast Reconstr Surg 1979; 63:641.
159. Robb RM. Refractive errors associated with hemangiomas of the eyelids and orbit in infancy. Am J Ophthalmol 1977; 83:52.
160. Malm M. Port-wine stain: laser treatment and evaluation of results. Stockholm: Kongl Carolinska Medico Chirargiska Institutet; 1987.
161. Healy GB et al. Treatment of subglottic hemangioma with the carbon dioxide laser. Laryngoscope 1980; 90: 809.
162. Kasabach HH, Merritt KK. Capillary hemangioma with extensive purpura. Am J Dis Child 1940; 59:1063.
163. McLean RH et al. Multinodular hemangiomatosis of the liver in infancy. Pediatrics 1972; 49:563.
164. Patel SD, Cohen BA, Kan JS et al. Extensive facial hemangiomas associated with cardiac and abdominal abnormalities. J Am Acad Dermatol 1997; 36:636.
165. Igarashi M, Uchida H, Kaji T. Supraumbilical midabdominal raphe and facial cavernous hemangiomas. Clin Genet 1985; 27:196.
166. Schneeweiss A, Blieden LC, Shem-Tov A et al. Coarctation of the aorta and congenital hemangioma of the face and neck and aneurysm or dilatation of a subclavian or innominate artery. Chest 1982; 82:186.
167. Reese V, Frieden IJ, Paller AS et al. Association of facial hemangiomas with Dandy–Walker and other posterior fossa malformations. J Pediatr 1993; 122:379.
168. Frieden IJ, Reese V, Cohen D. PHACE syndrome. Arch Dermatol 1996; 132:307.
169. Gorlin RJ, Kantaputra P, Aughton DJ et al. Marked female predilection in some syndromes associated with facial hemangiomas. Am J Med Genet 1994; 52:130.
170. Goldberg NS, Hebert AA, Esterly NB. Sacral hemangiomas and multiple congenital abnormalities. Arch Dermatol 1986; 122:684.
171. Albright AL, Gartner JC, Wiener ES. Lumbar cutaneous hemangiomas as indicators of tethered spinal cords. Pediatrics 1989; 83:977.
172. Enjolras O, Gelbert F. Superficial hemangiomas: associations and management. Pediatr Dermatol 1997; 14:173.
173. Finn MC, Glowacki J, Mulliken JP. Congenital vascular lesions: clinical applications of a new classification. J Pediatr Surg 1983; 18:894.
174. Tanner JL, et al. Growing up with a facial hemangioma: parent and child coping and adaptation. Pediatrics 1998; 101:446–52.
175. Modlin JJ. Capillary hemangiomas of the skin. Surgery 1955; 38:169.
176. Mulliken JB. Treatment of hemangiomas. In: Mulliken JB, Young AE, eds. Vascular birthmarks, hemangiomas and malformations. Philadelphia: WB Saunders; 1988.
177. Cherry GW. A review of the role of surgery in the treatment of hemangiomas and port-wine stains. In: Ryan TJ, Cherry GW, eds. Vascular birthmarks: pathogenesis and management. New York: Oxford University Press; 1987.
178. Bek V, Zahn K. Cataract as a late sequela of contract roentgen therapy of angiomas in children. Acta Radiol 1960; 54:443.
179. Tan OT, Gilchrest BA. Laser therapy for selected cutaneous vascular lesions in the pediatric population: a review. Pediatrics 1988; 82:652.
180. MacCollum DW. Treatment of hemangiomas. Am J Surg 1935; 29:32.
181. Brain RT, Calvan CD. Vascular naevi and their treatment. Br J Dermatol 1952; 64:147.
182. Matthews DN. Hemangiomata. Plast Reconstr Surg 1968; 41:528.
183. Scerri L, Navaratnam A. Basal cell carcinoma presenting as a delayed complication of thorium X used for treating a congenital hemangioma. J Am Acad Dermatol 1994; 31: 796.
184. Lomholt S. Alpha and beta ray therapy in dermatology. Br J Dermatol 1936; 48:567.
185. Bowers RE. Treatment of haemangiomatous naevi with thorium X. Br Med J 1951; 1:121.
186. Courtermarche AD. Thorium X induced BCC: a case report. Br J Plast Surg 1961; 14:254.
187. Caldwell JB, Ryan MT, Benson PM et al. Cutaneous angiosarcoma arising in the radiation site of a congenital hemangioma. J Am Acad Dermatol 1995; 33:865.
188. Dinehart S, Waner M, Flock S. The copper vapor laser for treatment of cutaneous vascular and pigmented lesions. J Dermatol Surg Oncol 1993; 19:370.
189. Sybert V. Personal communication, 1992.
190. George ME, Sharma V, Jacobson J, et al. Adverse effects of systemic glucocorticosteroid therapy in infants with hemangiomas. Arch Dermatol 2004; 140:963–9.
191. Kushner BJ. The treatment of periorbital infantile hemangiomas with intralesional corticosteroid. Plast Reconstr Surg 1985; 76:517.
192. Nelson LB, Melick JE, Harley RD. Intralesional corticosteroid injections for infantile hemangiomas of the eyelid. Pediatrics 1984; 74:241.
193. Ellis PO. Occlusion of the central retinal artery after retrobulbar corticosteroid injection. Am J Ophthalmol 1983; 85:352.
194. Chowdri NA, Darzi MA, Fazili Z et al. Intralesional corticosteroid therapy for childhood cutaneous hemangiomas. Ann Plast Surg 1994; 33:46.
195. Enjolras O, Mulliken JB. The current management of vascular birthmarks, Pediatr Dermatol 1993; 10:311.
196. Brousty-Brye D, Zelter BR. Inhibition of cell motility by interferon. Science 1980; 208:516.
197. Ezekowitz RA, Mulliken JB, Folkman J. Interferon alpha-2a therapy for life-threatening hemangiomas of infancy. N Engl J Med 1992; 326:1456.
198. Stratte EG, Tope WD, Johnson CL et al. Multimodal management of diffuse neonatal hemangiomatosis. J Am Acad Dermatol 1996; 34:337.
199. Apfelberg DB, Greene RA, Maser MR. Results of argon laser exposure of capillary hemangiomas of infancy: preliminary report. Plast Reconstr Surg 1981; 67:188.
200. Hobby LW. Further evaluation of the potential of the argon laser in the treatment of strawberry hemangiomas. Plast Reconstr Surg 1983; 71:481.
201. Achauer BM, VanderKam VM. Argon laser treatment of strawberry hemangioma in infancy. West J Med 1985; 143:628.
202. Apfelberg DB. Cases 5.6, 5.7, 5.9, 5.10, 5.11. In: Apfelberg DB, ed. Atlas of cutaneous laser surgery. New York: Plenum; 1992.
203. Shapshay SM, David LM, Zeitels S. Neodymium-YAG laser photocoagulation of hemangiomas of the head and neck. Laryngoscope 1987; 97:323.
204. Apfelberg DB. Cases 6.9, 6.10, 6.19, 6.20. In: Apfelberg DB, ed. Atlas of cutaneous laser surgery. New York: Plenum; 1992.
205. Preeyanont P, Nimsakul N. The Nd:YAG laser treatment of hemangioma. J Clin Laser Med Surg 1994; 12:225.

206. Burnstein FD, Simms C, Cohen SR et al. Intralesional therapy of extensive hemangiomas in 100 consecutive pediatric patients. Ann Plast Surg 2000; 44:188–94.
207. Apfelberg DB, Maser MR, Lash H. YAG laser resection of complicated hemangiomas of the hand and upper extremity. J Hand Surg 1990; 15A:765.
208. Apfelberg DB, Maser MR, Lash H. High- and low-tech solutions for massive cavernous hemangioma of the face. Lasers and leeches to the rescue. Ann Plast Surg 1989; 23:341.
209. Thompson HG, Lonigan M. The Cyrano nose: a clinical review of hemangiomas of the nasal tip. Plast Reconstr Surg 1979; 63:155.
210. Afpelberg DB. Argon and YAG laser photocoagulation and excision of hemangiomas and vascular malformations of the nose. West J Med 1995; 163:122.
211. Hoffman WL, Anvari B, Said S et al. Cryogen spray cooling during Nd:YAG laser treatment of hemangiomas. Dermatol Surg 1997; 23:635.
212. Groot D, Rao J, Johnston P, Nakatsui T. Algorithm for using a long-pulsed Nd:YAG laser in the treatment of deep cutaneous vascular lesions. Dermatol Surg 2003; 29:35–42.
213. Achauer BM, Vanderkam VM, Celikoz B. Intralesional bare fiber laser treatment of hemangioma. Lasers Surg Med 1997; Suppl 9:41.
214. Raulin C, Greve B. Retrospective clinical comparison of hemangiomas treatment by flashlamp-pumped (585 nm) and frequency-doubled Nd:YAG (532 nm) lasers. Lasers Surg Med 2001; 28:40–43.
215. Kaplan I, Sharon U. Current laser surgery. Ann NY Acad Sci 1976; 267:247.
216. Labandter H, Kaplan I. Experience with a continuous laser in the treatment of suitable cutaneous conditions. Preliminary report. J Dermatol Surg Oncol 1977; 3:527.
217. Apfelberg DB, Maser MR, Lash H et al. Benefits of carbon dioxide laser in oral hemangioma excision. Plast Reconstr Surg 1985; 75:46.
218. Apfelberg DB, Maser MR, Lash H. Review and usage of argon and carbon dioxide lasers for pediatric hemangiomas. Ann Plast Surg 1984; 12:353.
219. Scheepers JH, Quaba AA. Does the pulsed tunable dye laser have a role in the management of infantile hemangiomas? Observations based on 3 years' experience. Plast Reconstr Surg 1995; 95:305.
220. Morelli JG, Weston WL. Pulsed dye laser treatment of hemangiomas. In: Tan OT, ed. Management and treatment of benign cutaneous vascular lesions. Philadelphia: Lea & Febiger; 1992.
221. Morelli JG, Tan OT, Yohn JJ. Treatment of ulcerated hemangiomas in infancy. Arch Pediatr Adolesc Med 1994; 148:1104.
222. Garden JM, Babus AD, Paller AS. Treatment of cutaneous hemangiomas by the flashlamp-pumped pulsed dye laser: prospective analysis. J Pediatr 1992; 120:555.
223. Maier H, Neumann R. Treatment of strawberry marks with flashlamp-pumped pulsed dye laser in infancy. Lancet 1996; 347:131.
224. Barlow RJ, Walker NPJ, Markey AC. Treatment of proliferative haemangiomas with the 585 nm pulsed dye laser. Br J Dermatol 1996; 134:700.
225. West T, Fitzpatrick RE, Goldman MP, Alster T. Treatment of capillary hemangiomas with the Candela flashlamp-pumped pulsed dye laser and corticosteroids. Dermatol Surg 1998.
226. McDaniel DH, Mordon S. Hexascan: a new robotized scanning laser handpiece. Cutis 1990; 45:300.
227. Kauvar A. Long-pulse and high energy pulsed dye laser treatment of port-wine stains and hemangiomas. Presented at 24th Annual meeting of the American Society of Dermatologic Surgery, Boston, MA; May 1997.
228. Poetke M, Philipp C, Berlien HP. Flashlamp-pumped pulsed dye laser for hemangiomas in infancy. Arch Dermatol 2000; 136:628–632.
229. Hohenleutner S, Badur-Ganter E, Landthaler M, Hohenteutner U. Long-term results in the treatment of childhood hemangiomas with the flashlamp-pumped pulsed dye laser: An evaluation of 617 cases. Lasers Surg Med 2001; 28:273–277.
230. Foster TD, Gold MH. The successful use of the PhotoDerm VL in the treatment of a cavernous hemangioma in a dark-skinned infant. Minim Invas Nurs 1996; 10:102.
231. Fujino T. Microsurgical technique in resection of haemangioma in infants. Ann Plast Surg 1985; 13:190.
232. Argenta L. Controlled tissue expansion in reconstructive surgery. Br Plast Surg 1984; 37:520.
233. Grabb WC et al. Facial hamartomas in children: neurofibroma, lymphangioma and haemangioma. Plast Reconstr Surg 1980; 66:509.
234. Apfelberg DB, Lane B, Marx MP. Combined (team) approach to hemangioma management: arteriography with superselective embolization plus YAG laser/sapphire-tip resection. Plast Reconstr Surg 1991; 88:71.
235. Raulin C, Raulin SJ, Hellwig S, Schonermark MP. Treatment of benign venous malformation with an intense pulsed light source (Photoderm VL). Eur J Dermatol 1997; 7:279.
236. Frieden IJ, Eichenfield LF, Esterly NB et al. Guidelines of care for hemangiomas of infancy. J Am Acad Dermatol 1997; 37:631.
237. Pasyl KA. Classification and histopathological features of haemangiomas and other vascular malformations. In: Ryan TJ, Cherry GW, eds. Vascular birthmarks: pathogenesis and management. New York: Oxford University Press; 1987.
238. Bucci FA, Wiener BD. The pyogenic granuloma. Ariz Med 1984; WLI:794.
239. Cooper PH, Mills SE. Subcutaneous granuloma pyogenicum: lobular capillary hemangioma. Arch Dermatol 1982; 118: 30.
240. Patrice SJ, Wiss K, Mulliken JB. Pyogenic granuloma (lobular capillary hemangioma): a clinicopathologic study of 178 cases. Pediatr Dermatol 1991; 8:267.
241. Goldberg DJ, Sciales CW. Pyogenic granuloma in children. J Dermatol Surg Oncol 1991; 17:960.
242. Mills SE, Cooper PH, Fechner RE. Lobular capillary hemangioma: the underlying lesion of pyogenic granuloma, a study of 73 cases from the oral and nasal mucous membranes. Am J Surg Pathol 1980; 4:471.
243. Arndt KA. Argon laser therapy of small cutaneous vascular lesions. Arch Dermatol 1982; 118:220.
244. Blickenstaff RD et al. Recurrent pyogenic granuloma with satellitosis. J Am Acad Dermatol 1989; 21:1241.
245. Tan OT, Kurban AK. Noncongenital benign cutaneous vascular lesions: pulse dye laser treatment. In: Tan OT, ed. Management and treatment of benign cutaneous vascular lesions. Philadelphia: Lea & Febiger; 1992.
246. Glass AT, Milgram S. Flashlamp-pumped dye laser treatment for pyogenic granuloma. Cutis 1992; 49:351.
247. Gonzalez S, Vibhagool C, Falo LD Jr et al. Treatment of pyogenic granulomas with the 585-nm pulsed dye laser. J Am Acad Dermatol 1996; 35:428.
248. Merlen JF. Red telangiectasias, blue telangiectasias. Soc Franc Phlebol 1970; 22:167.
249. Goldman MP, Bennett RG. Treatment of telangiectasia: a review. J Am Acad Dermatol 1987; 17:167.

250. Redisch W, Pelzer RH. Localized vascular dilatations of the human skin: capillary microscopy and related studies. Am Heart J 1949; 37:106.
251. Kaplan I, Peled I. The carbon dioxide laser in the treatment of superficial telangiectases. Br J Plast Surg 1975; 28:214.
252. Achauer BM, VanderKam VM. Argon laser treatment of the face and neck: 5 years' experience. Lasers Surg Med 1987; 7:495.
253. Lyons GD, Owens RE, Moriney DF. Argon laser destruction of cutaneous telangiectatic lesions. Laryngoscope 1981; 91:1322.
254. Greenwald J et al. Comparative histological studies of the tunable dye (at 577 nm) laser and argon laser: the specific vascular effects of the dye laser. J Invest Dermatol 1981; 77:305.
255. Scheibner A, Wheeland RG. Argon-pumped tunable dye laser therapy for facial port-wine stain hemangiomas in adults: a new technique using small spot size and minimal power. J Dermatol Surg Oncol 1989; 15:277.
256. Scheibner A, Wheeland RG. Use of the argon-pumped tunable dye laser for port-wine stains in children. J Dermatol Surg Oncol 1991; 17:735.
257. Cosman B. Role of retreatment in minimal-power argon laser therapy for port-wine stains. Lasers Surg Med 1982; 2:43.
258. Fitzpatrick RE, Feinberg JA. Low dose argon laser therapy of port-wine stains. ICALEO '83 Proceedings; 1984; 6:47.
259. Rotteleur G et al. Robotized scanning laser handpiece for the treatment of port-wine stains and other angiodysplasias. Lasers Surg Med 1988; 8:283.
260. Orenstein A, Nelson JS. Treatment of facial vascular lesions with a 100 μm spot 577 nm pulsed continuous wave dye laser. Ann Plast Surg 1989; 23:310.
261. Apfelberg DB. Cases 7.6, 7.7, 7.22, 7.30. In: Apfelberg DB, ed. Atlas of cutaneous laser surgery. New York: Raven; 1992.
262. McDaniel DH, Mordon S. Hexascan: a new robotized scanning laser handpiece. Cutis 1990; 45:300.
263. Broska P, Martinho E, Goodman MM. Comparison of the argon tunable dye laser with the flashlamp pulsed dye laser in treatment of facial telangiectasia. J Dermatol Surg Oncol 1994; 20:749.
264. Waner M, Dinehart S. Lasers in facial plastic and reconstructive surgery. In: Davis RK, Shapstray S, eds. Lasers in otolaryngology/head and neck surgery. Philadelphia: WB Saunders; 1989.
265. Dinehart SM, Waner M. Comparison of the copper vapor and flashlamp-pulsed dye laser in the treatment of facial telangiectasia. J Am Acad Dermatol 1991; 24:116.
266. Neumann RA, Leonhartsberger H, Bohler-Sommereger K et al. Results and tissue healing after copper-vapour laser (at 578 nm) treatment of port-wine stains and facial telangiectasias. Br J Dermatol 1993; 128:306.
267. Thibault PK. Copper vapor laser and microsclerotherapy of facial telangiectases. J Dermatol Surg Oncol 1994; 20: 48.
268. Waner M, Dinehart SM, Wilson MB et al. A comparison of copper vapor and flashlamp pumped dye lasers in the treatment of facial telangiectasia. J Dermatol Surg Oncol 1993; 19:992.
269. McCoy SE. Copper bromide laser treatment of facial telangiectasia: results of patients treated over five years. Lasers Surg Med 1997; 21:329.
270. McCoy S, Hanna M, Anderson P et al. An evaluation of the copper-bromide laser for treating telangiectasia. Dermatol Surg 1996; 22:551.
271. Mordon SR et al. Comparison study of the 'point-by-point technique' and the 'scanning technique' for laser treatment of port-wine stain. Lasers Surg Med 1989; 9:398.
272. Cassuto DA, Ancona DM, Emanuelli G. Treatment of facial telangiectasias with a diode-pumped Nd:YAG laser at 532 nm. J Cutan Laser Ther 2000; 2:141–6.
273. Hevia O. New laser treatment for facial telangiectasias: a randomized study. Cosmetic Dermatol 1997; 10:53.
274. Goldberg DJ, Marcus J. The use of the frequency-doubled Q-switched Nd:YAG laser in the treatment of small cutaneous vascular lesions. Dermatol Surg 1996; 22:841.
275. Goldberg DJ, Meine JG. A comparison of four frequency-doubled Nd:YAG (532 nm) laser systems for treatment of facial telangiectases. Dermatol Surg 1999; 25:463–7.
276. Kauvar ANB, Frew KE, Friedman PM, Geronemus RG. Cooling gel improves pulsed KTP laser treatment of facial telangiectasia. Lasers Surg Med 2002; 30:149–53.
277. Fitzpatrick RE et al. Treatment of facial telangiectasia with the flash pump dye laser. Lasers Surg Med 1991; Suppl 3:70.
278. Rohrer TE, Chatrath V, Iyengar V. Does pulse stacking improve the results of treatment with variable-pulse pulsed-dye lasers? Dermatol Surg 2004; 30:163–7.
279. Alam M, Dover JS, Arndt KA. Treatment of facial telangiectasia with variable-pulse high-fluence pulsed-dye laser: comparison of efficacy with fluences immediately above and below the purpura threshold. Dermatol Surg 2003; 29:681–685.
280. Eremia S, Willoughby M. A prospective study of periocular reticular veins treated with a 940-nm diode pumped laser. Cosmet Dermatol 2002; 15:19–21.
281. Eremia S, Li CY. Treatment of face veins with a cryogen spray variable pulse width 1064 nm Nd:YAG laser: a prospective study of 17 patients. Dermatol Surg 2002; 28:244–247.
282. Sarradet DM, Hussain M, Goldberg DJ. Millisecond 1064-nm neodymium:YAG laser treatment of facial telangiectasia. Dermatol Surg 2003; 29:56–58.
283. Goldman MP. Optimal management of facial telangiectasia. Am J Clin Dermatol 2004; 5:423–434.
284. Bjerrimg P, Christian K, Troilius A. Intense pulsed light source for treatment of facial telangiectasias. J Cosmetic & Laser Ther 2001; 3:169–73.
285. Alderson MR. Spider naevi: their incidence in healthy school children. Arch Dis Child 1963; 38:286.
286. Wenzl JE, Burgert EO. The spider nevus in infancy and childhood. Pediatrics 1964; 33:227.
287. Oster J, Nielsen A. Nuchal naevi and intrascapular telangiectases. Acta Paediatr Scand 1970; 59:416.
288. Bean WB. Vascular spiders and related lesions of the skin. Springfield, IL: Thomas; 1958.
289. Geronemus RG. Treatment of spider telangiectases in children using the flashlamp pumped pulsed dye laser. Pediatr Dermatol 1991; 8:61.
290. Goldman MP, Fitzpatrick RE, Ruiz-Esparza J. Treatment of spider telangiectasia in children. Contemp Pediatr 1993; 10:16.
291. de Rooij MJM, Neumann HAM. Granuloma telangiectaticum after argon laser therapy of a spider nevus. Dermatol Surg 1995; 20:354.
292. Raulin C, Weiss RA, Schohermark MP. Treatment of essential telangiectasias with an intense pulsal light source (PhotoDerm VL). Dermatol Surg 1997; 23:941.
293. Wilkin JK. Rosacea: pathophysiology and treatment. Arch Dermatol 1994; 130:359.
294. Schmidt NF, Gans EH. Demodex and rosacea, I: the prevalence and numbers of Demodex mites in rosacea. Cosmetic Dermatol 2004; 17:497–502.

295. Hernandez-Perez E, Ibiett EV. Gross and microscopic findings in patients submitted to nonablative full face resurfacing using intense pulsed light. Dermatol Surg 2002; 28:651–5.
296. Prieto VG, Sadick NS, Lloreta J, et al. Effects of intense pulsed light on sun-damaged human skin, routine, and ultrastructural analysis. Lasers Med Surg 2002; 30:82–5.
297. Dahl MV, Ross AJ, Schlievert PM. Temperature regulates bacterial protein production: possible role in rosacea. J Am Acad Dermatol 2004; 50:266–72.
298. Fitzpatrick RE et al. Treatment of facial telangiectasia with the flash pump dye laser. Lasers Surg Med 1991; Suppl 3:70.
299. Lowe NJ et al. Flashlamp pumped dye laser for rosacea-associated telangiectasia and erythema. J Dermatol Surg Oncol 1991; 17:522.
300. Clark SM, Lanigan SW, Marks R. Laser treatment of erythema and telangiectasia associated with rosacea. Lasers Surg Med 2002; 17:26–33.
301. Jasim ZF, Woo WK, Handley JM. Long-pulsed (6-ms) pulsed dye laser treatment of rosacea-associated telangiectasia using subpurpuric clinical threshold. Dermatol Surg 2004; 30:37–40.
302. Tan SR, Tope WD. Pulsed dye laser treatment of rosacea improves erythema, symptomotology, and quality of life. J Am Acad Dermatol 2004; 51:592–9.
303. Lonne-Rahm S, Nordlund K, Edstrom DW, Ros AM. Laser treatment of rosacea: a pathoetiological study. Arch Dermatol 2004; 140:1345–9.
304. Berg M, Edstrom DW. Flashlamp pulsed dye laser did not cure papulpustular rosacea. Lasers Surg Med 2004; 34:266–8.
305. Silver BE, Livshots YL. Preliminary experience with the KTP/532 nm laser in the treatment of facial telangiectasia. Cosmetic Dermatol 1996; 9:61.
306. Mark K, Sparacio RM, Voigt A, et al. Objective and quantitative improvement of rosacea-associated erythema after intense pulsed light treatment. Dermatol Surg 2003; 9:600–4.
307. Schroeter CA, Below SH, Neumann HAM. Effective treatment of Rosacea using intense pulsed light systems. Dermatol Surg 2005 (in press).
308. Taub AF. Treatment of rosacea with intense pulsed light. J Drugs Dermatol 2003; 3:254–9.
309. Civatte A. Poikilodermie reticulae pigmentaire du visage et du col. Ann Derm Syph 1923; 6:605.
310. Batta K, Hindson C, Cotterill JA, Foulds IS. Treatment of poikiloderma of Civatte with the potassium titanyl phosphate (KTP) laser. Br J Dermatol 1999; 140:1191–2.
311. Wheeland RG, Applebaum J. Flashlamp-pumped pulsed dye laser therapy for poikiloderma of Civatte. J Dermatol Surg Oncol 1990; 16:12.
312. Haywood RM, Monk BE. Treatment of poikiloderma of Civatte with the pulsed dye laser: a series of seven cases. J Cutan Laser Ther 1999; 1:45–8.
313. Goldman MP, Weiss RA. Treatment of poikiloderma of Civatte on the neck with an intense pulsed light source. Plast Reconstr Surg 2001; 107:1376–81.
314. Weiss RA, Goldman MP, Weiss MA. Treatment of poikiloderma of Civatte with an intense pulsed light source. Dermatol Surg 2000; 26:823–8.
315. Zheng P, Lavker RM, Kligman AM. Anatomy of striae. Brit J Dermatol 1985; 112:185.
316. Arem AJ, Kischer CW. Analysis of striae. Plast Recontr Surg 1980; 65:22.
317. Bean WB, Walsh JR. Venous lakes. Arch Dermatol 1956; 74:459.
318. Lanthaler M, et al. Laser therapy of venous lakes (Bean–Walsh) and telangiectasia. Plast Reconstr Surg 1984; 73:78.
319. Pasyk KA. Case 5.27: venous lake at the lower lip. In: Apfelberg DB, ed. Atlas of cutaneous laser surgery. New York: Raven; 1992.
320. Orenstein A. Case 5.28: venous lake of the lip. In: Apfelberg DB, ed. Atlas of cutaneous laser surgery. New York: Raven; 1992.
321. Neumann RA, Knobler RM. Venous lakes (Bean–Walsh) of the lips: treatment experience with the argon laser and 18 months follow-up. Clin Exp Dermatol 1990; 15:115.
322. Alcalay J, Sandbank M. The ultrastructure of cutaneous venous lakes. Int J Dermatol 1987; 26:645.
323. Rosio TJ. Case 7.31: venous lake. In: Apfelberg DB, ed. Atlas of cutaneous laser surgery. New York: Raven; 1992.
324. Rowson KEK, Mahy BWJ. Human papova (wart) virus. Bacteriol Rev 1967; 31:100.
325. Lever WF, Schaumberg-Lever G. Diseases caused by viruses. In: Lever WF, ed. Histopathology of the skin. Philadelphia: Lippincott; 1983.
326. Nemeth AJ, Reyes BA. Copper vapor laser treatment of genital and body warts. Lasers Surg Med 1950; 10:52.
327. Webster GF, Satur N, Goldman MP et al. Treatment of recalcitrant warts using the pulsed dye laser. Cutis 1996; 56:230.
328. Tan OT, Hurwitz RM, Stafford TJ. Pulsed dye laser treatment of recalcitrant verrucae: a preliminary report. Lasers Surg Med 1993; 13:127.
329. Kauvar AB, McDanial DH, Geronemus RG. Pulsed dye laser treatment of warts. Arch Fam Med 1995; 4:1035.
330. Jacobsen E, McGraw R, McCagh S. Pulsed dye laser efficacy as initial therapy for warts and against recalcitrant verrucae. Cutis 1997; 59:206.
331. Jain A, Storwick GS. Effectiveness of the 585 nm flashlamp-pulsed tunable dye laser (PTDL) for treatment of plantar verrucae. Laser Surg Med 1997; 21:500.
332. Huilgol SC, Barlow RJ, Markey AC. Failure of pulsed dye laser therapy for resistant verrucae. Clin Exp Dermatol 1996; 21:93.
333. Ross BS, Levine VJ, Nehal K et al. Pulsed dye laser treatment of warts: an update. Dermatol Surg 1999; 25:377–80.
334. Stern P, Levine N. Controlled localized heat therapy in cutaneous warts. Arch Dermatol 1992; 128:945.
335. Diakuzono N, Joffe SN, Tajiri H et al. Laserthermia: a computer controlled contact Nd:YAG system for interstitial local hyperthermia. Med Instrum 1987; 21:275.
336. Pfau A, Abd-El-Raheem TA, Baumler W et al. Nd:YAG laser hyperthermia in the treatment of recalcitrant verrucae vulgares (Regensburg's technique). Acta Derm Venereol (Stockh) 1994; 74:212.
337. Pfau A, Abd-El-Raheem TA, Baumler W et al. Treatment of recalcitrant verrucae vulgares with Nd:Yag laser hyperthermia (Regensburg's technique): preliminary results in 31 cases. J Dermatol Treat 1995; 6:39.
338. Li Y, Yang K. Treatment of recalcitrant flat warts using frequency-doubled Q-switched Nd-YAG laser. Lasers Surg Med 2001; 29:244–247.
339. Tuncel A, Gorgu M, Ayhan M, et al. Treatment of anogenital warts by pulsed dye laser. Dermatol Surg 2002; 28:350–352.

Chapter 3
Treatment of Benign Pigmented Cutaneous Lesions

Divya Railan and Suzanne Kilmer

Introduction

Significant advances in laser technology have increased the options available for the treatment of benign pigmented lesions. Lasers were first used in the treatment of pigmented lesions by Leon Goldman in the 1960s when he used the ruby laser (694 nm) to treat nevi and tattoos. The focus then shifted to the use of continuous wave modalities such as the carbon dioxide laser (10,600 nm) and the argon laser (418 nm, 514 nm). These continuous-wave lasers were used to treat pigmented lesions via nonselective destruction. Due to the lack of selectivity, the results were often unpredictable, with frequent complications such as scarring and pigmentary changes. Further progress in the laser treatment of pigmented lesions was not made until the elucidation of Anderson and Parrish's theory of selective photothermolysis, which revolutionized cutaneous laser therapy.

Principle of Selective Photothermolysis

Selective destruction of human epidermis with lasers using melanin as the target chromophore was first demonstrated in the early 1960s[1,2] using a normal-mode ruby laser (wavelength 694 nm, pulse width 500 μs). Subsequent studies with the Q-switched ruby laser using a 50-ns pulse width showed the threshold radiant exposure to be 10 to 100 times lower, suggesting a more selective effect of the shorter pulse width.[3] For the next 20 years this work was largely overlooked, until the emergence of Anderson and Parrish's theory of selective photothermolysis.[4–9] The theory of selective photothermolysis redirected attention to the concept of treating a specific target or chromophore (melanin, hemoglobin) with specific laser parameters (wavelength, pulse width, and energy level).

Wavelength selectivity limits absorption to a specific target chromophore. Thermal damage is then confined to that target by limiting the pulse width to less than or equal to the thermal relaxation time of the target chromophore. Once the pulse width is determined, energy levels can be optimized to achieve a desired effect. Application of the theory of selective photothermolysis facilitates the selection of the most appropriate laser for various pigmented lesions, without the high rates of complications and recurrence noted with destructive, continuous wave modalities. For example, melanocytes or melanin-containing keratinocytes are best targeted with a Q-switched (QS) laser in the nanosecond (ns) domain, whereas longer pulse widths used in lasers for hair removal better target clumped melanin. In both cases, when appropriate settings are used the risk of dyspigmentation and scarring is rare.

Clinical Technique

Lasers and Light Sources

Continuous-wave Lasers

The continuous-wave lasers used include the argon (488, 514 nm) green light (532 nm), and CO_2 (10,600 nm) lasers. These continuous-wave lasers are useful only for epidermal lesions because the thermal injury that accompanies their use often leads to scarring when applied to dermal lesions. When each individual lesion is treated, nonspecific thermal damage results in its destruction with subsequent denuding of the epidermis. The lesion's destruction may be followed by erythema as well as pigmentary and textural changes, but generally heals with excellent cosmetic results.

Q-switched Lasers

The Q-switched laser systems used for the treatment of superficial pigmented lesions include the 532-nm frequency-doubled Q-switched Nd:YAG, the 694-nm ruby, and the 755-nm alexandrite lasers. Strong absorption of light at these wavelengths by melanin and the nanosecond pulse duration make these lasers an excellent treatment modality for superficial and some dermal pigmented lesions in which the melanin is finely distributed. The Q-switched ruby, alexandrite, and 1064-nm Nd:YAG lasers may be useful for treating deeper pigmented lesions such as nevi of Ota and tattoos.[10] The 1064-nm Q-switched Nd:YAG laser should be used when treating darker skin types, because it greatly reduces the risk of epidermal injury and pigmentary alteration.

Long-pulsed Lasers

To better target hair follicles (which are larger melanin-containing targets), lasers with longer (millisecond-range) pulse durations were developed. These systems include the long-pulsed ruby (694 nm), alexandrite (755 nm), diode (810 nm), and Nd:YAG (1064 nm) lasers. The millisecond (ms) pulse width more closely matches the thermal relaxation time of nested melanocytes, and collateral thermal damage provides a lethal injury to melanocytes that are adjacent to the target area but that might not actually contain melanin at the time of treatment.[8–11] Because scarring may result from thermal spread, care should be taken to minimize thermal damage to surrounding collagen. Scarring is a particular concern in treating large, deeply pigmented lesions such as large congenital nevi, where the bulk of the dermis is taken up by nested melanocytes and extensive collateral thermal damage can occur to the minimal normal dermis that remains.[11,12]

Intense Pulsed Light

The noncoherent, broadband, intense pulsed light (IPL) source has also demonstrated efficacy in the treatment of pigmented lesions. IPL is particularly effective in the treatment of epidermal pigmented lesions, such as lentigines. This modality can also be safely used on darker skin types when used in a double or triple pulsed mode that allows the epidermis to cool between light pulses as well as its low risk of postinflammatory hyperpigmentation.

Table 3.1 *Laser Selection for Different Types of Pigmented Lesions*

Pathology	Lesion Type	Preferred Laser Choices
Epidermal	Lentigo	FD QS Nd:YAG (532 nm)
	Café-au-lait macule	QS ruby (694 nm)
	Ephelide	QS alexandrite (755 nm)
	Junctional nevus	Long pulse alexandrite (755 nm)
	Nevus spilus	KTP (532 nm)
	Seborrheic keratosis	QS ruby (694 nm)
Epidermal–dermal	Melasma	QS ruby (694 nm) QS alexandrite (755 nm) FD QS Nd:YAG (532/1064 nm) Erbium (2940 nm) CO_2 (10 600 nm) IPL
	Becker's nevus	Combination of two lasers Hair removal laser appropriate for skin and hair type Pigment-specific laser such as QS ruby, alexandrite, or Nd:YAG
Dermal	Congenital nevus	Laser treatment should be undertaken with caution
	Acquired nevus	Laser treatment should be undertaken with caution QS ruby (694 nm) QS alexandrite (755 nm) FD QS ND:Yag (532/1064 nm) LP alexandrite (755 nm) Diode (810 nm)
	Nevus of Ito/nevus of Ota	QS ruby (694 nm) QS alexandrite (755 nm) QS Nd:YAG (532/1064 nm)
	Blue nevus	Laser treatment should be undertaken with caution QS ruby (694 nm) QS alexandrite (755 nm) QS Nd:YAG (1064 nm)

Lesion Classification

To effectively treat pigmented lesions, they must be categorized according to depth of targeted melanin distribution – epidermal, dermal, or combination of epidermal and dermal. The most suitable device can then be decided upon (Table 3.1).

Pigment Location

Epidermal pigmented lesions include lentigo, café-au-lait macule, ephelide, junctional nevus, nevus spilus, and seborrheic keratosis. Dermal pigmented lesions include blue nevus and nevus of Ota or Ito. Some pigmented lesions, such as melasma, Becker nevus, and compound nevus, have both an epidermal and a dermal component. For some pigmented lesions, the target is melanosomes in keratinocytes, whereas in most cases it is melanosomes in melanocytes or the whole melanocyte. In some cases, the spread of thermal damage from pigment containing melanocytes may be advantageous in targeting adjacent melanocytes lacking significant melanin content (i.e. dermal nevi or compound melanocytic nevi).

The success of the Q-switched lasers in the realm of pigmented lesions is based on the ability of these lasers to selectively target melanosomes situated within melanocytes and keratinocytes. The melanosome specific damage is due to the absorption of high-energy, nanosecond, laser pulses.[5,6] Long pulsed lasers in the millisecond domain were developed to target pigmented hair. These lasers can also be used to target epidermal and dermal pigment found in larger clumps such as those in nested melanocytes or confluent melanin in the epidermis.[7–11]

Pigmented Lesion History

A principle that must be strictly adhered to is that a pigmented lesion with atypical features should never be treated with laser. Atypical features can be summarized by the acronym ABCDE:

A = asymmetry
B = border
C = color
D = diameter
E = evolving.

Lesions with atypical features should *not* be treated with a laser, and should be evaluated by a dermatologist. In addition, hypopigmentation surrounding a pigmented lesion may signal the body's immunologic response against abnormal melanocytes, and should alert the clinician to the possibility of melanoma-associated leukoderma. A patient with a personal or family history of melanoma or dysplastic nevi should be advised against laser treatment of nevi.

The treatment of congenital melanocytic nevi remains controversial due to the inability of Q-switched lasers to target the more deeply seated nevomelanocytes, which generally lack melanin and are the target chromophore. Another concern raised is that the residual melanocytes may become activated on exposure to sublethal doses of energy, thereby potentially stimulating malignant transformation, although this has not been reported. The alternative view is that decreasing the number of nevomelanocytes decreases the overall risk of these cells becoming malignant.

Laser Treatment for Epidermal Lesions

Epidermal lesions are amenable to treatment with multiple modalities because of their superficial location; virtually all injuries confined to the epidermis heal without scarring. The 532-nm (frequency-doubled [FD] Nd:YAG), and 694-nm (ruby) wavelengths are most appropriate for epidermal lesions, followed by the 755-nm (alexandrite) and, least effective, the 1064-nm wavelength (long pulse Nd:YAG). Even though less penetrating, the shorter wavelengths are particularly useful because their greater melanin absorption best targets the superficial melanin in keratinocytes and melanocytes. In addition, lesions with less melanin can still be effectively targeted such as lighter lentigines, freckles, or CALMs.

Lentigines

Lentigines are small, irregular but sharply marginated brown macules. Solar lentigo (lentigo senilis) is an acquired lentigo resulting from sun exposure. These lesions increase in number with advancing age and are usually related to the extent of past sun exposure, but are not premalignant. Histologically these lesions have elongated rete ridges that extend into the underlying papillary dermis. The basal cell layer of the epidermis often shows hypermelanosis with an increased number of basal melanocytes.

Lentigines can also be a component of different cutaneous syndromes, including lentiginosis profusa, Peutz–Jeghers syndrome, Moynahan syndrome, and LEOPARD (multiple lentigines) syndrome. In these syndromes, the histology of the lentigo is identical to a normal lentigo simplex or slightly different, with the finding that basal melanocytes are not always increased in number as with other lentigines. In addition, in Peutz–Jeghers syndrome the melanosomes are deeply melanized. Giant macromelanosomes are found in the cells of the LEOPARD syndrome.

The three Q-switched lasers and 532 nm KTP laser have demonstrated efficacy in clearance of lentigines,[12–19] as well as the noncoherent, broadband, intense pulsed light (IPL) source.[20] For the Q-switched lasers, one should utilize a 2- to 4-mm spot with a fluence that produces brisk whitening without epidermolysis. Due to concomitant hemoglobin absorption when using the 532-nm wavelength, purpura may ensue. Although the purpura generally resolves, residual erythema may be noted for the first month postoperatively. The 532 nm KTP laser will immediately darken the lesion, which will then peel off approximately 7 days later if on the face, or 10–14 days later if on the body. Purpura is not a factor as the longer pulse width does not cause bruising. The IPL should be set so that normal skin pigment is protected, but the treated lesions darken with treatment.

Case 1

Lentigo

A 28-year-old woman presented with a lentigo over the left cheek, which had failed to improve with topical hydroquinone and liquid nitrogen treatment (Fig. 3.1A). The treatment plan included IPL, daily application of sunblock and nightly application of hydroquinone. The lesion was treated at the time of the initial visit with two passes of IPL, the 1st pass at 32 J/cm^2, and the 2nd pass at 36 J/cm^2. At the 5-week follow-up appointment, complete clearing of the lentigo was noted (Fig. 3.1B).

A B

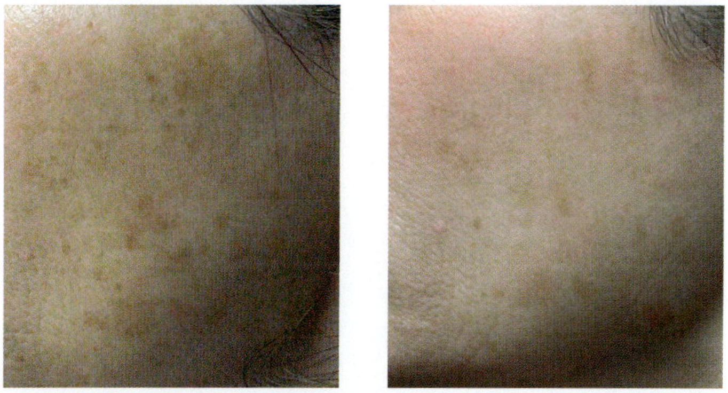

Figure 3.1 Lentigines. (A) Before and (B) 5 weeks after single intense pulsed light treatment.

Case 2
Lentigines

A 52-year-old man with numerous lentigines over bilateral dorsal forearms presented for discussion of treatment options (Fig. 3.2A). Treatment regimen included QS alexandrite (755 nm) treatment utilizing a 3 mm spot size at a fluence of 7 J/cm^2, in conjunction with strict sun protection. Dramatic clearing of lentigines over the right forearm were noted at 4-weeks posttreatment (Fig. 3.2B).

A

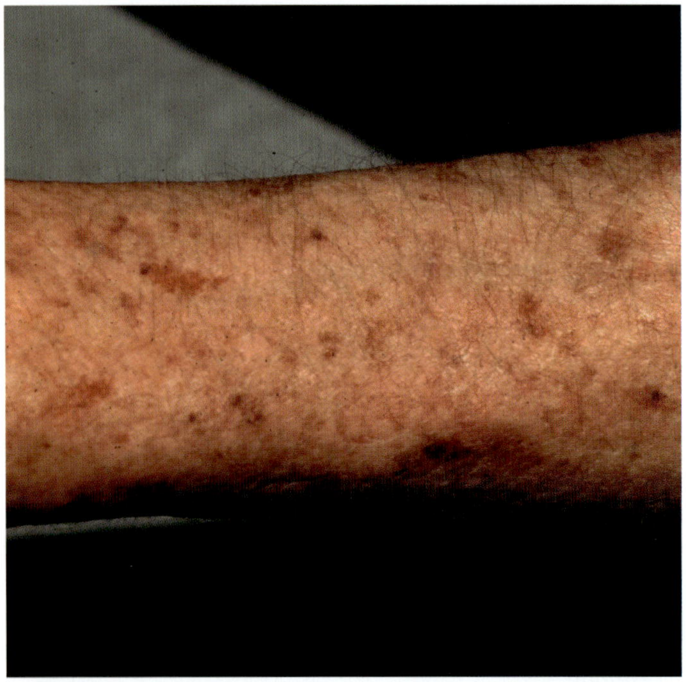

B

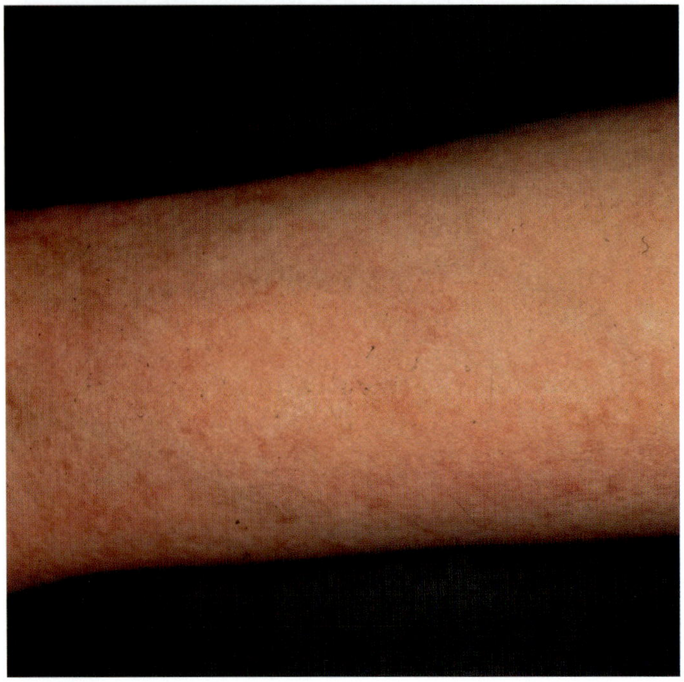

Figure 3.2 Lentigines. (A) Before and (B) 4 weeks after treatment with QS alexandrite (755 nm).

Case 3
Solar Lentigo

A 48-year-old women presents with multiple solar lentigos (Fig. 3.3A). Figure 3.3B shows the clinical appearance after one treatment with a Q-switched alexandrite laser at 9 J/cm^2. (Courtesy Mitchel P. Goldman, MD.)

Ephelides

Ephelides (commonly known as freckles) are well demarcated, tan- to dark-brown-colored macules that occur on sun-exposed skin and darken in response to sunlight. Ephelides appear early in childhood and increase in number during the summer. Their incidence decreases with age. Axillary freckling, the only type that appears in non-sun-exposed skin, is seen in von Recklinghausen disease (neurofibromatosis).

Histologically, ephelides show normal epidermis without elongation or branching of the rete ridges, as occurs in lentigines. Hypermelanization is generally confined to the basal cell layer. The total number of basal

A

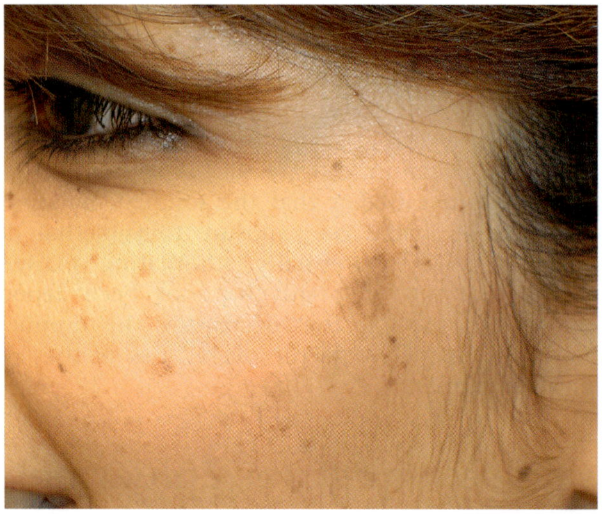

B

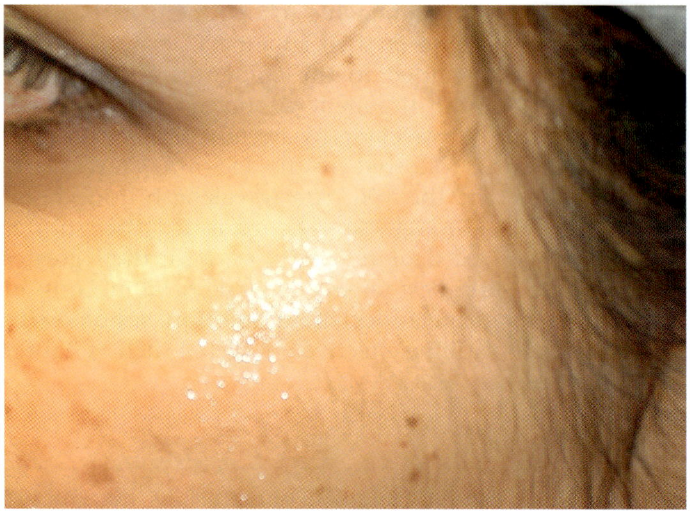

Figure 3.3 (A) Multiple solar lentigos. (B) Clinical appearance after treatment.

A B

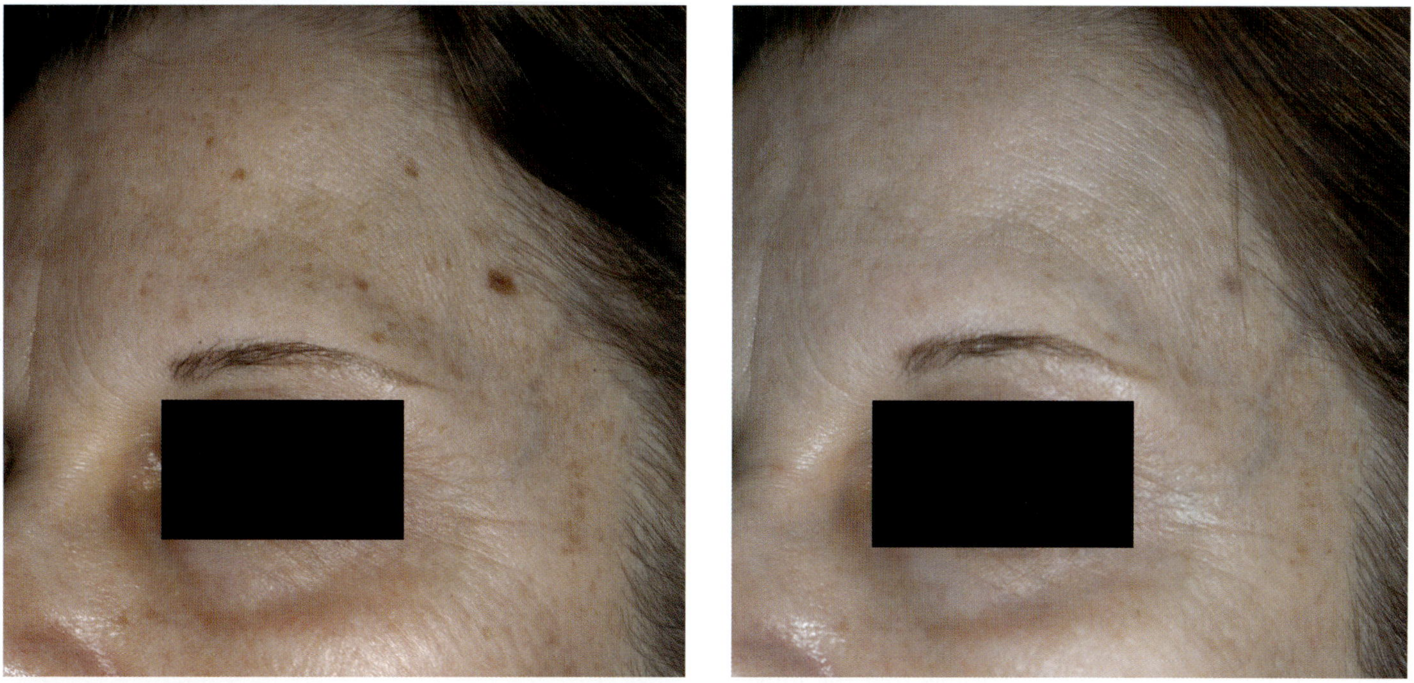

Figure 3.4 Ephelides (A) before and (B) 6 weeks after treatment with QS 532nm Nd:YAG.

melanocytes does not increase, but melanosomes and melanocytes are larger and more active.[15–17]

Treatment of ephelides usually consists of sunscreen application and sun avoidance. Hydroquinone, alpha-hydroxy acids and tretinoin can also diminish freckling if applied regularly. When requested for cosmetic purposes, similar to lentigines, the three Q-switched lasers (QS Ruby (694nm), QS alexandrite (755nm) and QS FD Nd:YAG (532nm) and KTP (532nm) can be used to treat these lesions.[18] Noncoherent, broadband IPL is also an effective modality in the treatment of ephelides.[20] Reexposure to ultraviolet light without adequate sun protection stimulates recurrence and new ephelides.

> ***Case 4***
> *Ephelides*
> A 54-year-old woman with numerous ephelides presented for evaluation and discussion of treatment options (Fig. 3.4A). The ephelides were treated with the QS 532nm Nd:YAG laser utilizing a 6-mm spot size and a fluence of 1.5 J/cm^2. Significant improvement was noted at 6-weeks follow-up (Fig. 3.4B).

Seborrheic Keratoses

Seborrheic keratoses are common benign epidermal proliferations that evolve from light-yellow, smooth macules to verrucous pigmented papules or plaques. Although there are several histopathologic variants of seborrheic keratoses, the acantholytic type is most common, consisting of interweaving bands of keratinocytes associated with variable amounts of increased epidermal pigmentation. Seborrheic keratoses respond similarly to the lasers discussed for lentigines, but thicker lesions may require additional treatments.[17–19] In addition, for thicker lesions, use of the longer pulsed alexandrite laser is more effective and

A B

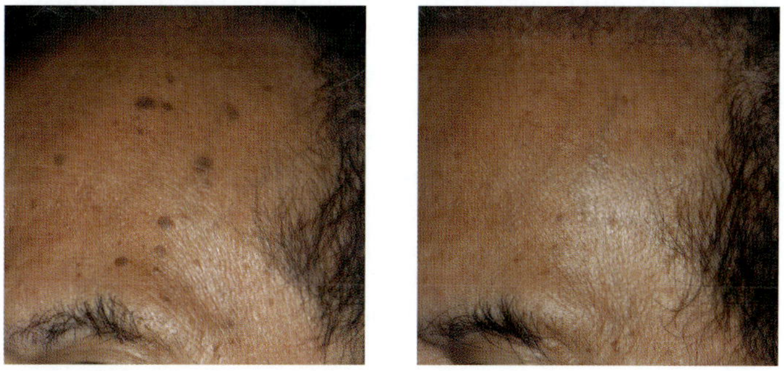

Figure 3.5 (A) Before and (B) 6 weeks after treatment with the QS Alexandrite laser (755nm).

requires fewer treatments. The long pulsed alexandrite laser can be utilized for this purpose with spot sizes ranging from 8 to 12mm, a fluence of 30–40J/cm^2, and cooling set at 20ms. Liquid nitrogen remains an excellent option.

> ***Case 5***
> *Seborrheic Keratoses*
> A 51-year-old man with history of numerous seborrheic keratoses scattered over the face, presented for discussion of treatment options (Fig. 3.5A). Options were discussed, including liquid nitrogen, electrocautery, and laser treatment. Risks of possible pigmentary change secondary to treatment were emphasized to the patient. A test spot was performed using the QS alexandrite laser at 6.5 J/cm^2 with a 3-mm spot size. When the patient returned 3 weeks later, the treated area was noted to have complete clearance without residual pigmentary change. A larger area over the left forehead was therefore treated at the same settings. Patient returned 6 weeks following treatment and was noted to have significant improvement in his seborrheic keratoses (Fig. 3.5B).

Café-au-lait Macules

Café-au-lait macules (CALMs) are light-tan to brown hypermelanotic flat lesions that are sharply demarcated from surrounding normal skin. Found in up to 13.8% of the population, CALMs may appear at birth or soon thereafter and increase in number over the first two decades of life. This lesion may be found in several syndromes, including von Recklinghausen disease, Albright syndrome, and Marfan syndrome.[21,22]

Histologically, hypermelanosis is present in the basal layer of the epidermis in melanocytes and keratinocytes. Giant melanosomes, present in keratinocytes and basal melanocytes of CALMs in patients with neurofibromatosis, have not been reported in other CALMs patients. These lesions are not associated with malignant potential and are commonly treated for cosmetic reasons.

The QS ruby (5.0- to 6.5-mm spot size with 5–8 J/cm^2), QS alexandrite (3- to 5-mm spot size with 6–9 J/cm^2) and FD QS Nd:YAG lasers (3- to 4-mm spot size with 1–4 J/cm^2) have been used to treat CALMs.[23,24] Longer pulsed alexandrite lasers have been used recently in hopes of decreasing the recurrence rate and also decreasing the number of treatment sessions required. It is possible that the longer pulse width allows for collateral thermal damage to non-pigment containing melanocytes. CALMs may recur weeks to months after laser treatment, but are often responsive to retreatment; in other cases, they can recur years later or can be very resistant to treatment. The variable behavior of CALMs implies a subset of lesions with unique biologic behavior. Repigmentation may occur from normal melanocytes in the normal surrounding skin or from melanocytes that were inactive at the time of treatment. Because the response of these lesions to laser treatment is unpredictable, it is advisable that a test spot be performed prior to treating the entire lesion.

Case 6

Café-au-lait

A 21-year-old woman with history of large café-au-lait on left anterior neck presented for evaluation (Fig. 3.6A). Treatment plan included monthly sessions of treatment with the alexandrite laser (755 nm). At the first treatment session, the lesion was treated with an 8-mm spot, and fluence of 50 J/cm^2, with multiple pulses. When she returned 6 weeks later, 50% clearance of the lesion was noted. The lesion was again treated with an 8-mm spot, 60 J/cm^2, no cooling. When she returned 3 months later, the lesion was noted to be 90% cleared (Fig. 3.6B). The café-au-lait was again treated with the alexandrite laser with an 8-mm spot, fluence of 60 J/cm^2, 50/20 cryogen cooling with three treatments approximately 6 weeks apart to treat the minimal amount of residual pigment.

A

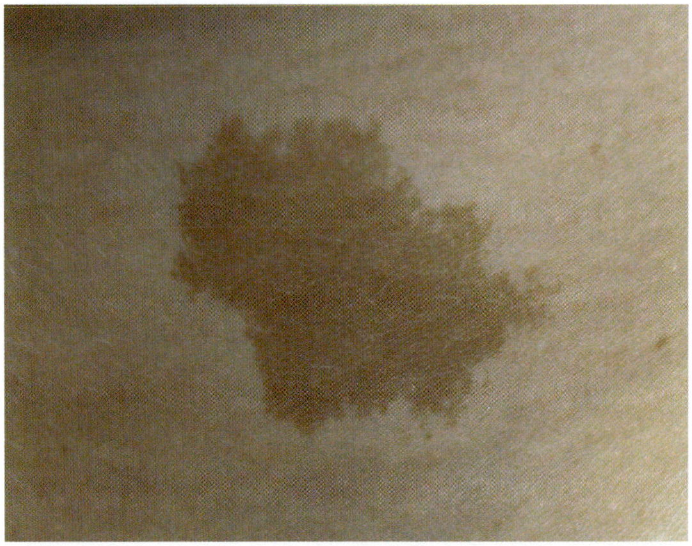

B

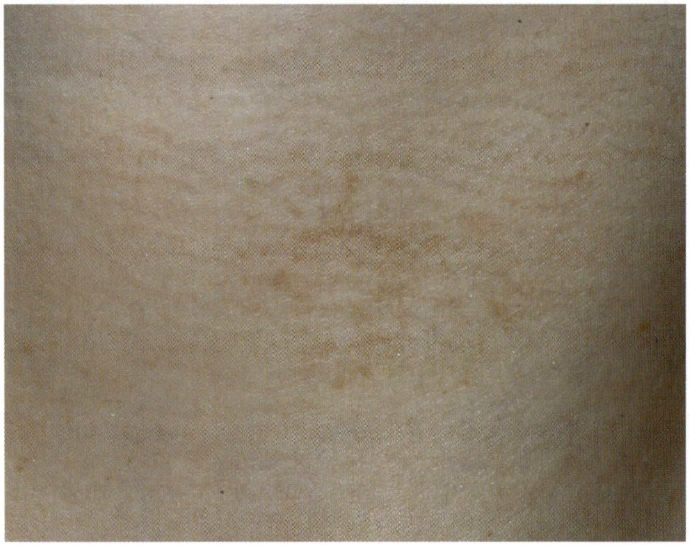

Figure 3.6 Café-au-lait. (A) Before and (B) after six treatment sessions with 755 nm alexandrite laser.

Nevi Spilus

Nevus spilus is a lesion in which darkly pigmented macules or papules lie within a typical CALM. Estimated to occur in 2.3% of patients (male and female equally) visiting a dermatology practice, nevi spilus seem to be concentrated on the trunk and lower extremities. Although nevus spilus is generally not considered to be a precursor of malignant melanoma, several studies have reported cutaneous melanomas within these nevi.

Histologically, these lesions are composed of a lentiginous elongation and hyperpigmentation of rete ridges with an increase in melanocytes. Often a nesting of nevus cells occurs within the lesion. The clinically darker speckled areas are either junctional nevi or compound nevi.

Although rare reports of nevus spilus undergoing malignant degeneration suggest exercising caution when treating them,[25–28] many report a good response to QS-ruby, QS-alexandrite and QS-FD 532 nm Nd:YAG lasers.[29,30] Unfortunately, some patients respond poorly, and complete resolution may require four or more treatments. In addition, the longer pulsed diode and alexandrite lasers in the millisecond domain can be used on the discrete nevi within the nevus spilus. The underlying biology may explain the poor responders; not all the involved melanocytes are targeted because of insufficient melanin. The histology of these lesions reveals nothing that would further explain those with a poor response. Treatment is the same as for CALM.

Laser Treatment for Epidermal–Dermal Lesions

Becker Nevus

Becker nevi usually appear in childhood or early adult life as a light-to-medium-brown patch ranging in size from as small as 2 cm to encompassing an entire shoulder. Lesions are variably hyperkeratotic, with an increase in coarseness of hair occurring during puberty. Incidence has been calculated to be 0.5% of the population. Histologically, these lesions show rete ridge elongation and basal layer hyperpigmentation with variable amounts of acanthosis and hyperkeratosis. Although no nevus cells are found, melanocytes appear to be increased, and the dermis tends to be thickened. In addition, hypertrophied sebaceous glands and bundles of smooth muscle fibers and enlarged pilar apparatus may be present. Therefore this lesion is more correctly considered an organoid hamartoma.[31,32]

Treatment of Becker nevus requires therapeutic consideration of its two pathologic components: (1) increased hair growth; and (2) increased pigmentation. The chromophore that must be targeted in its treatment is melanin. The fine clumping of melanin granules in the epidermis requires shorter pulse widths (nanosecond domain), than the larger hair follicles, which typically respond best to the millisecond pulse widths used in hair removal lasers.

Becker nevi are notoriously difficult to clear, possibly because of their hamartomatous pathophysiology. The Q-switched ruby, alexandrite, and FD Nd:YAG lasers can effectively target the increased pigmentation in Becker nevi, but recurrence is common.[33] The long pulsed alexandrite laser offers the best possibility for more permanent clearing of both the pigmentation and the increased hair growth. Settings are similar to CALM for the surrounding pigment and the hair removal lasers are used at their appropriate settings for hair color and shaft size (please refer to Chapter 5).

Melasma

Melasma is an acquired, usually symmetric, light-to-dark-brown facial hypermelanosis that develops slowly. It may be idiopathic or more often associated with pregnancy or ingestion of oral contraceptives. This disorder, with a reported incidence of 50% to 70% in pregnant women, usually occurs in the second and third trimesters. It has an incidence of 8% to 29% in women taking oral contraceptives. The etiology and pathogenesis of melasma are unknown, however, a genetic predisposition is supported by a 21% familial occurrence in one series.[34–36]

Two types of melasma exist on histologic examination. In the epidermal type the major sites of melanin deposition are in the basilar and suprabasilar layers. The melanocytes have been found to contain highly melanized melanosomes. The dermal type is characterized by melanophages in the superficial and deep dermis in addition to the epidermal hyperpigmentation. A simple clinical differentiation between the two types uses the long-wave UV Wood light examination, which shows enhancement of pigmentation in the epidermal type and not in the dermal type.

The pigmentation may be attributed to the inability to halt the underlying pathoetiologic mechanism, and therefore laser is only an option where topical regimens have failed. Repigmentation can be minimized by strict sun avoidance and sun protection, as well as regular use of hydroquinone. Strict sun avoidance and sun protection with UVA- and UVB-blocking sunscreens, is paramount. Treatment with Q-switched lasers (ruby, alexandrite, Nd:YAG), IPL, erbium, and CO_2 lasers is not satisfying and subsequent repigmentation is a common occurrence, as is postinflammatory hyperpigmentation. Test sites help to predict which patient will respond to Q-switched laser treatment. Those with a more superficial component are more likely to respond to the shorter wavelengths and those with a dermal component may respond better to longer wavelengths. A test site should be treated before undertaking treatment of the entire affected area, as some cases may be exacerbated by treatment. Superficial resurfacing with the erbium laser seems to provide the best chance for benefit, but is unpredictable, and recurrence is possible due to the condition's underlying etiology. In addition, it is difficult to treat discrete areas as concomitant actinic bronzing is removed and a relative hypopigmentation may be seen.

Laser Treatment for Dermal Lesions

Nevocellular Nevi

Common Acquired Nevi

Common acquired nevi appear after the first 6 to 12 months of life and enlarge with body growth, reaching a peak average count in the third or fourth decade. Although the exact factors that influence the natural history of common nevi are not yet fully understood, a relationship exists between sun exposure and the number of nevi. The number of nevi increases with a greater concentration in sun-exposed areas. In addition, environmental factors, such as a propensity to burn rather than tan, a history of sunburn, a tendency to freckle, and a lifestyle involving increased sun exposure, are also related to the number of benign pigmented nevi in children.

Unfortunately, the increased prevalence of benign melanocytic nevi in certain subgroups is a major predictor of malignant melanoma, with relative risks of 10 or more reported. In addition, small nevi, present from birth or in early childhood, may give rise to malignant melanomas, with approximately 44% of melanomas in the under-30 age group developing within a nevus of this type. Therefore any treatment of common acquired nevi without histologic evaluation should be undertaken cautiously.

The efficacy of Q-switched laser treatment of nevi is variable. Smaller and thinner nevi respond better; all three Q-switched laser systems (Q-switched ruby, alexandrite, and Nd:YAG lasers) are effective with minimal side effects. Unfortunately, many nevi recur or only partially respond. Long pulsed lasers (alexandrite, diode) have been shown to more effectively eradicate these nevi in fewer treatment sessions, using fluences of 40–60 J/cm^2, and 8- to 12-mm spot sizes. Cooling may be turned off for better efficacy as long as the surrounding skin is protected. Settings should be determined with consideration of the nevus color, in the context of the patient's skin type.

Case 7

Nevi

A 24-year-old man with type IV skin presented with history of dark compound melanocytic nevi over the face, and was initially interested in surgical treatment (Fig. 3.7A). He was interested in treatment but did not want to have the lesions excised due to risk of scarring. Treatment plan included monthly sessions with the diode (810 nm) laser. Lesions were treated at 1-month intervals as follows: session 1, 40 J/cm^2 and 20-ms pulse width; session 2, 40 J/cm^2 and 20-ms pulse width (double pulsed); session 3, 60 J/cm^2 and 30-ms pulse width (double pulsed). Cooling was left on due to the patient's type IV skin type. Dramatic clearing was noted on follow-up at 11 weeks after the initial visit (Fig. 3.7B).

A

B

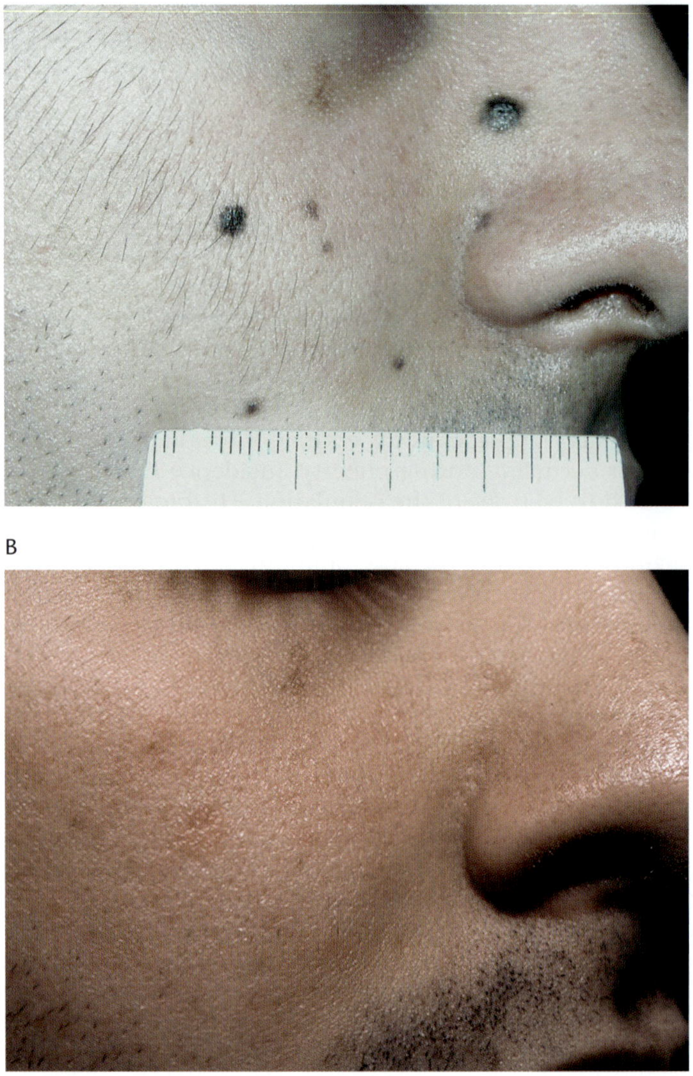

Figure 3.7 Nevi (A) Before and (B) 11 weeks after treatment with the diode (810 nm) laser.

Congenital Nevocellular Nevi

Note: Laser treatment of congenital nevi is rarely advised. Although the treatment may lighten areas of the nevus and improve its appearance, it does not remove the deeper pigment cells where malignant changes may also occur.

The prevalence of congenital nevocellular nevi ranges from 1% to 2.5% of newborns. The nevi are classified as small, intermediate or medium-sized, and large or giant. Small congenital nevi are <1.5 cm in greatest diameter, intermediate- or medium-sized congenital nevi range from 1.5 to 19.9 cm in greatest diameter, and large (or giant) congenital nevi are 20 cm or greater. The relative risk of melanoma associated with very large congenital nevocellular nevi has been estimated to be at least 17-fold, with a lifetime risk of 6.3%. Unfortunately, small congenital nevi are also infrequent precursors of melanoma. The proportion of melanomas reported to develop in association with small congenital nevi ranges from 3% to 15% and thus is several orders of magnitude greater than the expected rate based on chance occurrence.[37–43]

It is still not known whether laser treatment will increase or decrease the risk for malignant degeneration. It has been proposed that irritation of melanocytes may lead to increased risk of melanoma formation, but this is countered by the possibility that the decreased melanocytic load may in turn decrease this risk. In either case, removal of the superficial component may leave a deeper dermal component that may be changed, hidden, or not pigmented, making routine surveillance difficult. Therefore many recommend that small congenital nevi should be excised rather than undergo laser therapy whenever possible to prevent melanoma. Larger lesions, especially in cosmetically difficult areas, may be more amenable to treatment.

Laser treatment of congenital nevi with Q-switched lasers remains problematic due to the failure to destroy the deeply situated nevomelanocytes which lack pigment.[44–53] Studies by Grevelink et al[46] have demonstrated that Q-switched lasers may eliminate a number of nevus cells in the superficial and deep portions of the nevus, but many residual, deeply seated melanocytes remain unaffected by treatment. Although destruction of nevomelanocytes may decrease the risk of melanoma, sublethal doses of laser radiation may also have the potential to stimulate the growth activity of nevomelanocytes.

With these cautionary observations and background information, many patients choose to have common acquired nevi removed for cosmetic reasons. The ruby laser has been shown to be effective in removing only 12% (9 of 74) of pigmented nevi in a Japanese population.[52] In an effort to find reasons for this reported lack of efficacy, biopsies of 62 pigmented nevi were performed before and after laser treatment. Histologic examination demonstrated nevocellular nests in the mid-dermis in all the non-responding lesions and junctional nests in all successfully treated lesions. Although multiple treatments were not performed, lesions unresponsive to a single treatment might have lightened with additional therapy.

Because congenital nevocellular nevi extend into the deepest reticular dermis in many patients, it is unlikely that treatment even with a Q-switched ruby or alexandrite laser at 694 or 755 nm would destroy all these cells. A similar comparison would be the treatment of giant congenital nevi with dermabrasion. This technique, although improving the cosmetic appearance, does not remove most nevus cells and thus is not recommended as an effective treatment for the prevention of melanoma in these lesions. Laser treatment of congenital nevi, similar to dermabrasion, likely removes only the superficial pigment-bearing nevus cells, leaving residual dermal, subcutaneous, and even fascial nevus cells.[53] Some physicians accept laser removal of the superficial layer of nevus cells in congenital nevi not amenable to surgical excision because they believe removing a percentage of the potential precursors proportionately reduces the risk of melanoma and improves cosmetic appearance. This remains controversial, however, because other physicians are concerned that repeated laser injury to residual nevus cells may predispose them to malignant change, and laser-induced thermal scarring may conceal changes occurring deeper in the dermis. In addition, removal of the superficial protective pigment may make the deeper lying cells more vulnerable to ultraviolet rays. Cases must be reviewed on an individual basis with consideration of these factors.

Case 8

Congenital Nevus

This 7-year-old Asian girl presented with an unsightly nevus on the left upper lip. She was very self-conscious about its appearance. It measured 6 mm in diameter and was without any clinical atypicality (Fig. 3.8A). After a discussion with her mother regarding surgical excision and laser ablation, a decision was made to treat the lesion with a laser and watch it carefully for any atypical changes. The appearance after four monthly Q-switched ruby laser treatments given at 4–5 J/cm^2 is shown in Fig. 3.8B. Six months later (Fig. 3.8C), the lesion began to recur. After three separate Q-switched alexandrite laser treatments at 6–7 J/cm^2 given over 2 years, the lesion is almost totally resolved (Fig. 3.8D). Further treatments with the 5-ms long-pulsed alexandrite laser at 15–20 J/cm^2 was given to further improve the lesion and eliminate hairs within the lesion (Fig. 3.8E). The final appearance 6 years later – 15 years after first laser treatment – is shown in Fig. 3.8F. The lesion was treated with topical anesthetic cream (EMLA) prior to each treatment. (Courtesy of Mitchel P. Goldman, MD.)

A B C D E F

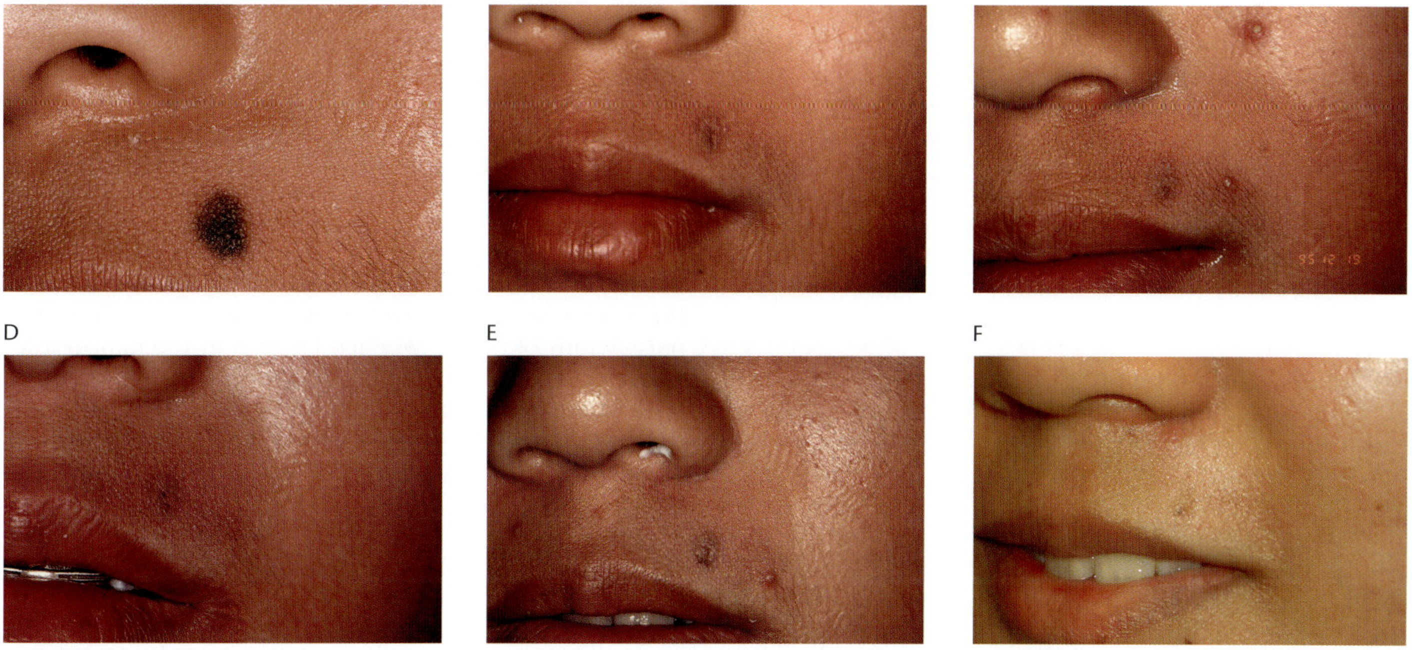

Figure 3.8 (A) Nevus on the left upper lip of a 7-year-old girl. (B) Appearance after 4-monthly Q-switched ruby laser treatments. (C) 6 months later the lesion began to recur. (D) After three separate Q-switched alexandrite laser treatments the lesion is almost totally resolved. (E) Further treatment with the 5-ms long-pulsed alexandrite laser further improved the lesion and eliminated hairs within the lesion. (F) The final appearance 10 years later.

A B

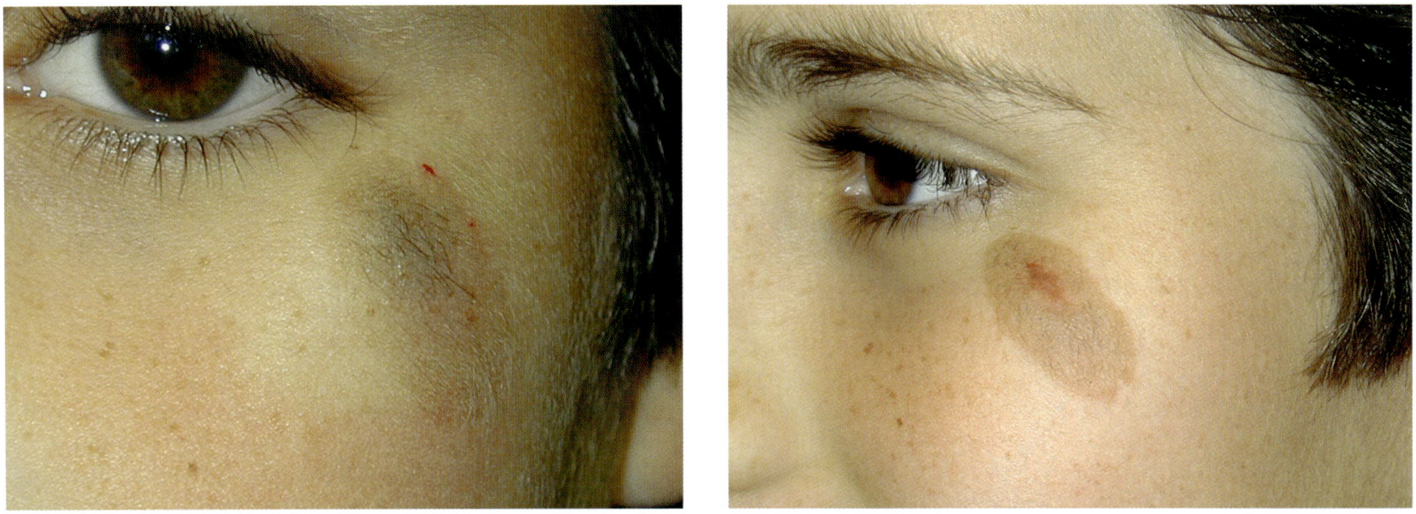

Figure 3.9 (A) A congenital hairy nevus on the left cheek of a 12-year-old girl. (B) Clinical appearance after 11 separate laser treatments.

Case 9

Congenital Hairy Nevus

This 12-year-old girl was concerned over the cosmetic appearance of a congenital hairy nevus on the left cheek (Fig. 3.9A). After a discussion with her parents regarding surgical excision versus laser treatment, a decision was made to treat the lesion with laser therapy and close clinical follow-up. Figure 3.9B shows the clinical appearance after 11 separate laser treatments consisting of: two Q-switched ruby laser treatments at 5 J/cm^2, one 510-nm 300-ms pigment lesion laser at 3 J/cm^2, one Q-switched 532-nm Nd:YAG treatment at 4 J/cm^2, three Q-switched alexandrite laser treatments at 7–8 J/cm^2, three treatments with the long-pulsed alexandrite laser at 5 ms and 20 J/cm^2, and one treatment with the Lumenis Vasculite IPL with a 640-nm cutoff filter and a double pulse of 3 ms and 3 ms, 10-ms delay between pulses at an energy of 40 J/cm^2. The lesion is lightened and there is no more hair but the color has not resolved. Local anesthesia with 1% lidocaine with epinephrine infiltrated into the lesion was performed prior to each procedure to minimize pain. (Courtesy of Mitchel P. Goldman, MD.)

Nevus of Ota, Nevus of Ito

Nevus of Ota consists of bluish gray patches on the areas of the face innervated by the first and second divisions of the trigeminal nerve. It is frequently associated with ipsilateral ocular pigmentation and has been associated with glaucoma. This nevus is most often found in Asians and people of African ancestry and has a strong predilection for females. Incidence in the Japanese population is estimated at 1% to 2%. Nevus of Ito has a similar clinical and histologic appearance to Nevus of Ota but is found in the areas innervated by the posterior supraclavicular and lateral brachial cutaneous nerves. The lesion is much rarer than nevus of Ota and the exact incidence is unknown. The clinical appearance resembles a powder blast, with poorly demarcated macules and patches blending readily with the normal surrounding skin. Lesions vary in color from brown to darker shades such as blue, gray, and purple.

Histologic examination of both lesions shows long, slender dermal melanocytes scattered largely in the upper half of the dermis. The normal dermal collagen architecture is well preserved. Although the epidermis is generally normal, focal basal hyperpigmentation may also be seen.

The lesions are usually benign, but rare cases of malignant melanoma arising in a nevus of Ota have been reported, and patients should be followed carefully. Development of new subcutaneous nodules within the lesion is particularly suggestive of malignant melanoma and the nodules should be biopsied. Ophthalmologic evaluation for possible glaucoma or ocular melanoma is necessary in patients with ocular involvement. The optimized ability of the Q-switched ruby (694 nm), alexandrite (755 nm), and Nd:YAG lasers (1064 nm), to target deeply situated melanocytes may be attributed to their longer wavelengths. Lesions containing more superficially located melanocytes may respond readily to treatment, whereas those that are deeper will likely be more resistant. The pulse width of the Q-switched lasers is in the nanosecond range, thereby effectively targeting melanocytes and minimizing thermal injury to the surrounding collagen. Lesion clearance is generally noted with fluences ranging from 6 to 10 J/cm^2, after one to seven treatments.[10,54] Start with a larger spot size at maximal fluence, then decrease spot size and retreat the area and maximal fluence available. More resistant lesions generally continue to demonstrate improvement with successive treatments, though more slowly.

Conflicting reports of fluences necessary for treatment, as well as the necessary number of treatments and treatment intervals, probably result from the variability in lesions and spot size used.[52–57] Treatments at 3-month intervals allow for macrophage engulfment, and then removal of pigment. Gradual clearing of lesions is noted after multiple treatments over several months. The optimal treatment interval between treatment sessions remains to be elucidated, however the current recommendation is to wait 3 months between treatment sessions to allow for pigment removal by melanophages and the resolution of all laser-induced hyperpigmentation, which can be facilitated by use of zinc oxide sunblock and a hydroquinone preparation.

Case 10

Nevus of Ota

An 18-year-old man with history of nevus of Ota presented for discussion of treatment options (Fig. 3.10A). He was treated with QS Nd:YAG (1064 nm) laser using a 4-mm spot, 8.7 J/cm^2 over the area with a total of four treatment sessions at 3-month intervals with significant improvement (Fig. 3.10B).

A

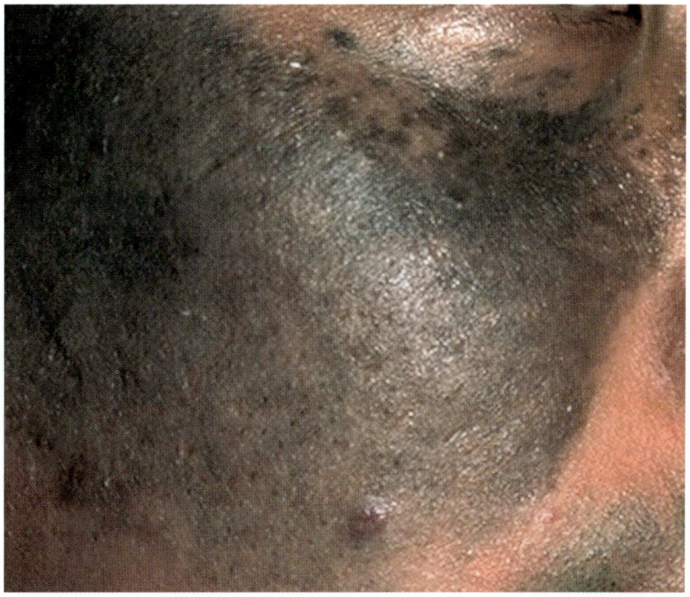

B

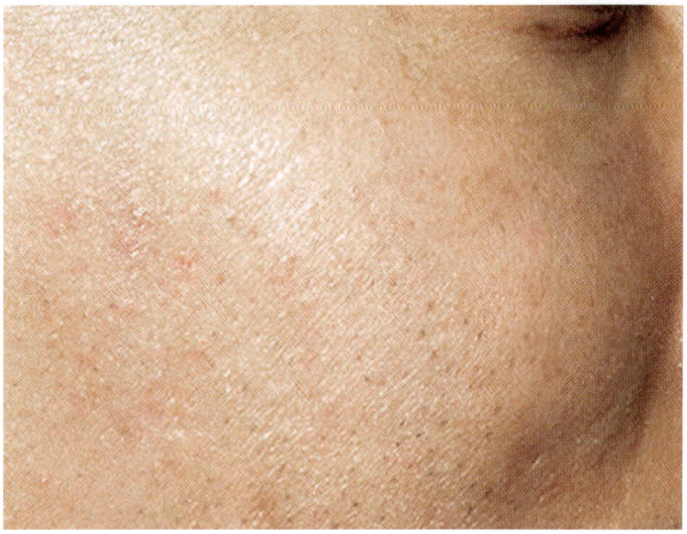

Figure 3.10 Nevus of Ota. (A) Before and (B) after four treatment sessions (at 3-month intervals) with QS Nd:YAG (1064 nm) laser.

Case 11

Nevus of Ota

This 26-year-old woman is concerned over the pigmented lesion above and below the left eyelid (Fig. 3.11A). Because of the close proximity of the lesion to the eye, an internal stainless steel eye-shield was inserted into the eye prior to treatment. The patient was required to have someone drive her to and from the office in case of any blurry vision from the use of the topical anesthetic and lubrication required for inserting the eye-shield. Local anesthesia with 1% lidocaine with epinephrine infiltrated into the lesion was performed prior to each procedure to minimize pain. Figure 3.11B shows the result after one treatment with the Q-switched alexandrite laser at 9 J/cm^2; there is 75% resolution of the lesion. Figure 3.11C shows the result 6 months after a second treatment with the Q-switched ruby laser at 5J/cm^2: there is complete resolution of the lesion. (Courtesy of Mitchel P. Goldman, MD.)

A

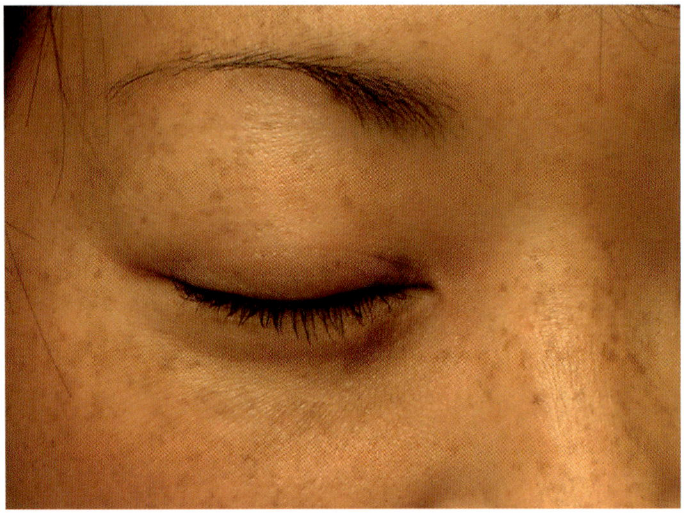

B

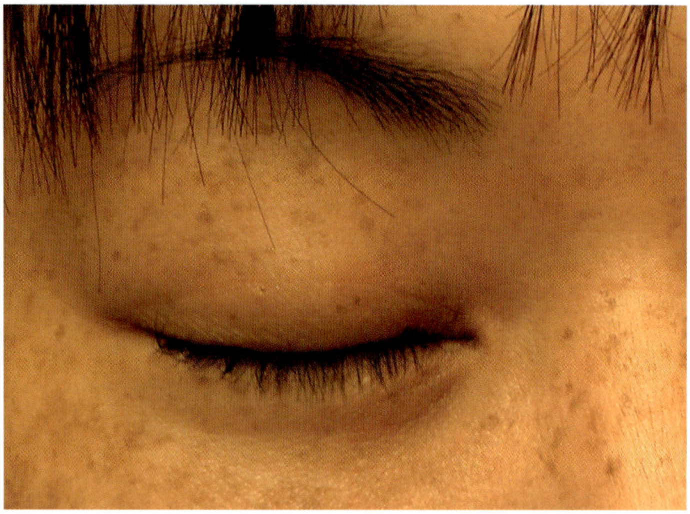

C

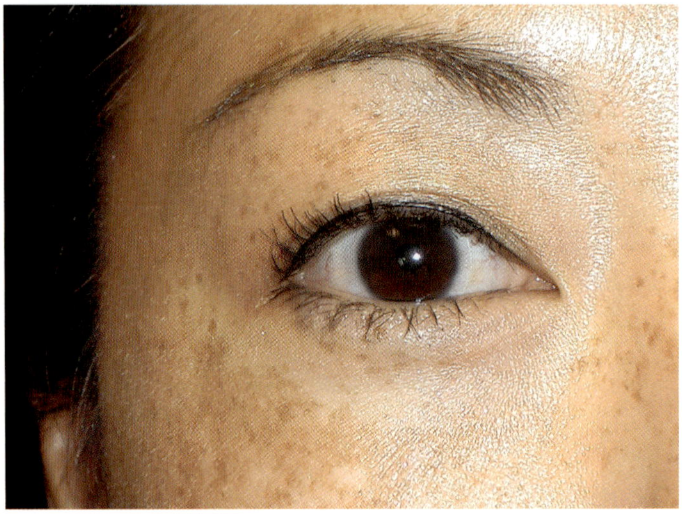

Figure 3.11 (A) Pigmented lesion above and below the left eyelid. (B) The result after one treatment with the Q-switched alexandrite laser at 9 J/cm^2; there is 75% resolution of the lesion. (C) 6 months after a second treatment with the Q-switched ruby laser at 5 J/cm^2.

Case 12

Nevus of Ito

This 3-year-old presented with a dark brown linear nevus on the lateral aspect of the neck extending to the left chin (Fig. 3.12A). Figure 3.12(B) shows the appearance 6 years after three monthly treatments with either a Q-switched ruby laser at 5 J/cm², Q-switched alexandrite laser at 8 J/cm² or Q-switched 1064 nm Nd:YAG laser at 10 J/cm². All treatments were given after topical anesthesia with EMLA cream supplemented with local infiltration with 1% lidocaine with epinephrine. The appearance 10 years after the sixth and last treatment with a Q-switched ruby laser at 5 J/cm²: the lesions is lighter but still persistent (Fig. 3.12C). (Courtesy of Mitchel P. Goldman, MD.)

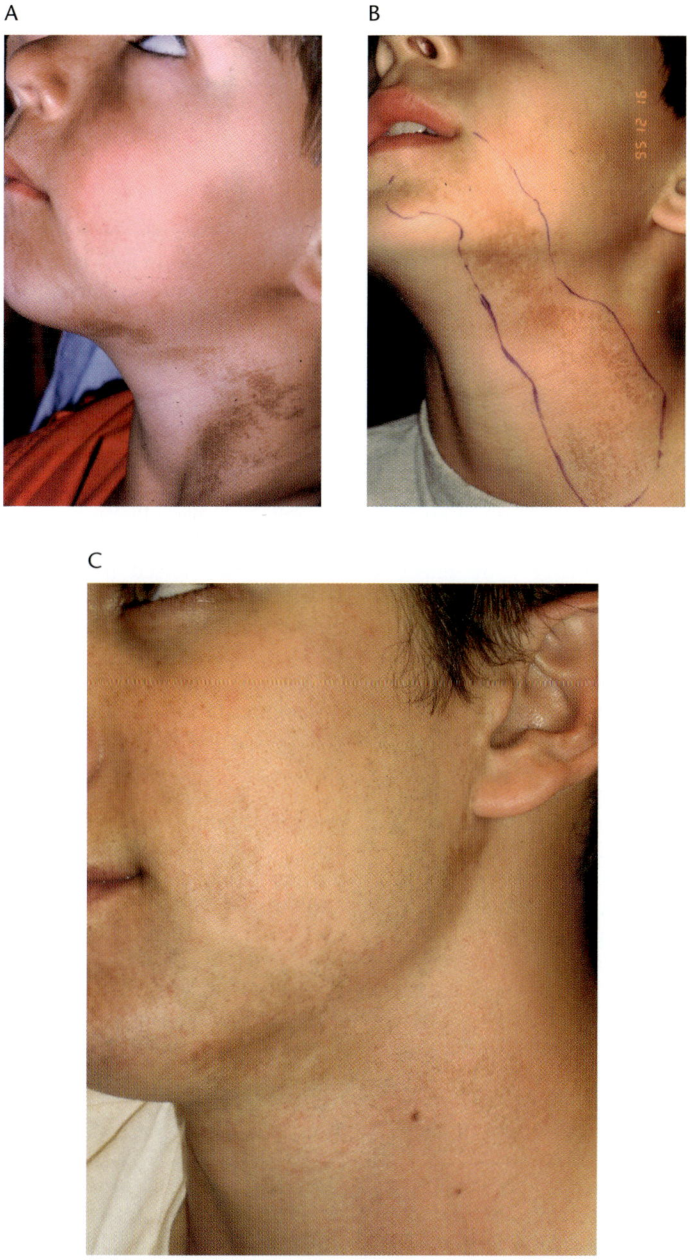

Figure 3.12 (A) A dark brown linear nevus on the lateral aspect of the neck of a 3-year-old. (B) Appearance 6 years after 3 monthly treatments. (C) Appearance 10 years after the last treatment with a Q-switched ruby laser at 5 J/cm².

Blue Nevus

Blue nevi are usually solitary, discrete, well-circumscribed papules 1 to 8 mm in diameter that arise spontaneously, most often in children and young adults. The male:female ratio is approximately 2:1. The melanin-producing cells are deep within the dermis and their blue–black color results from the Tyndall light-scattering effect of the overlying tissues.

Histologic examination shows an extensive number of spindle-shaped, elongated melanocytes within the middle and lower dermis, occasionally extending into the fat. These cells may be grouped in fascicles between collagen bundles and tend to aggregate around adnexal structures, nerves, and blood vessels.

Because of their benign nature, blue nevi are usually removed for cosmetic reasons. Although extremely rare, malignant blue nevi have been reported. The primary method of removal of these lesions is local excision. Similar to treatment of nevi of Ota and Ito, the Q-switched ruby, alexandrite, and Nd:YAG lasers should also be effective in removing these deep dermal melanocytes, as long as the lesion does not extend into the subcutaneous fat.[58–63] Biopsy should be strongly considered for lesions which are new, multinodular or plaque-like, or changing. Rare cases of malignant melanoma arising from cellular blue nevi have been reported. Cellular blue nevi should therefore be excised due to this rare but potential risk for malignant transformation.

The only mode of treatment mentioned in the literature is with the Q-switched ruby laser,[63] although all three Q-switched lasers are efficacious, similar to their use with nevus of Ota and Ito. Again, the longer-pulsed ruby and alexandrite lasers may prove effective.

Patient Selection

When determining if a patient with a pigmented lesion is appropriate for laser treatment, the patient's dermatologic history must be evaluated. Consideration must be given to the patient's Fitzpatrick skin type and their innate tendency to hyperpigment in response to inflammation.

Patients should be educated regarding the laser procedure so that they have realistic expectations. Patients should be advised of potential side effects, including hyperpigmentation, hypopigmentation, temporary or permanent textural change, scarring, or recurrence. Showing patients photographs of similar lesions, immediately post-treatment, after a few treatment sessions, and final clinical result, will increase their awareness of what to expect. It is also helpful to show examples of patients with average results, not complete clearing, so that patients are aware of the range of possible outcomes. It should be clearly stated that not all lesions can be removed completely and that successful lightening may require several treatment sessions at 6-week intervals. In addition, the unknown risk of melanoma formation must be addressed for all melanocytic lesions.

Laser Selection

Laser Technique

Most benign pigmented lesions respond fairly well to laser treatments. Those located more superficially can be treated with the shorter wavelengths of 510 and 532 nm, as well as 694 and even 755 nm. Deeper lesions require the longer wavelengths of 694, 755, and 1064 nm for better depth of penetration. Larger spot sizes also enhance the penetration depth. Unfortunately, pigmented lesions respond variably to lasers, and for any individual patient it is difficult to predict treatment outcome.

Epidermal lesions treated with the Q-switched lasers should have immediately visible superficial whitening, often associated with a slightly eroded surface, which heals over the course of approximately 7–10 days. The patient should be advised that the treated area may appear darker in color as it heals. If the lesion is treated with the QS Nd:YAG laser (532 nm), purpura may develop from the rupture of blood vessels due to the coincident absorption of hemoglobin and melanin at this wavelength. If an urticarial response to treatment is noted the patient may require oral antihistamines, and premedication with oral antihistamines should be considered prior to the next treatment session. The patient should be advised to wash the area daily with mild soap and water and cover with a layer of petrolatum or antibiotic ointment.

CLINICAL PEARLS

Atypical lesions should be carefully examined by a dermatologist and biopsied. When approaching pigmented lesions, a high level of suspicion should be maintained so that worrisome lesions are not overlooked, and appropriate treatment not delayed.

Management of Complications

The risks of laser surgery include transient hyperpigmentation or hypopigmentation, scarring, permanent hyperpigmentation, incomplete clearance of treated lesion and recurrence. Treatment of pigmented lesions is often done for cosmetic reasons. In selecting a therapeutic regimen, optimal esthetic result must be the goal in choosing the most appropriate treatment with minimal risk. Ideally, it must be both effective and free from the adverse sequelae of scarring and permanent pigmentary complications. This can be best achieved by selective targeting of pigment-containing cells. Should blistering of the treated area occur, local wound care should be administered. In an effort to minimize the risk of hyperpigmentation following laser treatment, the patient should be counseled on sun protection measures, including use of broad spectrum physical sunblock such as those containing micronized zinc dioxide.

If hyperpigmentation is noted within the healing irradiated sites, hydroquinone therapy should be used two times per day until the hyperpigmentation resolves. Avoidance of sun exposure and use of a UVA/UVB sunblock to minimize postinflammatory hyperpigmentation are recommended. If hypopigmentation does occur, it often resolves spontaneously with time. If not, the excimer laser or other narrow band ultraviolet source may be utilized. In the rare event of adverse sequelae such as scarring, it is best to implement early treatment with the pulsed dye laser.

Future Directions

The optimization of laser parameters, refinements in technique, and a better understanding of the underlying biology may further help clinicians to treat these lesions more effectively. The application of hair removal lasers in the treatment of pigmented lesions utilizes longer pulse widths. These longer pulse widths are better able to target clumped melanin and deeper lesions. In the future, we are likely to better understand the ability of hair removal lasers to treat other pigmented lesions.

References

1. Goldman L, Wilson R, Hornby P. Radiation from a Q-switched ruby laser: effect of repeated impacts of power output of 10 megawatts on a tattoo of man. J Invest Dermatol 1965; 44:69.
2. Goldman L, Rockwell J, Meyer R, et al. Laser treatment of tattoos: a preliminary survey of three years' clinical experience. JAMA 1967; 201:841.
3. Goldman L. Optical radiation hazards to the skin. In: Sliney D, Wolbarsht M, eds. Safety with lasers and other optical sources: a comprehensive handbook. New York: Plenum; 1983.
4. Anderson RR, Parrish JA. Selective photothermolysis: precise microsurgery by selective absorption of pulsed irradiation. Science 1983; 220:524.
5. Anderson RR, Parrish JA: The optics of human skin. J Invest Dermatol 1981 77:13.
6. Anderson RR, Margolis RJ, Watanabe S et al. Selective photothermolysis of cutaneous pigmentation by Q-switched Nd:YAG laser pulses at 1064, 532 and 355 nm. J Invest Dermatol 1989; 93:28.
7. Margolis RJ, Dover JS, Polla LL et al. Visible action spectrum for melanin-specific selective photothermolysis. Lasers Surg Med 1989; 9:389.
8. Kurban AK, Scearbo ME, Morrison P et al: Pulse duration effects on cutaneous pigment ablation. Lasers Surg Med 1990; Suppl 2:213A.
9. Parrish JA, Anderson RR, Harris T et al. Selective thermal effects with pulsed irradiation from laser: from organ to organelle. J Invest Dermatol 1983; 80:755.
10. Geronemus RG. Q-switched ruby laser therapy of nevus of Ota. Arch Dermatol 1992; 128:1618.
11. Kilmer SL, Chotzen VA, McClaren M et al. Diode (810 nm) laser treatment of pigmented lesions. Lasers Surg Med 2000; Suppl 12(23):55.
12. Kilmer SL, Garden JM: Laser treatment of pigmented lesions and tattoos. Semin Cutan Med Surg 2000; 19:232–244.
13. Kurban AK, Morrison PR, Trainor S et al. Pulse duration effects on cutaneous pigment. Lasers Surg Med 1992; 12:282.
14. Watanabe S, Anderson RR, Brorson S. Comparative studies of femtosecond to microsecond laser pulses on selective pig-

mented cell injury in skin. J Photochem Photobiol 1991; 53:757.
15. Goldberg DJ. Laser treatment of pigmented lesions. Dermatol Clin 1997; 15:397.
16. Kilmer SL, Wheeland RG, Goldberg DJ, Anderson RR. Treatment of epidermal pigmented lesions with the frequency-doubled Q-switched Nd:YAG laser: a controlled, single-impact, dose-response, multicenter trial. Arch Dermatol 1994; 130:1515.
17. Taylor CR, Anderson PR. Treatment of benign pigmented epidermal lesions by Q-switched ruby laser. Int J Dermatol 1993; 32:908.
18. Goldberg DJ. Benign pigmented lesions of the skin: treatment with the Q-switched ruby laser. J Dermatol Surg Oncol 1993; 19:376.
19. Tse Y, Levine VJ, McClain SA, Ashinoff R. The removal of cutaneous pigmented lesions with the Q-switched ruby laser and the Q-switched neodymium:yttrium-aluminum-garnet laser: a comparative study. J Dermatol Surg Oncol 1994; 20:795.
20. Kawada A. Shiraishi H. Asai M, et al. Clinical improvement of solar lentigines and ephelides with an intense pulsed light source. Dermatol Surg 2002; 28(6):504–8.
21. Crowe FW, Scnull WJ. Diagnostic importance of café-au-lait spot in neurofibromatosis. Intern Med 1953; 91:758.
22. Benedict PH, Szabo G, Fitzpatrick TB, Sinesi SJ. Melanotic macules in Albright's syndrome and in neurofibromatosis. JAMA 1968; 205:618–26.
23. Carpo GB, Grevelink JM, Grevelink SV. Laser treatment of pigmented lesions in children. Semin Cutaneous Med Surg 1999; 18:233.
24. Shimbashi T, Kamide R, Hashimoto T. Long-term follow-up in treatment of solar lentigo and café-au-lait macules with Q-switched ruby laser. Aesthetic Plast Surg 1997; 21:445–8.
25. Rhodes A, Mihm MC Jr. Origin of cutaneous melanoma in a congenital dysplastic nevus spilus. Arch Dermatol 19990; 126:500.
26. Rutten A, Goos M. Nevus spilus with malignant melanoma in a patient with neurofibromatosis. Arch Dermatol 1990; 126:539.
27. Cohen HJ, Minkin W, Frank S. Nevus spilus. Arch Dermatol 1970; 102:433.
28. Stewart DM, Altman J, Megregan AH. Speckled lentiginous nevus. Arch Dermatol 1978; 114:895.
29. Grevelink JM, Gonzalex S, Bonoan R et al. Treatment of nevus spilus with the Q-switched ruby laser. Dermatol Surg 1997; 23(5):365.
30. Miyasaka M, Tanino R, Morita T et al. Case 8.29: nevus spilus of the cheek; and case 8.30: nevus spilus of the left knee. In: Apfelberg DB, ed. Atlas of cutaneous laser surgery. New York: Raven; 1992.
31. Chapel TA, Tavafoghi V, Mehregan AH. Becker's melanosis: an organoid hamartoma. Cutis 1981; 27:405.
32. Haneke E. The dermal component in melanosis naeviformis Becker. J Cutan Pathol 1979; 6:53.
33. Raulin C, Schonermark MP, Greve B, Werner S. Q-switched ruby laser treatment of tattoos and benign pigmented skin lesions: a critical review. Ann Plastic Surg 1998; 41:555–65.
34. Gilchrest BA, Fitzpatrick TB, Anderson RR, Parvish JA. Localization of melanin pigmentation on the skin with Wood's lamp. Br J Dermatol 1977; 96:245.
35. Sanchez NP, Pathak MA, Sato S et al. Melasma: a clinical, light microscopic, ultrastructural and immunofluorescent study. J Am Acad Dermatol 1981; 4:698.
36. Resnick S. Melasma induced by oral contraceptive drugs. JAMA 1967; 199:95.
37. Buettner PG, Leiter U, Eigentler TK, Garbe C. Development of prognostic factors and survival in cutaneous melanoma over 25 years: an analysis of the Central Malignant Melanoma Registry of the German Dermatological Society. Cancer 2005; 103:616–24.
38. Betti R, Inselvini E, Vergani R, Crosti C. Small congenital nevi associated with melanoma: case reports and considerations. J Dermatol 2000; 27:583–90.
39. Swerdlow AJ, English JSC, Qiao Z. The risk of melanoma in patients with congenital nevi: a cohort study. J Am Acad Dermatol 1995; 32:595–9.
40. Rhodes AR. Congenital nevomelanocytic nevi: histologic patterns in the first year of life and evolution during childhood. Arch Dermatol 1986; 122:1257.
41. Marghoob AA, Schoenbach SP, Kopf AW, et al. Large congenital melanocytic nevi and the risk for the development of malignant melanoma. A prospective study. Arch Dermatol 1996; 132:170–5.
42. DeDavid M, Orlow SJ, Provost N, et al. A study of large congenital melanocytic nevi and associated malignant melanomas: review of cases in the New York University Registry and the world literature. J Am Acad Dermatol 1997; 36:409–15.
43. Dawson HA, Atherton DJ, Mayou B. A prospective study of congenital melanocytic naevi: progress report and evaluation after 6 years. Br J Dermatol 1996; 134:617–23.
44. Rosenbach A, Williams CM, Alster TS. Comparison of the Q-switched alexandrite (755 nm) and Q-switched Nd:YAG (1064 nm) lasers in the treatment of benign melanocytic nevi. Dermatol Surg 1997; 23:239.
45. Vibhagool C, Byers HR, Grevelink J. Treatment of small nevomelanocytic nevi with a Q-switched ruby laser. J Am Acad Dermatol 1997; 36(5, pt 1):738.
46. Grevelink JM, van Leeuwen RL, Anderson RR, Byers HR. Clinical and histological responses of congenital melanocytic nevi after single treatment with Q-switched lasers. Arch Dermatol 1997; 133(3):349.
47. Waldorf HA, Kauvar AN, Geronemus RG. Treatment of small and medium congenital nevi with the Q-switched ruby laser. Arch Dermatol 1996; 132(3):301.
48. Illig L, Weidner F, Hundeiker M et al. Congenital nevi 10 cm as precursors to melanoma: 52 cases, a review, and a new conception. Arch Dermatol 1985; 121:1274.
49. Rhodes AR, Sober AJ, Day CL et al. The malignant potential of small congenital nevocellular nevi: an estimate of association based on a histologic study of 234 primary cutaneous melanomas. J Am Acad Dermatol 1982; 6:230.
50. Rhodes AR, Melski JW. Small congenital nevocellular nevi and the risk of cutaneous melanoma. J Pediatr 1982; 100:219.
51. Rhodes AR. Congenital nevi: should these be excised? JAMA 1989; 262:1696.
52. Nakoaka H, Ohtsuka H. Ruby laser treatment of pigmented nevi: a histological analysis of ineffective cases. Jpn J Plast Surg 1992; 35:25.
53. Ueda S, Imayama S. Normal-mode ruby laser for treating congenital nevi. Arch Dermatol 1997; 133:355.
54. Rompel R, Moser M, Petres J. Dermabrasion of congenital nevocellular nevi: experience in 215 patients. Dermatol 1997; 194:261–7.
55. Lowe NJ, Wieder JM, Sawcer D, Burrows P. Nevus of Ota: treatment with the high energy fluences of the Q-switched ruby laser. J Am Acad Dermatol 1993; 29:997.
56. Taylor CR, Flotte TJ, Gange RW, Anderson RR. Treatment of nevus of Ota by Q-switched ruby laser. J Am Acad Dermatol 1994; 30:743.

57. Alster TS, Williams CM. Treatment of nevus of Ota by the Q-switched alexandrite laser. Dermatol Surg 1995; 21:592.
58. Patel BC, Egan CA, Lucius RW, et al. Cutaneous malignant melanoma and oculodermal melanocytosis (nevus of Ota): report of a case and review of the literature. J Am Acad Dermatol 1997; 38:862.
59. Balmaceda CM, Fetell RM, O'Brian JL, Housepian EH. Nevus of Ota and leptomeningeal melanocytic lesions. Neurology 1993; 43:381.
60. Chan HH, Leung RS, Ying SY, et al. A retrospective analysis of complications in the treatment of nevus of Ota with the Q-switched Alexandrite and Q-switched Nd:YAG lasers. Dermatol Surg 2000; 26:1000.
61. Rodriguez HA, Ackerman LV. Cellular blue nevus: clinicopathologic study of 45 cases. Cancer 1968; 21:393.
62. Rubenstein N, Kopolovic J, Wexler MR et al. Malignant blue nevus. J Dermatol Surg Oncol 1985; 11:921.
63. Milgraum SS, Cohen ME, Auletta MJ. Treatment of blue nevi with the Q-switched ruby laser. J Am Acad Dermatol 1995; 32:307.

Chapter 4

Treatment of Tattoos

Mitchel P. Goldman, Michelle Ehrlich and Suzanne Linsmeier Kilmer

Overview

Tattooing is an ancient art, the origins of which have been traced as far back as the Stone Age (12,000 before the common era [BCE]).[1] Primitive humans slashed their skin during bereavement ceremonies and rubbed ash into the cuts as a sign of grief. Decorative tattooing has been traced to the Bronze Age (8000 BCE) by the circumstantial evidence of crude needles and pigment bowls found in caves in France, Spain, and Portugal.[2] People of this age decorated animal skins worn for warmth with ochre and plant pigments. This may have led to decorative tattooing of their own skin, because mummies dating from 4000 BCE had crude tattoos.[3] Tattooing also thrived throughout ancient China, Japan, and North Africa, areas isolated by geography and absence of communication, suggesting that tattooing represents a response to an inherent human need.

Although most psychologic studies of persons with tattoos have been restricted to psychiatric inpatients,[4–6] prisoners in correctional institutions,[4–9] and military personnel,[10–12] and as such reflect only specific populations, one common conclusion of these studies is that, of all the various motives for obtaining a tattoo, the quest for personal identity is central. The skin serves as a useful canvas to portray statements of individuality, sexuality, belonging, machismo, frustration, boredom, and anger. The most commonly stated reasons for obtaining a first tattoo are 'to try something new or experimental' or 'peer pressure'.[13] The mid-1980s began a surge in tattooing popularity in the United States and recent surveys from this millennium find that 3–8% of the general population, 10–13% of adolescents, 19–35% of individuals in the 16–35-year-old age group, 11–28% of the 36–50-year-old age group, and 5–6% of Americans over age 50 have tattoos.[14–17] The average age of acquisition of a professional tattoo is 18 years[18] and that of a self-inflicted amateur tattoo 14 years.[19–21] However, one's quest for identity at ages 14 to 18 is often irrelevant or embarrassing at age 40, and 50% or more of individuals regret their tattoos.[12,17] Even Egyptian mummies from 4000 BCE show evidence of attempts at tattoo removal.[22] Motivation for tattoo removal may encompass not only internal regret and desire for more mature identity and self-expression but may be driven by external societal pressure. Tattoos may become a significant barrier to employment, social status or religious acceptance.[23,24] Because most people live in the present rather than in anticipation of future endeavors, however, tattoos remain popular.[25] Significantly, smokers are almost three times more likely than non-smokers to have tattoos, and slightly more women than men on college campuses and entering military service have tattoos.[14,16,17] In a recent study of professional women with tattoos, 94% were pleased with the tattoo,[25] although a potential bias exists in that those who were pleased may have been more likely to respond; 55% had friends with tattoos, a known influential factor. Despite this bias and stated satisfaction, 38% mentioned significant problems with having a tattoo and 28% were considering tattoo removal. In general, tattoos are not well received by the public and tattooed individuals may be perceived as antisocial, aggressive, or immature and unable to accept controls and authority.

Histology

As Ross and Anderson discuss in the introductory chapter to this text, tattoos are constituted by intracellular,

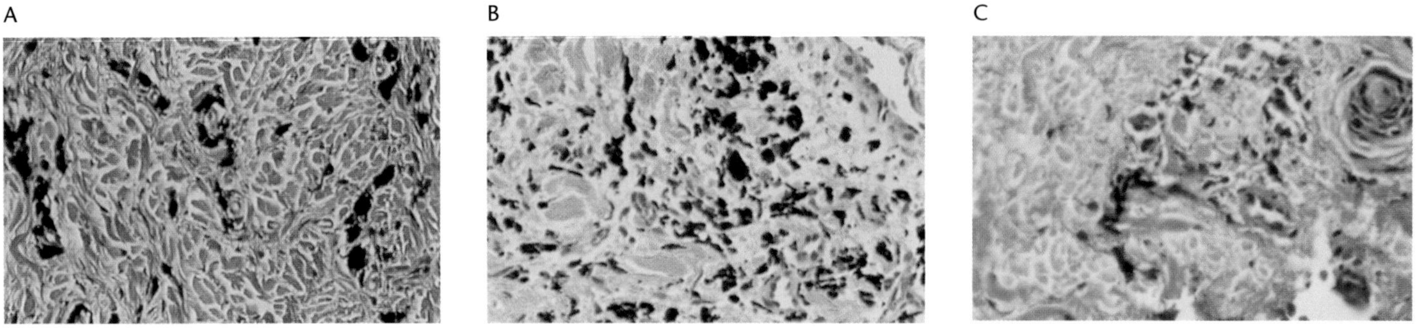

Figure 4.1 (A) Black tattoo ink in dermis. (B) Red tattoo ink in dermis. (C) Green tattoo ink in dermis (all magnification ×40).

submicrometer-sized insoluble ink particles that have been ingested by phagocytes after intradermal injection. Most amateur tattoos employ carbon-based inks such as India ink, graphite or ash, whereas professional tattoo pigments represent a wide variety of insoluble metal salts, oxides or organic compounds. Very little is known regarding the natural history of an intradermally placed tattoo. A report of serial biopsy examinations of tattoos placed 24 hours; 1, 2, and 3 months; and 40 years previously has given some insight into this process,[26] as has an electron microscopic study of tattoos treated with the Q-switched ruby,[27] argon, and tunable dye lasers.[28] Initially, ink particles are found within large phagosomes in the cytoplasm of both keratinocytes and phagocytic cells, including fibroblasts, macrophages, and mast cells.[29–31] The epidermis, epidermal–dermal junction, and papillary dermis appear homogenized immediately after tattoo injection. At 1 month the basement membrane is reforming and aggregates of ink particles are present within basal cells. In the dermis, ink-containing phagocytic cells concentrate along the epidermal–dermal border below a layer of granulation tissue closely surrounded by collagen. Pigment is not seen within mast cells, endothelial cells, pericytes, Schwann cells, in the lumina of blood and lymphatic vessels, or extracellularly. At 1 month, transepidermal elimination of ink particles through the epidermis is still in progress, with ink particles present in keratinocytes, macrophages, and fibroblasts.

Reestablishment of an intact basement membrane prevents further transepidermal loss. In biopsies obtained at 2–3 months and 40 years, ink particles are found only in dermal fibroblasts, predominantly in a perivascular location beneath a layer of fibrosis, which had replaced the granulation tissue.[32] Rabbit studies support that the fibroblast is responsible for the stable intracutaneous lifespan of the tattoo.[31] Ink particle aggregates were usually surrounded by a single membrane, suggesting they were partially free in the dermis; however, they were not found free in several studies[26,27,31] and in one study[28] were present both extracellularly as well as within fibroblasts. The interpretation of free extracellular tattoo pigment may be a consequence of the difficulty in detecting the single membrane seen by some investigators.[26,27,31] Tattoo pigment has been reported both intracellularly and extracellularly[33–39] and with mild fibrosis and occasional foreign body giant cell reactions,[32] allergic granulomas,[33,34,40–42] and sarcoid reactions.[32,43–45] Infections through cutaneous inoculation secondary to tattooing such as tuberculosis, atypical mycobacteria, veruccae and zygomycosis, and coincidental lesions including sarcoidosis, B-cell lymphoma, non-Hodgkin lymphoma, pseudolymphoma, melanoma, basal cell carcinoma and squamous cell lymphoma have been detected histologically in biopsy specimens from tattoos.[46,47]

Tattoo particles are initially dispersed diffusely as fine granules in the upper dermis as well as in vertical foci at sites of injection but aggregate to a more focal concentrated appearance between 7 and 13 days.[26,31] Black ink granules have a mean diameter of 4.42 ± 0.72 μm[26] as compared to a mean particle diameter of 4.024 ± 0.76 μm when embedded in agar. Taylor and colleagues[27] found black pigment granules in tattoos to be polymorphous, varying from 0.5 to 4.0 μm in diameter. Turquoise and red pigment particles are approximately twice as large as black granules. In both amateur and professional tattoos, pigment ink depth and density are highly variable, although greater variability of size, shape, and location is noted with amateur tattoos. However, despite the diverse origins of tattoo pigment, the light and electron microscopic appearances of all pigments are remarkably similar, except for their color (Fig. 4.1).

Tattoo pigment granules are composed of three kinds of loosely packed particles, ranging from 2 to 400 nm in diameter,[27] most often 40 nm, much less often 2 to 4 nm and slightly more electron dense, and least frequently 400 nm and very electron dense with a crystalline structure. A study of freshly implanted eyeliner tattoo ink revealed particle size in the extracellular matrix to be 0.1–1.0 μm, even though the average particle size in the pigment vial before implantation was 0.25 μm.[48] A prominent network of connective tissue surrounds each of the fibroblasts containing ink particles, effectively entrapping and immobilizing the cell. The lifespan of these fibroblasts is unknown and may persist for the individual's life.

Although these studies give considerable detail regarding the architectural morphology and physiology, they do not fully explain the natural history of dermal tattoo ink. It is common to observe that a tattoo becomes duller, bluer, more indistinct, and blurred with time, presumably a consequence of ink particles moving deeper into the dermis, by the action of mobile phagocytic cells. Indeed, random biopsies of older tattoos demonstrate pigment in the deep

Box 4.1 *Pigments Used by Tattoo Artists*[50,51]

Black
- Carbon
- Iron oxide
- Logwood (extract from logwood tree)

Blue
- Cobaltic aluminate (azure blue)

Green
- Chrome oxide (Casalis green)
- Hydrated chromium sesquioxide (Guignet green)
- Malachite green
- Lead chromate
- Ferro-ferric cyanide
- Curcumin green
- Phthalocyanine dyes (copper salts with yellow coal tar dyes)

Red
- Mercury sulfide (cinnabar)
- Cadmium selenide (cadmium red)
- Sienna (ochre: ferric hydrate and ferric sulfate)

Yellow
- Cadmium sulfide (cadmium yellow)
- Ochre
- Curcumin yellow

Brown
- Ochre

Violet
- Manganese violet

White
- Titanium dioxide, zinc oxide

Flesh
- Iron oxides (variant of ochre)

dermis as opposed to a more superficial location of newer tattoos.[49] Eventually tattoo ink appears in regional lymph nodes of tattooed patients.[49,50] After laser treatment, as Ross and Anderson discuss, tattoo ink is only partially extruded through the scale crust that forms following epidermal injury. A greater proportion of the ink particles may be fragmented, released into the extracellular space and eliminated into the lymphatics or rephagocytosed as laser-altered residual tattoo particles, perhaps with altered optical properties.

Tattoo ink is remarkably nonreactive histologically, even though many different pigments, often of unknown purity and identity, are used by tattoo artists (Box 4.1).[17,48,50–52]

Amateur tattoo inks consist of simple carbon particles from burnt wood, cotton, plastic, or paper or from a variety of inks, including India ink, various pen inks, and even vegetable matter. Although rare, red (mercury),[37,38,51,53,54] yellow (cadmium),[50,55–57] green (chromium),[51,54,57,58] and blue (cobalt)[59] tattoo pigments have elicited a persistent localized allergic or photoallergic dermatitis, and, more rarely, systemic reactions.[60–63] Laser tattoo removal has rarely been reported to cause delayed local and systemic hypersensitivity reactions and, to date, in one instance has reportedly caused immediate cutaneous hypersensitivity reaction.[64] Interestingly, the colors most often involved in allergic reactions (red and yellow) often spontaneously disappear from a tattoo, even without any clinical signs of reaction[55] (Fig. 4.2).

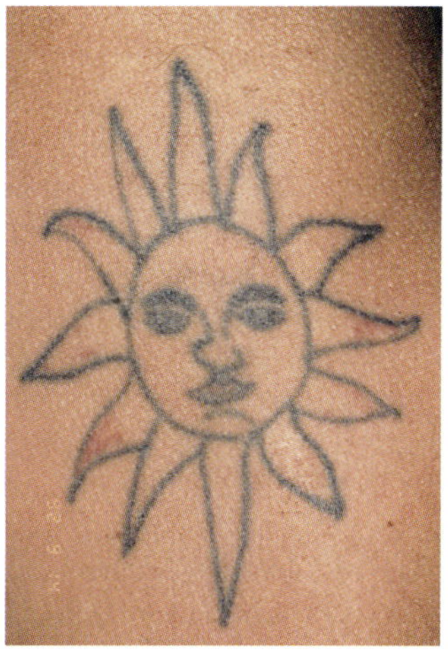

Figure 4.2 This tattoo has been present for 20 years. The original tattoo consisted of red 'flames' from the sun with yellow tips. Over the years the yellow has faded completely and the red has faded away by more than 95%.

Tattoo Removal Techniques

With the advent of Q-switched lasers operating in the nanosecond (ns) range and the future development of picosecond lasers, the promise of scarless tattoo removal has become a reality. Over centuries past, many different methods for tattoo removal have been explored. We present an overview of these techniques for historical interest.

The earliest documented report of tattoo removal was by Aetius, a Greek physician, who described salabrasion in AD 543.[65] Older tattoo removal techniques involve destruction or removal of the outer skin layers by mechanical, chemical, or thermal means, accompanied by inflammation. Transepidermal elimination of pigment occurs through denuded skin[66–69] and via an exudative phase that allows tattoo pigment to migrate to the wound surface to be absorbed into the dressing. The inflammatory response may also promote macrophage activity with increased phagocytosis, enabling additional pigment loss during the healing phase.

Mechanical Tissue Destruction

Salabrasion

This – the oldest method of physical tissue destruction – involves abrading the superficial dermis past the point of bleeding with coarse granules of common table salt and a moist gauze pad.[65] Salt is then applied to the wound surface and left in place under the surgical dressing for 24 hours. Although some authors are very enthusiastic about this procedure,[70–74] residual tattoo pigment often remains after the wound heals.

The primary method of mechanical tissue destruction is dermabrasion. To remove as much of the tattoo pigment as possible, a rapidly spinning diamond fraise wheel or a wire brush abrades skin that has usually been frozen with a skin refrigerant such as Frigiderm to produce a hard surface.[66,69] This tends to be bloody with tissue and blood particulates of a size that can access the pulmonary and mucosal surfaces, aerosolized in the operative suite,[75] with potentially infectious agents.

Subsequent scarring is worse if complete pigment removal is attempted in one session by creating a deep wound to the full depth of the tattoo pigment. Removing tissue only to the depth of the papillary dermis[67] (Fig. 4.3) minimizes scarring but leaves significant tattoo pigment, requiring additional procedures, thereby increasing the potential for scarring. To enhance the efficacy of the procedure, gentian violet[76,77] or tannic acid and silver nitrate[67] have been applied to the superficially abraded surface, and exposed pigment has been curetted[78] or removed with fine tweezers.[79,80] Other mechanical treatments include linear incisions, scratches, punctures,[76] and a grid of crisscross abrasions followed by application of a caustic chemical.[79]

The primary disadvantage of all these mechanical destructive modalities is the high risk of scarring; hypertrophic scars are very common when the removal of tissue is performed deeply in an attempt to remove all tattoo pigment. In addition, residual tattoo pigment is common (Fig. 4.4), and postoperative pain can be significant.

Surgical excision of skin containing tattoo pigment is also common but often results in incomplete tattoo removal, tissue distortion, and scarring because of limitations in wound closure and healing (Fig. 4.5). Small tattoos located in areas of adequate skin laxity allowing primary closure without excessive tension can be removed very satisfactorily with simple excision.[73] However, this situation does not occur often and complex wound closures,[72,76] skin grafting,[76,81] multistage excision,[69,73,76,79,82] and the use of tissue expanders[81] are often necessary to repair the tissue defect created by excision of the tattoo. These techniques typically result in scarring and tissue changes that are unacceptable to the patient. Split-thickness tangential excision without grafting has been reported as well[83] but has the same limitations as dermabrasion.

Chemical Tissue Destruction

Variot first described the use of caustic chemicals (tannic acid and silver nitrate) after disruption of the skin surface with punctures and incisions in 1888.[84] This technique, known as the French method, results in a less coarse scar than that which would occur from the application of more destructive chemicals[79] but often has variable amounts of residual tattoo. A combination of superficial dermabrasion and application of tannic acid also resulted in hypertrophic scarring in 34% of patients and residual tattoo in cases with deep tattoo pigment.[85]

Intradermal injection of tannic acid with the use of reciprocating needles results in epidermal and superficial dermal slough and has the same risks as other destructive modalities[65] (Fig. 4.6). Phenol solution, used in the same manner as for facial peels,[72] and trichloroacetic acid (TCA) used in a 95% solution[86,87] have been used to remove tattoos but result in hypopigmented scars. Repeat application is hazardous and may result in a full-thickness burn requiring skin grafting.

A

B

C

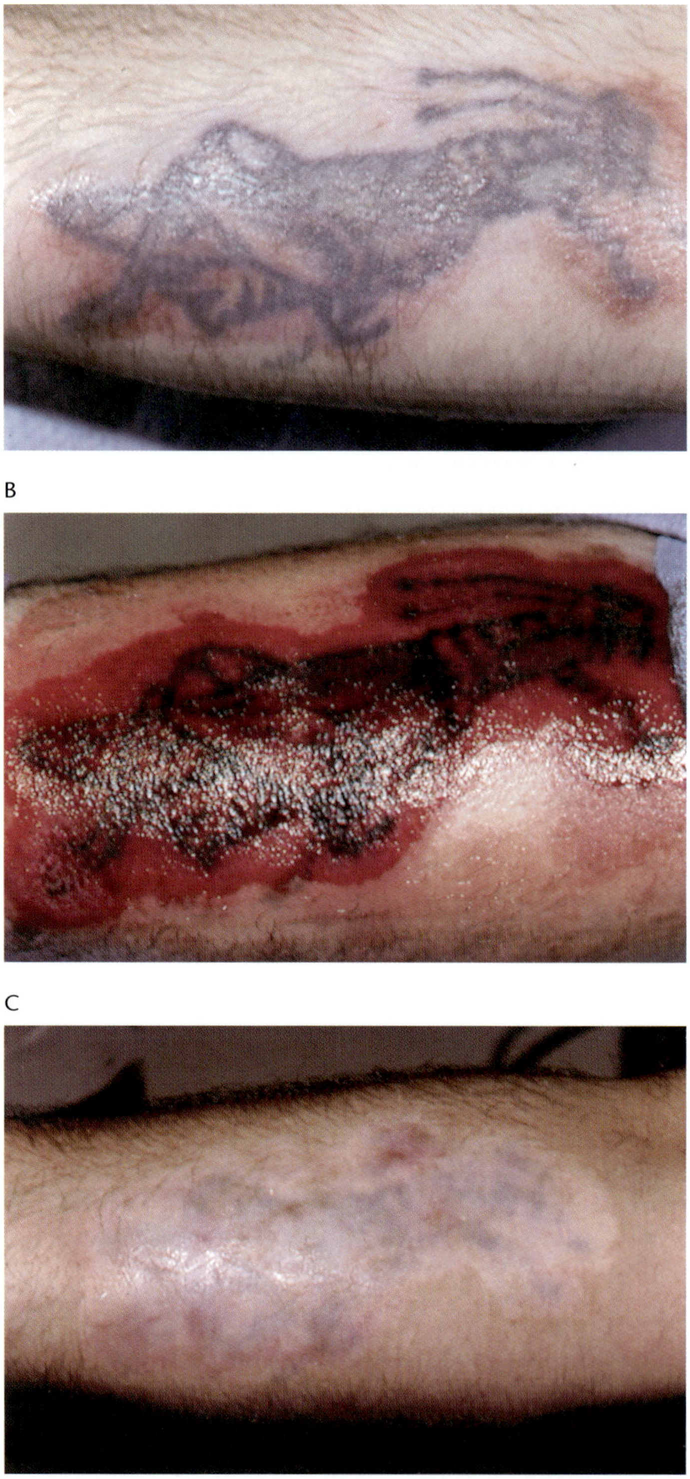

Figure 4.3 (A) Tattoo of forearm 1 month after one session of superficial dermabrasion. (B) Immediately after dermabrasion session number two. (C) Scarring and residual tattoo are evident 6 months after fourth dermabrasion session.

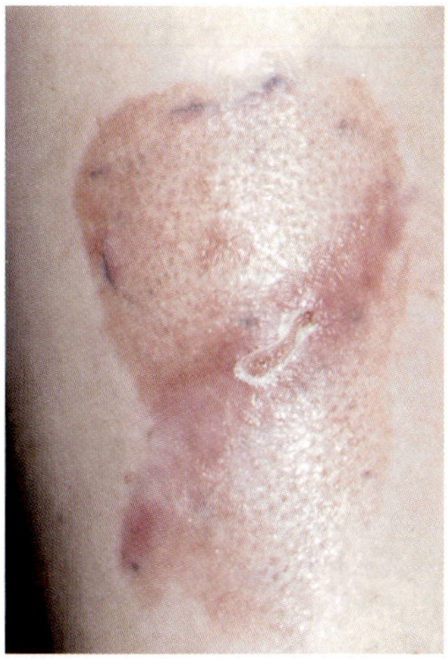

Figure 4.4 Hypertrophic scar is present in central aspect of this tattoo, as well as residual pigment at superior aspect 1 month after dermabrasion.

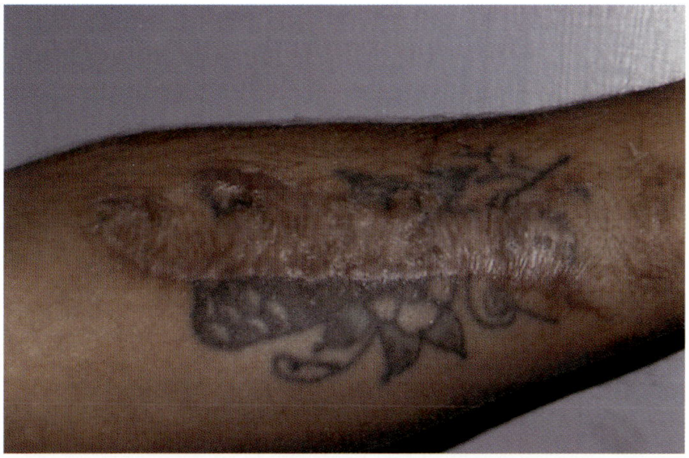

Figure 4.5 Staged linear excisions of this tattoo had been planned but were abandoned because of difficulty in wound closure. Incomplete tattoo removal and widely stretched unsightly scar are end result of procedure performed.

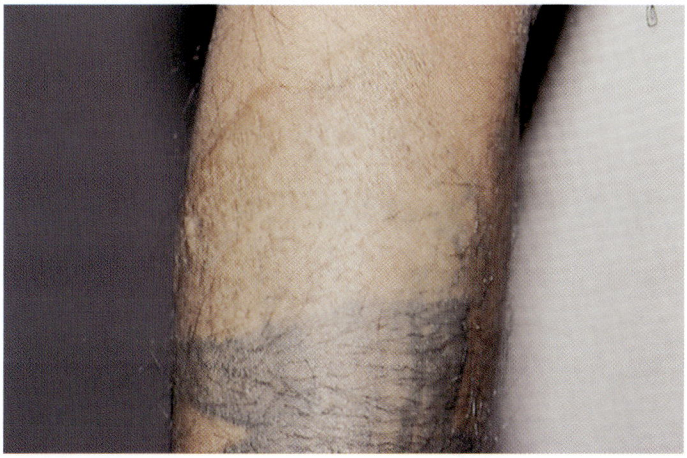

Figure 4.6 Upper portion of this tattoo was removed by injection of tannic acid into skin by a tattoo needle, which induced tissue necrosis and slough followed by hypertrophic scarring.

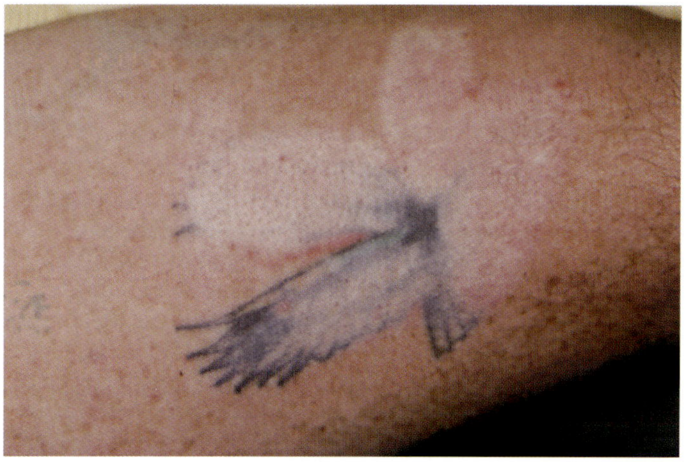

Figure 4.7 Patient attempted to remove this tattoo from his arm by heating a butter knife with a cigarette lighter flame and applying the hot knife blade to his skin. Resultant scarring and tattoo removal are comparable to other nonspecific tissue-destructive treatment modalities.

Thermal Tissue Destruction

Thermal injury, via fire, hot coals, and cigarettes, has been used for centuries in an attempt to remove unwanted tattoos, usually with significant scarring. Thermal cautery, with the use of a glowing soldering iron or an electrical spark for electrodesiccation or electrocautery, is equally crude and unpredictable (Fig. 4.7).

The infrared coagulator, developed in West Germany in 1979, delivers a noncoherent, multispectral light with preset pulses triggered by an electronic timer. This instrument is used in an attempt to produce a more controlled cutaneous thermal injury[88] for treatment of cutaneous vascular lesions[89–91] and tattoos.[91–94] A tungsten halogen light is used as the energy source and emits light with wavelengths of 400–2700 nm and a maximum emission near the infrared (IR) range at 900–960 nm. The primary tissue chromophores at this range are water and oxygenated hemoglobin, but when exogenous black and blue tattoo pigments predominate as target chromophores, a nonspecific thermal burn from heat absorption and diffusion into tissue would be expected. Pulse duration can be varied from 0.8 to 1.5 s; pulses of 1.25 and 1.5 s have been reported,[92–95] with use of a 1.125-s pulse achieving coagulation to a depth of 1 mm.[95] These pulse durations are far in excess of the thermal relaxation time of tattoo particles, blood vessels, and other dermal structures and thus produce nonspecific damage. A quartz-like guide is used to transmit light to a 6-mm sapphire tip, which is placed on the skin surface. This technique has little advantage over the other nonspecific methods reviewed, because scarring is inevitable, and incomplete tattoo removal is common. Amateur tattoos have been more responsive than professional tattoos, particularly those on the fingers.[95]

Although the use of liquid nitrogen (–196°C) to destroy superficial cutaneous lesions is commonly used in general dermatology,[96,97] it has not proved very useful in tattoo removal because the nonspecific destruction leads to prolonged healing and unpredictable results.[76,82,98] However, successful treatment has been described,[99–101] particularly the use of two 30-s freeze–thaw cycles for the treatment of digital tattoos.[101]

Thermal Tissue Destruction with Lasers

Early on, it was hoped that lasers would provide a precise means of inducing predictable thermal necrosis to tattoo-containing tissue in a manner that would eliminate scarring. With the advent of Q-switched lasers operating in the nanosecond range and the further new development of picosecond lasers, scarless tattoo removal has become a reality. Tattoo removal with the ruby and argon laser was first proposed by Goldman et al in 1963,[102] and a relatively enthusiastic report of the normal-mode ruby laser[103] was soon followed by one using the Q-switched ruby laser.[104] Goldman's initial report of successful tattoo removal using ruby (694 nm) and neodymium:yttrium-aluminum-garnet (Nd:YAG) (1060 nm) lasers appeared in 1967.[105] A study of Q-switched ruby laser interaction with tattoo pigment appeared the same year,[106] and further studies[107,108] confirmed this specific laser-tissue interaction. Unfortunately, these early reports were largely ignored for 15 years, and attention was focused on the newly emerging field of laser surgery using the argon and carbon dioxide (CO_2) lasers.

Argon Laser

The first report of the use of the argon laser for tattoo removal in 28 patients appeared in 1979.[109] Although hypertrophic scarring occurred in 21% and half of the patients had residual tattoo pigment, the complete removal of tattoo pigment in eight patients (29%) with acceptable, reportedly scarless, cosmetic results led the authors to recommend this laser enthusiastically for tattoo removal. In their subsequent study, 20 of 60 patients had complete removal of tattoo pigment without scarring, with amateur tattoos responding slightly better than professional tattoos (42% versus 29%).[110] However, hypertrophic scarring occurred in 35% of patients, and residual tattoo pigment remained in 67%. Biopsy studies showed obliteration of the dermis to a depth of 1 mm, and the authors stressed the preservation of adnexal structures to aid wound healing and avoid scarring.[109–111]

The initial use of the argon laser for treatment of tattoos was based on selective absorption of energy with vaporization from its 488- and 514-nm wavelengths by complementary tattoo pigment colors.[110,112] However, the clinical usefulness of this factor is severely limited by melanin and hemoglobin absorption of laser energy, resulting in unwanted thermal damage to tissue.[28,112] It was also originally thought that selective heating of tattoo pigments and their immediate surroundings would elicit an inflammatory response and help remove or obscure the pigment. Although nonspecific heat absorption resulted in diffuse tissue necrosis, this was thought to be necessary for successful pigment removal.[28]

A histologic study was performed to determine if it was possible to oxidize or fragment tattoo pigment, confining thermal necrosis to a zone immediately adjacent to tattoo particles and thus avoiding widespread thermal necrosis of the dermis.[28] The argon laser was used with powers ranging from 1.0 to 3.5 W and shuttered pulses of 0.2 s and 50 ms in addition to a continuous beam, using a 1-mm spot size. At 48 hours, subepidermal blisters overlying necrotic papillary dermal collagen appeared with all treatment parameters. At 3 months, fibrosis was present in the papillary and upper reticular dermis. Pigment-laden macrophages were present at the junction of fibrotic and nonfibrotic dermis, with pigment present at a deeper level within the dermis. Thus, even though these authors were able to demonstrate somewhat selective absorption of laser energy by tattoo pigment (the threshold being 6.25 J/cm^2 for black and red tattoos, compared with 20 J/cm^2 for injury to normal skin), the 50- to 200-ms pulses allowed extensive diffusion of heat from all absorbing chromophores, resulting in nonselective thermal destruction. The inflammatory response was found to be a minor factor; clinical improvement depended on widespread necrosis removing pigment and resultant fibrosis altering light transmission through the dermis to obscure underlying residual pigment. Fitzpatrick et al[113] confirmed these results and the lack of a specific laser-induced change in tattoo pigment particles as a result of argon laser therapy (Fig. 4.8). Although Apfelberg and

A

B

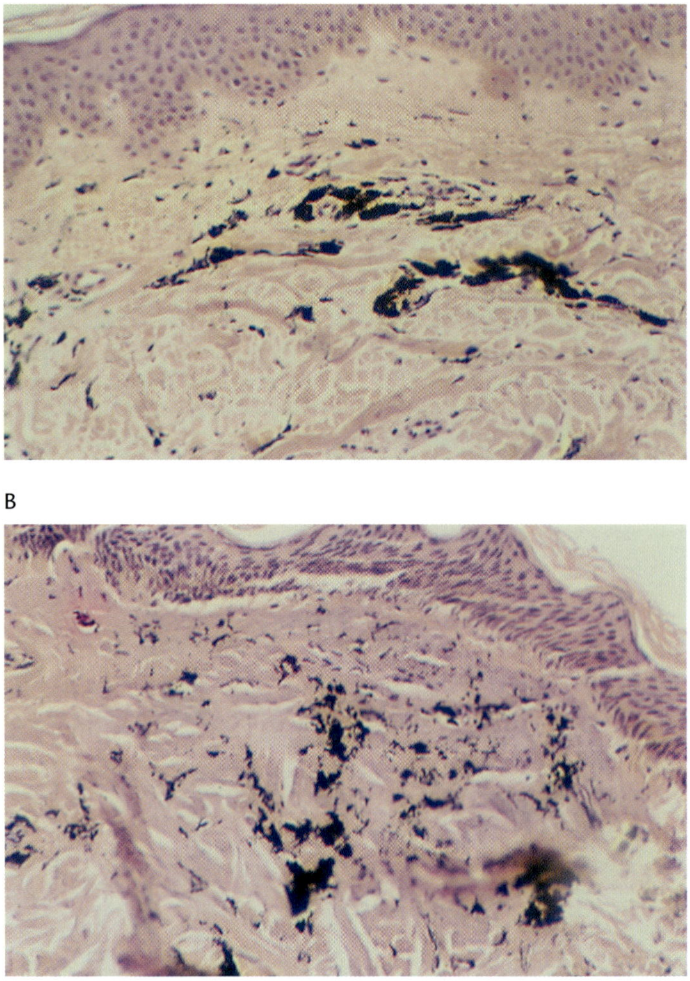

Figure 4.8 Nonspecific thermal damage of dermis and epidermis after treatment of tattoo using the argon laser at 1.2 W with a continuous beam (×40). (A) Before treatment. (B) After treatment.

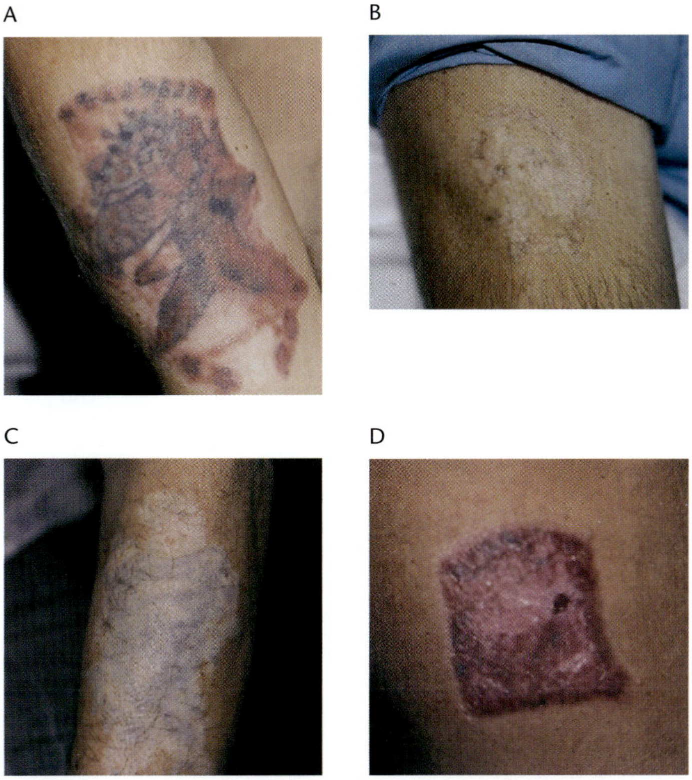

Figure 4.9 Spectrum of results of tattoo removal using argon laser. (A) Incomplete tattoo removal 1 month after single treatment session. (B) Mild scarring and minimal residual tattoo 1 year after third treatment session with argon laser. (C) Atrophic scarring, hypopigmentation, and residual pigment 6 months after seven treatment sessions with argon laser. (D) Hypertrophic scar and residual tattoo pigment after treatment with argon laser.

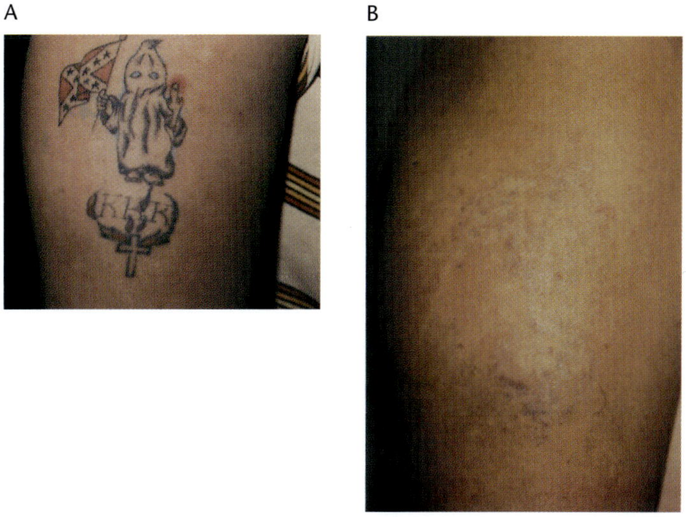

Figure 4.10 Complete removal of tattoo present less than 72 hours with two treatments of argon laser. (A) Before treatment. (B) Six months after second argon laser treatment.

colleagues[114] reported the argon laser to be comparable to the CO_2 laser for tattoo removal, the relatively low power emission of the argon laser results in inefficient removal of tattoo pigment, requiring multiple treatment sessions, and a high incidence of hypertrophic scarring (Fig. 4.9).

Carbon Dioxide Laser

Initial reports of the successful removal of tattoos with the CO_2 laser appeared in 1978,[112,115,116] and other reports followed soon thereafter.[117–120] The CO_2 laser emits a continuous beam at 10,600 nm, a wavelength completely absorbed by water, limiting penetration to a depth of 0.1 to 0.2 mm. Instantaneous transfer of heat from laser absorption by tissue (cellular) water results in immediate vaporization. The physics of this interaction were initially misinterpreted to imply that this always results in confinement of thermal damage to the 30- to 50-µm layer of laser impact. In reality, thermal diffusion can be quite extensive when a continuous beam is used. Even with pulses of 50 to 200 ms, great caution must be used to avoid unwanted thermal necrosis.

The original objective in CO_2 treatment of tattoos was to vaporize tissue containing tattoo pigment, using visual control to remove all tattoo pigment in one treatment session. Attempts were made to confine the depth of tissue vaporization to the precise level of tattoo pigment, which often varies from one portion of the tattoo to another, resulting in a variable wound depth. Histologic evaluation of the created wounds revealed loss of dermis and subcutaneous tissue up to a depth of 5 mm.[117] Because of the slow healing time (4.5 ± 1.5 weeks)[112] and resultant thick, unsightly scars, most did not attempt complete pigment removal in one session and instead treated more conservatively, relying on macrophage engulfment and transepidermal removal of tattoo pigment during the healing phase.[117] Residual pigment is retreated after healing is complete. Recently applied tattoos respond more readily to treatment with the CO_2 and argon lasers, presumably because pigment is more uniformly superficial in the papillary dermis, lying free rather than within dermal fibroblasts, particularly during the first month after application (Fig. 4.10).

Originally used as a continuous beam, repetitive pulses of 50 to 200 ms or superpulsed CO_2 lasers became more acceptable, with reports of good results in 29 of 30 tattoos after an average of 2.4 treatments. Although only a 7% incidence of hypertrophic scarring was noted, vaporization confined to the tattoo may result in a scar in its original shape; therefore feathering into normal tissue is recommended. Power settings of 8 to 25 W were common for repetitive treatments, with higher powers more rapidly vaporizing tissue.

Because of the common occurrence of residual tattoo pigment after more superficial CO_2 laser vaporization, together with the increasing risk of hypertrophic scarring with subsequent treatments, methods to improve the results of a single treatment were explored. Although the concomitant use of 2% gentian violet to prolong the exudative phase following superficial CO_2 laser vaporization did not increase efficacy, 50% urea paste did improve results,[121] as previously reported in conjunction with the argon laser.[122] Tissue is vaporized only to the papillary dermis. A generous application of 50% urea in hydrophilic ointment is applied to the wound and covered with a nonstick dressing. The dressing is changed daily with reapplication of the urea ointment for 1 to 2 weeks, until tattoo pigment is no longer seen on the bandage. This usually removes more than 95% of the tattoo pigment in a single treatment. Hypertrophic scarring depends more on anatomic location than operative technique (25% incidence for deltoid and chest areas, 10% for other locations), and although excellent results can be obtained, the cosmetic results are unpredictable and some scarring usually occurs.

In summary, the CO_2 laser removes tattoo pigment in much the same way as the argon laser, although with higher fluences, tissue vaporization with the CO_2 laser is significantly more efficient. Tattoo pigment is removed by direct tissue vaporization, as well as by thermal necrosis of adjacent tissue and through loss of pigment in the exudative healing phase. Dermal tissue is reconstituted by fibrosis and scar tissue.

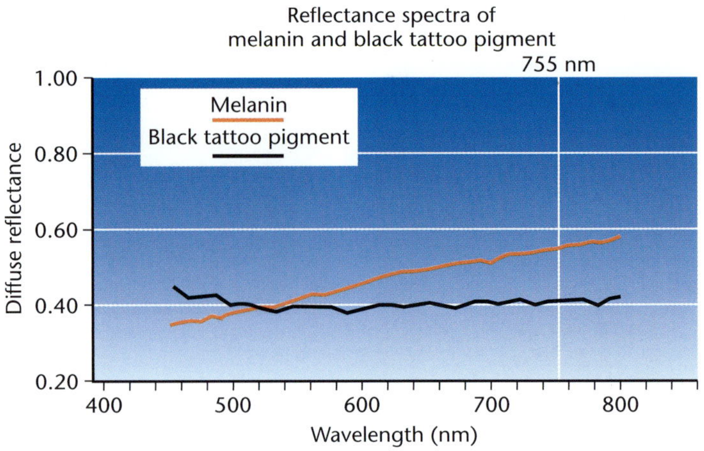

Figure 4.11 Diffuse reflectance spectra of black tattoo pigment and melanin. (Courtesy Candela Laser Corp.)

Pulsed Laser Treatment of Tattoos

Anderson and Parrish's principle of selective photothermolysis revolutionized the treatment of tattoos.[123] They proposed that if a wavelength was well absorbed by the target and the pulse width was equal to or shorter than the target's thermal relaxation time, the heat generated would be confined to the target. To target tattoos specifically, laser wavelength and pulse duration must be appropriately chosen. In one of the earliest studies, Diette et al[28] examined the effects of a tunable dye laser at three wavelengths (505, 577, and 680 nm) using a 1-µs pulse to remove black, blue, red, and white tattoo pigment. They found that the threshold dose to induce the same histologic changes was much less than that required for the argon laser, and that each wavelength reacted only with complementary colors of tattoo pigment. However, despite the short 1-µs pulse, widespread tissue necrosis was observed, and tattoo lightening occurred only as a result of significant dermal necrosis and resultant fibrosis. The authors postulated that an even shorter pulse in the nanosecond domain would interact best with the micrometer-sized pigment granule's approximate thermal relaxation time.

To destroy tattoo ink selectively, the best wavelength is chosen to achieve selective absorption for that ink color while minimizing the nonspecific thermal effects from the primary endogenous chromophores, hemoglobin and melanin. Black ink is by far the most common color seen in tattoos, followed by blue, green, red, then yellow and orange. More recently applied tattoos have an even greater range of colors, including various shades of pink, brown, purple, and even fluorescent colors. Reflectance spectra data for tattoo ink colors may aid in choosing the best available wavelength.[124,125]

Because of difficulties with absorption spectroscopy, diffuse reflectance spectroscopy was studied to model dermal tattoo ink using 17 different tattoo ink colors and six different variants of black tattoo ink mixed with gelatin

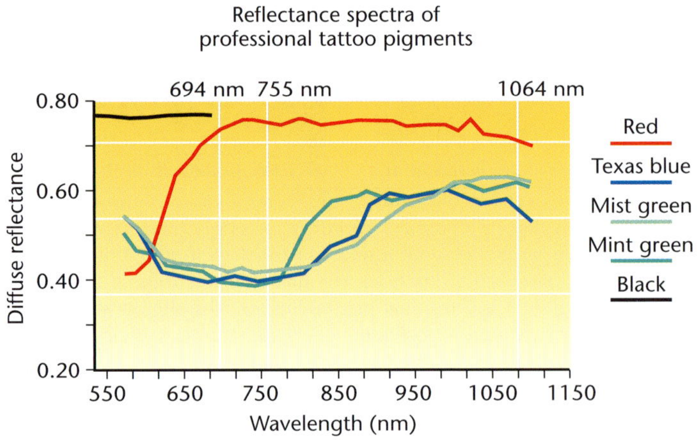

Figure 4.12 Diffuse reflectance spectra of black, blue, green, and red tattoo pigments. (Courtesy Candela Laser Corp.)

(Candela, unpublished data, 1991). Reflectance spectra were obtained from 450 to 1000 nm for each pigment and used to provide information on their absorption properties.

Figures 4.11 and 4.12 show that black pigment would be expected to be absorptive at all wavelengths (having minimal reflectance), and that competition from melanin absorption in the epidermis decreases gradually as wavelength increases. Absorption for blue and green is greatest for wavelengths of 625 to 755 nm, whereas red absorbs best below 575 nm (Figures 4.12 and 4.13). Yellow is primarily reflective above 520 nm, orange above 560 nm, and violet is very similar to red in its absorption and reflectance properties (Fig. 4.13). Tan pigment is most absorptive below 560 nm and flesh-colored pigment below approximately 535 nm (Fig. 4.14). These observations for optimal wavelength absorption for different tattoo ink colors were corroborated by Kilmer et al[124] and Hodersdal et al.[125]

Many tattoo inks are mixtures of colors with a wide range of tint (blues, greens, violets, oranges) and are difficult to classify as a single pigment. When a color is a

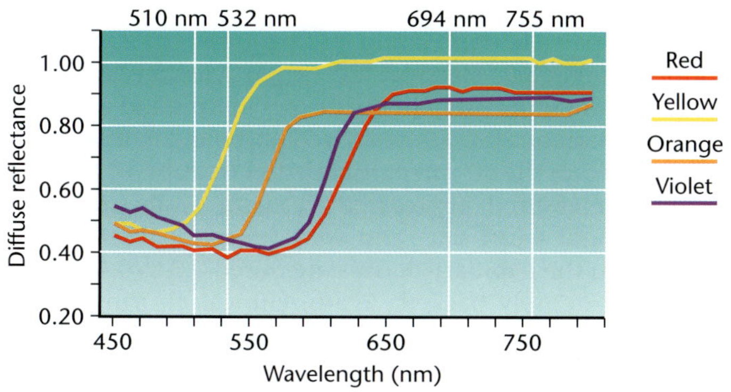

Figure 4.13 Diffuse reflectance spectra of yellow, red, violet, and orange tattoo pigments. (Courtesy Candela Laser Corp.)

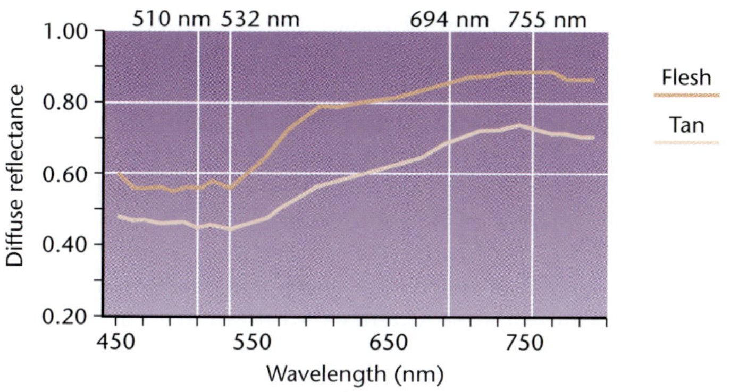

Figure 4.14 Diffuse reflectance spectra of tan and flesh-colored tattoo pigments. (Courtesy Candela Laser Corp.)

mixture of two or more pigments (one of which is reflective and one absorptive), some of the reflected light from nonabsorbing pigment will reach the absorbing pigment, causing plasma formation. The resultant reaction may be adequate to affect both pigments because of the proximity of the two pigments in the mixture.

The differing composition of amateur (elemental carbon) and professional (organic dyes mixed with metallic elements) tattoos may in part explain why the latter respond less favorably. However, the primary difference between amateur and professional tattoos may simply be the former's usual paucity of pigment granules.[126] Of 25 tattoos studied, five of eight amateur tattoos were among the ten with the lowest volume of pigment granules and cleared rapidly, and overall, tattoos responded according to their total pigment volume.

Q-switched Ruby Laser

The earliest reports of tattoo-pigment interaction with short-pulsed lasers were by Goldman et al in 1965,[103,104] who compared the reaction of a dark-blue tattoo to a Q-switched ruby laser with nanosecond pulses with a microsecond-pulsed ruby laser. They found nonspecific thermal necrosis with microsecond impacts, whereas nanosecond impacts produced only transient edema accompanied by a peculiar whitening of the impact area, lasting about 30 minutes. No thermal necrosis was present but tattoo fragments remained in the dermis. The mechanism of this reaction was unknown but was not thought to be thermal because of normal measurements taken with a thermistor. Because of the reported retention of tattoo pigment, this modality was originally interpreted as a failure. Goldman, however, followed the patient's progress and noted continued fading of the treated area. Unable to continue this work because his engineer was fatally electrocuted, Goldman abandoned the project. Only 3 years later, however, other investigators confirmed and expanded these results,[107,108] using a Q-switched ruby laser (694 nm, 20 ns) to remove blue and black tattoo pigment successfully without tissue damage. Biopsies performed after 3 months showed absence of tattoo pigment and no evidence of thermal damage. These effects were dose dependent, with fluences of 5.6 J/cm^2 or less showing absence of thermal damage but incomplete pigment removal. Higher fluences led to subepidermal blisters similar to a second-degree burn and dermal fibrosis at 3 months, although pigment removal was more complete. Subsequent studies[127,128] concluded that this treatment modality was impractical because of the small target areas and the risk of coagulation necrosis of tissue surrounding the tattoo pigment.

Reid and coworkers[129] continued to study the Q-switched ruby laser and in 1983 published an additional report on removal of black pigment in professional and amateur tattoos. They reported good results, particularly with amateur tattoos, but noted several disadvantages, including the need for multiple treatments, often six or more, for complete pigment removal. They also reported scarring in two patients and emphasized the need to use relatively low powers (but above the threshold to produce immediate tissue whitening) and the importance of the treatment interval. At least 3 weeks between treatments was necessary for tissue healing and pigment removal by macrophages. In vitro tests showed an immediate reaction in ink that could be explained only by a chemical reaction. Biopsy specimens revealed evidence of fragmentation of ink into smaller particles, which were then phagocytized by macrophages. These two phenomena correspond with the clinical observations of an immediate reduction in pigment observable the first week after treatment, followed by gradual fading over the next several weeks without further therapy.

Stimulated by studies of the Q-switched ruby laser preferentially damaging melanized cells in animal skin[130,131] and the tattoo studies previously cited, researchers at the Wellman Laboratories of Photomedicine at Harvard Medical School completed a detailed dose-response study of Q-switched ruby laser in 1990.[132] Using a 40- to 80-ns pulse, they treated 41 tattoos five times at doses of 1.5 to 4.0 J/cm^2. Of 27 amateur tattoos, eight cleared by more than 75% (all of which had been treated at 4 J/cm^2) in an average of 2.6 treatments. None of the 14 professional tattoos reached this level of clearing within five treatment sessions, and frequent purpura and rare punctate bleeding occurred. Twenty-eight tattoos with residual pigment were treated an additional five sessions at fluences of 5 to 8 J/cm^2 with more tissue damage, frequent purpura, and occasional superficial erosions noted. At the completion of this phase an additional ten amateur tattoos cleared over 75%, requiring an average of an additional 3.5 treatments. Three professional tattoos achieved this degree of clearing after an additional single high-dose treatment at 7 J/cm^2. Overall results were excellent in 78% of amateur tattoos, but only 23% of professional tattoos.

Despite these rather discouraging statistics, the authors were optimistic that the Q-switched ruby laser would develop into a preferred treatment for tattoos, because of the rare scarring. In addition, the authors stressed the competitive absorption by melanosomes leading to vacuolization of melanocytes and keratinocytes, with hypopigmentation noted in 39% (low fluences) to 46% (higher fluences) of cases. Normal pigmentation was progressively reestablished over a 4- to 12-month period; however, four of ten tattoos examined 1 year after treatment still had confetti-like hypopigmentation.

The authors agreed with previous investigators that the immediate whitening seen represents rapid localized heating with steam or gas formation resulting in dermal and epidermal vacuolization. They noted an unexplained brief emission of white light as the laser pulse struck the tattoo pigment. Interestingly, histologic persistence of altered tattoo pigment in areas of clinical clearing was noted, suggesting a change in the optical properties of the tattoo pigment.

This study was not able to establish an optimal treatment interval. Although the mean interval was 3 weeks, intervals of 1 to 5 weeks were used, and no statistical difference in responses was noted. Blue and black pigments were most responsive, whereas green and yellow responded less well, and red was poorly responsive if at all. Purpura and punctate bleeding most likely represent indirect vascular injury from photoacoustic waves generated by laser interaction with tattoo pigment. A study by Scheibner and coworkers[133] reported preliminary results of treatment of 101 amateur and 62 professional tattoos using fluences of 2 to 4 J/cm^2 with a 40-ns pulse width, spot sizes of 5 and 8 mm, and a treatment interval of 5 to 6 weeks. Although details of response are lacking, after an average of four treatments, 87% of amateur tattoos were greater than 80% clear, whereas of 62 professional tattoos, only 11% were greater than 80% clear. Treated areas required 10 to 14 days to heal and remained erythematous for an additional 1 to 3 weeks, and most patients developed hypopigmentation lasting 2 to 6 months. Skin textural changes resolved over 6 to 8 weeks, with no scarring reported. Tattoos of the face and neck responded sooner but were more sensitive to tissue damage, necessitating the use of lower fluences. Interestingly, a better response was noted with older professional tattoos and blue inks than with other colors.

As stated earlier, Taylor and colleagues[27] reported on light and electron microscopic analysis of Q-switched ruby laser-treated tattoos. After irradiation, all three previously described particle types could still be found, in addition to round, lamellated, electron-lucent particles measuring 25 to 40 nm and more often in the deeper dermis and even into the subcutaneous fat. These altered particles are thought to originate from the 40-nm particle. After treatment, pigment granules measured approximately 1 μm (compared with their original 4-μm size) and were loosely packed. Those granules in the papillary dermis measured 0.2 to 0.4 μm and were very densely packed. Again, clinical clearing poorly correlated with histologic clearing, because tattoos responding well often had residual pigment.

The mechanism of action of the Q-switched ruby laser is through photon absorption by tattoo pigment within fibroblasts. During the 40-ns pulse, temperatures exceeding 1000°C can occur. Gaseous products of pyrolysis or pores created by superheated steam may account for the lamellated appearance of the granules after laser exposure. The reduction in pigment particle size and fragmentation of pigment-containing cells probably result from rapid thermal expansion, shock waves, and potentially localized cavitation. Fluence-dependent thermal damage to collagen immediately surrounding the irradiated tattoo pigment also occurs. Computer simulation models confirm that the breakup of tattoo particles is photoacoustic, and the optimal pulse duration for photoacoustic destruction of tattoo particles with minimal non-specific damage to the surrounding tissue would be in the 10–100 picosecond range.[134]

Newer ruby lasers with a shorter pulse duration (approximately 25 ns), higher fluences (8–10 J/cm^2), and better beam quality more rapidly clear tattoos.[135,136] Lowe et al[137] reported similar results using 10 J/cm^2 at 6- to 8-week intervals and after five treatment sessions reported 22 of 28 professional tattoos as having excellent results (greater than 75% improvement) (Fig. 4.15). Levins and coworkers'

A B

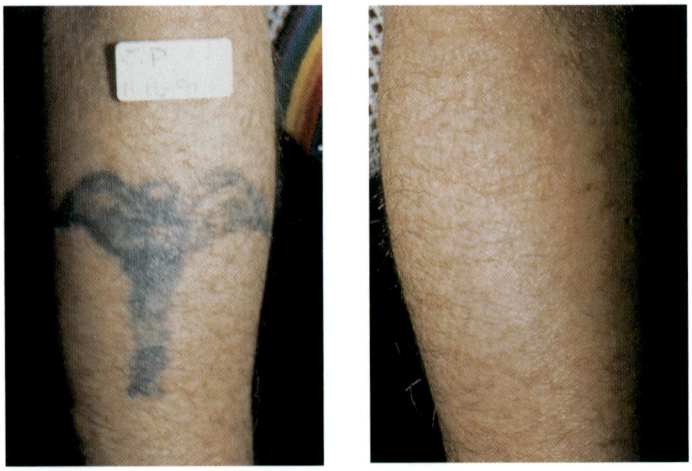

Figure 4.15 Virtually complete tattoo pigment removal after two treatments with ruby laser at 10 J/cm^2 with 8 weeks between treatments. (A) Before treatment. (B) Approximately 6 months after second treatment. (Courtesy Dr Nicholas Lowe, Santa Monica, CA.)

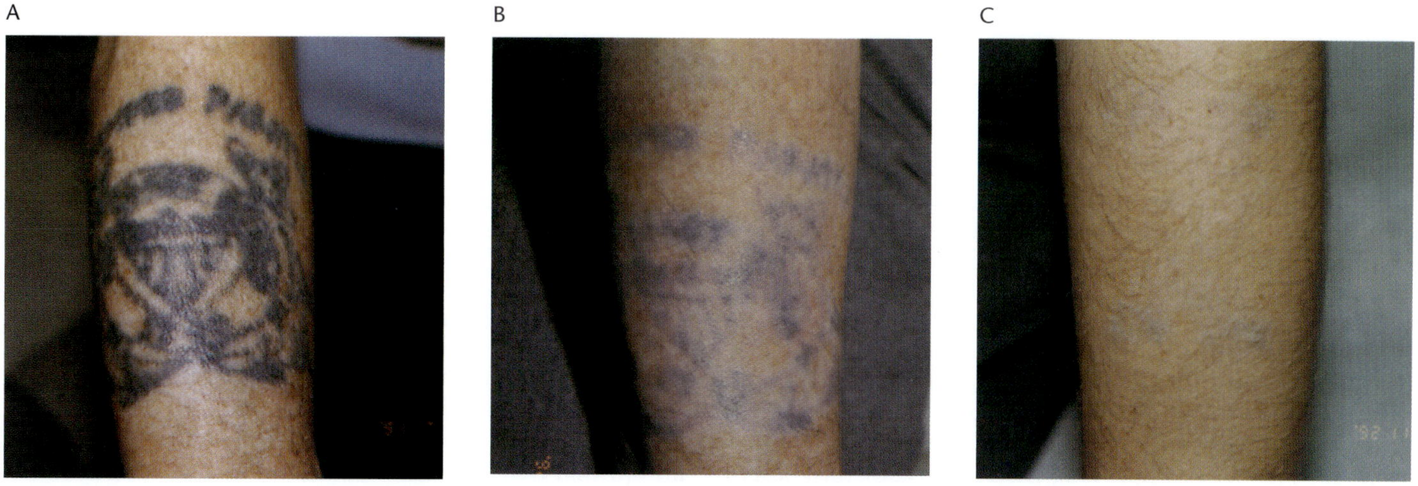

Figure 4.16 (A) Tattoo before treatment. (B) Tattoo after four treatments with the ruby laser. (C) Tattoo after five treatments with ruby laser. Green pigment remains. (Courtesy Dr Joop Grevelink, Massachusetts General Hospital Laser Center.)

preliminary report was similar, with excellent results and minimal side effects.[138] In addition to amateur and professional tattoos, cosmetic, iatrogenic, traumatic and mucosal amalgam tattoos have been removed without scarring using Q-switched ruby lasers.[66,139–141]

Kilmer and Anderson[142] initiated treatment at a fluence of 6 to 8 J/cm^2 with a 40- to 80-ns pulse width and reported black and green ink to be most responsive, with other colors requiring significantly more treatments. Amateur tattoos usually required four to six treatment sessions and professional tattoos six to ten sessions, but in some instances up to 20 treatment sessions were needed. The authors noted several trends: professional, distally located, recently placed, or deeply placed tattoos may be difficult to remove, requiring more treatment sessions to eradicate them completely. Acceptable clearing varied greatly from patient to patient, with some individuals more accepting of vague residual pigment.

In summary, the Q-switched ruby laser is remarkably effective in removing tattoos with minimal scarring, although multiple treatment sessions are necessary (Fig. 4.16). Hypopigmentation is common (more than 50% of patients), and although usually transient (2 to 6 months), it may be permanent[142] (Fig. 4.17). Transient hyperpigmentation is also common and seems to be related more to skin type than laser treatment (Fig. 4.18). Scarring and textural changes occur more rarely. The risk of adverse tissue response and speed of clearing both appear to be related to fluence and pulse width, with higher fluences and shorter pulses being more effective but causing more nonspecific tissue damage as well. These high-energy short pulses cause a pressure shock wave that ruptures blood vessels and aerosolizes tissue with potentially infectious particles, requiring the use of a protective barrier or a plastic tube to protect the operator from tissue and blood contact. The use of lower fluences eliminates this problem to a large degree but results in the need for more treatment sessions. The occurrence of scarring or tissue textural changes has also been attributed to hot spots within the

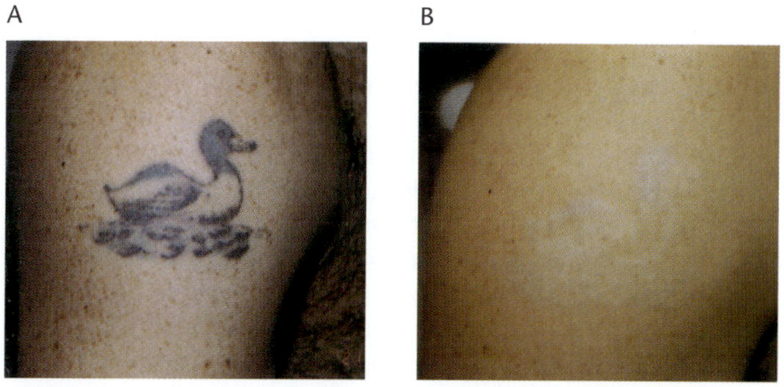

Figure 4.17 (A) Tattoo before treatment. (B) Tattoo after eight treatments with ruby laser. Mild hypopigmentation and persistence of some green pigment are visible. (Courtesy Dr Joop Grevelink, Massachusetts General Hospital Laser Center.)

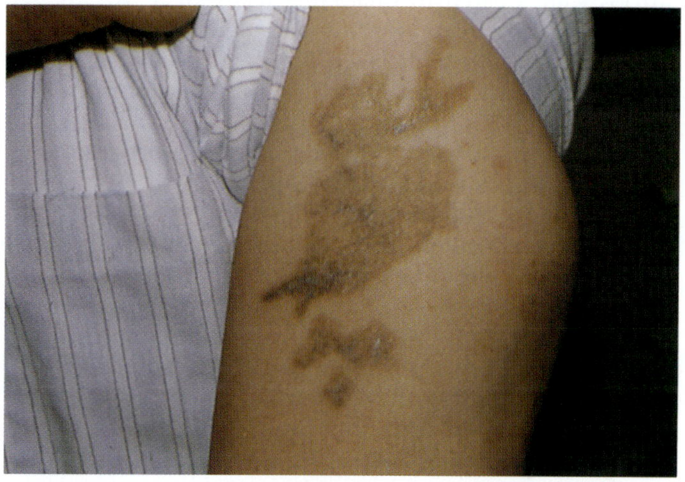

Figure 4.18 Transient hyperpigmentation of area treated with Q-switched ruby laser. (Courtesy Dr Joop Grevelink, Massachusetts General Hospital Laser Center.)

beam and pulse-to-pulse variability. The ruby laser is very effective for removing black, blue-black, and green ink; green ink can be difficult, even though reflectance spectra predict that it should respond to a 694-nm wavelength. Other colors are poorly responsive. The ruby laser has a repetitive rate of 1 pulse every 1 to 2 s, but no aiming beam to assist in proper alignment. Bleeding and tissue splatter can be cumbersome, but use of cone devices protect the operator from exposure.

Q-switched Nd:YAG Laser

The Q-switched Nd:YAG laser was then explored in anticipation that its longer wavelength (1064 nm) would increase dermal penetration and decrease melanin absorption (see Fig. 4.11), improving the response of ruby laser-resistant tattoos and avoiding pigmentary changes. An initial report of 20 professional and three amateur tattoos in four treatment sessions showed the Nd:YAG laser to be equal to the ruby laser in removal of blue–black tattoos at 6 J/cm^2. Hypopigmentation and skin texture change were more common with the ruby laser. Green and red pigment were not removed with the Nd:YAG laser, whereas some green pigment was removed with the ruby laser.[143]

The ability of the Q-switched Nd:YAG laser (1064 nm, 10 ns, 5 Hz) to remove pigment in ruby laser-resistant tattoos was assessed in the treatment of 28 tattoos (23 professional, five amateur) using fluences of 6 to 12 J/cm^2 with a 2.5-mm-diameter spot size. In most cases, greater than 50% lightening of residual tattoo ink was noted with the first treatment, with the greatest improvement seen with higher fluences.[144] Unfortunately, the higher fluences (12 J/cm^2) and shorter pulses (10 ns) resulted in more tissue debris and bleeding, necessitating the use of a plastic shield or transparent membrane to promote laser operator safety.[145]

Kilmer et al[146] investigated both ruby laser-resistant and untreated tattoos in a prospective, blinded, dose-response study using the Q-switched Nd:YAG laser (2.5-mm spot size). Twenty-five professional tattoos and 14 amateur tattoos were treated in quadrants using 6, 8, 10, and 12 J/cm^2. Four treatment sessions were performed at 3- to 4-week intervals. Greater than 75% ink removal was seen in 77% of black tattoos and over 95% ink removal in 28% of tattoos (11 of 39) treated at 10 to 12 J/cm^2. There was no significant difference in the response of previously untreated tattoos and ruby laser-resistant tattoos. Treatment at the highest fluence (12 J/cm^2) proved to be significantly more effective ($p < 0.01$) at removing black tattoo ink than the lower doses of 6 and 8 J/cm^2. Green, yellow, white, and red inks were virtually resistant to treatment and cleared 25% or less after four treatment sessions. Purple and orange inks responded minimally. Although textural changes were noted during the course of treatment, these cleared with time, and only 2 of 39 tattoos were graded as having trace textural changes. No hypopigmentation and a single case of hyperpigmentation were noted. These results were similar to those reported by Ferguson and August.[147]

Biopsy of treated tattoos revealed fragmentation of black ink particles up to 1.5 mm below the surface. This may prove advantageous for the treatment of deeply implanted traumatic tattoos.[148–150] There was little if any fibrosis in the superficial dermis. In addition, biopsies demonstrated that even with clinical clearing of the tattoo, ink remained in the dermis, as reported with the Q-switched ruby laser.[145]

Kilmer et al[146] noted that the lack of scarring both clinically and histologically, despite the increased bleeding and tissue splatter seen, is most likely caused by the lack of thermal injury to collagen. The dermis and epidermis sustain mechanical injury from the photoacoustic wave, but this trauma is apparently highly reparable. Textural changes generally resolve within 4 to 6 weeks, suggesting an optimal treatment interval of 6 weeks or longer.

The authors[146] also noted a bright flash of white light from the tattoo during laser exposure, as mentioned with the ruby laser. Because 1064-nm light is not visible, this flash must result from either laser-stimulated plasma or incandescence of tattoo ink particles. These both imply extreme temperatures greater than 500°C.

The Q-switched Nd:YAG laser has a great advantage for treating darker-skinned patients (Fig. 4.19). Both Jones et al[151] and Grevelink et al[152] demonstrated effective tattoo removal with minimal hypopigmentation or hyperpigmentation. This provides a significant benefit over the Q-switched ruby laser for darker-skinned patients in whom melanin absorption is a hindrance, and for cosmetic eyeliner tattoos, where care must be taken not to damage the eyelashes or retinal melanin.[153] In addition, the smaller spot size available with most Q-switched Nd:YAG lasers (1.5-mm diameter) allows for more accurate distinction of tattoo in sensitive areas (Figs 4.20 and 4.21).

In summary, the Q-switched Nd:YAG laser has proved to be somewhat more effective in removal of black ink,

A B

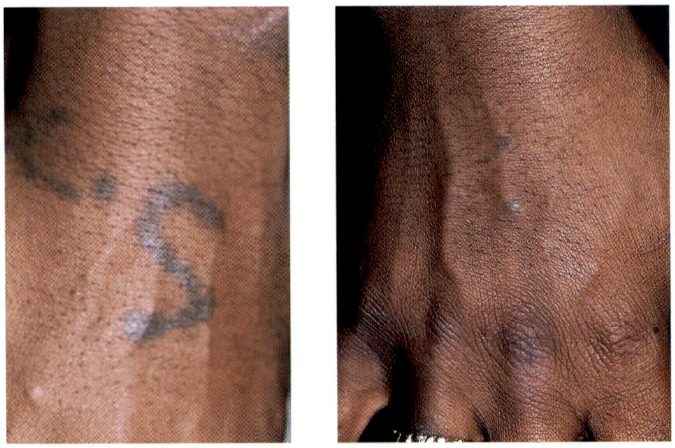

Figure 4.19 (A) Amateur tattoo on dorsal palm of 40-year-old black male for more than 20 years. (B) Six months after second treatment with Nd:YAG laser using 3-mm-diameter spot size at 6 to 7 J/cm^2.

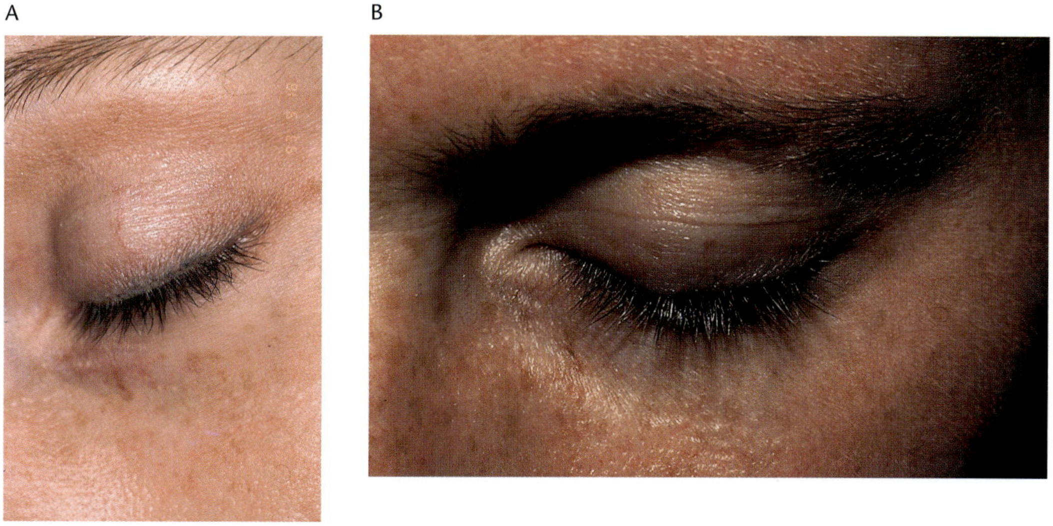

Figure 4.20 (A) Misplaced tattoo eyeliner. (B) Complete removal 3 weeks after single treatment with Nd:YAG laser at 10 J/cm^2 through 1.5-mm-diameter spot.

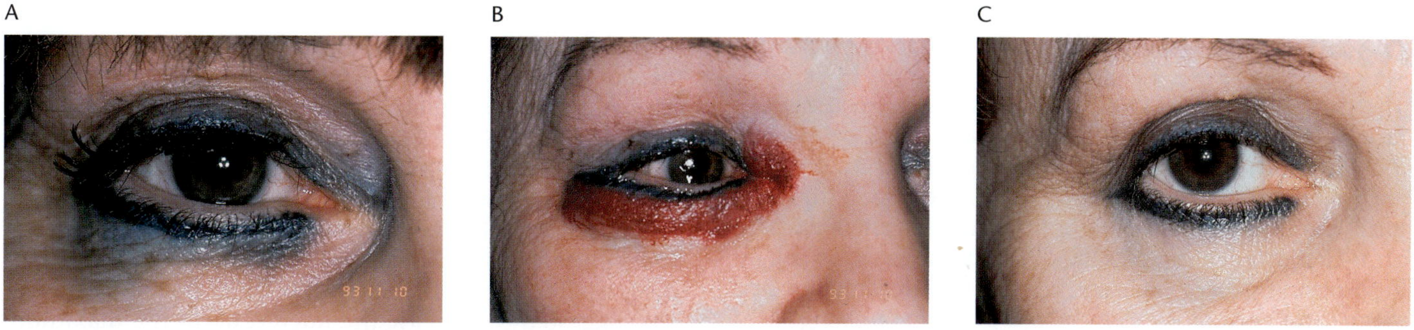

Figure 4.21 (A) Spread of tattoo pigment 1 month after placement. (B), Immediately after treatment with Nd:YAG laser using 2-mm-diameter spot at 10 J/cm^2. (C) Five months after single treatment showing tattoo the patient wanted to receive.

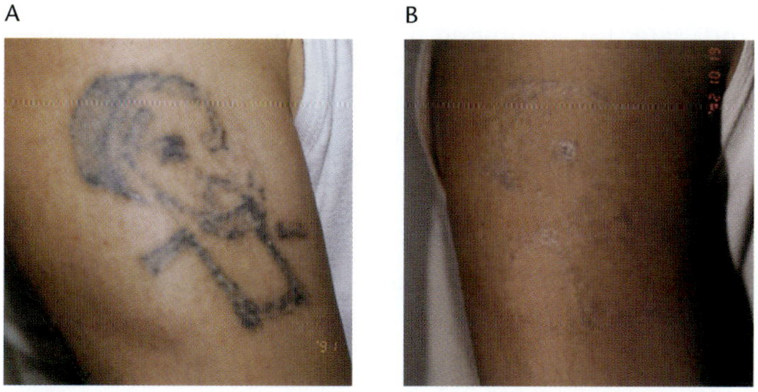

Figure 4.22 (A) Amateur tattoo after 10 Q-switched ruby laser treatments. (B) Near-complete removal after five treatments with Q-switched Nd:YAG laser. Treatment sessions were performed using 10 J/cm^2 and with 3 to 4 weeks between treatments.

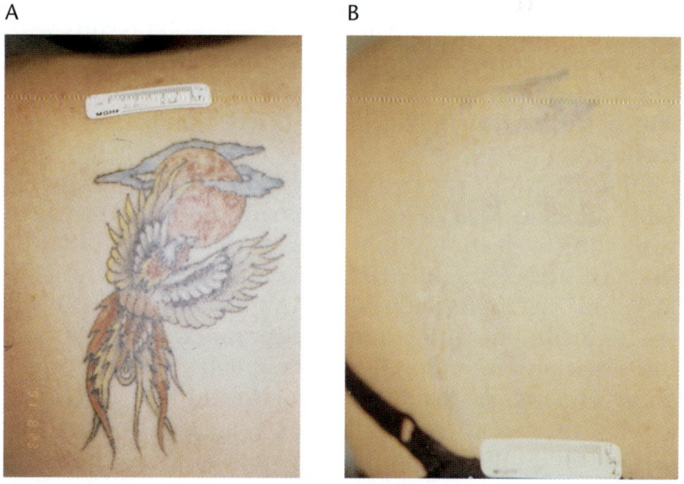

Figure 4.23 (A) Professional multicolored tattoo before treatment with Nd:YAG laser. (B) After four treatment sessions using 1064-nm wavelength and four treatment sessions using 532-nm wavelength, only small amount of blue pigment persists.

with rare textural changes and almost no hypopigmentation (Figs 4.22 and 4.23). These improvements are attributed to the longer wavelength, higher fluence, and shorter pulse width. These same factors cause more bleeding and tissue splatter during treatment, making the treatment itself more cumbersome. However, the faster repetition rate (1–10 Hz) shortens the treatment session, although this is somewhat counterbalanced by the use of a smaller beam size (2–4 mm versus 5–6.5 mm for the ruby laser). Larger spot sizes up to 6 mm are now available with new, higher-powered Nd:YAG laser systems, enabling deeper penetration and more effective treatment of deeper, denser tattoos.[154] Better beam profiles have minimized epidermal damage, decreasing bleeding, tissue splatter, and transient textural changes. Often, little wound care is needed.

The primary disadvantage of 1064 nm is its limited color range, basically restricted to black and dark-blue/black tattoo pigment. However, a frequency-doubling crystal is a feature of this laser, which allows the use of the 532-nm wavelength to treat red ink effectively. Greater than 75% removal of red ink has been reported with three treatment sessions, and orange and some purples respond almost as well; however, yellow ink responds poorly, presumably because of its dramatic drop in absorbance between 510 and 520 nm, as do green and blue inks, where absorption is greater at 600 nm or longer.[124]

Because of absorbance of 1064-nm light by melanin and hemoglobin, blistering and purpura frequently occur.

Q-switched Alexandrite Laser

The third Q-switched laser developed for the treatment of tattoos, the alexandrite laser, has a wavelength of 755 nm, a pulse width of 100 ns (50 ns available in newer models), and a repetition rate of 1 Hz.[155–158] The 3-mm-diameter beam is delivered via a fiberoptic system or an articulated arm. Reflectance studies at 755 nm suggest excellent absorption by black pigment, good absorption by blue and green, and poor absorption by red pigments (see Figs 4.11 to 4.13), as confirmed by preliminary studies performed on tattooed guinea pigs and harvested human skin.[159] This corroborates previous findings from preliminary trials on Yucutan minipigs, where one treatment session provided excellent results in removal of black ink, good results with blue and green, and poor results with red ink. Efficacy was fluence related; 8 J/cm^2 was more effective than 6 J/cm^2, which was more effective than 4 J/cm^2, and 2 J/cm^2 was ineffective.[113]

In contrast to previous reports using the Q-switched ruby and Nd:YAG lasers, histologic clearing correlated with clinical clearing. Similar to reports with the other Q-switched lasers, fragmentation of tattoo pigment was followed by macrophage engulfment and gradual clearing of the pigment, but with clinically clear tattoos devoid of ink histologically. Interestingly, tattoo pigment became progressively altered during this process, initially appearing as very sharp-bordered grains of pigment in clumps and taking on a progressively more amorphous form and lighter color within the macrophages (Fig. 4.24). No clinical or histologic reaction in collagen, scarring, or atrophy was seen in laser-treated sites.

The Q-switched alexandrite laser was initially studied with 30 tattoos using fluences of 4.5 to 8.0 J/cm^2. Test sites using three fluences up to 6 J/cm^2 were evaluated at 4 weeks. The appropriate fluence was then selected and treatment begun. A second test was done if none of the previous fluences revealed significant lightening. Fluences of 6 J/cm^2 or higher were used once the tattoo had lightened by 20% to 50%. Approximately 25% clearing of tattooed pigment required 1.7 treatments, 50% clearance 2.8 treatments; 75% clearance 5 treatments, 90% clearance 6.4 treatments, and total clearance 10.4 treatments (range 4 to 16) (Fig. 4.25). Professional tattoos, cosmetic tattoos, traumatic tattoos and amalgam tattoos cleared as well as amateur tattoos, although the latter were more rapidly responsive, requiring approximately three fewer treatments to reach complete clearance (Fig. 4.26), although some professional tattoos responded rapidly as well.[126,160–164]

Transient hypopigmentation is common (50% of patients), but often is not apparent until after five to seven treatment sessions, and usually resolves gradually over 1 to 12 months (Fig. 4.27). As with the other Q-switched lasers, hyperpigmentation is more dependent on skin type and clears with hydroquinone and sunscreen. Transient surface textural changes have been noted in about 10% of patients, but all resolved within 3 to 9 months, although one patient developed a small scar (2 × 7 mm) secondary to excoriating a treated area.

On laser impact, the immediate flash of white light from the tattoo is followed by epidermal whitening and slight edema, as seen with both the Q-switched ruby and the Q-switched Nd:YAG lasers. When higher fluences are used, purpura is noticed, and pinpoint bleeding may occur. Tissue splatter and erosions were not seen at any of the fluences used with the 100-nsec pulse width, but the shorter 50-ns pulse width, which reportedly increases tattoo clearance, is associated with more epidermal debris. Therefore it is suggested to increase the fluence up to the maximum available without causing pinpoint bleeding to prevent the problems of working in a bloody field and possible tissue trauma.

In summary, the Q-switched alexandrite laser is effective and safe for removing blue, black, and green tattoo pigment (Fig. 4.28). Four to 10 treatments performed at 1- to 2-month intervals usually clears the tattoo without scarring; however, half of patients develop transient hypopigmentation.

Q-switched Laser Treatment in General

Treatment Intervals

In early studies of Q-switched lasers, patients were treated every 4 weeks. In the alexandrite study, of the four patients unable to return for their scheduled treatment, two went 3 months and two went 5 months between treatments. Two of these four patients reported progressive and gradual clearing of their tattoo during this prolonged interval between treatment sessions, whereas two patients noticed only immediate improvement and then stabilization without further clearing. To study different treatment intervals, one group of patients received three treatments within 7 to 10 days and then no treatment for 3 months,

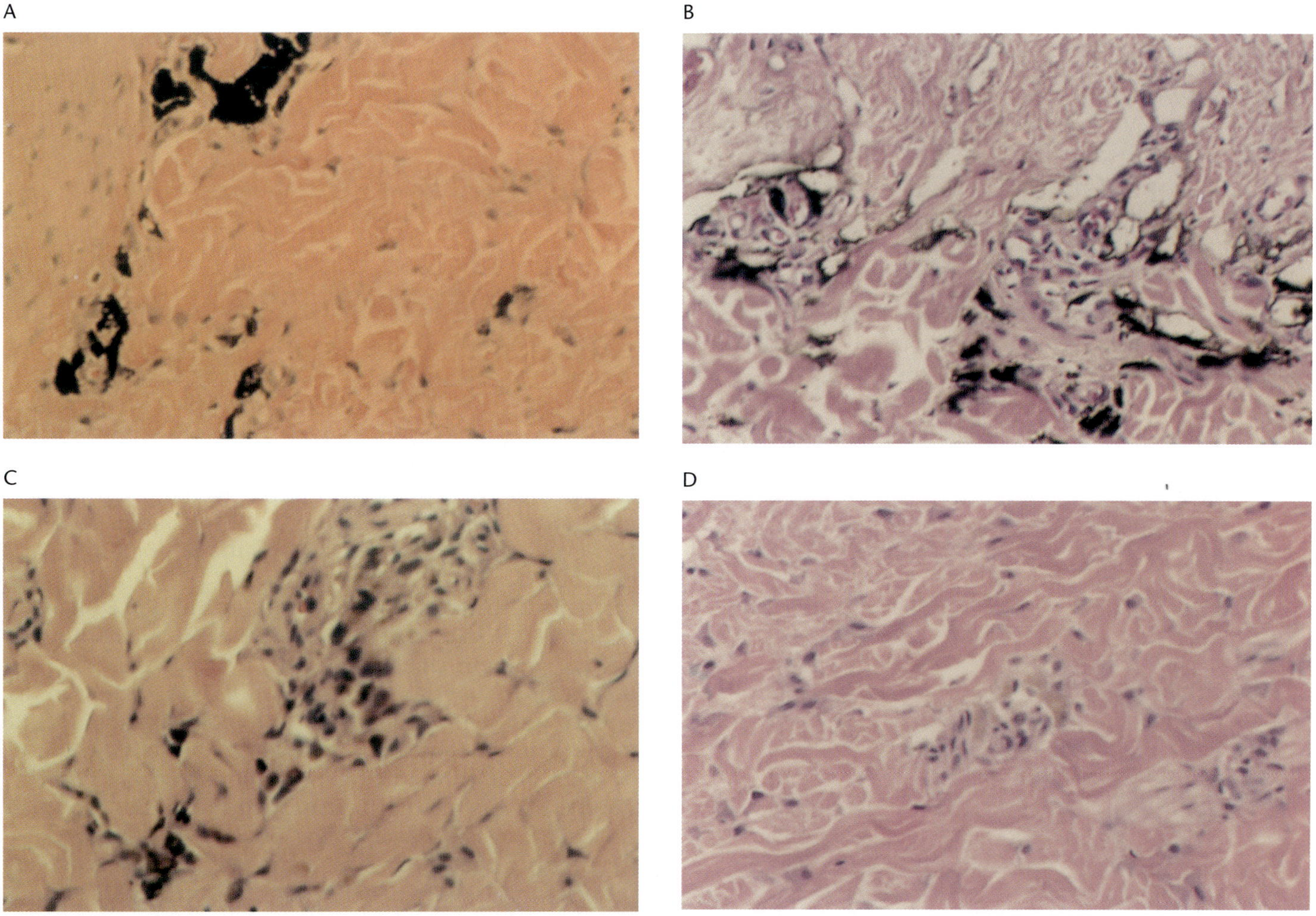

Figure 4.24 (A) Tattoo granules present in dermis before treatment. (B) Tattoo pigment fragmentation and dermal lacunae formation 1 hour after treatment with alexandrite laser. (C) One week after treatment, tattoo pigment is intracellular within macrophages. (D) One month after treatment, total amount of pigment present is greatly decreased and much more amorphous within macrophages. (Fig. 4.24A: Reprinted from Fitzpatrick RE, Goldman MP, Ruiz-Esparza J. Journal of the American Academy of Dermatology 28:745 © 1993, with permission from the American Academy of Dermatology, Inc.)

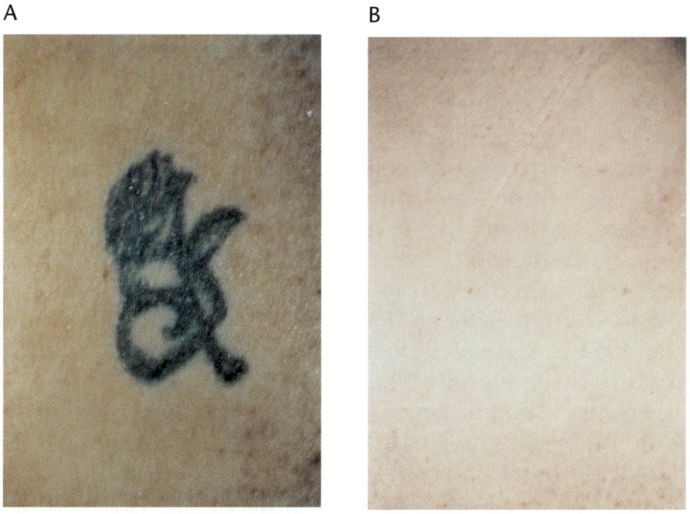

Figure 4.25 (A) Tattoo before treatment. (B) Complete clearance after six treatment sessions with alexandrite laser.

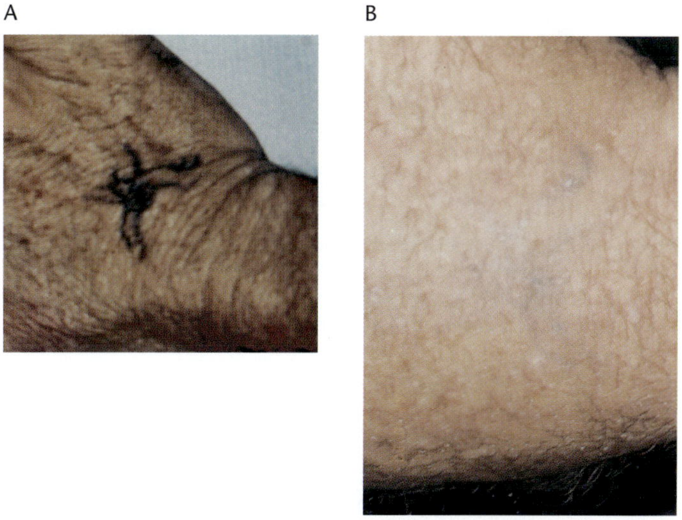

Figure 4.26 (A) Amateur tattoo before treatment. (B) Almost complete clearing after two treatment sessions with alexandrite laser.

A B C

Figure 4.27 (A) Tattoo before treatment. (B) Hypopigmentation of treated area after nine treatment sessions. (C) Gradual improvement of hypopigmentation after additional 3 months of healing.

A

B

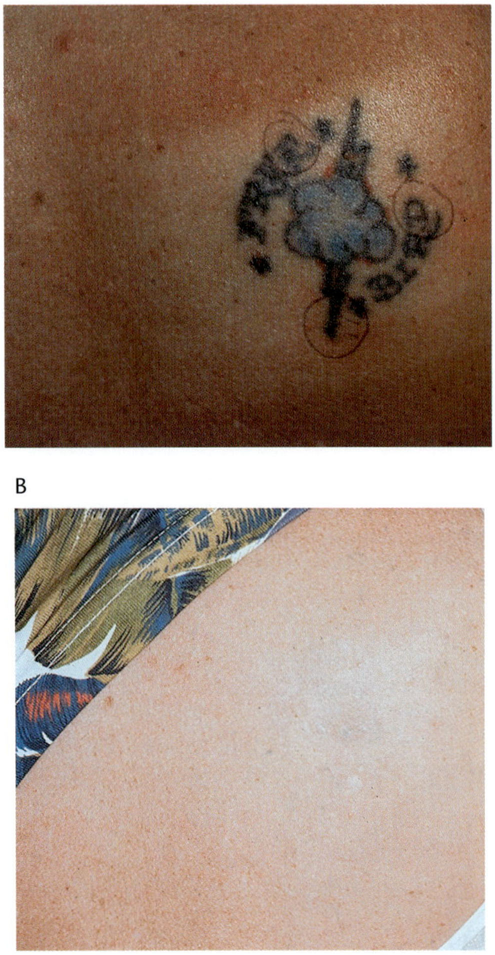

Figure 4.28 (A) Black, blue, and red tattoo before treatment. (B) Six months after total of 25 monthly treatments with Q-switched alexandrite laser at 8.0 J/cm^2 with 3-mm spot size. Complete clearing of all pigments was achieved without textural change in skin.

a second group had a single treatment at 2-month intervals, and the third group had a single treatment at 1-month intervals.

Appropriate treatment interval is critical and yet poorly understood. It had been hoped that rapid fragmentation of tattoo pigment by condensing three treatment sessions within a 7- to 10-day period, followed by adequate time for macrophage activity (3 months), would result in more rapid tattoo removal with fewer total treatments required. However, the condensed treatment protocol did not enhance clearing. Treatment intervals of 1 month could interfere with macrophage activity, because the pigment-containing macrophages are laser targets as well as the stationary pigment-laden fibroblasts.[112,148] By extending the treatment interval to 2 and 3 months, essentially no difference was seen in the rate of tattoo clearing, because all three treatment intervals resulted in approximately 50% clearing after three treatment sessions. However, as the number of treatments increases, the potential for tissue reaction increases as well. Occasional rest periods or longer treatment intervals of 2 to 3 months allow recovery of melanin and normalization of any transient textural changes, which may be beneficial for avoiding unwanted adverse tissue response. Higher fluences and shorter pulse widths appear to remove tattoo pigment more rapidly but have the potential of inducing excessive shock wave tissue reaction and therefore must be balanced with the desire to remove pigment without scarring or hypopigmentation. Therefore the current recommendation is to treat at 6- to 8-week intervals unless a longer period is needed for tissue recovery.

Recommended Treatment Parameters

The main parameters to be chosen include pulse duration, wavelength, fluence, and spot size. All the Q-switched lasers are in the nanosecond domain, and the pulse width is predetermined by the laser used. The wavelength is chosen based on the best available wavelength for the tattoo ink color to be treated. In other words, red ink by a green wavelength (510 or 532 nm)[135] and green ink by a red wavelength (694 or 755 nm). When melanin is present, the 1064-nm wavelength is the best choice to avoid disrupting the epidermis (Fig. 4.29).[165–168]

Fluence should be sufficient to produce immediate whitening, but immediate bleeding or blistering should be avoided. Larger spot sizes allow deeper penetration and should be used as long as sufficient fluence can be obtained. This will maximize distribution of laser light to the dermal pigment and minimize cutaneous injury.

A B

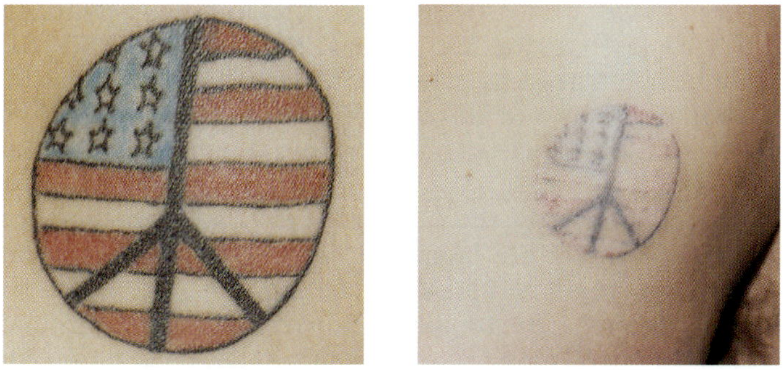

Figure 4.29 (A) Tattoo before treatment. (B) Removal of red tattoo pigment after three treatment sessions with 510-nm, 300-nsec, flashlamp-pumped pulsed dye laser (FLPD laser).

A B

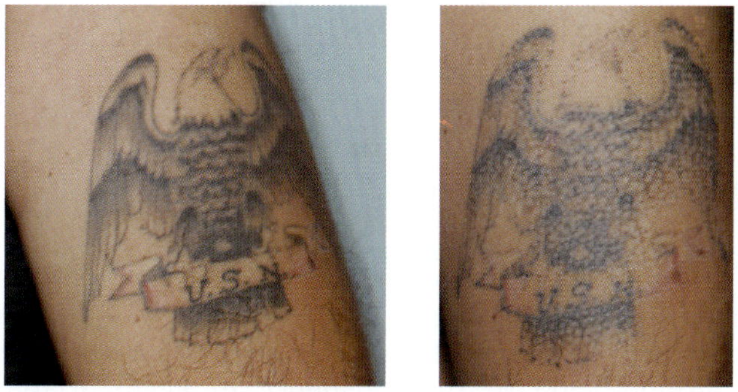

Figure 4.30 (A) Tattoo before treatment. (B) From 40% to 50% improvement after single treatment session with alexandrite laser.

Table 4.1 *Q-Switched Laser Treatment: Tattoo Pigment Depth Effect*

Tattoo pigment maximum depth (mm)	No. patients	Average improvement (%)	Average No. treatments
<0.92 (average 0.58)	4	87.5	7
>1.78 (average 2.19)	4	81.3	9.3

Table 4.2 *Q-Switched Laser Treatment: Tattoo Pigment Surface Area Effect*

Tattoo pigment surface area (cm^2)*	No. patients	Average improvement (%)	Average No. treatments
<4.3 (average 2.56)	7	92.1	7
>16.7 (average 24.7)	5	89.0	10.4

*Mean: $10.5 \pm 6.2\,cm^2$.

Table 4.3 *Q-Switched Laser Treatment: Tattoo Pigment Volume Effect*

Tattoo pigment volume (mm^3)*	No. patients	Average improvement	Average No. treatments (%)
>2644 (average 4040)	4	91.3	12.5
<442 (average 328)	6	90.8	7.5

*Mean: $1543 \pm 1011\,mm^3$.

It is difficult to predict the number of treatment sessions necessary for tattoo removal. Frequently the initial treatment session produces a more dramatic response than subsequent sessions. Very definite sites of clearing, corresponding to laser impacts, are often visible (Fig. 4.30). Other tattoos are strongly unresponsive during early treatment phases, even though biopsies reveal fragmentation of tattoo granules. The explanation of these differences in response from one patient to another is likely to involve the efficiency of mobile macrophages in removal of fragmented tattoo pigment debris, as well as the density and amount of tattoo pigment present. The speed of the macrophage response, as well as the maximum amount of pigment removed per session, likely varies from patient to patient and to some extent from treatment to treatment.

To evaluate the effects of pigment placement and volume, treatment response in relation to: (1) maximum pigment depth; (2) pigment surface area; and (3) total pigment volume (the product of these first two figures) was examined. As expected, the more superficial the tattoo pigment and the lesser the total volume of pigment, the fewer were the number of treatments necessary to remove the pigment; this was particularly apparent at the extremes (upper and lower 15% of values). When tattoo pigment was less than 0.92 mm in depth, seven treatments resulted in an average of 87.5% improvement, whereas pigment greater than 1.78 mm in depth required 9.3 treatments to achieve an average of 81.3% improvement (Table 4.1). In addition, smaller (Table 4.2) and lower-volume (Table 4.3) tattoos cleared with fewer treatments. Analysis of these values reveals that response rate is a function of pigment depth and total pigment volume, as well as surface area.

In contrast to anecdotal reports with the ruby and Nd:YAG lasers, new tattoos treated with Q-switched alexandrite lasers cleared faster, possibly because of the more superficial location of a new tattoo. New tattoos have sharp lines with bright colors, whereas older tattoos are blurred with indistinct lines and duller, bluer colors presumably from the ink moving deeper into the dermis. Further studies to explore these observations are underway.

Side Effects

Unlike previous modalities, the Q-switched lasers are much more effective with very few side effects. Hypopigmentation is more a function of the wavelength used. Repigmentation of postlaser hypopigmentation can be promoted with phototherapy or ultraviolet-range lasers. Increased melanin absorption seen with shorter wavelengths increases the risk for hypopigmentation, which completely resolves in most patients.

Hyperpigmentation, is related more to the patient's skin type. Those with darker skin are more prone to this no matter which wavelength is used. Treatment with hydroquinone and broadspectrum sunscreens will resolve the hyperpigmentation within a few months, although in some patients it can be more prolonged.

Textural changes or scars are – luckily – very rare. Scarring has been reported following Q-switched laser treatment of combustible materials in the case of traumatic gunpowder tattooing and with dense pigment deposition in the case of 'double tattoos' where a pre-existing tattoo is overlaid with a second tattoo.[169,170] Transient textural changes are often noted but resolve within 1 to 2 months. If a patient is more prone to this, longer treatment intervals are recommended.

Allergic reactions to tattoo pigment after Q-switched laser treatment are possible.[171] Unlike the destructive modalities previously described, Q-switched lasers mobilize the ink and may generate a systemic allergic response. If an allergic reaction to the ink has been noted, Q-switched laser treatment is not advised. There is no evidence, to date, of systemic toxicity reactions in vivo following laser treatment of tattoos, however chemical and photophysical analysis studies do find some evidence that potentially hazardous compound can be liberated from laser treatment of tattoo pigment in vitro.[172,173]

Finally, tattoo ink darkening has been noted. Although this can occur with any colored ink, it is more common with red, white, and flesh-toned inks, although darkening of yellow ink has also been reported.[174] This is a particular concern with cosmetic tattoos and is discussed at length in a later section.

Comparative Studies of Q-Switched Lasers

Direct comparison studies are difficult, because varying treatment parameters including spot sizes and fluences are difficult to standardize and results are therefore often inconclusive. Several comparative studies have been done using different lasers on the same tattoos. A comparison of the ruby and Nd:YAG lasers[146] found them to be equally effective in removal of black ink, but the ruby laser was more effective for green ink. A second comparison of the ruby and Nd:YAG lasers was limited to one treatment session,[175] and a similar response was noted. After 1 month the Nd:YAG was judged to cause more textural change and hyperpigmentation than the ruby laser, possibly related to the smaller spot size used and the ruby laser causing more hypopigmentation. One report comparing the Q-switched Nd:YAG laser to the alexandrite laser found the former achieved better results, whereas a comparison between the Q-switched ruby and alexandrite lasers for amateur tattoos revealed the ruby laser to remove more pigment after two sessions.[176]

In a similar study, the ruby laser removed more pigment than the alexandrite laser and resulted in more textural change, hypopigmentation, and hair loss. A comparison at two or three treatment sessions may not be optimal because only 50% to 60% of the tattoo has been removed, and speed and efficacy of tattoo removal as well as the avoidance of textural changes, scarring, hair loss, and pigment alterations must be examined. In addition, the range of colors responsive to laser systems is important. Whereas all three Q-switched lasers can effectively treat black tattoos, QS-alexandrite lasers are more effective for blue and green pigment, QS-ruby lasers are more effective for purple and violet pigment, and 532 nm frequency-doubled QS-Nd:YAG lasers are more effective for removing red pigment.[165–168]

Laser Ablation of Facial Cosmetic Tattoos

The use of facial cosmetics for ornamental purposes and attraction of the opposite sex is an ancient art, first traced to around 3500 BC from evidence in Egyptian tombs and limestone caves.[177] The merger of this art form with tattooing occurred in 1984, when Angres[178] popularized tattoo blepharopigmentation (permanent eyeliner). Although originally promoted as an alternative to eyeliner application for women crippled with arthritis or other physical impairments, it has become a popular procedure for general cosmetic purposes.[179] In addition, tattooing of eyebrows, lip lines, and cheeks to simulate facial cosmetics was introduced in 1987.[180] The public's acceptance of the cosmetic use of facial tattoos to simulate makeup application has been surprising and has stirred medical controversy.[177–179] It has led to the use of the technique by estheticians, tattoo artists, and nurse practitioners, as well as physicians. In 1987 it was estimated that more than 75,000 persons had undergone various types of cosmetic dermal pigmentation procedures.[180]

Pigment Placement

The black dye used is primarily ferric oxide and is relatively inert. Tissue examined 6 weeks after blepharopigmentation revealed an absence of inflammation.[181] Carbon and titanium oxide are often present as well,[182] and numerous other metals have been detected in the dyes by X-ray microanalysis.

Many of the dyes used have been supplied by a variety of sources, some unlicensed. Fortunately, complications have been rare. One allergic granuloma has been reported,[33] as has one case of eyelid margin necrosis with

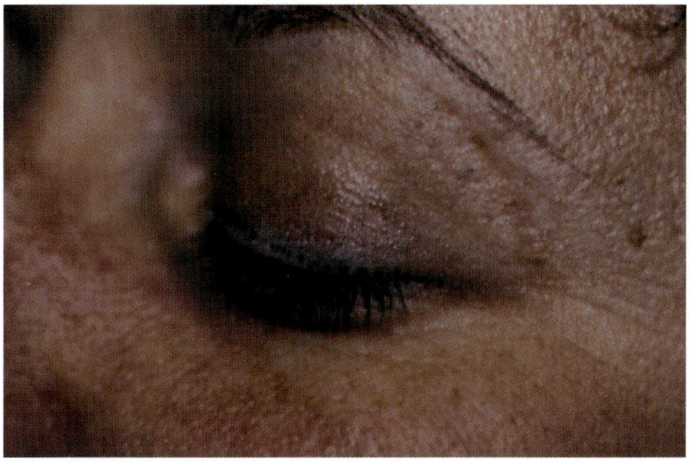

Figure 4.31 Misapplication of eyeliner tattoo pigment has been the most common complication of cosmetic blepharopigmentation.

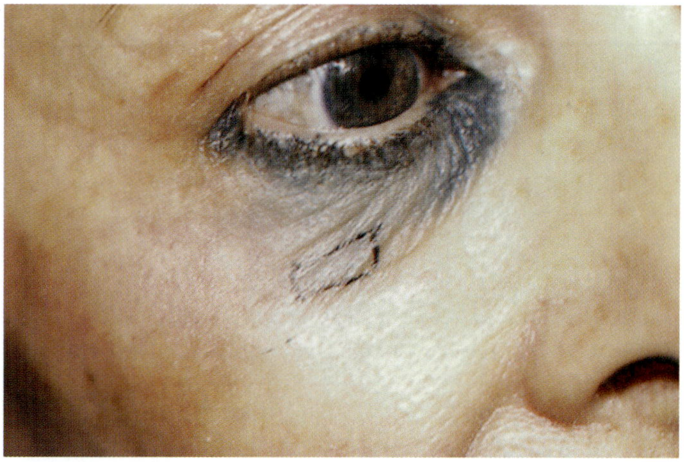

Figure 4.32 Pigment fanning after blepharopigmentation is thought to occur from tattoo pigment spreading in plane of tarsal fibrous tissue of lid.

loss of lashes and secondary cicatricial entropion.[183] By far the most common complication has been misapplication of the pigment[182,184] (Fig. 4.31). A survey of members of the American Society of Ophthalmic Plastic and Reconstructive Surgery reported improper pigment placement in 4% of patients who had undergone blepharopigmentation.[182] Angres[180] noted an increasing number of patients who were dissatisfied with the positioning of the pigment placed during blepharopigmentation and expressed concern over the confusion among practitioners as to the ideal cosmetic result. He further commented that proper pigment placement is directly in the lash line between the base of the lash follicles and not above the lash line.

Pigment placement is accomplished with an instrument using oscillating disposable needles, which penetrate to a fixed depth of 1.2 mm. Microscopic examination of eyelid tissue previously tattooed reveals pigment granules extending to a depth of 1.5 mm in the dermis and connective tissue of the muscle fibers of the orbicular ocular muscle.[185] Virtually all implanted pigment has been shown to be within the cytoplasm of macrophages, which persist at the site of injection. Pigment migration has been reported in 5% of patients[182] and is thought to be secondary to loss of pigment placed too superficially in the epidermis. A particularly disastrous complication, referred to as pigment fanning, is thought to be the result of tattoo pigment placed so deep that it enters the tarsal fibrous tissue of the lid and spreads in this tissue plane, causing a fan-shaped pigmentation of the entire lid[184,186] (Fig. 4.32). Fortunately, all the Q-switched lasers can effectively treat this condition.

Pigment Removal

Traditional techniques reported for removal of permanent cosmetic tattoos include surgical excision,[187,188] scraping the pigment off with a chelation curette,[187] ablation of the tattoo with an argon laser,[177] and injection of tannic acid with a tattoo needle.[189]

Surgical excision of a few misplaced dots is feasible and can be accomplished with a punch excision or a tiny ellipse or curettage of spots.[187] However, excision of an entire line of pigment is complicated by the presence of eyelashes within the tattoo with possible postoperative entropion or ectropion or unacceptable scarring or distortion of the vermilion border with removal of a lip line tattoo. Bleaching of unwanted tattoo pigment by injection of alcohol is suggested by the manufacturer of Accents, but this is an unproven technique in these locations and would be expected to produce inflammation, ulceration, and superficial tissue necrosis if effective, as reported with the injection of tannic acid.[189] Removal of any tattoo pigment is a difficult procedure, and most of the currently used tissue-destructive techniques are not appropriate for removal of facial cosmetic tattoos.

Vaporization of tattoo pigment with an argon laser has been successful. It is difficult, however, and thermal damage to cilial follicles results in loss of eyelashes.[181]

In one study, five different lasers were used to remove: (1) midcheek rouge; (2) eyelid; (3) eyebrow; (4) lipliner; and (5) tattoos.[190] The superpulsed CO_2 laser (10,600 nm, continuous wave), a very controlled, precise instrument, provides a dry surgical field and precise removal of tattoo pigment in delicate areas such as the eyelid and eyebrow.

The superpulsed CO_2 laser was used in the SP3 under continuous mode (pulse parameters: 400 μs, 250 Hz, 80-W peak power) and in the conventional continuous mode with a 50-ms shuttered pulse and power settings of 1 to 2 W. The beam diameter was varied between 0.1 and 1.5 mm, depending on the width of the tattoo being vaporized. When possible, individual dots of pigment were vaporized, using a beam size to correspond to the pigment dot. When the tattoo was a more uniform line, the laser was swept across the tattoo pigment, vaporizing the outer layer of skin overlying the tattoo. Repeated passes (three or four) resulted in a 1.5- to 2-mm incisional groove replacing the line of tattoo if complete removal of tattoo pigment was attempted, as in removing eyeliner tattoo. However, when the CO_2 laser was used for removal of lipliner tattoo

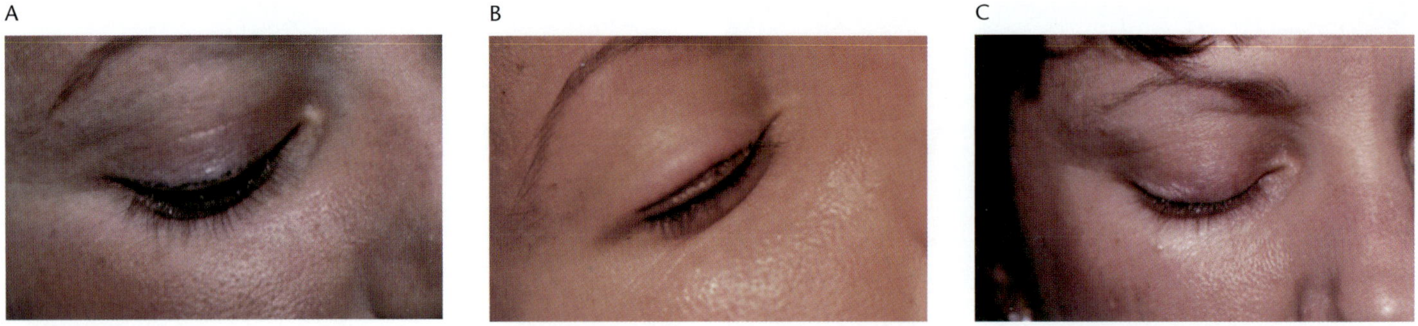

Figure 4.33 (A) Eyeliner tattoo before treatment. (B) Wound resulting from CO_2 laser ablation was allowed to heal by secondary intention. (C) Final result 1 year after procedure.

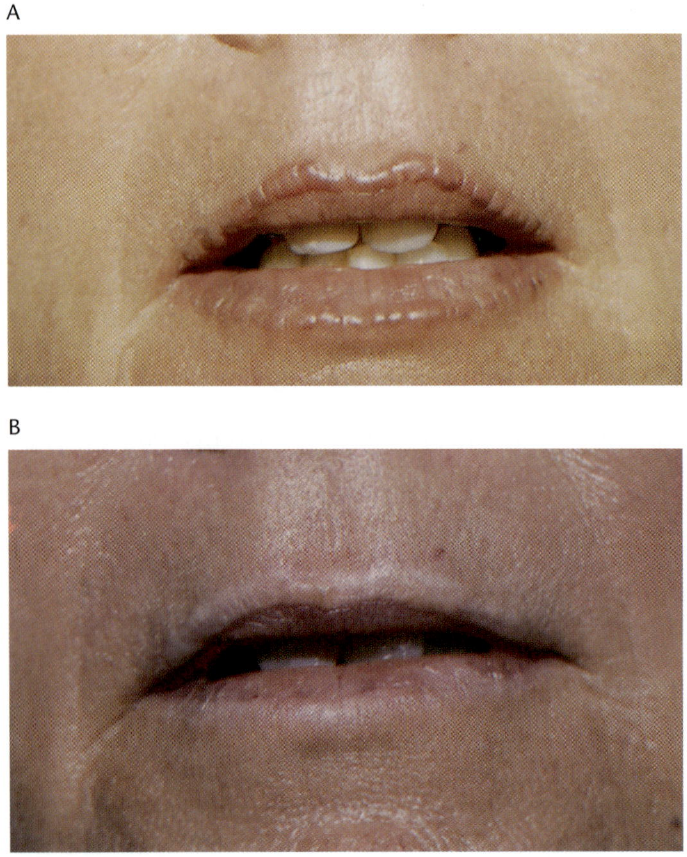

Figure 4.34 (A) Allergic granulomatous dermatitis in red lipliner tattoo. (B) Hypopigmented scar tissue remains after obliteration of tattoo pigment and granulomas with superpulse CO_2 laser.

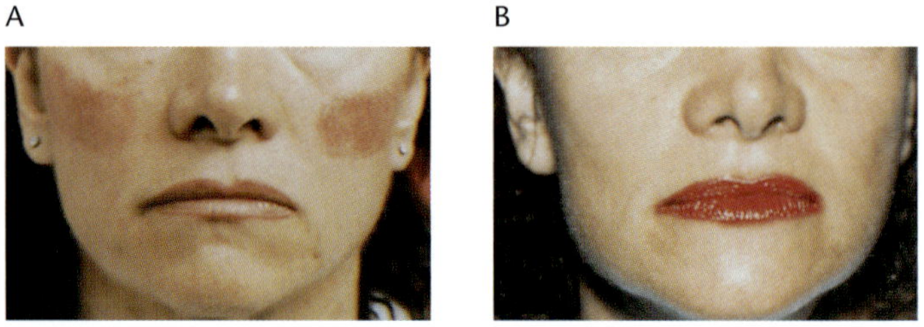

Figure 4.35 (A) Before laser treatment, red tattoos intended to simulate rouge. (B) Complete tattoo removal was achieved with 510-nm, 300-nsec pulsed dye laser.

and eyebrow tattoo, only the outer superficial tissue was vaporized, leaving an open superficial dermal wound containing tattoo pigment. As the wound healed, residual tattoo pigment would seep out onto the bandage, which was changed daily.

Before laser treatment, the skin containing tattoo pigment was infiltrated with lidocaine 1% with 1:100,000 epinephrine (adrenaline). During the procedure the eye was protected with a metallic scleral contact lens after instillation of topical proparacaine hydrochloride 0.5% drops in the conjunctival cul-de-sac. When vaporizing tattoo pigment adjacent to eyelashes, the beam is pulsed in short bursts of 0.05 to 0.1 s to achieve better control and avoid damaging the cilia follicles. Although it can be very difficult to differentiate between tattoo pigment and small fragments of charred tissue at the edges of the laser impact crater, all eyeliner tattoos cleared completely. The wounds healed by secondary intention with imperceptible scars within 6 months and no distortion of lid margins or loss of eyelashes (Fig. 4.33). One eyebrow tattoo was completely removed without scarring using the CO_2 laser, but a hypopigmented scar was seen in one lipliner tattoo (Fig. 4.34). The UltraPulse CO_2 ($UPCO_2$) laser further minimizes thermal damage and thereby decreases the risk of scarring and dyspigmentation.[191]

In one patient with red lipliner tattoo and one patient with cheek rouge tattoo, the FLPD laser (585 nm, 450 s, 3- to 5-mm beam, power density of 7.5 J/cm^2, 20% overlap) was used. Both tattoos responded with 20% to 30% improvement with a single treatment. More encouraging, the FLPD laser (510 nm, 300 ns, 5-mm spot size, energy density of 3.5 J/cm^2) completely cleared two red tattoos in five treatments at 4-week intervals without residual scarring (Fig. 4.35). The frequency-doubled (fd) Nd:YAG laser (532 nm, 5 ns) is equally effective.[192]

The argon laser with a continuous beam of 0.1 mm and power of 2.2 W (Model 1000, Coherent Medical, Palo Alto, CA) minimally improved two lipliner tattoos. The Q-switched alexandrite and ruby lasers are also appropriate for removal of facial tattoos, as is the Q-switched Nd:YAG laser for black ink tattoos.[192]

A lipliner tattoo overtattooed with flesh tones in an attempt to cover the unwanted pigment was initially treated with the FLPD laser and irreversibly darkened to a dark slate gray (Fig. 4.36). Flesh-tone, red, and white tattoo ink darkening with Q-switched ruby, Q-switched Nd:YAG, and Q-switched alexandrite laser treatment has been reported. Attempts to remove the darkened ink with

A B C

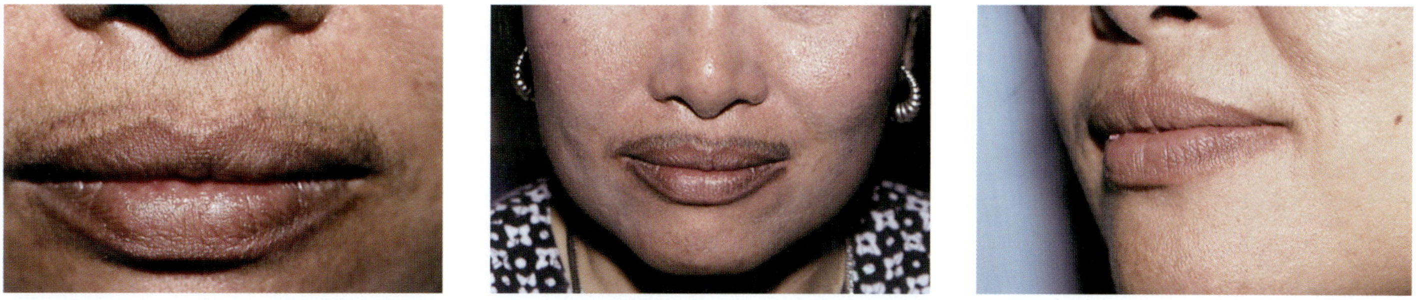

Figure 4.36 (A) Unwanted lipliner tattoo had been overtattooed with flesh tones in attempt to cover red pigment. (B) After single treatment with 510-nm, 300-nsec pulsed dye laser, flesh-tone pigment irreversibly changed to black. (C) Unwanted pigment was removed after six treatments with alexandrite laser (755 nm, 100 ns).

A B C

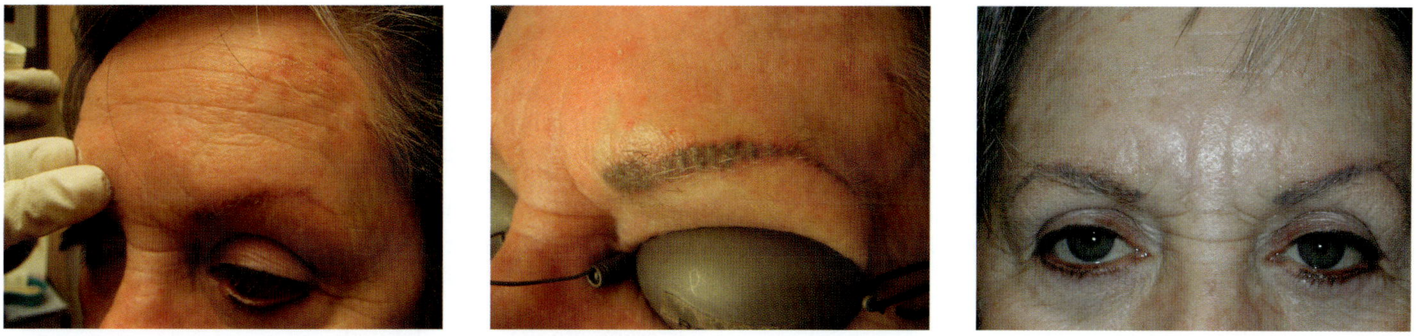

Figure 4.37 (A) Red-brown eyebrow tattoos prior to treatment. (B) After a single treatment with Q-switched ruby laser, red pigment immediately blackens. (C) Dark gray pigment remains after 3 months.

further laser treatment failed in two cases, and surgical excision was necessary. In the other cases, subsequent laser treatments successfully removed the darkened ink.

In vitro tests with various tattoo pigments in agar have found that a surprising number of pigments (most containing iron oxide) will change color when irradiated with Q-switched laser energy.[193,194] Iron oxide changes color from brown to black when raised to a temperature above 1400°C as ferric oxide is ignited.[195] In clinical practice multiple colors, including flesh tones, red, white, and brown, containing pigments (nonoxide, titanium dioxide) have been reported to change color on laser impact. Even several green and blue tattoo pigments have changed to black when irradiated with the Q-switched alexandrite laser. The chemical mechanism of tattoo ink darkening remains unknown. It likely involves the conversion of ferric oxide (Fe_2O_3) to ferrous oxide (FeO) by reduction or the strong ignition of ferric oxide above 1400°C. Crystalline ferrous oxide is unstable and tends to convert to ferric oxide or iron. Ferric oxide has a rust color and occurs in nature as the mineral hematite; ferrous oxide is black, as is Fe_3O_4, which occurs in nature as a black crystal of the mineral magnetite. The ability of each of these iron oxides to alter its composition without any structural change accounts for their ready interconvertibility.[195] These reactions may require extreme temperatures known to be generated during the very short pulse of Q-switched lasers, estimated at several hundreds to thousands of degrees Celsius.

Laser treatment of flesh-tone, pink, red and brown tattoos must be approached with caution. The resultant gray–black or other color change of the tattoo may be difficult to remove and is certainly more visible than the original cosmetic tone; therefore test sites are recommended.[196–199] The Q-switched lasers appear to be ideal for removal of large areas of black facial tattoos (tarsal fanning of pigment, eyebrow tattoo). However, the beam size (2–6.5 mm) may make removal of small dots of precisely confined tattoo pigment, as found in eyeliner tattoo, technically difficult without temporary or permanent hair loss from heat damage to the terminal hair. Because of the facial location of these tattoos, avoidance of scarring secondary to treatment is essential. The use of high fluences and very short pulses with the Q-switched lasers may increase the risk of tissue reaction and should be approached with caution.

Under certain circumstances the potential for tattoo ink darkening with Q-switched lasers can be used to therapeutic advantage. One patient who had auburn hair in her youth received red-brown eyebrow tattoos at age 30. Her hair color grayed and at age 55 she presented for tattoo treatment (Fig. 4.37). To change the tattoo color to match her hair, we employed the Q-switched ruby laser at fluence of $5\,J/cm^2$. Our patient had immediate pigment darkening, healing to a permanent gray-black color matching her hair.

In summary, the removal of unwanted facial cosmetic tattoos can be accomplished with the use of various lasers. For removal of black, red, green, or blue pigments, the appropriate Q-switched laser is best. Removal of red tattoo pigment is best accomplished with a short wavelength and a rapid pulse (510 nm, 300-ns pigment laser) or the fre-

A B C

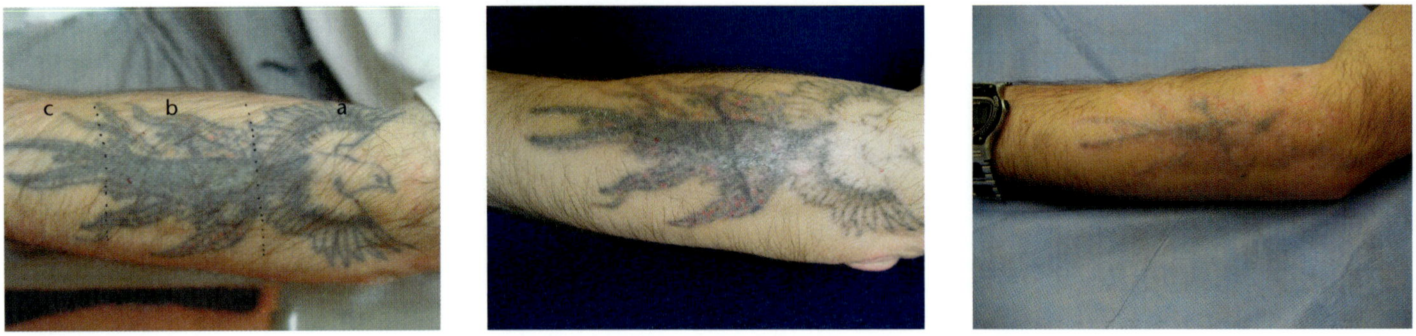

Figure 4.38 (A) Prior to treatment, this tattoo was divided into three test sections: 'a' laser followed by imiquimod cream, 'b' imiquimod pretreatment followed by laser, and 'c' imiquimod cream alone. (B) After 6 weeks, section 'a' cleared more than section 'b', whereas section 'c' did not clear significantly. (C) After two Q-switched alexandrite and four Q-switched ruby laser treatments, all followed by regimen 'a' with imiquimod cream, the overlaid tattoo is completely removed and only the older, underlying tattoo remains.

quency doubled Nd:YAG laser (532 nm, 10 ns). Treatment of cosmetic tattoos should be approached with caution because of the potential irreversible pigment darkening induced by laser interaction with iron oxide pigments or titanium dioxide. However, selected cases of eyeliner tattoo removal can be achieved with use of the $UPCO_2$ laser or other similarly engineered superpulsed CO_2 lasers because of the extreme precision obtainable.

Present and Future Developments in Tattoo Removal

Q-switched lasers provide a dramatic improvement over previous modalities for tattoo removal, and scarless tattoo removal has become the expected therapeutic outcome. Appropriate wavelength choice will facilitate clearing of multicolored tattoos, and current goals include more efficient specific targeting of tattoo pigment over a shorter number of treatment sessions. Exploration into the use of picosecond lasers is underway and may further enhance our ability to remove tattoos rapidly without damaging surrounding tissue.[193,195,200–202]

As Cohen and Goldman first hypothesized in 1994, macrophage stimulating factors can be used for adjuvant therapy with laser tattoo removal.[203] With the advent of Imiquimod, the first of a new class of topical immune response modifier drugs, such adjuvant therapy is readily accomplished. Non-surgical tattoo removal in animal models has been demonstrated using topical imiquimod cream.[204–206]

One of our patients volunteered for a trial of imiquimod cream and Q-switched laser, treating separate portions of his tattoo for comparison. As a teenager, he had a small blue-black tattoo of a bird, which was later covered with a second, larger tattoo of another bird. Initially, the tattoo was divided into three sections (Fig. 4.38). Section 'a' was treated with Q-switched alexandrite laser followed by imiquimod cream. Section 'b' was pretreated with imiquimod prior to laser, without subsequent imiquimod. Section 'c' was treated with imiquimod cream alone, without laser. The 6-week follow-up demonstrates section 'a' cleared more than section 'b,' whereas section 'c' did not clear significantly.

In our clinical experience, tattoos treated with Q-switched laser in conjunction with at home imiquimod therapy during the interval between laser sessions yields more rapid visible clearance of the tattoo than either laser or Imiquimod treatment alone. Newer topical immune response modifier molecules are under development and optimal therapeutic parameters for this class of adjuvant therapy are yet to be defined.

Acknowelgement

This chapter has been modified from Goldman MP, Fitzpatrick RE: Ch 4 in Cutaneous Laser Surgery: The Art and Science of Selective Photothermolysis 2nd Ed. Goldman MP, Fitzpatrick RE (eds) Mosby, St. Louis, 1999.

References

1. Grumet GW. Psychodynamic implications of tattoos. Am J Orthopsychiatry 1983; 53:482.
2. Scutt R, Gotch C. Art, sex and symbol: the mystery of tattooing. Cranbury, NJ: Barnes; 1974.
3. Ebensten H. Pierced hearts and true love. London: Verschoyle; 1953.
4. Pers M, von Herbst T. Tatovering af umyndige. Ugeskr Laeg 1965; 31:973.
5. Pers M, von Herbst T. The demand for removal of tattoos: a plea for regulations against tattooing of minors. Acta Chir Scand 1966; 131:201.
6. Gittleson N, Wallen G, Dawson-Butterworth K. The tattooed psychiatric patient. Br J Psychiatry 1969; 115:1249.
7. Taylor A. A search among Borstal girls for the psychological and social significance of their tattoos. Br J Criminol 1968; 8:170.
8. Hamburger E, Lacovara D. A study of tattoos in inmates at a federal correctional institution: its physical and psychological implications. Milit Med 1963; 128:1205.
9. Roe A, Howell R, Payne I. Comparison of prison inmates with and without juvenile records. Psychol Rep 1974; 34:1315.
10. Lander J, Kohn A. A note on tattooing among selectees. Am J Psychiatry 1943; 100:326.

11. Youniss R. The relationship of tattoos to personal adjustment among enlisted submarine school volunteers. US Naval Med Res Lab 1959; Report no 319; 18:1.
12. Goldstein N. Psychological implications of tattoos. J Dermatol Surg Oncol 1979; 5:883.
13. Smith SR, Matheson BK, Riffenburgh RH. Trends in tattooing. Dermatol Surg 1996; 22:485–6.
14. Stephens MB. Behavioral risks associated with tattooing. Fam Med 2003; 35(1):52–4.
15. Carroll ST, Riffenburgh RH, Roberts TA, Myhre EB. Tattoos and body piercings as indicators of adolescent risk-taking behaviors. Pediatrics 2002; 109(6):1021–7.
16. Forbes GB. College students with tattoos and piercings: motives, family experiences, personality factors, and perception by others. Psychol Rep 2001; 89(3):77486.
17. Rooks JK, Roberts DJ, Scheltema K. Tattoos: their relationship to trauma, psychopathology, and other myths. Minn Med 2000; 83(7):247.
18. Hellgren L. Tattooing: the prevalence of tattooed persons in a total population. Stockholm: Almquist & Wiksell; 1967.
19. Hamburger E. Tattooing as a psychic defence mechanism. Int J Soc Psychiatry 1966; 12:60.
20. Lepine A. Tattooing in approved schools and remand homes. Health Trends 1969; 1:11.
21. Scutt RWB. The chemical removal of tattoos. Br J Plast Surg 1972; 25:189.
22. Cohen M. Tattooing: some medical and psychological aspects. Br J Dermatol 1927; 39:290.
23. Armstrong ML et al. Motivation for tattoo removal. Arch Dermatol 1996; 132:412–16.
24. Lapidoth M, Aharonowitz G. Tattoo removal among Ethiopian Jews in Israel: tradition faces technology. J Am Acad Dermatol 2004; 51(6):906–9.
25. Armstrong ML. Career-oriented women with tattoos. J Nurs Schol 1991; 23:215.
26. Lea PJ, Pawlowski A. Human tattoo: electron microscopic assessment of epidermis, epidermal–dermal junction, and dermis. Int J Dermatol 1987; 26:453.
27. Taylor CR, Anderson R, Gange W et al. Light and electron microscopic analysis of tattoos treated by Q-switched ruby laser. J Invest Dermatol 1991; 97:131.
28. Diette KM, Bronstein BR, Parrish JA. Histologic comparison of argon and tunable dye lasers in the treatment of tattoos. J Invest Dermatol 1985; 85:368.
29. Patipa M, Jakobiec FA, Krebs W. Light and electron microscopic findings with permanent eyeliner. Ophthalmology 1986; 93(10):1361.
30. Christensen HE, Schmidt H. The ultrastructure of tattoo marks. Pathol Microbiol Scand 1972; 80A:573.
31. Mann R, Klingmuller G. Electron-microscopic investigation of tattoos in rabbit skin. Arch Dermatol Res 1981; 271:367.
32. Goldstein AP. Histologic reactions in tattoos. J Dermatol Surg Oncol 1979; 5:896.
33. Yang DS, Kim SC, Lee S et al. Foreign body epithelioid granuloma after cosmetic eyebrow tattooing. Cutis 1989; 43:224.
34. Ravits HG. Allergic tattoo granuloma. Arch Dermatol 1962; 86:287.
35. Guillaume AC. Recherches sur le mechanisme du tatouage et enseignements qui en resultent au point de vue des fonctions de la peau. Bull Med Paris 1927; 41:1399.
36. Guillaume AC. Quelques particularites des fonctions de la peau qui sont enseignes par l'etude des tatouages. Bull Med Paris 1927; 41:1457.
37. Silberberg I, Leider M. Studies of a red tattoo. Arch Dermatol 1970; 101:299.
38. Abel EA, Silberberg I, Queen D. Studies of chronic inflammation in a red tattoo by electron microscopy and histochemistry. Acta Dermatol Venereol (Stockh) 1972; 52:453.
39. Olander K, Kanai A, Kaufman HE. An analytical electron microscopic study of a corneal tattoo. Ann Ophthalmol 1983; 15:1046.
40. Tope WD, Arbiser JL, Duncan LM. Black tattoo reaction: the peacock's tale. J Am Acad Dermatol 1996; 35(3):477–9.
41. Duke D et al. A reaction to a red lip cosmetic tattoo. J Am Acad Dermatol 1998; 39(3):488–90.
42. Schwarze HP et al. Delayed-hypersensitivity granulomatous reaction induced by blepharopigmentation with aluminum-silicate. J Am Acad Dermatol 2000; 42(5):888–91.
43. Dickinson JA. Sarcoidal reaction in tattoos. Arch Dermatol 1969; 100:315.
44. Farzan S. Sarcoidal reaction in tattoos. NY State J Med 1977; 77:1477.
45. Jones MS, Maloney ME, Helm KF. Systemic sarcoidosis presenting in the black dye of a tattoo. Cutis 1997; 59:113–15.
46. Jacob CI. Tattoo-associated dermatoses: a case report and review of the literature. Dermatol Surg 2002; 28(10):961–5.
47. Wolf R, Wolf D. A tattooed butterfly as a vector of atypical Mycobacteria. J Am Acad Dermatol 2003; 48(S)73–4.
48. Tse T, Folberg R, Moore K. Clinicopathologic correlate of a fresh eyelid pigment implantation. Arch Ophthalmol 1985; 103:1515.
49. Goldstein N, Sewell M. Tattoos in different cultures. J Dermatol Surg Oncol 1979; 5:857.
50. Everett MA. Tattoos: abnormalities of pigmentation. In: Clinical dermatology, vol 2, units 11–21. Hagerstown, MD: Harper & Row; 1980.
51. Rostenberg A, Brown RA, Caro MR. Discussion of tattoo reactions with report of a case showing a reaction to a green color. Arch Dermatol Syph 1950; 62:540.
52. Anderson RR. Tattooing should be regulated. N Engl J Med 1992; 326:207.
53. Ballin DB. Cutaneous hypersensitivity to mercury from tattooing: report of case. Arch Dermatol Syph 1933; 27:292.
54. Bonnell JA, Russell B. Skin reactions at sites of green and red tattoo marks. Proc R Soc Med 1956; 49:823.
55. Bjornberg A. Reactions to light in yellow tattoos from cadmium sulfide. Arch Dermatol 1963; 88:267.
56. Tindall JP, Smith JG Jr. Unusual reactions in yellow tattoos: microscopic studies on histologic sections. South Med J 1962; 55:792.
57. Loewenthal LJA. Reactions in green tattoos: the significance of valence state of chromium. Arch Dermatol 1960; 82:237.
58. Bjornberg A. Allergic reactions to chrome in green tattoo markings. Acta Derm Venereal 1959; 39:23.
59. Tazelaar DJ. Hypersensitivity to chromium in a light-blue tattoo. Dermatologiea 1970; 141:282.
60. Rorsman H, Dahlquist I, Jacobsson S et al. Tattoo granuloma and uveitis. Lancet 1969; 11:27.
61. Swinny B. Generalized chronic dermatitis due to tattoo. Ann Allergy 1946; 4:295.
62. Novy FG. A generalized mercurial (cinnabar) reaction following tattooing. Arch Dermatol 1944; 49:172.
63. Goldstein N. Complications for tattoos. J Dermatol Surg Oncol 1979; 5:869.
64. England RW, Vogel P, Hagan L. Immediate cutaneous hypersensitivity after treatment of tattoo with Nd:YAG laser: a case report and review of the literature. Ann Allergy Asthma Immunol 2002; 89(2):215–17.

65. Rudlinger R. Successful removal by ruby laser of darkened ink after ruby laser treatment of mismatched tattoos for acne scars. J Cut Laser Ther 2000; 2:37–9.
66. Boo-Chai K. The decorative tattoo: its removal by dermabrasion. Plast Reconstr Surg 1963; 32:559.
67. Clabaugh W. Removal of tattoos by superficial dermabrasion. Arch Dermatol 1968; 98:515.
68. Clabaugh W. Tattoo removal by superficial dermabrasion. Plast Reconstr Surg 1975; 55:401.
69. Bunke HJ, Conway H. Surgery of decorative and traumatic tattoos. Plast Reconstr Surg 1957; 20:67.
70. Crittenden FM. Salabrasion: removal of tattoos by superficial abrasion with table salt. Cutis 1971; 7:295.
71. Koerber WA, Price NM. Salabrasion of tattoos. Arch Dermatol 1978; 114:884.
72. Lindsay DG. Tattoos. Dermatol Clin 1989; 7:147.
73. Morgan BDG. Tattoos. Br Med J 1974; 3:34.
74. Strong AMM, Jackson JT. The removal of amateur tattoos by salabrasion. Br J Dermatol 1979; 101:693.
75. Wentzell JM, Robinson JK, Wentzell JM et al. Physical properties of aerosols produced by dermabrasion. Arch Dermatol 1989; 125:1637.
76. Goldstein N. Tattoo removal. Dermatol Clin 1987; 5:349.
77. Bailey BN. Treatment of tattoos. Plast Reconstr Surg 1976; 40:361.
78. Ceilley RI. Curettage after dermabrasion: techniques of removal of tattoos. J Dermatol Surg Oncol 1979; 5:905.
79. Goldstein N, Penoff J, Price N et al. Techniques of removal of tattoos. J Dermatol Surg Oncol 1979; 5:901.
80. Robinson J. Tattoo removal. J Dermatol Surg Oncol 1985; 11:14.
81. Apfelberg DB, Manchester GH. Decorative and traumatic tattoo biophysics and removal. Clin Plast Surg 1987; 14:243.
82. Gupta SC. An investigation into a method for the removal of dermal tattoos: a report on animal and clinical studies. Plast Reconstr Surg 1965; 36:354.
83. Wheeler ES, Miller TA. Tattoo removal by split thickness tangential excision. West J Med 1976; 124:272.
84. Variot G. Nouveau procede de destruction des tatouages. Compte Rendu Societe Biologie (Paris) 1888; 8:836.
85. Penoff JH. The office treatment of tattoos: a simple and effective method. Plast Reconstr Surg 1987; 79:186.
86. Piggot TA, Norris RW. The treatment of tattoos with trichloroacetic acid: experience with 670 patients. Br J Plast Surg 1988; 41:112.
87. Hudson DA, Lechtape-Gruter RU. A simple method of tattoo removal. S Afr Med J 1990; 78:748.
88. Colver GB, Jones RL, Cherry GW et al. Precise dermal damage with an infrared coagulator. Br J Dermatol 1986; 114:603.
89. Colver GB, Cherry GW, Dawber RPR et al. The treatment of cutaneous vascular lesions with the infrared coagulator: a preliminary report. Br J Plast Surg 1986; 39:131.
90. Colver GB, Hunter JAA. Venous lakes: treatment by infrared coagulation. Br J Plast Surg 1987; 40:451.
91. Dorn B, Christophers E, Kietzmann H. Treatment of port-wine stains and haemangiomas by infrared contact coagulation. 17th World Congress of Dermatology Abstracts 1987; 2:3071987.
92. Groot DW, Arlett JP, Johnston PA. Comparison of the infrared coagulator and the carbon dioxide laser in the removal of decorative tattoos. J Am Acad Dermatol 1986; 15:518.
93. Colver GB, Cherry GW, Dawber RPR et al. Tattoo removal using infrared coagulation. Br J Dermatol 1985; 112:481.
94. Venning VA, Colver GB, Millard PR et al. Tattoo removal using infrared coagulation: a dose comparison. Br J Dermatol 1987; 117:99.
95. Colver GB. The infrared coagulator in dermatology. Dermatol Clin 1989; 7:155.
96. Leopold PJ. Cryosurgery for facial skin lesions. Proc R Soc Med 1975; 68:606.
97. Zacarian SA. Cryosurgery for cutaneous carcinoma. Dermatol Dig 1970; 9:49.
98. Ruiz-Esparza J, Fitzpatrick RE, Goldman MP. Tattoo removal: selecting the right alternative. Am J Cosmetic Surg 1992; 9:171.
99. Colver GB, Dawber RPR. Tattoo removal using a liquid nitrogen cryospray. Clin Exp Dermatol 1984; 9:364.
100. Dvir E, Hirshowitz B. Tattoo removal by cryosurgery. Plast Reconstr Surg 1980; 66:373.
101. Colver GB, Dawber RPR. The removal of digital tattoos. Int J Dermatol 1985; 24:567.
102. Goldman L, Blaney DJ, Kindel DJ et al. Effect of the laser beam on the skin: preliminary report. J Invest Dermatol 1963; 40:121.
103. Goldman L, Blaney DJ, Kindel DJ et al. Pathology of the effect of the laser beam on the skin. Nature 1965; 197:912.
104. Goldman L, Wilson RG, Hornby P et al. Radiation from a Q-switched ruby laser. J Invest Dermatol 1965; 44:69.
105. Goldman L et al. Laser treatment of tattoos: a preliminary survey of three years' clinical experience. JAMA 1967; 201:841.
106. Goldman L, Rockwell RJ, Meyer R et al. Laser treatment of tattoos. JAMA 1967; 201:163.
107. Yules RB, Laub DR, Honey R et al. The effect of Q-switched ruby laser radiation on dermal tattoo pigment in man. Arch Surg 1967; 95:179.
108. Laub DR, Yules RB, Arras M et al. Preliminary histopathological observation of Q-switched ruby laser radiation on dermal tattoo pigment in man. J Surg Res 1968; 5(8):220.
109. Apfelberg DB, Maser MR, Lash H. Argon laser treatment of decorative tattoos. Br J Plast Surg 1979; 32:141.
110. Apfelberg DB, Rivers J, Maser MR et al. Update on laser usage in treatment of decorative tattoos. Lasers Surg Med 1982; 2:169.
111. Apfelberg DB, Laub DR, Maser MR et al. Pathophysiology and treatment of decorative tattoos with reference to argon laser treatment. Clin Plast Surg 1967; 7:369.
112. Reid R. Tattoo removal with laser. Med J Aust 1978; April 8 (letter).
113. Fitzpatrick RE, Goldman MP, Ruiz-Esparza J. The use of the alexandrite laser (755 nm, 100 μsec) for tattoo pigment removal in an animal model. J Am Acad Dermatol 1993; 28:7451993.
114. Apfelberg DB, Maser MR, Lash R et al. Comparison of argon and carbon dioxide laser treatment of decorative tattoos. a preliminary report. Ann Plast Surg 1985; 14:61985.
115. McBurney EI. Carbon dioxide laser treatment of dermatologic lesions. South Med J 19778; 71:795.
116. Brady SC, Blokmanis A, Jewett L. Tattoo removal with the carbon dioxide laser. Ann Plast Surg 1978; 2:482.
117. Beacon JP, Ellis H. Surgical removal of tattoos by carbon dioxide laser. J R Soc Med 1980; 73:298.
118. Bailin PL, Ratz JL, Levine HL. Removal of tattoos by CO_2 laser. J Dermatol Surg Oncol 1980; 6:997.
119. Reid R, Muller S. Tattoo removal by CO_2 laser dermabrasion. Plast Reconstr Surg 1980; 65:717.
120. Dixon J. Laser treatment of decorative tattoos. In: Arndt KA, Noe JM, Rosen S, eds. Cutaneous laser therapy: principles and methods. New York: John Wiley & Sons; 1983.
121. Ruiz-Esparza J, Goldman MP, Fitzpatrick RE. Tattoo removal with minimal scarring: the chemo-laser technique. J Dermatol Surg Oncol 1989; 14:1372.

122. Dismukes DE. The 'chemo-laser technique' for the treatment of decorative tattoos: a more complete dye-removal procedure. Lasers Surg Med 1986; 6:59.
123. Anderson RR, Parrish JA. Selective photothermolysis: precise microsurgery by selective absorption of pulsed irradiation. Science 1983; 220:524.
124. Kilmer SL, Lee MS, Anderson RR. Treatment of multi-colored tattoos with the frequency-doubled Q-switched Nd:YAG laser (532 nm): a dose-response study with comparison to the Q-switched ruby laser. Lasers Surg Med 1993; Suppl 5:54.
125. Hodersdal M, Bech-Thomsen N, Wulf HC. Skin reflectance-guided laser selections for treatment of decorative tattoos. Arch Dermatol 1996; 132:403.
126. Fitzpatrick RE, Goldman MP. Tattoo removal using the alexandrite laser (755 nm, 100 ns). Arch Dermatol 1994; 130:1508.
127. Goldman L. Laser surgical research. Ann NY Acad Sci 1970; 168:649.
128. Reid RI, Muller S. Tattoo removal with laser. Med J Aust 1978; 1:389.
129. Reid WH, McLeod PJ, Ritchie A et al. Q-switched ruby laser treatment of black tattoos. Br J Plast Surg 1983; 36:455.
130. Polla LL, Margolis RJ, Dover JS et al. Melanosomes are a primary target of Q-switched ruby laser irradiation in guinea pig skin. J Invest Dermatol 1987; 89:281.
131. Dover JS, Margolis RJ, Polla LL et al. Pigmented guinea pig skin irradiated with Q-switched ruby laser pulses: morphologic and histologic findings. Arch Dermatol 1989; 125:43.
132. Taylor CR, Gange RW, Dover JS et al. Treatment of tattoos by Q-switched ruby laser: a dose–response study. Arch Dermatol 1990; 126:893.
133. Scheibner A, Kenny G, White W et al. A superior method of tattoo removal using the Q-switched ruby laser. J Dermatol Surg Oncol 1990; 16:1091.
134. Darwin D, et al. Laser-tattoo removal – a study of the mechanism and the optimal treatment strategy via computer simulations. Lasers Surg Med 2002; 30:389–97.
135. Geronemus RG, Ashinoff R. Use of the Q-switched ruby laser to treat tattoos and benign pigmented lesions of the skin. Lasers Surg Med 1991; Suppl 3:64.
136. Ashinoff R, Geronemus RG. Rapid response of traumatic and medical tattoos to treatment with the Q-switched ruby laser. Plast Reconstr Surg 1993; 91:841.
137. Lowe NJ, Luftman D, Sawcer D. Q-switched ruby laser: further observations on treatment of professional tattoos. J Dermatol Surg Oncol 1994; 20:307.
138. Levins PC, Grevelink JM, Anderson RR. Q-switched ruby laser treatment of tattoos. Lasers Surg Med 1991; Suppl 3:63.
139. Bernstein LJ et al. Tattoo formation from absorbable synthetic suture and successful removal with Q-switched ruby laser. Dermatol Surg 1996; 22:1040–2.
140. Ashinoff R, Tanenbaum D. Treatment of an amalgam tattoo with the Q-switched ruby laser. Cutis 1994; 54:269–70.
141. Achauer BM et al. Treatment of traumatic tattoos by Q-switched ruby laser. Plastic Reconstr Surg 1994; 93(2):318–23.
142. Kilmer SL, Anderson RR. Clinical use of the Q-switched ruby and the Q-switched Nd:YAG (1064 nm and 532 nm) lasers for treatment of tattoos. J Dermatol Surg Oncol 1993; 19: 330.
143. DeCoste SD, Anderson RR. Comparison of Q-switched ruby and Q-switched Nd:YAG laser treatment of tattoos. Lasers Surg Med 1991; Suppl 3:64.
144. Kilmer SL, Lee M, Farinelli W et al. Q-switched Nd:YAG laser (1064 nm) effectively treats Q-switched ruby laser resistant tattoos. Lasers Surg Med 1992; Suppl 4:72.
145. Pay AD, Kenealy JM. Laser transmission through membranes using the Q-switched Nd:YAG laser. Lasers Surg Med 1999; 24:48–54.
146. Kilmer SL, Lee MS, Grevelink JM et al. The Q-switched Nd:YAG laser (1064 nm) effectively treats tattoos: a controlled, dose–response study. Arch Dermatol 1993; 129:971.
147. Ferguson JE, August PJ. Evaluation of the Nd/YAG laser for treatment of amateur and professional tattoos. Br J Dermatol 1996; 135:586.
148. Naverson DN, Igelman JD. Q-switched laser management of an explosion tattoo. J Am Adac Dermatol 2004; 50:479–80.
149. Suzuki H. Treatment of traumatic tattoos with the Q-switched Neodynium:YAG laser. Arch Dermatol 1996; 132:1226–9.
150. Wong SS, Goh KS. Successful treatment of traumatic tattoos with the Q-switched neodymium:YAG laser: a report of two cases. J Dermatol Treatment 1998; 9:193–5.
151. Jones A, Roddey P, Orengo I, Rosen T. The Q-switched Nd:YAG laser effectively treats tattoos in darkly pigmented skin. Dermatol Surg 1996; 22:999.
152. Grevelink JM, Duke D, Van Leeuwen RL et al. Laser treatment of tattoos in darkly pigmented patients: efficacy and side effects. J Am Acad Dermatol 1996; 34:653.
153. Geronemus RG. Surgical pearl: Q-switched Nd:YAG laser removal of eyeliner tattoo. J Am Adac Dermatol 1996; 35:101–2.
154. Kilmer SL, Farinelli WF, Tearney G, Anderson RR. Use of a larger spot size for the treatment of tattoos increases clinical efficacy and decreases potential side effects. Lasers Surg Med 1994; Suppl 6:51.
155. Fitzpatrick RE, Goldman MP. Tattoo removal using the alexandrite lasers. Arch Dermatol 1994; 130:1508.
156. Alster TS. Q-switched alexandrite laser treatment (755 nm) of professional and amateur tattoos. J Am Acad Dermatol 1995; 33:69.
157. Stafford TJ, Lizek R, Tan OT. Role of the alexandrite laser for removal of tattoos. Lasers Surg Med 1995; 17:32.
158. Garcia C, Clark RE. Tattoo removal using the alexandrite laser. NC Med J 1995; 56:336.
159. Dozier Se et al. The Q-switched alexandrite laser's effects on tattoos in guinea pigs and harvested human skin. Dermatol Surg 1995; 21:237–40.
160. Shah G, Alster TS. Treatment of an amalgam tattoo with a Q-switched alexandrite (755nm) laser. Dermatol Surg 2002; 28:1180–1.
161. Moreno-Arias GA, Camps-Fresneda A. The use of Q-switched alexandrite laser (755nm, 100ns) for eyeliner tattoo removal. J Cut Laser Ther 1999; 1:113–15.
162. Moreno-Arias GA, Camps-Fresneda A. Cosmetic tattoo refractive to Q-switched alexandrite laser. J Cut Laser Ther 1999; 1:117–19.
163. Moreno-Arias GA, Camps-Fresneda A. Use of the Q-switched alexandrite laser (755nm, 100ns) for eyebrow tattoo removal. Lasers Surg Med 1999; 25:123–5.
164. Moreno-Arias GA, Casals-Andreu M, Camps-Fresneda A. Use of Q-switched alexandrite laser (755nm, 100ns) for removal of traumatic tattoo of different origins. Lasers Surg Med 1999; 25:445–50.
165. Leuenberger ML, et al. Comparison of the Q-switched alexandrite, Nd:YAG, and ruby lasers in treating blue-black tattoos. Dermatol Surg 1999; 25(1):10–14.
166. Goyal S et al. Laser treatment of tattoos: a prospective, paired, comparison study of the Q-switched Nd:YAG (1064 nm), frequency-doubled Q-switched Nd:YAG (532nm), and Q-switched ruby lasers. J Am Acad Dermatol 1997; 36:122–5.

167. Zelickson BD et al. Clinical, histologic, and ultrastructural evaluation of tattoos treated with three laser systems. Lasers Surg Med 1994; 15:364–72.
168. Boehncke WH, Hibst R, Kaufman R. Within-individual comparison of Q-switched Nd:YAG and alexandrite lasers in the treatment of monochromatic black amateur tattoos. J Dermatol Treatment 1994; 5:29–32.
169. Fusade et al. Treatment of gunpowder traumatic tattoo by Q-switched Nd:YAG laser: an unusual adverse effect. Dermatol Surg 2000; 26:1057–9.
170. Alora MB et al. Scarring following Q-switched laser treatment of 'double tattoos.' Arch Dermatol 2000; 136:269–70.
171. Ashinoff R, Levine VJ, Soter NA. Allergic reactions to tattoo pigment after laser treatment. Dermatol Surg 1995; 21:291.
172. Naarman VR et al. Tattoo pigments are cleaved by laser light – the chemical analysis in vitro provide evidence for hazardous compounds. Photochem Photobiol 2004; 80(2):185–90.
173. Baumler W et al. Q-switch laser and tattoo pigments: first results of the chemical and photophysical analysis of 41 compounds. Lasers Surg Med 2000; 26:13–21.
174. Swanson VS. Tattoo ink darkening of a yellow tattoo after Q-switched laser treatment. Clin Exp Dermatol 2002; 27(6):461–3.
175. Levine V, Geronemus R. Tattoo removal with the Q-switched ruby laser and the Q-switched Nd:YAG laser: a comparative study. Cutis 1995; 55:291.
176. McMeekin TO, Goodwin DP. A comparison of the alexandrite laser (755 nm) with the Q-switched ruby laser (694 nm) in the treatment of tattoos. Lasers Surg Med 1993; Suppl 5:43.
177. Balsam MS, Sagarin E, eds. Cosmetics: science and technology, 2nd edn. New York: Wiley-Interscience; 1974.
178. Angres GA. Angres permalid-liner method: a new surgical procedure. Am J Ophthalmol 1984; 16:145.
179. Farber MG, Lamberg RC, Smith ME. A histologic study of eyelid pigment eight weeks after implantation (eyelid tattoo). Arch Ophthalmol 1986; 104:1434.
180. Angres GG. Blepharo and dermapigmentation techniques for facial cosmesis. Ear Nose Throat J 1987; 66:344.
181. Tanenbaum M, Karas S, McCord CD. Laser ablation of blepharopigmentation. Ophthal Plast Reconstr Surg 1988; 4:49.
182. Wilkes TD. The complications of dermal tattooing. Ophthalmic Surg 1986; 2:1.
183. Goldberg RA, Shorr N. Complications of blepharopigmentation. Ophthalmic Surg 1989; 20:420.
184. Angres FF. Blepharopigmentation procedure guidelines. Plast Reconstr Surg 1986; 77:338.
185. Hurwitz JJ, Brownstein S, Mishkin SK. Histopathological findings in blepharopigmentation (eyelid tattoo). Can J Ophthamol 1988; 23:267.
186. Lee IW et al. Complications of eyelash and eyebrow tattooing: reports of two cases of pigment fanning. Cutis 2001; 68:53–5.
187. Putterman AM, Migliori ME. Elective excision of permanent eyeliner. Arch Ophthalmol 1988; 106:1034.
188. Dedio RM, Henry WJ, Scipione CR. Surgical removal of blepharopigmentation. Am J Cosmetic Surg 1990; 7:93.
189. Fogh H, Wulf HC, Poulsen T et al. Tattoo removal by overtattooing with tannic acid. J Dermatol Surg Oncol 1989; 15:1089.
190. Fitzpatrick RE, Goldman MP, Dierickx C. Laser ablation of facial cosmetic tattoos. Aesthetic Plast Surg 1994; 18:91–98.
191. Herbich GJ. Ultrapulse carbon dioxide laser treatment of an iron oxide flesh-colored tattoo. Dermatol Surg 1997; 23: 60.
192. Kilmer SL, Fitzpatrick RE, Da Silva LB et al. Picosecond and femtosecond laser treatment of tattoo ink. Lasers Surg Med 1996; Suppl 8:36.
193. Cotton FA, Wilkinson G, eds. The transition elements. In: Cotton FA, Wilkinson G, eds. Advanced inorganic chemistry. New York: Interscience; 1972.
194. Anderson RR, Geronemus R, Kilmer SC et al. Cosmetic tattoo ink darkening: a complication of Q-switched and pulsed-laser treatment. Arch Dermatol 1993; 8:1010.
195. Ross V, Naseef G, Lin G et al. Comparison of responses of tattoos to picosecond and nanosecond Q-switched neodymium:YAG lasers. Arch Dermatol 1998; 134: 167.
196. Jimenez G, Weiss E, Spencer JM. Multiple color changes following laser therapy of cosmetic tattoos. Dermatol Surg 2002; 28:177–9.
197. Chang SE et al. Areolar cosmetic tattoo ink darkening: a complication of Q-switched alexandrite laser treatment. Dermatol Surg 2002; 28:95–6.
198. Casparian JM, Krell J. Using a side effect to therapeutic advantage: the darkening of red eyebrow tattoo pigment following Q-switched laser treatment. Dermatol Surg 2000; 26:255–7.
199. Fitzpatrick RE, Lupton JR. Successful treatment of treatment-resistant laser-induced pigment darkening of a cosmetic tattoo. Lasers Surg Med 2000; 27:358–61.
200. Herd RM et al. A clinical and histologic prospective controlled comparative study of the picosecond titanium:sapphire (795nm) laser versus the Q-switched alexandrite (752nm) laser for removing tattoo pigment. J Am Acad Dermatol 1999; 40(4):603–6.
201. Aschwanden A et al. 2.1 picosecond passively mode-locked external-cavity semiconductor laser. Opt Lett 2005; 1;30(3):272–4.
202. Audebert P et al. Picosecond time-resolved X-ray absorption spectroscopy of ultrafast aluminum plasmas. Phys Rev Lett 21; 94(2):025004, Epub 2005.
203. Cohen PR, Goldman MP. The adjuvant use of macrophage colony stimulating factor in tattoo removal using laser. Medical Hypotheses 1995; 45:83–5.
204. Magee NS et al. Triweekly topical 5% imiquimod cream fades experimental tattoos in guinea pigs. Cosmetic Dermatol 2005; 18(20):155–61.
205. Solis B et al. Experimental nonsurgical tattoo removal in a guinea pig model with topical imiquimod and tretinoin. Dermatol Surg 2002; 28:83–7.
206. Berman B, Poochareon VN, Villa AM. Novel dermatologic uses of the immune response modifier imiquimod 5% cream. Skin Therapy Lett 2002; 7(9):1–6.

Chapter 5

Hair Removal by Lasers and other Light Sources

Christine C. Dierickx

Introduction

The first laser-assisted hair removal device was marketed in 1996. Today such hair removal devices include ruby, alexandrite, diode and neodymium:yttrium aluminum garnet (Nd:YAG) lasers and intense pulsed light (IPL) sources. With the numerous lasers and nonlaser light sources available today, one is faced with the question which hair removal device to use. This article explains the mechanisms of using light to remove hair, examines the attributes of specific light devices systems and focuses on treatment protocol for the various systems in order to provide a safe and effective treatment.

Mechanisms of Hair Follicle

There are three means by which light can destroy hair follicles: thermal (due to local heating), mechanical (due to shockwaves or violent cavitation) and photochemical (due to generation of toxic mediators like singlet oxygen or free radicals). Removal of hair has been attempted by all three means.

Photothermal Destruction

Photothermal destruction is based on the principle of selective photothermolysis. The principle states that by choosing an appropriate wavelength, pulse duration, and fluence, thermal injury can be confined to a target chromophore.[1] In the visible to near infrared region, melanin is the natural chromophore for targeting hair follicles. It is found in the hair shaft, the outer root sheath of the infundibulum and the matrix area.[2] Lasers or light sources that operate in the red or near-infrared wavelength region (694 nm ruby laser, 755 nm alexandrite laser, 800 nm diode laser, 1064 nm Nd:YAG laser and noncoherent light sources with cutoff filters), all lie in an optical window of the electromagnetic spectrum, where selective absorption by melanin is combined with deep penetration into the dermis.[3] Deep, selective heating of the hair shaft, hair follicle epithelium and the heavily pigmented matrix is therefore possible in the 600–1100 nm region.

However, melanin in the epidermis presents a competing site for absorption. Selective cooling of the epidermis has been shown to minimize epidermal injury. Cooling can be achieved by various means including ice,[4] a cooled gel layer,[5] a cooled glass chamber,[6] cooled sapphire window,[7] a pulsed cryogen spray,[8] or cold air flow.[9]

Laser pulse width also appears to play an important role, as suggested by thermal transfer theory.[10] Thermal conduction from the melanin-rich shaft and matrix will heat surrounding follicular structures. To obtain spatial confinement of thermal damage, the pulse duration should be shorter than or equal to the thermal relaxation time of the hair follicle. Thermal relaxation of human terminal hair follicles has never been measured but is estimated to be about 10 to 100 ms,[1,10,11] depending on size. Therefore, devices for hair removal have pulse durations in the millisecond domain region. The normal mode 694 nm ruby,[12–14] normal mode 755 nm alexandrite,[15–17] 800 nm pulsed diode,[18–22] and long pulsed Nd:YAG lasers,[22,23] as well as filtered flashlamp technology,[24,25] all have pulse durations in the millisecond range.

However, sometimes the actual target is not pigmented and is at some distance from a pigmented structure. For example, the follicular stem cells, which line the outer root sheath, in an area called the bulge, near the attachment of the arrector pili muscle, are not pigmented and at some distance from the pigmented hair shaft. These cells appear to be an important target for permanent hair destruction. The concept of thermal damage time (TDT) has therefore been proposed.[26] Pulses longer than the thermal relaxation time of the hair shaft allow propagation of the thermal damage front through the entire volume to better damage the follicular stem cells. Super long pulse heating (>100 ms) appears to allow for long-term hair removal.[27]

Finally, hair removal is also dependent on fluence. Careful studies with computerized hair counts have demonstrated that greater hair loss was achieved at the higher fluences tested.[28,29] However, a patient's skin color will determine the highest tolerated fluence.

Photomechanical Destruction

Photomechanical destruction of hair has been attempted with very short nanosecond pulses by Q-switched 1064 nm Nd:YAG lasers, with or without carbon suspension.[30–33] However, when these very short pulses are used to target hair follicles, there is extremely rapid heating of the chromophore (melanin). This generates photoacoustic shock waves that cause focal photomechanical disruption of the melanocytes[34] but no complete follicular disruption, leading in animals to leukotrichia but not to hair loss.[35] Consistent with this behavior, temporary hair loss with an absence of permanent hair loss has been reported in humans, despite a decade of using Q-switched lasers widely for tattoo removal.

Photochemical Destruction

Photodynamic therapy is the use of light and a photosensitizer to produce a targeted photochemical reaction and therapeutic effect. Hair removal with topical Aminolevulinic Acid (ALA) has been reported in a pilot study.[36] ALA is a precursor in the porphyrin synthesis and is rapidly and selectively converted to protoporphyrin IX (PPIX) by cells derived from the epidermis and follicular epithelium. On absorption of a photon, PPIX efficiently crosses into an excited triplet state, which in turn generates singlet oxygen by collision with ground-state oxygen. Singlet oxygen is a potent oxidizer that damages cell membranes and protein. This is a so-called photodynamic reaction. A mean hair loss of 40% was reported in 12 volunteers after a single exposure to 630 nm light, 3 hours after application of 20% ALA to the skin. A host of other porphyrins, chlorins, phthalocyanines, purpurins and phenothiazine dyes can act as photodynamic agents and are under development as drugs for photodynamic therapy. It is likely that ALA or one of these other drugs will prove useful for hair removal.

Clinical Technique

Patient Selection

The individual's skin type, hair color and coarseness will determine which device is the most appropriate as well as predict response to treatment. The ideal patient has realistic expectations, normal endocrine status, with thick dark hair and light skin tones. Current techniques are not generally successful in permanently removing white hairs or fine vellus hairs. Laser treatment is much more effective when the pigmented hair shaft is present within the follicle. Patients should therefore not pluck or wax for at least 6 weeks prior to treatment. Shaving, bleaching, or use of chemical depilatories are acceptable alternatives for patients awaiting laser treatment. Due to increased risk for eye injury, patients should not be treated within the orbital rim. Certain medications and hormonal imbalances may inhibit permanent hair removal due to hair stimulation. While treatment can be safely performed with a shorter wavelength device (e.g. ruby laser) in fair patients, it is preferable to utilize a longer wavelength device in darker patients. Further epidermal protection is also afforded by utilizing longer pulse durations and active cooling. When assessing individuals with a suntan, it is usually prudent to delay treatment until fading of the tan occurs. Recent reports indicate the induction of hair growth after laser hair removal. This usually occurs in young female patients with skin types III–VI, who present with fine dark hairs on the lateral face. Laser-induced hypertrichosis is observed in the treated areas as well as in the adjacent non treated zones.[37,38] Although the exact mechanism for this observation is not known, patients should be made aware of this before starting.

Laser Selection

Endogenous Chromophore

694 nm Ruby Lasers

Of the original five normal-mode, 694 nm ruby lasers, only two are still commercially available for hair removal: the RubyStar and Sinon (Table 5.1). Because of high melanin absorption at 694 nm, the ruby lasers are best indicated in light skinned (Fitzpatricks's skin type I–III) individuals with dark hairs.

The E2000 (Palomar) uses a sapphire cooled handpiece (Epiwand™) to protect the epidermis.[7] The sapphire lens is actively cooled to 0 or −10°C and put in direct contact with the skin. Compared to air as an external medium, the sapphire provides heat conduction away from the epidermis before, during and after each laser pulse. It permits beam coupling with the skin and internal reflection reduction by index matching. In addition to surface cooling, the Epiwand™ sapphire handpiece has other distinct advantages. The sapphire lens provides a convergent beam to maximize delivery of light into the dermis. Its surface allows for application of pressure on the skin surface, which deforms the dermis and decreases the distance from the epidermis to the deeper follicular structures. In addition, the pressure blanches the underlying blood vessels, minimizing absorption of laser energy by hemoglobin. Light is delivered through a fiber and two different spot sizes are available (10 and 20 mm). A retroreflector is build into the handpiece, which allows for photon recycling and therefore sufficient energy delivery.[39,40] Depending on skin type or hair thickness, a single pulse (3 ms) or twin pulse (100 ms, i.e. two 3-ms pulses, delivered with a delay of 100 ms) can be chosen.[41]

The EpiTouch™ long-pulsed Ruby (Sharplan, Yokneam, Israel) employs a triple-pulse technology with a 10-ms interval between pulses. It keeps the follicle temperature at a sufficient level to cause destruction while the epidermis temperature remains below damage threshold. This synchronized pulsing technology should make treatment of darker skin types possible. Cooling of the epidermis is achieved by applying a thick layer of cooled transparent gel on the skin. A thin, patented, laser-aligning sheet can be placed on top of the cooling gel, which enables proper positioning of the laser beam and helps to insure uniform laser application to all intended areas.[42]

The RubyStar (Aesculap-Meditec, Jena, Germany) and the Sinon ruby laser (Wavelight, Erlangen, Germany) are

Table 5.1 *Hair Removal Lasers*

Light source	Wavelength (nm)	System name	Pulse duration	Fluence (J/cm^2)	Spot size (mm)	Repetition rate	Other features
Long pulse ruby	694	Ruby Star (Aesclepion-Meditec)	4 ms	Up to 24	Up to 14	1 Hz	Dual mode: may also be Q-switched
		Sinon (Wavelight)	4 ms	Up to 30	5, 7, 9	0.5–2 Hz	Cold air unit: may also be Q-switched
		E2000 (Palomar)	3, 100 ms	10–40	10, 0	1 Hz	Cooling handpiece 0–10°C Fiber delivery Photon recycling
		Epitouch Ruby (Sharplan)	1.2 ms	10–40	3–6	1.2 Hz	Triple pulse technology
		Chromos (Mehl Biophile)	800 μs	10–25	7	0.4–0.6 Hz	
Long pulse alexandrite	755	Apogee (Cynosure)	0.5–300 ms	25–50	5, 10, 12, 15	3 Hz	Cold air or integrated cooling
		Gentlelase (Candela)	3 ms	10–100	6, 8, 10, 12, 15, 18	Up to 1.5 Hz	Dynamic cooling device
		Epitouch ALEX (Sharplan)	2–40 ms	Up to 50	5, 7, 10	1 Hz	Scanner option
		Ultrawave II–III (Adept Medical)	5–50 ms	5–55	8, 10, 12	1–2 Hz	Available with 532 nm and/or 1064 nm Nd:YAG
		Epicare (Light Age)	3–300 ms	25–40	7, 9, 12, 15	1–3 Hz	
		Arion (WaveLight)	1–50 ms	Up to 40	6, 8, 10, 12, 14	Up to 5 Hz	Cold air unit
Diode laser	800	LightSheer (Lumenis)	5–400 ms	10–100	9 × 9, 12 × 12	Up to 2 Hz	Cooling handpiece
		Apex-800 (Iridex)	5–100 ms	5–60 (600 W)	7, 9, 11	Up to 4 Hz	Cooling handpiece
		SLP1000™ (Palomar)	5–1000 ms	Up to 575	12	Up to 3 Hz	SheerCool™ triple contact cooling, photon recycling
		MedioStar (Aesclepion-Meditec)	50 ms	Up to 64	10, 12, 14	Up to 4 Hz	Integrated scanner with cold air cooling device
		F1 Diode Laser (Opusmed)	15–40 ms	10–40	5, 7	4 Hz	
		EpiStar (Nidek)	5–700 ms	0.12–400	2, 3, 4, 5	1–15 Hz	
Q-switched Nd:YAG	532/1064	Softlight (Telsar)	12–18 ns	2.5–3	7	Up to 10 Hz	Only 1064 nm
		MedLite C6 (Hoya/ConBio)	<20 ns	Up to 12	3, 4, 6, 8	Up to 10 Hz	532 and 1064 nm
Long-pulsed Nd:YAG	1064	CoolGlide (Cutera)	0.1–300 ms	Up to 300	3, 5, 7, 10	Up to 2 Hz	Contact precooling
		Lyra/Gemini (Laserscope)	20–100 ms	5–900	10		Contact cooling
		Ultrawave (Adept Medical)	5–100 ms	5–500	2, 4, 6, 8, 10, 12	1–2 Hz	Photon recycling available with 532 nm and/or 755 nm
		Athos (Quantel)	3.5 ms	Up to 80	4	Up to 3 Hz	
		Gentle Yag (Candela)	0.25–300 ms	Up to 600	1.5, 3, 6, 8, 10, 12, 15, 18	Up to 10 Hz	Cryogen spray optional

Continued

Table 5.1 *Continued*

Light source	Wavelength (nm)	System name	Pulse duration	Fluence (J/cm²)	Spot size (mm)	Repetition rate	Other features
		Varia (CoolTouch)	300–500 ms	Up to 500	3–10		Pulsed cryogen cooling with thermal quenching
		Acclaim 7000 (Cynosure)	0.4–300 ms	300	3, 5, 7, 10, 12	5 Hz	Cold air or integrated cooling
		Smartepil II (Cynosure)	Up to 100 ms	16–200	2.5, 4, 5, 7, 10	6 Hz	Smart cool scanner
		Dualis (Fotona)	5–200 ms	Up to 600	2–10		
		Vasculight Elite (Lumenis)	2–16 ms	70–150 J	6	0,33 Hz	Combined with IPL
		Profile (Sciton)	0.1–200 ms	Up to 400			Combined with erbium
		Mydon (WaveLight)	5–90 ms	10–450	1.5, 3,5, 7, 10	1–10 Hz	Contact or air cooling
Intense pulsed broadband light source	590–1200	EpiLight (Lumenis)	15–100 ms	Up to 45	10 × 45, 8 × 35	0.5 Hz	Contact cooling Multiple pulsing
	695–1200	Quantum HR (Lumenis)	15–100 ms	25–45	34 × 8 mm	0.5 Hz	
	400–950	Ellipse (DDD)	0.2–50 ms	Up to 21	10 × 48	0.25 Hz	Dual mode filtering technique
	400–1200	PhotoLight (Cynosure)	5–50 ms	Up to 16	46 × 18		Xenon pulsed lamp
	500–1200	Estelux (Palomar)	10–100 ms	4–40	16 × 46	Up to 1	Fast coverage rate Coolroller™ cooling
	550–900	ProLite (Alderm)		10–50	10 × 20, 20 × 25	0.5 Hz	FLP (Fluorescent pulsed light
	400–1200	Spatouch (Radiancy)	35 ms	Up to 7	22 × 55	0.25 Hz	Light heat energy (LHE)
	510–1200	Quadra Q4 (Derma Med USA)	48	10–20	33 × 15		Quad pulsed light system
	510–1200	SpectraPulse (Primary Technology)	3 × 12 Pulse delay: 4 and 5 resp.	10–20	15 × 33		Light energy recycling (LER)
IPL + Nd:YAG	515–1200	VascuLight Elite (Lumenis)	0.5–25	3–90	35 × 8		Contact cooling/ combined with 1064
	400–1200	StarLux (Palomar)	5–500	Up to 30	16 × 46		
ELOS technology	Optical energy (580–980 nm) combined with electrical energy radiofrequency)	Aurora DS (Syneron)		Light energy: 10–30 RF energy: 5–20 J/cm³	12 × 25	0.7 Hz	Cooling (5–20°C on skin surface) combined with skin impedance control

dual-mode ruby lasers. They can operate in the conventional Q-switched mode for the treatment of tattoos and pigmented lesions, as well as in the normal mode for hair removal. An integrated cooling device consisting of a cooled contact handpiece (RubyStar) or cold air cooling (Sinon), precools the skin prior to laser pulse delivery.

Grossman et al initially reported selective injury to hair follicles by a long pulse ruby laser.[14] Thirteen patients with fair skin and dark hair were treated once on the thighs or back at fluences of 20–60 J/cm² with spot size of 6 mm. Hair growth delay was induced for 1–3 months in all subjects at all fluences. Biopsies obtained immediately after treatment showed selective thermal damage to pigmented hair follicles, with vaporization of the hair shafts, large patches of necrosis in the follicular epithelium, and occasional rupture with perifollicular dermal injury suggestive of steam vents. Transient pigmentary changes occurred in several patients but scarring was not observed. At one to two years follow-up, four of 7 recalled patients had persistent hair loss, which was greatest in sites treated at the highest fluence.[12] Biopsies from one patient showed a reduced number of terminal hairs with a reciprocal increase in small vellus-like hairs, but no evidence of fibrosis or destruction of hair follicles. It was suggested that permanent hair loss after 0.3-ms ruby laser treatment results from miniaturization of the follicular bulb and papilla, alike to the mechanism of androgenetic alopecia.

Additional studies with larger numbers of patients have confirmed that hair counts are reduced by approximately 30% after a single treatment with the ruby laser.[43] The effects of multiple treatment sessions are additive, as hair counts are reduced by approximately 60% after three or four treatment sessions.[44–47]

755 nm Alexandrite Lasers

Several long pulsed alexandrite lasers (755 nm) have been recently introduced for hair removal. At this longer wavelength, the ratio of energy deposited in the dermis to the epidermis is greater because of greater depth of penetration. The risk for epidermal damage in darker skin types is therefore reduced. Five different alexandrite lasers are available (Table 5.1): Apogee (Cynosure, Chelmsford, MA), Epitouch Alex (Lumenis, Santa Clara, CA) and GentleLase (Candela, Wayland, MA), Ultrawave II–III (Adept Medical, Rancho Santa Margarita, CA) and Epicare (LightAge, Somerset, NJ).

The Apogee laser provides pulse durations between 5 and 40 ms and fluences up to 50 J/cm^2. A cooling handpiece (SmartCool™) allows a continuous flow of chilled air to the treatment area. Epitouch Alex has a rapid repetition rate (5 Hz), and a scanner that can cover a $40 \times 40\,mm^2$ area within 6 seconds. GentleLase employs a dynamic cooling device (DCD) to protect the epidermis. This DCD cooling method uses short (5- to 100-ms) cryogen spurts, delivered on the skin surface through an electronically controlled solenoid valve; the quantity of cryogen delivered is proportional to the spurt duration. The liquid cryogen droplets strike the hot skin surface and undergo evaporation. Skin temperature is reduced as a result of supplying heat for vaporization. This cooling method allows for fast and selective cooling of the epidermis.[48] The UltraWave II–III offers the convenient combination of 755 and 1064 nm wavelength in a single device and is well suited for removing unwanted hair in all skin types. Epicare laser has a cold air cooling option and a Smartscreen software package that assists in record keeping, protocols, and even practice mangement.

McDaniel et al showed after one treatment with the variable pulse alexandrite laser on the lip, leg and back a 40–56% reduction of hair growth at 6 months[49] and Touma et al demonstrated a 70% decrease in hair counts at 60 months after a single treatment on the forearm with a 3-ms alexandrite laser.[50] Goldberg and Ahkami compared both the 2- and 10-ms pulse durations on 14 subjects who ranged in phototypes from I to III. At 6 months, hair counts did not show a statistically significant difference between the two pulse widths.[51] Nanni and Alster, in 36 subjects at 6 months, showed equivalent long-term hair removal with the long pulsed alexandrite at pulse durations of 5, 10, and 20 ms. Postinflammatory hyperpigmentation occurred in 3% of patients. It was generally less severe and resolved quicker in the test spots treated with the 20-ms pulse durations in comparison to the 5- and 10-ms pulse widths.[52] From these studies, it is uncertain that pulse durations of 2, 5, 10 and 20 ms show a significant clinical difference in terms of efficacy. However, the longer pulse durations provided better protection to the epidermis.

800 nm Diode Lasers

An extremely high-powered (2900 W) diode laser (LightSheer, Lumenis, Santa Clara, CA) is a popular laser hair removal device. Long-term results suggest that the pulsed, 800 nm diode laser is very effective for removal of dark, terminal hair: permanent hair reduction can be obtained in 89% of patients.[18–21,53] This laser operates at 800 nm, has pulse widths between 5 and 400 ms, a 12×12 mm spot, a 2 Hz repetition rate, fluences between 10 and 60 J/cm^2, and a patented contact cooling device (ChillTip™). Because of the longer wavelength, the active cooling and the longer pulse widths, darker skin types can be treated more safely.[54]

Several other 800 nm diode lasers are available (see Table 5.1): Apex-800 (Iridex, Mountain View, CA), F1 diode laser (Opus Medical Inc, Montreal, Canada), Mediostar (Asclepion-Meditec, Jena, Germany), SLP1000 (Palomar, Burlington, MA), and EpiStar (Nidek, Gamagori, Japan).

Q-switched 1064 nm Nd:YAG Laser

A high-powered, 1064 nm Q-switched Nd:YAG laser (MedLite IV, Conbio, Santa Clara, CA) is available for hair removal.[31,32] This laser has a very short pulse duration in the nanosecond range, a 4-mm spot, a repetition rate of 10 Hz and fluences up to 8–10 J/cm^2. The high repetition rate (10 Hz) delivers the laser pulses very rapidly and therefore larger areas can easily be covered and operative time is significantly shortened. The longer wavelength (1064 nm) makes it useful for darker skin types. Although capable for inducing a growth delay it appears to be ineffective for long-term hair removal.

Long-pulsed 1064 nm Nd:YAG Lasers

Several long-pulsed Nd:YAG lasers (1064 nm wavelength), that deliver pulses in the millisecond domain, are now available for hair removal laser treatment on all skin types (see Table 5.1). These lasers include: Lyra or Gemini (Laserscope, San Jose, CA), CoolGlide (Cutera, Brisbane, CA), Ultrawave (Adept Medical, Rancho Santa Margarita, CA), Profile (Sciton, Palo Alto, CA), VascuLight (Lumenis, Santa Clara, CA), SmartEpilI and Acclaim (Cynosure, Chelmsford, MA), Athos (Quantel, Les Ulis Cedex, France), Dualis (Fotona, Ljubljana, Slowenie), Varia (CoolTouch, Roseville, CA), Mydon (Wavelight, Erlangen, Germany) and GentleYAG (Candela, Wayland, MA).

The long-pulsed Nd:YAG have deeply penetrating 1064 nm wavelengths. The reduced melanin absorption at this wavelength necessitates the need for high fluences to adequately damage hair. However, the poor melanin absorption at this wavelength coupled with epidermal cooling makes the long pulsed Nd:YAG a potential safe laser treatment for darker skin types up to VI.[55–62] The Nd:YAG laser is also often used for treatment of pseudofollicultis barbae, a skin condition commonly seen in darker skin types.[63–65]

Pulsed, Noncoherent Broadband Light Sources

For several years, intense pulsed, nonlaser light sources, emitting noncoherent, multiwavelength light have also been used for hair removal: EpiLight (Lumenis, Santa Clara, CA), Ellipse (Danish Dermatologic Development, Hørsholm, Denmark).[66,67] By placing appropriate filters on the light source, wavelengths ranging from 590 to 1200 nm can be generated. Cutoff filters are used to eliminate short wavelengths so that only the longer, more deeply penetrating wavelengths are emitted. Pulse durations vary in the millisecond domain. A single- or multiple-pulse mode (two to five) with various pulse delay intervals, can be chosen. The wide choice of wavelengths, pulse durations and delay intervals makes this device potentially effective for a wide range of skin types. The devices come with software that guides the operator in determining treatment parameters depending on the patient's skin type, hair color and coarseness.

One of the newest emerging hair removal technologies are the lower-price, small, pulsed-light hair removal systems. These include the IPL Quantum HR (Lumenis, Santa Clara, CA), the ProLite (Alderm, Irvine, CA), the SpaTouch photoepilation system (Radiancy, Orangeburg, NY),[68,69] PhotoLight (Cynosure, Chelmsford, MA), Quadra Q4 (DermaMed USA, Lenni, PA), SpectraPulse (Primary Technology, Tampa, FL), and the Estelux (Palomar, Burlington, MA). These systems have been optimized for hair removal with wavelengths preferentially absorbed by melanin, long pulse widths and large spot sizes.

Recently, IPL systems have been developed that are combined with 1064 nm laser light: VascuLight (Lumenis, Santa Clara, CA) and Starlux (Palomar, Burlington, MA). These devices should allow for treatment of a wide spectrum of hair and skin colors.

Electro-optical Synergy (ELOS™) Technology

ELOS™ technology utilizes a synergy between electrical (conducted radiofrequency) and optical (laser or light) energies. The electrical energy causes heat, which is focused on the hair follicle and the bulge area, while the optical energy heats mainly the hairshaft. When combined, a uniform temperature distribution across the hairshaft and the follicle should be obtained to achieve effective hair removal. Based on this ELOS™ technology, Syneron (Yokneam Illit, Israel) has developed a system (Aurora) that combines RF energy with IPL and is equipped with cooling. The use of the RF energy should also allow for treatment of all skin types, since this form of energy is not absorbed by epidermal melanin.[70]

Exogenous Chromophore

Rather than targeting endogenous melanin, an exogenous chromophore can be introduced into the hair follicle and then irradiated with light of a wavelength that matches its absorption peak. This eliminates the problem of competition by epidermal melanin. The main problem is finding a reliable method for the chromophore to penetrate into all depths of the hair follicle.

Carbon Suspension-Q-switched Nd:YAG Laser

In this method, an exogenous chromophore (carbon suspension) with a peak absorption in the near infrared portion of the spectrum, is used in combination with a Q-switched Nd-YAG laser. The Softlight system (Telsar, Wood River, IL) uses a proprietary suspension of 10-μm diameter carbon particles applied to wax-epilated skin. The skin, after being wiped clean of the topical carbon material, is irradiated with relatively low energies (2–3 J/cm^2) of Q-switched Nd:YAG laser light (1064 nm, 10 Hz, 10 ns pulse duration, 7-mm spot size).[30,33] However, the short pulse duration of the laser used in this technique limits the extent of follicular damage. This technique therefore can successfully induce a delay in hair growth, but fails to produce long-lasting hair removal. However, when compared to laser treatment alone, no added benefit is obtained with waxing or carbon suspension application.[33]

Meladine™

Meladine™ is a topical, melanin-encased, phosphatidylcholine-based liposome solution that, when sprayed on the desired area, supposedly selectively deposits melanin directly into the hair follicle without staining surrounding skin. The proprietary liposome molecules are small enough to potentially penetrate the infundibulum. The result should be temporarily melanin-rich follicles, which allows patients with lighter hair colors to benefit from laser hair removal.

In European clinical studies, 90% of the patients with light colored hairs that were pretreated with Meladine™ experienced permanent hair reduction of 75% or more, compared with 0% of patients who did not receive Meladine™ treatment. The effectiveness of the treatment was directly proportional to the amount of Meladine™ used. In fact, those patients who used 86 mL or more in their pretreatment regimen experienced hair reduction of 95% (J De Leeuw, findings presented at the 2002 EADV meeting). Conversely, a study by Drs Tanzi and Alster using Meladine™ found growth delay, but not permanent hair loss, in subjects treated (findings presented at the 2003 American Society for Dermatologic Surgery meeting).

Aminolevulinic Acid

Photodynamic therapy (PDT) involves the use of a photosensitizer and light to produce therapeutic effects. The mechanism of action is presumed to involve the generation of toxic reactive oxygen species, subsequent to the photochemical activation of the photosensitizer by light.[71,72] The recent introduction of 5-aminolevulinic acid (5-ALA) as a topical photosensitizer has opened up a variety of potential therapeutic options. Selective protoporphyrin IX (PPIX) synthesis in pilosebaceous units is a unique feature of ALA over other photosensitizers and topical application circumvents the photosensitivity that is induced by systemic agents.[73–75]

In a small pilot study of 12 subjects, 5-ALA was applied topically to hair bearing skin after wax epilation. Test sites were irradiated 3 hours later with 630 nm light from an argon-pumped tunable dye laser. At 6 months after a single treatment, a dose-dependent decrease in hair regrowth was observed, with the greatest loss (40%) occurring in areas that received the highest doses of light (200 J/cm^2).[36] Temporary hyperpigmentation was the only adverse effect noted.

Preliminary reports from a recent study including 30 patients, examined the ability of Levulan® Herastick with either a proprietary nonlaser light source compared to a laser to remove human hair. The nonlaser light plus Levulan® did not result in more significant hair loss than placebo plus light. However, Levulan® plus laser light appears to prevent approximately 30% of the hair from regrowing with one treatment (unpublished data from DUSA Pharmaceuticals).

Photodynamic therapy may be a useful approach for hair removal. As photosensitizers tend to localize in the follicular epithelium, photochemical destruction of all hair follicles, no matter what hair color or growth cycle, could potentially be obtained. Long-term data and large-scale studies are needed to determine the safety and long-term efficacy of this modality.

Actual Technique

The numerous lasers and nonlaser light sources available today, provide clinicians with multiple options. Several variables need to be considered when determining whether or not laser or light-assisted hair removal is appropriate for a particular patient and which technique to use. These include a patient's hair color, hair type, hair density, skin color, hormonal factors and anatomical location. In order to determine the various critical factors for this procedure, the following general approach is used:

- a history is taken for appropriate patient selection
- a physical examination is performed to evaluate skin color and skin condition, hair color, hair diameter and hair density
- instructions are given to the patient concerning pre-treatment hair management and skin care
- treatment guidelines are determined by skin and hair properties
- appropriate post-treatment care is provided.

Patient interviews

When obtaining a patient history, one wishes to obtain information that will enable the best results. It is important to discuss patient expectations, medications, history of scarring, local infections, previous hair removal strategies, endocrine status, recent sun exposure and the patient's habits (i.e. sports, hot-tub use). A careful history is taken on the onset of hair growth and patients are screened for underlying conditions that may cause hypertrichosis, like hormonal disturbances, familial predisposition, drug intake, or underlying tumors. Patients on hormonal therapy or with underlying endocrine abnormalities are alerted to the potential limitations of hair removal treatment. Patients with active cutaneous infections are not treated. Patients with a history of recurrent staphylococcal and herpes simplex infections are started on appropriate prophylaxis to diminish the likelihood of an outbreak. Although a history of keloids or hypertrophic scarring is not an absolute contra-indication to treatment, individuals with these conditions are treated less aggressively. Attention must be paid to avoid treating naevi and moles in the hair-bearing areas. Although it has been reported that laser treatment of individuals who are taking isotretinoin is safe, the issue remains controversial.[76,77] Caution should be exercised when treating patients who are on gold therapy with Q-switched lasers[78] because of a risk of a blue–gray skin discoloration immediately after Q-switched laser exposure. Patients with skin diseases such as vitiligo and psoriasis should be warned of the risk of koebnerization following laser surgery. Clinically this problem is rarely seen. The Q-switched lasers should be avoided in the hair bearing areas that overly tattoos. A listing of previous hair removal treatment modalities as well as response to this treatment modality should be recorded at the time of the initial consultation.

CLINICAL PEARL: PERTINENT HISTORY FOR LASER/PULSED LIGHT HAIR REMOVAL

- Presence of conditions that may cause hypertrichosis:
  - hormonal
  - familial
  - drug
  - tumor
- History of local or recurrent skin infection
- History of herpes simplex, especially perioral
- History of herpes genitalis, important when treating the pubic or bikini area
- History of keloids/hypertrophic scarring
- History of koebnerizing skin disorders such as vitiligo and psoriasis
- Previous treatment modalities – method, frequency and date of last treatment, as well as response
- Recent suntan or exposure to tanning or light cabinet
- Presence of tattoos or nevi
- Patient's expectations
- Present medications:
  - photosensitizing medications
  - Accutane intake within the past year
  - gold therapy

Clinical examination

When seeing a patient for the first time, the individual's skin type, hair color and coarseness are noted. This will determine which device is most ideal as well as predict response to treatment (Table 5.2). Location and density of excess hair should also be taken into consideration.

Treatment Techniques

Preoperative Care

6 Weeks Before Laser Treatment

Research has shown greater hair loss results at shaven rather than epilated sites, suggesting that light absorption by the pigmented hair shaft itself plays an important role. Patients who seek optimal results should therefore avoid plucking, waxing or electrolysis. Shaving and the use of depilatory creams will not interfere with laser hair removal results.

Use of a broadspectrum sunscreen is recommended. Sun avoidance must be practiced if hair removal is planned on

Table 5.2 *Indications and Expected Efficacy for Different Hair Removal Devices*

Laser or light source	Skin type	Hair color	Hair diameter	Expected efficacy
Normal mode ruby	I–III	Dark to light brown	Fine and coarse	Long-term hair removal
Normal mode alexandrite	I–IV	Dark to light brown	Fine and coarse	Long-term hair removal
Pulsed diode	I–VI	Dark to light brown	Coarse	Long-term hair removal
Normal mode Nd:YAG	I–VI	Dark	Coarse	Long-term hair removal
Q-switched Nd:YAG	I–VI	Dark to light brown	Fine and coarse	Temporary hair removal
Intense pulsed light	I–VI	Dark to light brown	Coarse	Long-term hair removal

sun-exposed sites. A bleaching cream such as 3% hydroquinone, retinoic acid 0.025% and hydrocortisone 2% can be prescribed to patients with darker skin types or who have received recent sun exposure.

Day Before Laser Treatment

The patient is instructed to shave the area to be treated. If the patient is uncomfortable with the idea of shaving the area, a depilatory cream can be used instead. Use of prophylactic antibiotic or antiviral agents such as valacyclovir, famciclovir or aciclovir may be started, when indicated.

Day of Treatment

Make-up and skin cream must be removed from the treatment site. Although less-sensitive areas (back, legs, arms) can frequently be treated without anesthesia, topical anesthesia is generally used on more sensitive areas: Emla (Astra-Zeneca, Wilmington, DE), LMX (Ferndale Laboratories, Ferndale, MI) or Topicaine (ESBA Laboratories, Mountain View, CA). When treating the upper lip, local or regional anesthesia with lidocaine is sometimes required. Alternatively, if shaving is done on the day of treatment, it should precede application of topical anesthetic.

CLINICAL PEARL: PREOPERATIVE CARE

6 weeks before laser treatment:

- Sunscreen: a broadspectrum sunscreen is recommended and sun avoidance must be practiced if hair removal is planned in exposed sites.
- Bleaching cream: a bleaching cream can be prescribed to patients with darker skin types or a suntan.
- No plucking, waxing or electrolysis
- Shaving and depilatory creams: may be used

Day before laser treatment:

- The patient is instructed to shave the area to be treated. If the patient is uncomfortable with the idea of shaving the area, a depilatory cream can be used instead.
- Start prophylactic antiviral or antibiotic treatment when indicated.

Day of treatment:

- Area to be treated should be clean and free of make-up
- If needed, apply a thick layer of a topical anesthetic cream as recommended before the scheduled laser treatment.

Treatment guidelines

The procedure for hair removal is similar using any of the devices previously described. A treatment grid can be applied to provide the operator with an outline of the area to be treated. In the absence of a grid, careful attention must be paid to prevent double treatment and skipped areas. Visibility can also be increased by the Syris™ Vizualisation system, a polarized headlamp with magnifying loupe (Syris Scientific,Gray, MA).

The ideal treatment parameters must be individualized for each patient. If needed, test sites can be placed at inconspicuous sites in the area to be treated. The treatment fluence is carefully increased while the skin is observed for signs of acute epidermal injury, such as whitening, blistering, ablation or Nikolsky's sign. Slightly overlapping laser pulses should be delivered with a predetermined spot size. It is recommended that the largest spot size and the highest tolerable fluence be used to obtain the best results.[79]

If the device is not equipped with a cooling device, a thick layer of cooled gel is applied before delivery of the laser pulses. With the Dynamic Cooling Device™ (Gentlelase, Candela), short bursts of cryogen spurts (5 to 80 ms) are delivered automatically onto the skin surface, immediately prior to delivery of the laser pulse. The Apogee laser (Cynosure) uses a cooling handpiece (SmartCool™) that allows a continuous flow of chilled air to the treatment area. The Coolglide uses a copper plate that precools the area to be treated. The Epilaser, LightSheer, and Lyra/Gemini use a sapphire-cooled handpiece (Epiwand™, Chilltip™, and Versasat™, respectively) that is placed in direct contact with the skin. Prior to pulse delivery, the handpiece is pressed firmly against the skin. After delivery, the handpiece is picked up and placed firmly on an adjacent site, until the entire area is covered. The sapphire contact cooling tip should be wiped clean every 5 to 10 pulses to remove debris. Between patients, disinfection of the handpiece is mandatory.

The ideal immediate response is vaporization of the hair shaft with no other apparent effect. After a few minutes, perifollicular edema and erythema may appear. The intensity and duration depends on the hair color and hair density. If there is a sign of epidermal damage, the fluence should be reduced.

CLINICAL PEARL: TREATMENT TECHNIQUE

- Skin preparation: remove the anesthetic cream, make-up or skin creams
- Anesthesia: use if necessary
- Visibility: a treatment grid can be applied in order to provide the operator with an outline of the area to be treated. Visibility can also be increased by the Syris light™, a polarized headlamp with magnifying loupe
- Treatment fluence: the ideal treatment parameters must be individualized for each patient. The ideal fluence should cause a perifollicular erythema and edema reaction without any signs of acute epidermal injury.
- Cooling of the epidermis:
  - cooling gel
  - dynamic cooling
  - contact cooling
  - air cooling
- Technique: slightly overlapping laser pulses are delivered with a predetermined spot size. It is recommended that the largest spot size and the highest tolerable fluence are used to obtain the best results

Post-operative considerations

Ice packs reduce postoperative pain and minimize edema. Analgesics are not usually required unless extensive areas have been treated. Prophylactic courses of antibiotics or antivirals should be completed when indicated. Topical antibiotic ointment applied twice daily is indicated if any epidermal injury occurred. Mild topical steroid creams may be prescribed to reduce posttreatment edema and erythema. Trauma (e.g. picking or scratching) to the treated area should be avoided. During the first week of healing, direct sun exposure should be avoided or sunblocks used. Make-up may be applied on the day following treatment unless blistering or crusts develop. The damaged hair is often shed during the first few weeks after treatment. Patients should be reassured that this is not a sign of hair regrowth.

CLINICAL PEARL: POSTOPERATIVE CARE

- Ice packs: reduce postoperative pain and minimize swelling
- Analgesics: are not usually required unless extensive areas are treated
- Prophylactic courses of antibiotic or antiviral: should be completed
- Topical antibiotic ointment: applied twice daily is indicated if epidermal injury occurred
- Mild topical steroid creams: may be prescribed to reduce swelling and erythema
- Avoid any trauma such as picking or scratching of the area
- Avoid sun exposure: use sunblock
- Make-up may be applied on the next day unless blistering or crusts developed
- Shedding of hair casts: especially on the face. The damaged hair follicle is often shed during the first week after treatment. Patients should be re-assured that this is not a sign of hair regrowth.

Subsequent Treatments

Research has shown that laser hair removal requires the presence of a pigmented hair shaft.[80–82] Retreatment can therefore be performed as soon as regrowth appears. Regrowth is based on the natural cycle, which varies by anatomic location, but on average, the timing is 6 to 8 weeks.

Expected Benefits

The concept of hair removal has been defined as follows:[12]

- Temporary hair loss: a delay in hair growth, which usually lasts for 1–3 months, consistent with the induction of telogen.
- Permanent hair reduction: refers to a significant reduction in the number of terminal hairs after a given treatment, which is stable for a period of time longer than the complete growth cycle of hair follicles at the given body site.

Recently, it has been suggested that another 6 months are added to this posttreatment observation time, i.e. the time it takes for a damaged follicle to recover from the laser injury and reenter a normal growth cycle.[83]

A distinction needs also to be made between permanent and complete hair loss. Complete hair loss refers to a lack of regrowing hairs (i.e. a significant reduction in the number of regrowing hairs to zero). Complete hair loss may be either temporary or permanent. Laser treatment usually produces complete but temporary hair loss for 1–3 months, followed by partial but permanent hair loss.

Patients have different expectations of treatment (e.g. temporary versus permanent, partial versus complete hair removal). All responses are clinically significant and may be separately desirable for different patients. Growth delay that provides a few months of hairless skin is far more reliably achieved than permanent hair loss. All laser systems have been shown to temporarily reduce hair growth for all hair colors (except white) and at all fluences. Except for one report,[84] blonde, red or gray-haired patients are unlikely to experience a permanent reduction, but hair loss in these patients can be maintained by treatment at approximately 1- to 3-month intervals.

Effectiveness for permanent hair reduction is strongly correlated with hair color and fluence. Long-term, controlled hair counts indicate an average of 20 to 30% hair loss with each treatment, indicating the need for multiple treatments to obtain near complete hair removal. Research also shows that in the ideal patient with fair skin and dark hair, the probability for long-term hair removal is about 80 to 89%, depending on the device used. Long-term comparison of different lasers (ruby, alexandrite, diode, Nd:YAG) and light sources (intense pulsed light) indicates that effective long-term hair removal can be achieved with all systems.[85–87]

The maximum fluence tolerated is determined by the epidermal pigmentation. Fair-skinned dark-haired patients are most easily treated. Dark-skinned patients pose a greater challenge. Any of the hair removal devices are safe and effective in light-skinned patients and longer wavelengths (near-infrared) and longer pulse durations, have been shown to treat darker skin types more safely when combined with cooling devices.[88–93] A Q-switched Nd:YAG laser, with or without an external chromophore, has been shown to be very useful for treatment of dark skin types but appears to be ineffective for permanent hair removal. For patients presenting with recent sun exposure, pretreatment with a bleaching agent, sunscreen and/or sun avoidance is recommended prior to laser treatment.

The number of treatments needed to obtain the best results for different anatomical sites is unknown. Generally, the average number of hair removal treatments to achieve a significant reduction of excess hair is between five and seven treatments performed at 1- to 3-month intervals. A rare patient can obtain long-term complete hair removal after a single treatment whereas others may respond poorly, for yet unknown reasons. However, most patients (80 to 89%) respond favorably.

Often, regrowing hairs are thinner and lighter in color, as indicated by measurements of diameter and color of regrowing hairs. This also contributes to the overall cosmetic outcome because the clinical impression of hairiness is not only defined by the absolute number of hairs but also by the color, the length and the diameter of the hairs. The range of outcomes can be summarized as absolute hair number reduction, finer, lighter regrowing hair and slower regrowth.

Animal studies have shown that the hair growth cycle affects the hair follicle destruction by ruby laser pulses: actively growing and pigmented anagen stage hair follicles were sensitive to hair removal by normal mode ruby laser exposure, whereas catagen and telogen stage hair follicles were resistant to laser irradiation.[80] However, in humans, the efficacy of laser hair removal does not appear to always be influenced by the hair growth cycle.[81,82] Unlike the animal model, there is enough melanin present in each growth cycle of the human hair follicle to obtain selective damage to the hair.

Case Studies

Case 1

This 37-year-old women is diagnosed with polycystic ovary syndrome (PCOS). Her symptoms of PCOS are: infrequent menstrual periods, increased growth of hair on the face, fingers and toes, oily skin and acne, obesity, and type 2 diabetes. Current therapy consists of maintaining a healthy weight and treatment of her diabetes with insulin. Although the male hormones are elevated, she refuses to take any androgen-blocking drugs. She consulted for treatment of her facial hirsutism, characterized by increased growth of black terminal hairs in the submandibular area, that she shaves daily (Fig. 5.1A). She was looking for a more efficient treatment modality of hair removal. As this patient was diagnosed with an underlying endocrine abnormality, she was alerted to the potential limitations of laser hair removal treatment. Initially, she was treated with a 800 nm diode laser (LightSheer, Lumenis) at 30–35 J/cm^2, 30 ms and a 12 × 12 mm spot. Once the regrowing hairs became lighter and finer, treatment was continued with a 3 ms, 755 nm alexandrite laser (GentleLase, Candela) 8 mm, at 40 J/cm^2 for an 8 mm spot with DCD cooling (30 ms on, 30 ms off time).

The patient underwent eight treatments sessions in total, at 2- to 3-month intervals. A very satisfying result with 90% reduction of the hair regrowth was obtained (Fig. 5.1B). Because of the continued hormonal stimulation, she continues to be treated once a year for the few regrowing hairs.

A

B

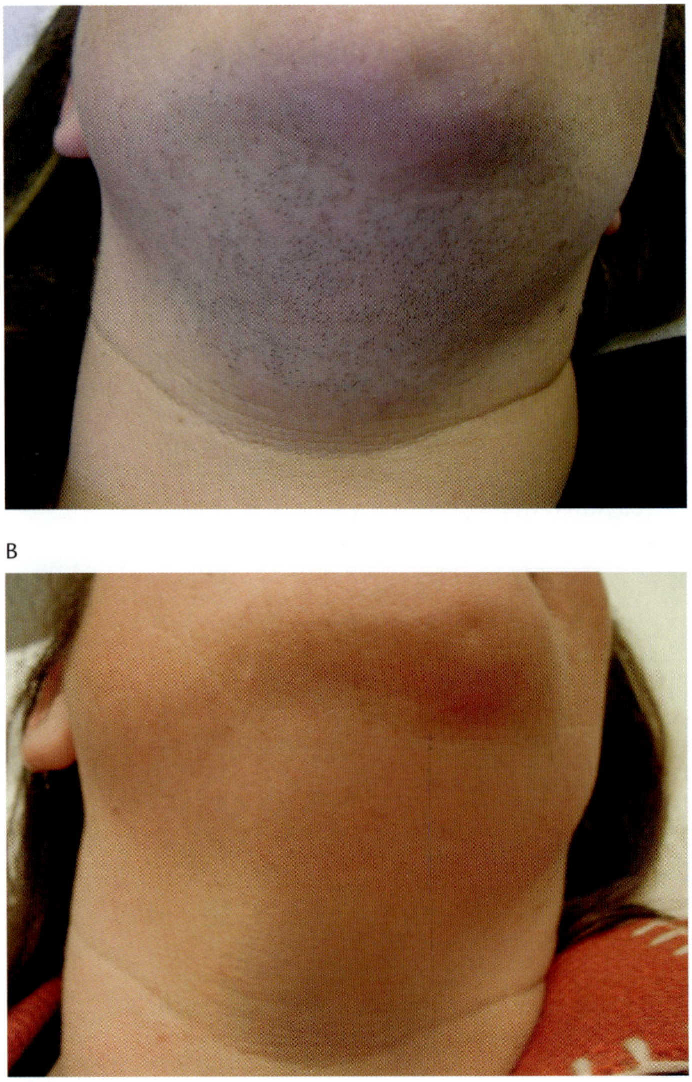

Figure 5.1 (A) Patient with hirsutism due to polycystic ovary syndrome. (B) Significant reduction of hair growth at 9 months after the eighth laser hair removal treatment.

Case 2

A 44-year-old female patient consulted for laser hair removal of her axillae (Fig. 5.2A). Previous treatment modality consisted of shaving or the use of depilatory creams. She received four treatments with a 800 nm LightSheer diode laser (30 ms, 30 J/cm^2, 12 × 12 mm) and one final treatment of the remaining fine, regrowing hairs with a 3-ms, 755 nm GentleLase, alexandrite laser (40 J/cm^2, 8-mm spot, 30/30 DCD cooling). Except for a few occasional regrowing hairs, a very satisfactory result was obtained 5 years after the last treatment (Fig. 5.2B).

Case 3

A 23-year-old male patient consulted for laser hair removal on his back (Fig. 5.3A). Previous treatment modalities consisted of shaving or waxing. He received seven treatments with an intense pulsed light source (Estelux, Palomar). This device produces smooth (nonspiky) pulses very broad in range from 0.5 ms to 500 ms. The spectrally filtered light is delivered through a LuxY handpiece (530–1200 nm), optimized for hair removal. The handpiece has a built-in photon recycling system, which returns photons that are reflected from the skin back to the treatment target. The gain factor of photon recycling is in the range of 1.1–1.5. With a large spot size (12 × 28 mm) and a repetition rate of 2 Hz, a covering rate can achieve 12 cm^2/s. A fluence of 24 J/cm^2 at a 20-ms pulse was used. A gradual decrease of the regowing hairs was obtained (Fig. 5.3B) until a very nice result at 8 months after the last treatment was obtained (Fig. 5.3C).

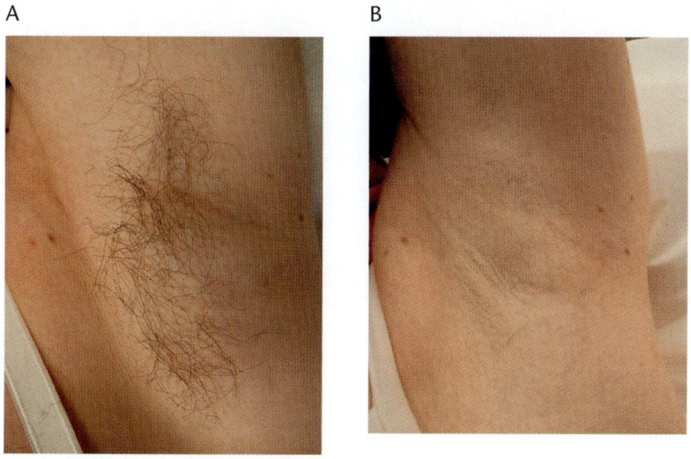

Figure 5.2 (A) Patient consulting for laser hair removal of axillary hair. (B) Result at 5 years after the fourth laser hair removal treatment.

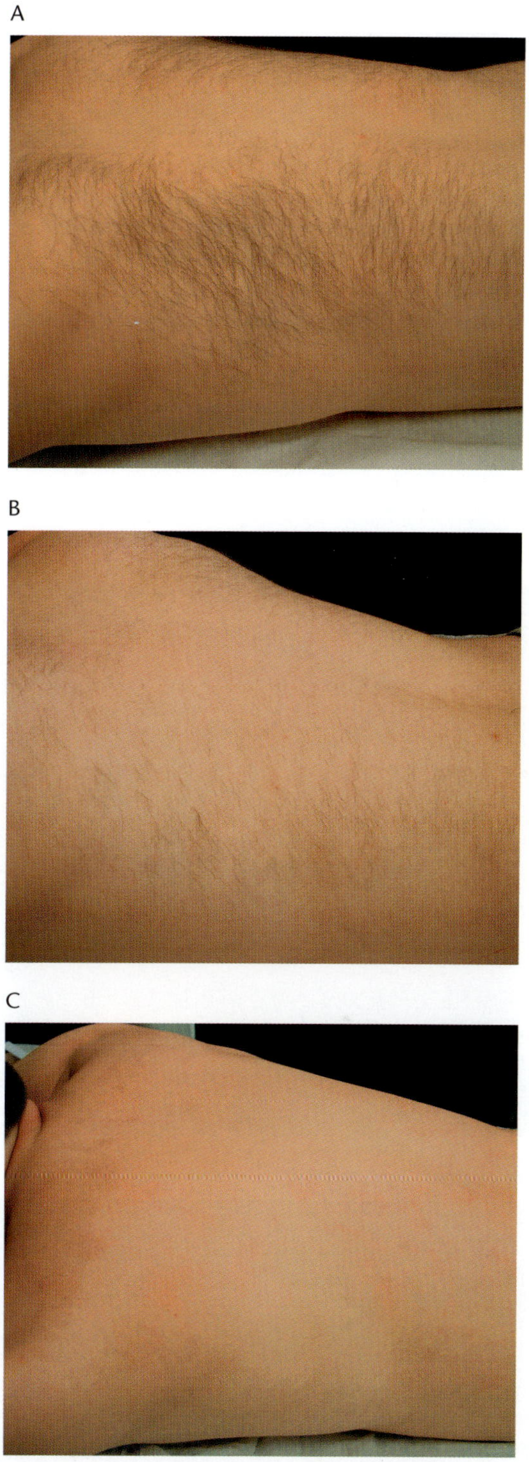

Figure 5.3 (A) Patient with hairy back before intense pulsed light (IPL) treatment. (B) Result at 4 months after fourth IPL hair removal treatment. (C) Result at 8 months after seventh IPL hair removal treatment.

Case 4

A 38-year-old male patient consulted with a minor form of spina bifida occulta. This condition is characterized by the failure of the plates of bone that form the spinal arch to fuse completely. This variation generally only affects one vertebra, particularly the vertebra lying lowest in the back. Because there are no associated abnormalities of the spinal cord or nerve roots, there are no leg, bladder or bowel problems. His symptoms consisted only of a small dimple with numerous hairs growing out of it (Fig. 5.4A). Because the hairs were fine and lighter, treatment was performed with a 3-ms, 755 nm GentleLase alexandrite laser (40 J/cm^2, 8-mm spot, 30/30 DCD cooling). Six months after treatment, a very satisfactory result was obtained, as shown in Fig. 5.4B.

Case 5

Three years earlier, this 42-year-old male patient was victim of a burn injury. His burn wounds healed with conventional wound care, causing scarring in his beard area. Since then a problem of recurrent ingrowing hairs occurred, which caused deep folliculitis (Fig. 5.5A). Because the hairs were coarse and dark, he was treated with a 800 nm LightSheer laser, at 30–35 J/cm^2, 30 ms and a 12 × 12 mm spot. After seven treatments, the ingrowing hairs were removed and the problem of recurrent deep folliculitis improved substantially. We also noted a pronounced, textural improvement of the scarred skin after diode treatment (Fig. 5.5B).

A

B

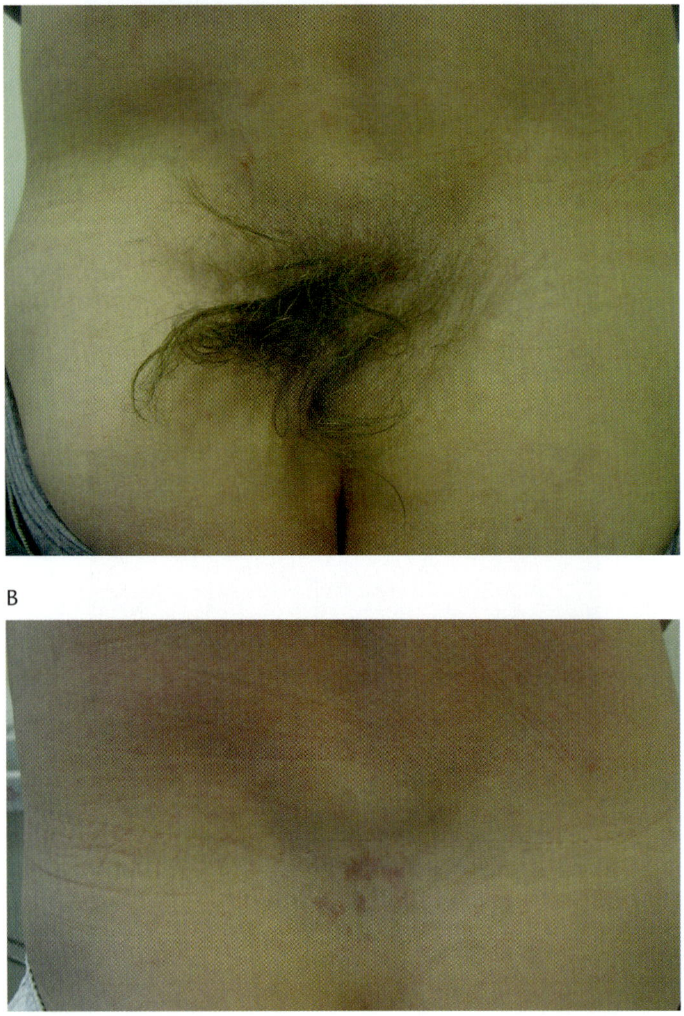

Figure 5.4 (A) Patient with hypertrichosis over spina bifida occulta area on lower back. (B) Result at 6 months after sixth laser hair removal treatment.

A

B

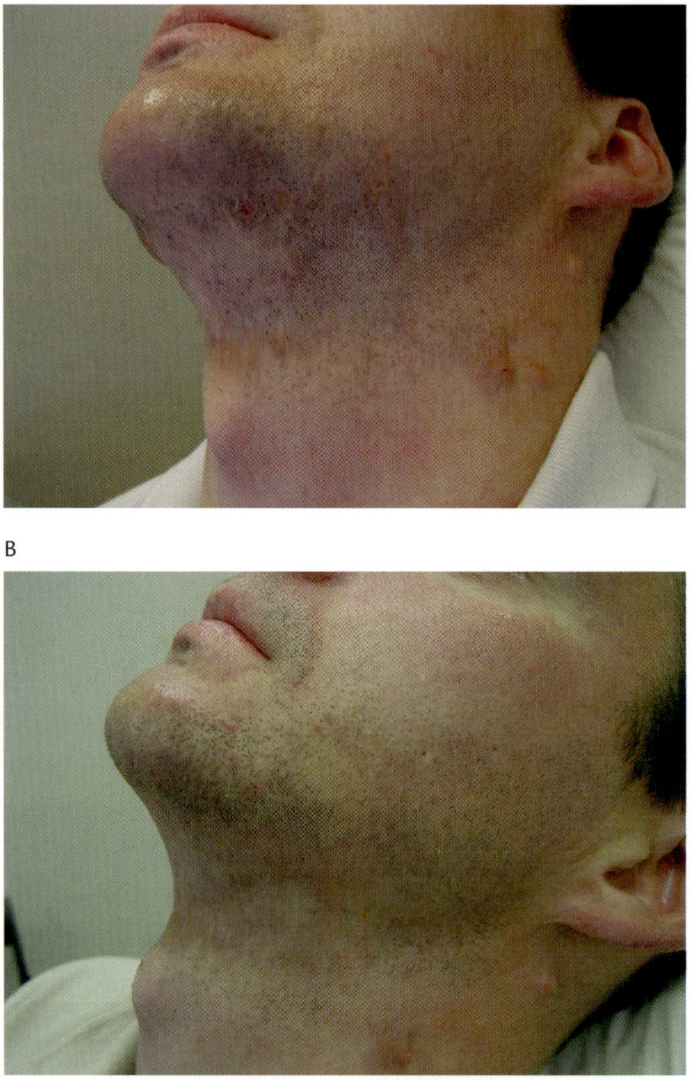

Figure 5.5 (A) Patient with recurrent folliculitis due to burn scars. (B) Result after seventh laser hair removal treatment with substantial improvement of skin texture.

Case 6

This 56-year-old female patient was diagnosed with a hairy nevus of Becker of her left hand (Fig. 5.6A). The presence of dark, terminal hairs in the brown pigmented plaque, was of great cosmetic concern to her. She received treatment with a 800 nm LightSheer laser, at 40 J/cm^2, 30 ms and a 12 × 12 mm spot. After three treatments, there was a significant reduction in the number of regrowing hairs (Fig. 5.6B). The patient was satisfied with this result and requested no further treatments. Note also that the hyperpigmented plaque remained unchanged despite laser treatment.

Case 7

This 18-year-old female patient was diagnosed with vaginal atresia. In this case, the congenital anomaly of the female genitourinary tract included an absence of the vagina (vaginal atresia or agenesis), with normal ovaries and normal external genitalia (Fig. 5.7A). The anomaly was detected at adolescence because of abdominal pain from an obstructed uterovaginal tract. Reconstruction of the vagina was scheduled to be done using a pudendal thigh flap. Because this fasciocutaneous flap uses hair-bearing skin, laser hair removal of the pudendal donor skin was performed prior to surgery. After six treatments with a 755 nm GentleLase alexandrite laser, hairfree donor skin could be used to reconstruct a vagina without hair growth (Fig. 5.7B).

Case 8

A 13-year-old girl consulted for improvement of a posttraumatic scar on the lateral part of her thigh. The scar was hypopigmented and spread. Because she did not want any major surgical intervention, a noninvasive approach to induce neocollagenesis was attempted. She received seven treatments at low dose, with a long-pulsed 1064 nm Nd:YAG laser (Lyra, Laserscope), at 30 ms, 24 J/cm^2 for a 10-mm spot size. After the last treatment, she noticed the appearance of black terminal hair around the treated scar (Fig. 5.8). Conversion of fine vellus hair to dark, coarse terminal hair in the immediate vicinity of the treatment area had occurred. Currently, she is being treated for hair removal with a 800 nm diode laser at high dose (12 × 12 mm, 45 J/cm^2 and 30 ms).

A B

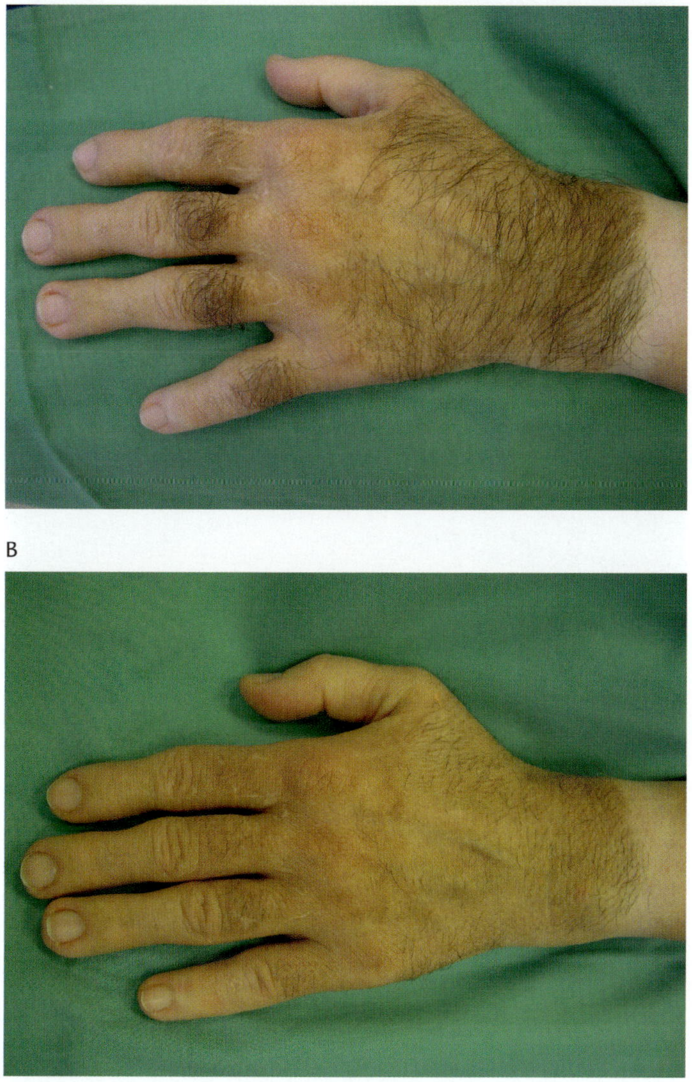

Figure 5.6 (A) Female patient with hairy nevus of Becker on back of her hand. (B) Result at 5 months after third laser hair removal treatment.

A B

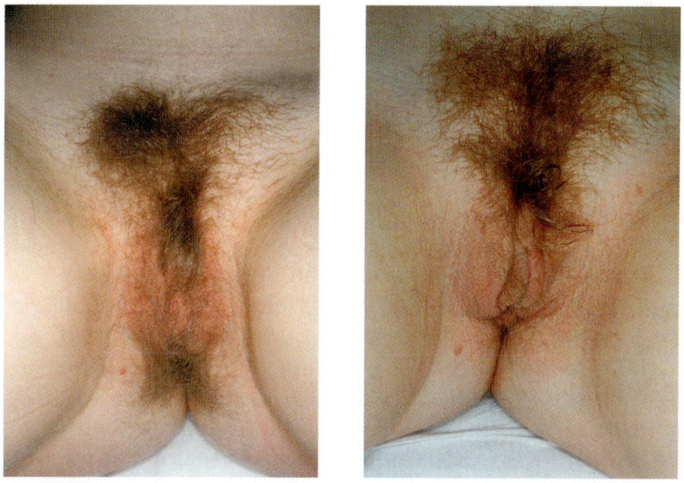

Figure 5.7 (A) Donor site (pudendal skin) for reconstructive surgery of vaginal atresia before laser hair removal. (B) Result at 5 months after sixth laser hair removal treatment.

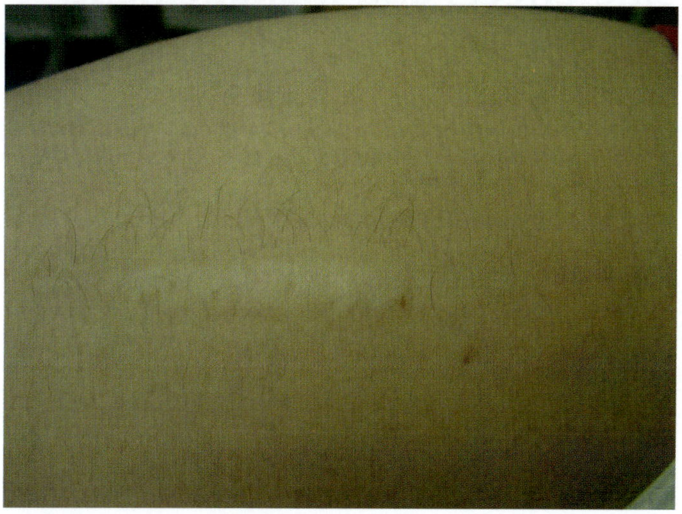

Figure 5.8 Hypertrichosis induced by 1064 nm long-pulsed Nd-YAG laser at low fluence for scar improvement.

A

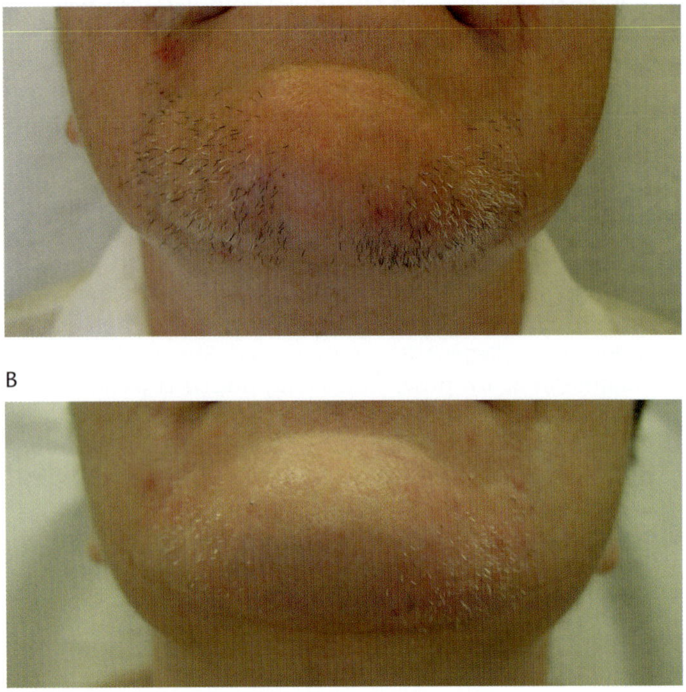

B

Figure 5.9 (A) Postmenopausal patient with hyperthrichosis on chin before laser hair removal. (B) Pigmented terminal hairs were successfully removed but white terminal hairs were resistant to treatment.

Case 9

A 56-year-old postmenopausal woman consulted for hair removal of the hypertrichosis on her chin. This was composed of 50% dark, coarse terminal hairs and 50% coarse white hairs (Fig. 5.9A). Laser hair removal with a 800 nm diode laser (12 × 12 mm, 35 J/cm^2 and 30 ms) successfully removed the black hairs, but left the white hairs untouched (Fig. 5.9B). Currently, no light-based techniques are available to induce long-term hair removal of white hairs.

Side Effects and Management of Complications

Laser hair removal was FDA cleared in 1996 and has an excellent safety and efficacy profile. Complications are rare if treatments are done carefully and with the patient's skin type in mind.

Laser hair removal is not a painless procedure. Most patients experience some discomfort during and immediately after treatment. A topical or local anesthetic can be used before treatment to reduce this effect. Perifollicular erythema and edema are expected in many patients treated with significant laser fluences. The intensity and duration depend on hair color and hair density. This usually lasts a few hours (Fig. 5.10).

Epidermal damage occurs if excessive fluences are used (Fig. 5.11). It is also more common in patients with a tan. Herpes simplex outbreaks are uncommon but may occur.

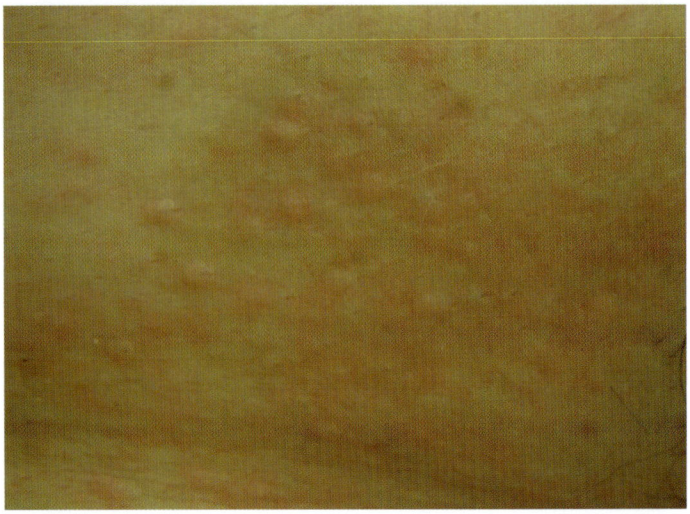

Figure 5.10 Transient perifollicular eythema and edema is a desired side effect to occur immediately after hair removal treatment.

A

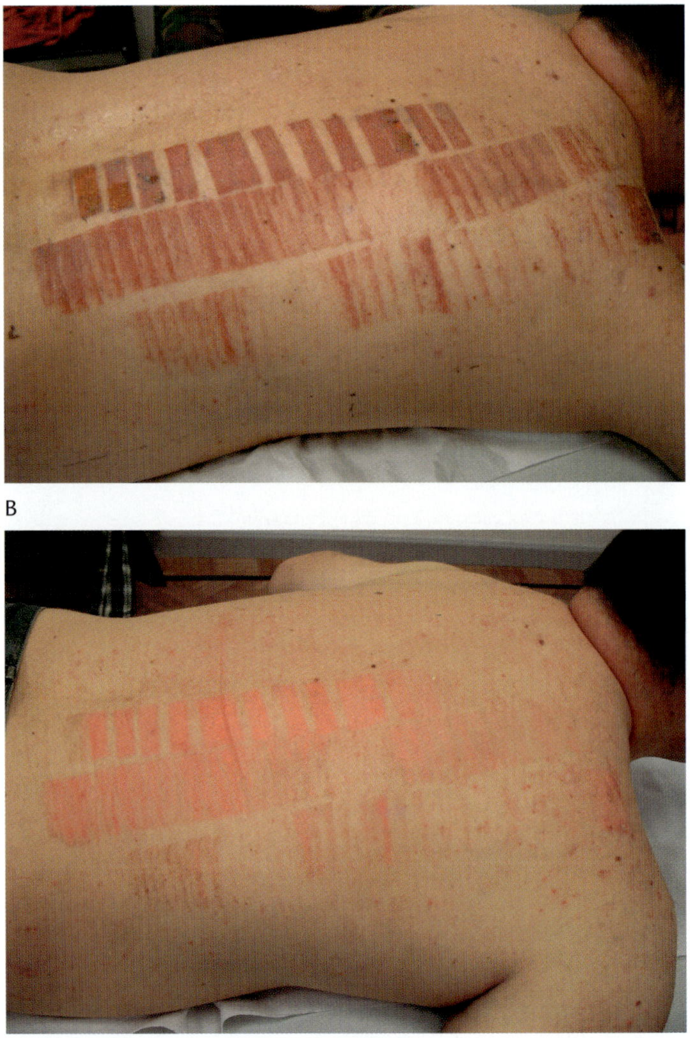

B

Figure 5.11 (A) Incorrect use of treatment parameters (fluence too high for particular skin type) caused epidermal damage with subsequent superficial erosions. (B) Complete healing with postinflammatory erythema and initial post-inflammatory hyperpigmentation at 2 weeks.

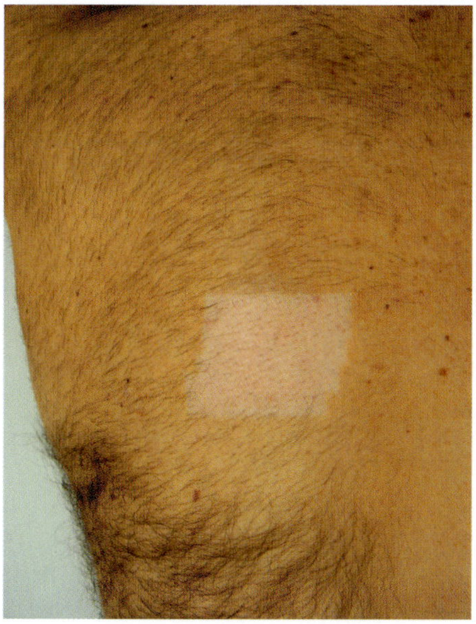

Figure 5.12 Treatment of recently tanned skin caused hypopigmentation.

There is a higher risk among patients with a previous history of herpes simplex and when the perioral, pubic, or bikini area are treated. The risk of bacterial infection is extremely low. However, it may occur following epidermal damage.

Folliculitis may occur in areas treated after excessive sweating or vigorous exercise. An additional risk is posed by swimming or using a hot-tub around treatment sessions.

The most common side effects are transient pigmentary changes such as hypopigmentation (Fig. 5.12) or hyperpigmentation (Fig. 5.13). It can be prevented if the appropriate treatment fluences are chosen for a certain skin type. This problem is mostly seen in patients with darker skin types or when patients have had a recent tan.[94–97] Permanent pigmentary changes are unlikely except in dark-skinned individuals.[98]

Scarring is unlikely except in cases of over-aggressive treatment or postoperative infection.

Loss of freckles or lightening of tattoos or pigmented lesions is not uncommon. Patients should be aware of this possibility.

Temporary or permanent leukotrichia has been said to develop following laser or IPL hair removal.[99] This finding may be explained by the difference in the thermal

A B C

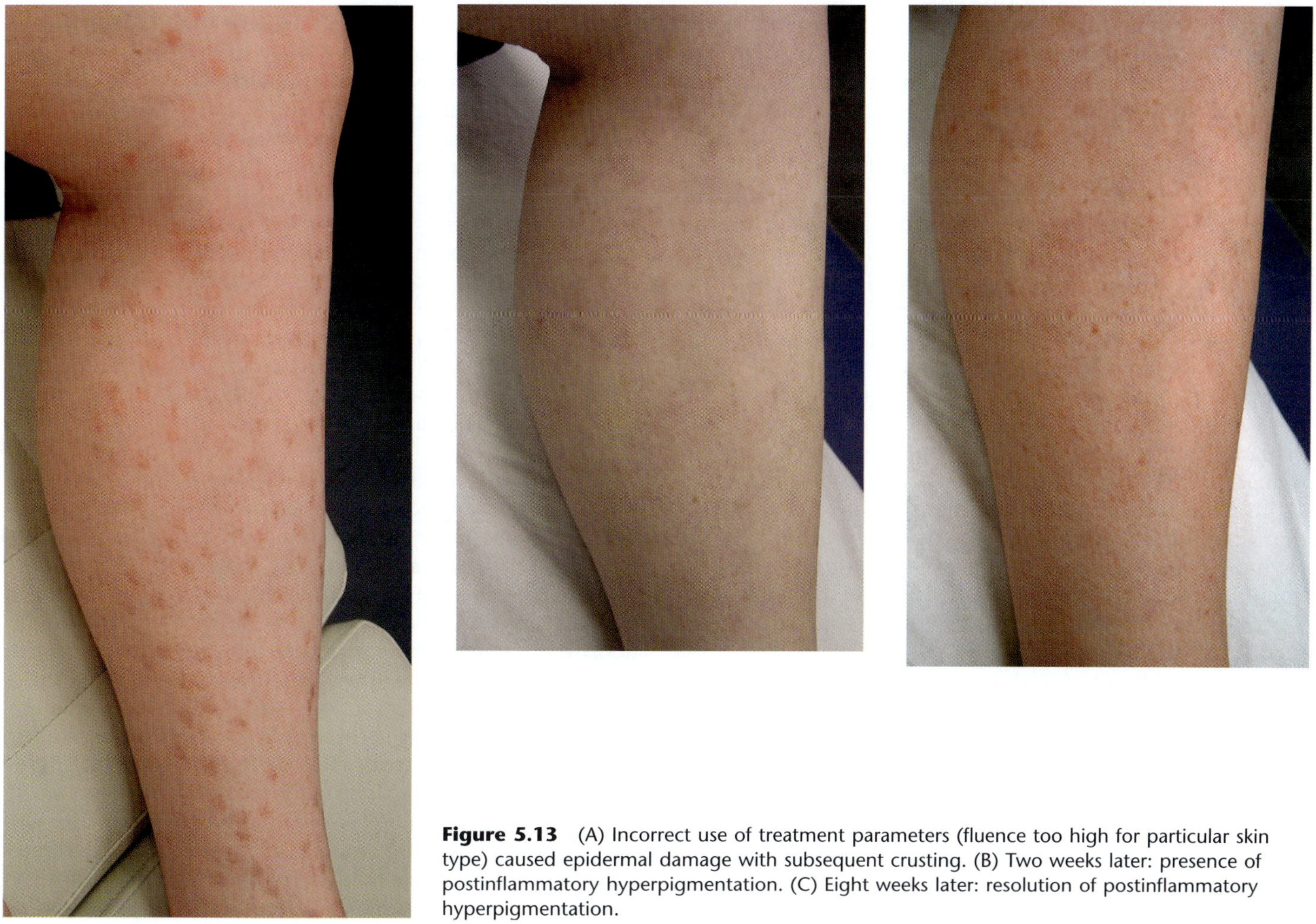

Figure 5.13 (A) Incorrect use of treatment parameters (fluence too high for particular skin type) caused epidermal damage with subsequent crusting. (B) Two weeks later: presence of postinflammatory hyperpigmentation. (C) Eight weeks later: resolution of postinflammatory hyperpigmentation.

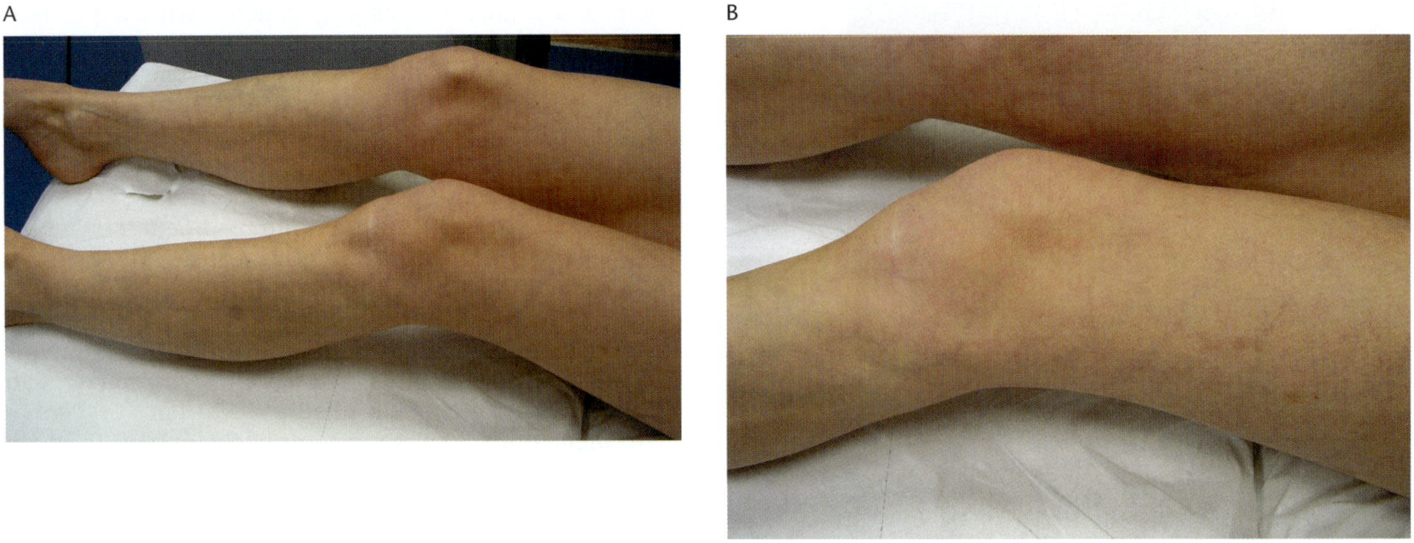

Figure 5.14 Induction of reticulate erythema on upper leg after a single treatment with an 800 nm diode laser (fluence 50 J/cm^2). Note the difference with the lower leg where no treatment was administered.

relaxation times of melanocytes and germinative cells. The light absorbed and the heat produced by melanin may be sufficient enough to destroy or impair the function of melanocytes but insufficient to damage the hair follicle cells.

A case of lichen planus triggered by long-pulsed ruby-laser treatment for hair removal has been reported.[100] Logic would suggest that all patients with a history of skin diseases known to show a Koebner phenomenon, such as psoriasis vulgaris, vitiligo, lichen planus, and Darier disease, should be informed about this possible adverse effect of treatment; clinically this is rarely seen.

Livedo reticularis[101] (Fig. 5.14), intense pruritus and urticaria[102] have been reported, including a case of intense swelling and erythema. The pathophysiology of these phenomena is not known. Management included topical corticosteroids, antihistamines, and discontinuing treatment. Several cases of induction of hair growth following laser hair removal in young female patients with darker skin types have been reported.[37] Two different phenomena have been observed: Either conversion of fine vellus hair to dark, coarse terminal hair at the site of treatment or induction of growth of long fine hairs in the immediate vicinity of the treatment area. Repetitive, low-fluence treatments with hair removal devices have also been reported to induce hair growth (see Fig. 5.8). Further study is ongoing to assess the mechanisms for this response. Treatment of this side effect has included continued treatment in some cases.

Light-based hair removal devices are designed for strong absorption by melanin and deep tissue penetration. These systems are therefore capable of causing retinal injury and proper eye protection must be worn by the patient and operating personnel. Treatment near or on the surface of an eye is not recommended. All other body sites can be treated safely.

The 'plume' generated by the vaporized hair shafts has a typical sulfuric smell and in large quantities, can be irritating to the respiratory tract. A smoke evacuator is recommended.

Future Directions

Research has shown that the average long-term hair loss per treatment is about 20–30%. Multiple treatment sessions are therefore usually required to achieve the maximal level of hair reduction. Attempts have been made to increase the efficacy of each treatment session, in an attempt to reduce the total numbers of treatments. A new, FDA approved patented technology, called Photopneumatic Therapy and developed by Aesthera Corp. (Livermore, CA.) has recently been introduced.[103,104] It combines the properties of broadband light with pneumatic energy. Photopneumatic technology results in the elevation of the hair follicle, bringing it closer to the surface of the skin, while melanin and blood concentration are greatly reduced. As a result, more effective photons should impact the hair follicles, making hair removal potentially more efficient.

The role of lasers and filtered flashlamps in hair removal has been determined over the last few years. Several controlled studies have demonstrated the efficacy and safety of light-based hair removal. The procedure is also very attractive because of its noninvasive nature, the ability to cover a large treatment area and the speed of treatment. Recently, smaller and less expensive light-based devices have become available for self treatment in home-like environment following instructions and guidance provided by a physician.[105] Studies showed that with adequate training and instruction, patients may administer self-treatments for hair removal with this small light based unit in a safe and effective manner. Recent studies have shown that CW laser systems that emit long laser pulses can potentially result in long-term hair removal after repeated treatments at low energy.[106–108] This has stimulated the research to develop portable, light-based hair-removal devices that women can buy and use at home, rather than having to visit a clinic for treatment. If research studies meet the regulatory requirements, product commercialization of these so-called laser-razors could potentially become a fact. One has to stay cautious and see how this area evolves.

References

1. Anderson R, Parrish J. Selective photothermolysis: precise microsurgery by selective absorption of pulsed radiation. Science 1983; 220:524–6.
2. Anderson RR, Parrish JA. The optics of human skin. J Invest Dermatol 1981; 77:13–19.
3. Ross V, Laden Z, Kreindel M, Dierickx C. Theoretical considerations in laser hair removal. Dermatol Clin 1999; 17(4):333–55.
4. Gilchrest BA, Rosen S, Noe JM. Chilling portwine stains improves the response to argon laser therapy. Plast Reconstr Surg 1982; 69:278–83.
5. Lask G, Elman M, Slatkine M, Waldman A, Rozenberg Z. Laser-assisted hair removal by selective photothermolysis. Dermatol Surg 1997; 23:737–9.
6. Alster TS, Lupton JS, Russo ML. Clinical and histologic efficacy of depilase long-pulsed Nd-YAG laser for hair removal in dark skin phototypes. Lasers Surg Med 2001; S13:196.
7. Altshuler GB, Zenzie HH, Erofeev AV, Smirnov MZ, Anderson RR, Dierickx C. Contact cooling of the skin. Phys Med Biol 1999; 44:1003–23.
8. Anvari B, Milner TE, Tanenbaum BS, Nelson JS. A comparative study of human skin thermal response to sapphire contact and cryogen spray cooling. IEEE Trans Biomed Eng 1998; 45(7):934–41.
9. Raulin C, Greve B, Hammes S. Cold air in laser therapy: first experiences with a new cooling system. Lasers Surg Med 2000; 27(5):404–10.
10. Van Gemert MJC, Welch AJ. Time constants in thermal laser medicine. Lasers Surg Med 2989; 9:405–21.
11. Anderson RR. Laser–tissue interactions. In: Goldman MP, Fitzpatrick RE, eds. Cutaneous laser surgery: the art and science of selective photothermolysis. St Louis: Mosby-Year Book; 1994:1–18.
12. Dierickx CC, Grossman MC, Farinelli WA, Anderson RR. Permanent hair removal by normal-mode ruby laser. Arch Dermatol 1998; 134(7):837–44.
13. Dierickx CC, Grossman MC, Farinelli WA, Manuskiatti W, Anderson RR. Long pulsed ruby laser hair removal. Lasers Surg Med 1997; S9:167.
14. Grossman MC, Dierickx C, Farinelli W, Flotte T, Anderson RR. Damage to hair follicles by normal-mode ruby laser pulses. J Am Acad Dermatol 1996; 35(6):889–94.
15. Eliezri YD. Fifteen-month clinical trial of hair removal with alexandrite laser. Lasers Surg Med 1998; S10:200.
16. Laughlin SA, Dudley DK. Long-term hair removal using a 3-millisecond alexandrite laser. J Cutan Med Surg 2000; 4:83–8.
17. Narukar V, Miller HM, Seltzer R. The safety and efficacy of the long pulse alexandrite laser for hair removal in various skin types. Lasers Surg Med 1998; S10:189.
18. Dierickx CC, Grossman MC, Farinelli WA, Manuskiatti W, Duque V, Lin D, Anderson RR. Hair removal by a pulsed, infrared laser system. Lasers Surg Med 1998; S10:198.
19. Dierickx CC, Grossman MC, Farinelli WA, Manuskiatti W, Duque V, Lin D, Anderson RR. Comparison between a long pulsed ruby laser and a pulsed infrared laser system for hair removal. Lasers Surg Med 1998; S10:199.
20. Grossman MC, Dierickx CC, Quintana A, Geronemus RG, Anderson RR. Removal of excess body hair with a 800 nm pulsed diode laser. Lasers Surg Med 1998; S10:201.
21. Lou WW, Quintana AT, Geronemus RG, Grossman MC. Prospective study of hair reduction by diode laser (800 nm) with long-term follow-up. Dermatol Surg 2000; 26:428–32.
22. Tanzi EL, Alster TS. Long-pulsed 1064-nm Nd:YAG laser-assisted hair removal in all skin types. Dermatol Surg 2004; 30(1):13–17.
23. Raff K, Landthaler M, Hohenleutner U. Optimizing treatment parameters for hair removal using long-pulsed Nd:YAG-lasers. Lasers Med Sci 2004; 18(4):219–22. Epub 2004 February 24.
24. Fodor L, Menachem M, Ramon Y, Shoshani O, Rissin Y, Eldor L, Egozi D, Peled IJ, Ullmann Y. Hair removal using intense pulsed light (EpiLight): patient satisfaction, our experience, and literature review. Ann Plast Surg 2005; 54(1):8–14.
25. Bedewi AF. Hair removal with intense pulsed light. Lasers Med Sci 2004; 19(1):48–51.
26. Altshuler GB, Anderson RR, Manstein D, Zenzie HH, Smirnov MZ. Extended theory of selective photothermolysis. Lasers Surg Med 2001; 29(5):416–32.
27. Rogachefsky AS, Silapunt S, Goldberg DJ. Evaluation of a new super-long-pulsed 810 nm diode laser for the removal of unwanted hair: the concept of thermal damage time. Dermatol Surg 2002; 28(5):410–14.
28. Rogachefsky AS, Becker K, Weiss G, Goldberg DJ. Evaluation of a long-pulsed Nd:YAG laser at different parameters: an analysis of both fluence and pulse duration. Dermatol Surg 2002; 28(10):932–5.
29. Kato T, Omi T, Naito Z, Hirai T, Kawana S. Histological hair removal study by ruby or alexandrite laser with comparative study on the effects of wavelength and fluence. J Cosmet Laser Ther 2004; 6(1):32–7.
30. Goldberg DJ, Littler CT, Wheeland, RG. Topical suspension-assisted Q-switched Nd:YAG laser hair removal. Dermatol Surg 1997; 23:741–5.
31. Kilmer SL, Chotzen VA, Calkin J. Hair removal study comparing the Q-switched Nd-YAG and long pulse ruby and alexandrite lasers. Lasers Surg Med 1998; S10:203.
32. Kilmer SL, Chotzen VA. Q-switched Nd-YAG laser (1064 nm) hair removal without adjuvant topical preparation. Lasers Surg Med 1997; S9:145.
33. Nanni CA, Alster TS. Laser-assisted hair removal: optimizing treatment parameters for hair removal using a topical carbon-based solution and 1064 nm Q-switched neodymium: YAG laser energy. Arch Dermatol 1997; 133:1546–9.
34. Anderson RR, Margolis RJ, Watenabe S, Flotte T, Hruza GJ, Dover JS. Selective photothermolysis of cutaneous pigmentation by Q-switched Nd-YAG laser pulses at 1064, 532 and 355 nm. J Invest Dermatol 1989; 93(1):28–32.
35. Dover JS, Margolis RJ, Polla LL, Watanabe S, Hruza GJ, Parrish JA, Anderson RR. Pigmented guinea pig skin irradiated with Q-switched ruby laser pulses: morphologic and histologic findings. Arch Dermatol 1989; 125(1):43–9.
36. Grossman MC, Wimberley J, Dwyer P, Flotte T, Anderson RR. PDT for hirsutism. Lasers Surg Med 1995; S7:205.
37. Moreno-Arias G, Castelo-Branco C, Ferrando J. Paradoxical effect after IPL photoepilation. Dermatol Surg 2002; 28(11):1013–16.
38. Alajlan A, Shapiro J, Rivers JK, MacDonald N, Wiggin J, Lui H. Paradoxical hypertrichosis after laser epilation. J Am Acad Dermatol 2005; 53:85–8.
39. Anderson RR, Dierickx CC, Altshuler G, Zenzie HH. Photon recycling: a new method of enhancing hair removal. Lasers Surg Med 1999; S11;190.

40. Ross EV, Rathyen JS, Gaudet T, Farinelli WA, Naseef G, DiMarizio C, Anderson RR. Recycling wasted photons: a device to increase laser energy used in surgery. Lasers Surg Med 1996; S8;87.
41. Campos V, Dierickx C, Alora B, Suthamjariya K, Palli K, Farinelli W, Anderson R. Hair removal by a pulsed, ruby laser system (E2000) with a twin pulse mode and photon recycling. Lasers Surg Med 2000; S12:78.
42. Lask G, Elman M, Noren P, Lee P, Nowfar-Rad M. Hair removal with the Epitouch ruby laser – a multicenter study. Laser Surg Med 1997; S9:147.
43. Williams R, Havoonjian H, Isagholian K, Menaker G, Moy R. A clinical study of hair removal using the long-pulsed ruby laser. Dermatol Surg 1998; 24:837–42.
44. Sommer S, Render C, Burd R, Sheehad-Dare R. Ruby laser treatment for hirsutism: clinical response and patient tolerance. Br J Dermatol 1998; 138:1009–14.
45. Topping A, Linge C, Gault D, Grobbelaar A, Sanders R. A review of the ruby laser with reference to hair depilation. Ann Plast Surg 2000; 44(6):668–74.
46. Polderman MC, Pavel S, le Cessie S, Grevelink JM, van Leeuwen RL. Efficacy, tolerability, and safety of a long-pulsed ruby laser system in the removal of unwanted hair. Dermatol Surg 2000; 26(3):240–3.
47. Gault DT, Grobbelaar AO, Grover R, Liew SH, Philp B, Clement RM, Kiernan MN. The removal of unwanted hair using a ruby laser. Br J Plast Surg 1999; 52(3):173–7.
48. Nelson JS, Milner TE, Anvari B, Tanenbaum BS, Kimel S, Svaasand LO, Jacques SL. Dynamic epidermal cooling during pulsed laser treatment of port-wine stain. A new methodology with preliminary clinical evaluation. Arch Dermatol 1995; 131:695–700.
49. McDaniel DH, Lord J, Ash K, Newman J, Zukowski M. Laser hair removal: a review and report on the use of the long-pulsed alexandrite laser for hair reduction of the upper lip, leg, back, and bikini region. Dermatol Surg 1999; 25:425–30.
50. Touma DJ, Rohrer TE. Persistent hair loss 60 months after a single treatment with a 3-millisecond alexandrite (755 nm) laser. J Am Acad Dermatol 2004; 50(2):324–5.
51. Goldberg DJ, Ahkami R. Evaluation comparing multiple treatments with a 2 msec and 10 msec alexandrite laser for hair removal. Laser in Surg Med 1999; 25:223–8.
52. Nanni CA, Alster TS. Long pulsed alexandrite laser assisted hair removal at 5, 10 and 20 millisecond pulse durations. Laser Surg Med 1999; 24:332–7.
53. Campos VB, Dierickx CC, Farinelli WA, Lin TY, Manuskiatti W, Anderson RR. Hair removal with an 800-nm pulsed diode laser. J Am Acad Dermatol 2000; 43(3):442–7.
54. Battle E, Suthamjariya K, Alora B, Palli K, Anderson RR. Very long-pulsed diode laser for hair removal on all skin types. Lasers Surg Med 2000; S12:85.
55. Rogachefsky AS, Becker K, Weiss G, Goldberg DJ. Evaluation of a long-pulsed Nd:YAG laser at different parameters. an analysis of both fluence and pulse duration. Dermatol Surg 2002; 28(10):932–5.
56. Kilmer S, Chotzen V, Calkin J, Silva S, McClaren M. Laser hair removal with a long-pulsed 1064 nm coolglide laser. Lasers Surg Med 2000; S12:84.
57. Lorenz S, Brunnberg S, Landthaler M, Hohenleutner U. Hair removal with the long pulsed Nd:YAG laser. A prospective study with one year follow-up. Lasers Surg Med 2002; 30(2):127–34.
58. Alster TS, Bryan H, Williams CM. Long-pulsed Nd:YAG laser-assisted hair removal in pigmented skin: a clinical and histological evaluation. Arch Dermatol 2001; 137(7):885–9.
59. Goldberg DJ, Silapunt S. Hair removal using a long-pulsed Nd:YAG laser: comparison at fluences of 50, 80, and 100 J/cm^2. Dermatol Surg 2001; 27(5):434–6.
60. Goldberg DJ, Silapunt S. Histologic evaluation of a millisecond Nd:YAG laser for hair removal. Lasers Surg Med 2001; 28(2):159–61.
61. Goldberg DJ, Samady JA. Evaluation of a long-pulse Q-switched Nd:YAG laser for hair removal. Dermatol Surg 2000; 26(2):109–13.
62. Bencini PL, Luci A, Galimberti M, Ferranti G. Long-term epilation with long-pulsed neodymium:YAG laser. Dermatol Surg 1999; 25(3):175–8.
63. Kauvar AN. Treatment of pseudofolliculitis with a pulsed infrared laser. Arch Dermatol 2000; 136(11):1343–6.
64. Ross EV, Cooke LM, Timko AL, Overstreet KA, Graham BS, Barnette DJ. Treatment of pseudofolliculitis barbae in skin types IV, V, and VI with a long-pulsed neodymium:yttrium aluminum garnet laser. J Am Acad Dermatol 2002; 47(2):263–70.
65. Ross EV, Cooke LM, Overstreet KA, Buttolph GD, Blair MA. Treatment of pseudofolliculitis barbae in very dark skin with a long pulse Nd:YAG laser. J Natl Med Assoc 2002; 94(10):888–93.
66. Fodor L, Menachem M, Ramon Y, Shoshani O, Rissin Y, Eldor L, Egozi D, Peled IJ, Ullmann Y. Hair removal using intense pulsed light (EpiLight): patient satisfaction, our experience, and literature review. Ann Plast Surg 2005; 54(1):8–14.
67. Troilius A, Troilius C. Hair removal with a second generation broad spectrum intense pulsed light source – a long-term follow-up. J Cutan Laser Ther 1999; 1(3):173–8.
68. Goldberg DJ, Silapunt S. Hair removal with a combined light/heat based photo-epilation system. J Cutan Laser Ther 2001; 3(1):3–7.
69. Adatto M. Hair removal with a combined light/heat-based photo-epilation system: a 6-month follow-up. J Cosmet Laser Ther 2003; 5(3–4):163–7.
70. Sadick NS, Shaoul J. Hair removal using a combination of conducted radiofrequency and optical energies – an 18-month follow-up. J Cosmet Laser Ther 2004; 6(1):21–6.
71. Henderson BW, Dougherty TJ. How does photodynamic therapy work? Photochem Photobiol 1992; 55:145–157.
72. Weishaupt KR, Gomer CJ, Dougherty TJ. Identification of singlet oygen as the cytotoxic agent in photo-inactivation of a murine tumor. Cancer Res 1976; 36:2326–9.
73. Divaris DXG, Kennedy JC, Poittier RH. Phototoxic damage to sebaceous glands and hair follicles of mice after systemic administration of 5-aminolevulinic acid correlates with localized protoporphyrin IX fluorescence. Am J Pathol 1990; 136:891–7.
74. Kennedy JC, Pottier RH. Endogenous protoporphyrin IX, a clinically useful photosensitizer for photodynamic therapy. J Photochem Photobiol B 1992; 14:275–92.
75. Kennedy JC, Pottier RH, Pross DC. Photodynamic therapy with endogenous protoporphyrin IX: basic principles and present clinical experience. J Photochem Photobiol B 1990; 6:143–8.
76. Khatri KA. Diode laser hair removal in patients undergoing isotretinoin therapy. Dermatol Surg 2004; 30(9):1205–7.
77. Cassano N, Arpaia N, Vena GA. Diode laser hair removal and isotretinoin therapy. Dermatol Surg 2005; 31(3):380–1.
78. Trotter MJ, Tron VA, Hollingdale J, Rivers JK. Localized chrysiasis induced by laser therapy. Arch Dermatol 1995; 131(12):1411–14.
79. Nouri K, Chen H, Saghari S, Ricotti CA Jr. Comparing 18- versus 12-mm spot size in hair removal using a gentlease

755-nm alexandrite laser. Dermatol Surg 2004; 30:494–7.
80. Lin TY, Manuskiatti W, Dierickx CC, Farinelli WA, Fisher ME, Flotte T, Baden HP, Anderson RR. Hair growth cycle affects hair follicle destruction by ruby laser pulses. J Invest Dermatol 1998; 111(1):107–13.
81. Dierickx CC, Campos VB, Lin DT, Farinelli, WA, Anderson RR. Influence of hair growth cycle on efficacy of laser hair removal. Lasers Surg Med 1999; S11:84.
82. Liew SH, Grobbelaar AO, Gault D, Green C, Linge C. Ruby laser-assisted hair removal: a preliminary report of the correlation between efficacy of treatment and melanin content of hair and the growth phases of hair at a specific site. Ann Plast Surg 1999; 42(3):255–8.
83. Olsen EA. Methods of hair removal. J Am Ac Derm 1999; 40:143–55.
84. Sadick NS, Laughlin SA. Effective epilation of white and blonde hair using combined radiofrequency and optical energy. J Cosmet Laser Ther 2004; 6(1):27–31.
85. Bouzari N, Tabatabai H, Abbasi Z, Firooz A, Dowlati Y. Laser hair removal: comparison of long-pulsed Nd:YAG, long-pulsed alexandrite, and long-pulsed diode lasers. Dermatol Surg 2004; 230:498–502.
86. Handrick C, Alster TS. Comparison of long-pulsed diode and long-pulsed alexandrite lasers for hair removal: a long-term clinical and histologic study. Dermatol Surg 2001; 27(7):622–6.
87. Bjerring P. Clinical comparison of hair reduction using the newest generation IPL and a first generation ruby laser. J Cutan Laser Ther 2000; 2(4):211.
88. Battle EF Jr, Hobbs LM. Laser-assisted hair removal for darker skin types. Dermatol Ther 2004; 17(2):177–83.
89. Smith EP, Winstanley D, Ross EV. Modified superlong pulse 810nm diode laser in the treatment of pseudofolliculitis barbae in skin types V and VI. Dermatol Surg 2005; 31(3):297–301.
90. Galadari I. Comparative evaluation of different hair removal lasers in skin types IV, V, and VI. Int J Dermatol 2003; 42(1):68–70.
91. Goh CL. Comparative study on a single treatment response to long pulse Nd:YAG lasers and intense pulse light therapy for hair removal on skin type IV to VI – are longer wavelengths lasers preferred over shorter wavelengths lights for assisted hair removal. J Dermatolog Treat 2003; 14(4):243–7.
92. Nahm WK, Tsoukas MM, Falanga V, Carson PA, Sami N, Touma DJ. Preliminary study of fine changes in the duration of dynamic cooling during 755-nm laser hair removal on pain and epidermal damage in patients with skin types III–V. Lasers Surg Med 2002; 31(4):247–51.
93. Johnson F, Dovale M. Intense pulsed light treatment of hirsutism: case reports of skin phototypes V and VI. J Cutan Laser Ther 1999; 1(4):233–7.
94. Campos VB, Dierickx CC, Farinelli WA, Lin TY, Manuskiatti W, Anderson RR. Ruby laser hair removal: evaluation of long-term efficacy and side effects. Lasers Surg Med 2000; 26(2):177–85.
95. Nanni CA, Alster TS. Laser assisted hair removal: side effects of Q-switched Nd:YAG, long-pulsed ruby and alexandrite lasers. J Am Acad Dermatol 1999; 141:165–71.
96. Haedersdal M, Egekvist H, Efsen J, Bjerring P. Skin pigmentation and texture changes after hair removal with the normal-mode ruby laser. Acta Derm Venereol 1999; 79(6):465–8.
97. Hasan AT, Eaglstein W, Pardo RJ. Solar-induced postinflammatory hyperpigmentation after laser hair removal. Dermatol Surg 1999; 25(2):113–15.
98. Moreno-Arias GA, Tiffon T, Marti T, Camps-Fresneda A. Long-term hypopigmentation induced by diode laser photo-epilation. J Cutan Laser Ther 2001; 3(1):9–10.
99. Radmanesh M, Mostaghimi M, Yousefi I, Mousavi ZB, Rasai S, Esmaili HR, Khadivi HA. Leukotrichia developed following application of intense pulsed light for hair removal. Dermatol Surg 2002; 28(7):572–4.
100. Wimmershoff MB, Hohenleutner U, Landthaler M. Isomorphic phenomenon: adverse effect after epilation with the long-pulsed ruby laser. Arch Dermatol 2000; 136(12):1570–1.
101. Lapidoth M, Shafirstein G, Ben Amitai D, Hodak E, Waner M, David M. Reticulate erythema following diode laser-assisted hair removal: a new side effect of a common procedure. J Am Acad Dermatol 2004; 51(5):774–7.
102. Moreno-Arias GA, Tiffon T, Marti T, Camps-Fresneda A. Urticaria vasculitis induced by diode laser photo-epilation. Dermatol Surg 2000; 26(11):1082–3.
103. Narukar VA. Photopneumatic pixilation: demonstration of a novel approach to light based hair reduction. Lasers Surg Med 2005; S17:245.
104. Kilmer SL. Validation of a radically new technology for permanent hair reduction. Lasers Surg Med 2005; S17: 284.
105. Rohrer TE, Chatrath V, Yamauchi P, Lask G. Can patients treat themselves with a small novel light based hair removal system? Lasers Surg Med 2003; 33(1):25–9.
106. Manstein D, Poureshagh M, Zenzie H, Altshuler G, Anderson R. Photoepilation with a new CW-diode laser with intradermal focusing optics in continuous contact scanning mode. Lasers Surg Med 2001; S13:87.
107. Zenzie H, Katri K, Stoll M, Manstein D, Altshuler G, Anderson G. Long-term hair reduction from multiple treatments with continuous-wave dode laser. Lasers Surg Med 2003; S15:281.
108. Manstein D, Bowes L, Rius F, Poureshagh M, Anderson R. Hair growth management with a low-dose, continuous-wave diode laser used in scanning mode. Laser Surg Med 2004; S16:69.

Chapter 6

Carbon Dioxide and Erbium:YAG Laser Ablation

Robert J. Willard, Brent R. Moody and George J. Hruza

Historical Perspective

The first medical lasers emitted wavelengths only in the visible spectrum and therefore initially targeted pigmented tissue to achieve specific thermal destruction of the intended structures. Indeed, the first patient treated with a laser in 1962 had malignant melanoma; it was treated with the ruby and neodymium pulsed laser prior to excision.[1] However, in 1964 the carbon dioxide (CO_2) laser with a wavelength of 10,600 nm in the far-infrared region (FIR) of the electromagnetic spectrum was developed.[2] This wavelength targets water, and surgical applications for this laser were first tested in 1967.[3]

The high absorption of the 10,600 nm wavelength by intracellular water led to the development of a number of applications, including the use of the CO_2 laser as a scalpel for excisional surgery, as a destructive instrument for cutaneous malignancies (similar to electrodesiccation and curettage), in cutaneous laser resurfacing, and in the ablation of various dermal and epidermal lesions. In surgery, the continuous wave CO_2 laser became more convenient than a cold steel scalpel in certain instances where there was a greater need for hemostasis, since the laser instantly coagulates blood vessels up to 0.5 mm in diameter. A very small spot size (0.1–0.2 mm) is needed to use the laser in this manner. In addition to the coagulation and sealing of small vessels, small cutaneous nerve endings and lymphatics are also sealed, offering a distinct advantage with less postoperative pain[4] and edema.[5] For use as an ablative instrument, a larger spot size is required and this is usually achieved through the use of a defocused mode by moving the laser handpiece farther away from its original focal point on the skin surface (Fig. 6.1).

Because the first CO_2 lasers were continuous wave with a beam of light that was constantly on, thermal damage beyond the zone of ablation or destruction was often unpredictable and difficult to control, resulting in unwanted scarring. The solution to this problem was the development of pulsed CO_2 lasers. The technology behind pulsed lasers varies from mechanically shuttering or chopping a continuous wave beam with a fan-like device, to electronically pumping a laser tube to deliver extremely high energy short pulsed bursts of light. Superpulsed and ultrapulsed lasers will be discussed in the next section. It is worth first defining the most commonly used terms when speaking about the delivery of laser energy.

Definition of Terms

Energy

Energy is the ability to do work and is equal to force times the distance over which the force is exerted. Newton's second law states that force is equal to mass times acceleration. This is expressed in units as kg × m/s^2. One kg·m/s^2 is equal to one Newton (N). Units of energy are expressed as force (N) times distance (m), or in Newton-meters (Nm). One Nm is defined as 1 joule (J) of energy. Energy is also the product of power × time. This is relevant to laser surgery in that the power of the laser beam multiplied by the pulse duration determines the total energy delivered to the target.

Power

Power is the rate of energy delivery (energy/time). The unit of power is defined as the Watt, and is equal to 1 joule per second. This is not as relevant to laser surgery as the power density.

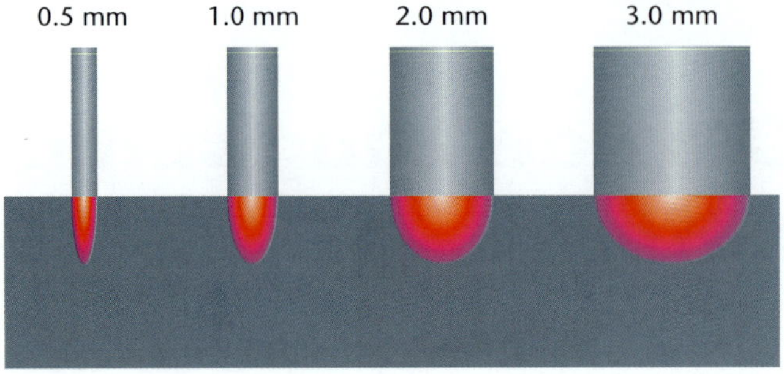

Figure 6.1 Larger spot size requires higher laser energy. As spot size increases, volume of tissue heated instantly by laser increases. This increases energy required to vaporize that volume of tissue. If laser energy is not changed, there is a decrease in thermal damage. (Courtesy Coherent Laser Corp., Palo Alto, CA.)

Power Density

Also termed 'irradiance', the power density is equal to power (W) per unit area (cm^2). Irradiance is calculated as the power of the laser beam divided by its surface (cross-sectional) area. Thus, for a circular beam of spot size (diameter) d, with power P, the irradiance is equal to $P/\pi(d/2)^2$, or $4P/\pi d^2$. It is obvious from this equation that a two-fold change in d produces a four-fold change in irradiance, while changes in P result in a corresponding linear change in irradiance. In practical terms, irradiance is the single-most important determinant of the rate of vaporization or ablation of tissue.

Although irradiance expresses the rate of energy delivery for a given area of tissue, it says nothing of the dose of energy given. The amount or dose of energy per unit area depends on the time over which a beam of a particular irradiance is delivered. 'Fluence' is the term used to express this latter concept.

Fluence

Fluence is best described as the energy density. It is equal to the energy in joules divided by the surface area of the beam (cm^2). This expresses the dose of energy delivered to the site of laser impact and incorporates the concepts of irradiance and time (fluence = irradiance × pulse width). It has been estimated that when irradiance is greater than $100\,W/cm^2$, the degree of tissue damage depends directly on time of application (pulse width) and not on irradiance.[6] It is important to remember that irradiance determines rate of tissue vaporization but that fluence determines the amount of energy deposited and thus the amount of vaporization. The minimum fluence needed to effect pure vaporization of tissue with a CO_2 laser is $5\,J/cm^2$. This is discussed in greater detail in the section on laser–tissue interaction.

Spot Size

The cross-sectional diameter of the laser beam or spot size can be controlled by focusing lenses or by varying the distance that the handpiece is held away from the skin surface. There is a Gaussian distribution of irradiance across the beam, with peak intensity in the center and minimal intensity at the beam edges. Therefore, the smaller the beam, the less even is the vaporization due to a very sharp drop in irradiance from center to edge. A larger spot size allows for a more gradual drop in irradiance from center to edge, and thus for more even vaporization (Fig. 6.2). However, as spot size increases, the volume of tissue heated increases and thus the energy required to heat that volume also increases. Therefore, higher-power lasers must be used to achieve the minimum fluence ($5\,J/cm^2$) needed for vaporization with larger spot sizes. If one increases spot size without a concomitant increase in power, then slow heating of tissue occurs with less vaporization and greater thermal injury leading to scarring.

Duty Cycle

For lasers used in a repetitive pulsed mode, the total amount of time that the laser is actually *on* divided by the total time of the cycle is the duty cycle, expressed as a percentage. It is also equal to pulse width times repetition rate. The usual range is 2–50%. As the repetition rate increases, the average power of the laser also increases (i.e. a more rapid rate of delivery of energy) while the irradiance remains constant. Average power can also be increased by keeping repetition rate constant and increasing pulse width.

Thermal Relaxation Time

The thermal relaxation time (τ_r) is the amount of time required for a material to lose 63% (1/e) of its heat by thermal diffusion. If energy is delivered to a target in a period of time faster than the time it takes for the target to lose its heat by conduction to its surroundings, then no (or minimal) thermal damage will occur beyond the target. This concept is discussed in more detail below with selective photothermolysis.

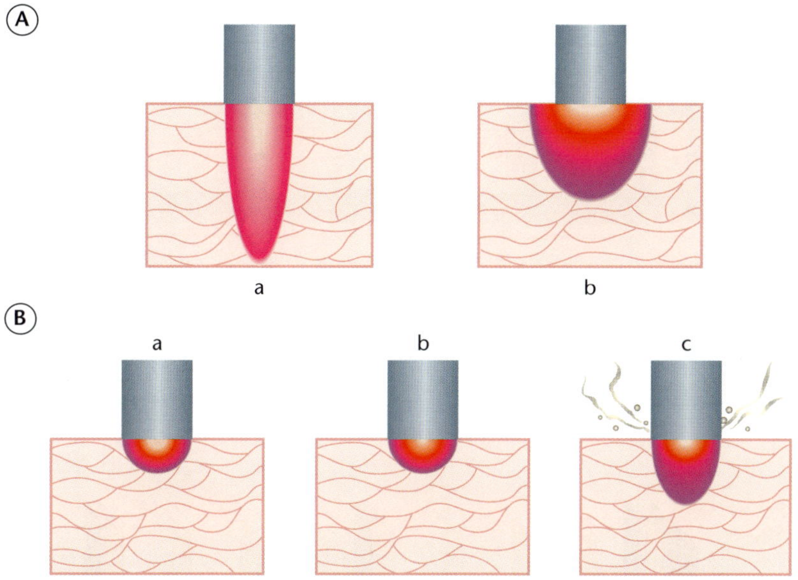

Figure 6.2 (A) Laser energy is transmitted through skin by transmission and conduction. (a) Laser instantly heats tissue to a depth determined by absorption length. (b) Heat flows from region heated by laser into adjacent tissue by conduction. (B) Laser light is absorbed by tissue. (a) Water temperature is raised to approximately 100°C. (b) Intercellular water boils. (c) Heat is carried away as steam and plume. (Courtesy Coherent Laser Corp., Palo Alto, CA.)

Laser Pulse

To achieve heating and destruction of target tissue in a period of time that is shorter than τ_r, the laser beam must be pulsed such that it is only on for a time $t < \tau_r$. The earliest forms of pulsed lasers were simply chopped beams of continuous wave energy. The peak power of each individual pulse was no different than the power of the continuous wave beam. However, the first truly pulsed laser was the 'superpulse' waveform, which was achieved through radiofrequency excitation of the lasing medium. This mode of pulsing ensures that the pulse energy is maintained well above the ablation threshold throughout the entire pulse duration. The pulse width of this waveform varies from 100 to 900 μs with repetition rates from 1 to 5000 pulses per second.[7] Peak powers of this laser are two to ten times higher than the continuous wave CO_2. The superpulse CO_2 can also be mechanically shuttered to yield short bursts of a series of 10 or more pulses depending on the repetition rate and shutter speed.

A further improvement in technology came in the form of the Ultrapulse CO_2 by Coherent (now Lumenis). This laser provides five to seven times the peak power per pulse as the superpulse CO_2 (>450 W, 250 mJ per pulse, 100 W average power, pulse width <1 ms). For a spot size of 2.5 mm and pulse energy of 250 mJ, the fluence would be $(0.25\,J/p[0.125\,cm]^2)$, or $5.1\,J/cm^2$, the minimum fluence necessary to achieve vaporization and ablation of tissue while minimizing thermal injury (see below). Figure 6.3 compares the power versus time profiles for the chopped, superpulse, and ultrapulse lasers.

Physics and Laser–Tissue Interaction

When a photon of energy strikes a material such as tissue, it can be either absorbed or scattered. It is the absorption by different chromophores in the skin that allows selective targeting by various wavelength lasers for specific intended purposes. According to the Beer–Lambert Law, absorbance is directly proportional to the concentration of the absorbing chromophore. The major chromophores in skin are melanin, oxy- and deoxyhemoglobin, and water. Laser energy that is absorbed by biological molecules is converted into heat energy, which may result in vaporization of tissue, coagulation necrosis, or submicroscopic cavitations. Because heat in the temperature range of 40–100°C can result in denaturation of proteins, unwinding of DNA, and disruption of cell membranes, a state incompatible with cell function is created and necrosis ensues.[8] With both the 10,600 nm carbon dioxide (CO_2) laser and the 2940 nm erbium:yttrium, aluminum, garnet (Er:YAG) lasers, the chromophore for absorbance is water. The epidermis is composed of 80% water. At the energies used for resurfacing, instant heating of water to 100°C occurs and vaporization of tissue ensues. Because the heating and thermal expansion are so rapid, explosions and cavitation of structures on a microscopic level occur, and a plume of water and tissue components is released upon impact. A zone of coagulation beyond the vaporization zone results with the CO_2 laser to a variable depth depending on the mode of use. The Er:YAG laser produces such a minimum

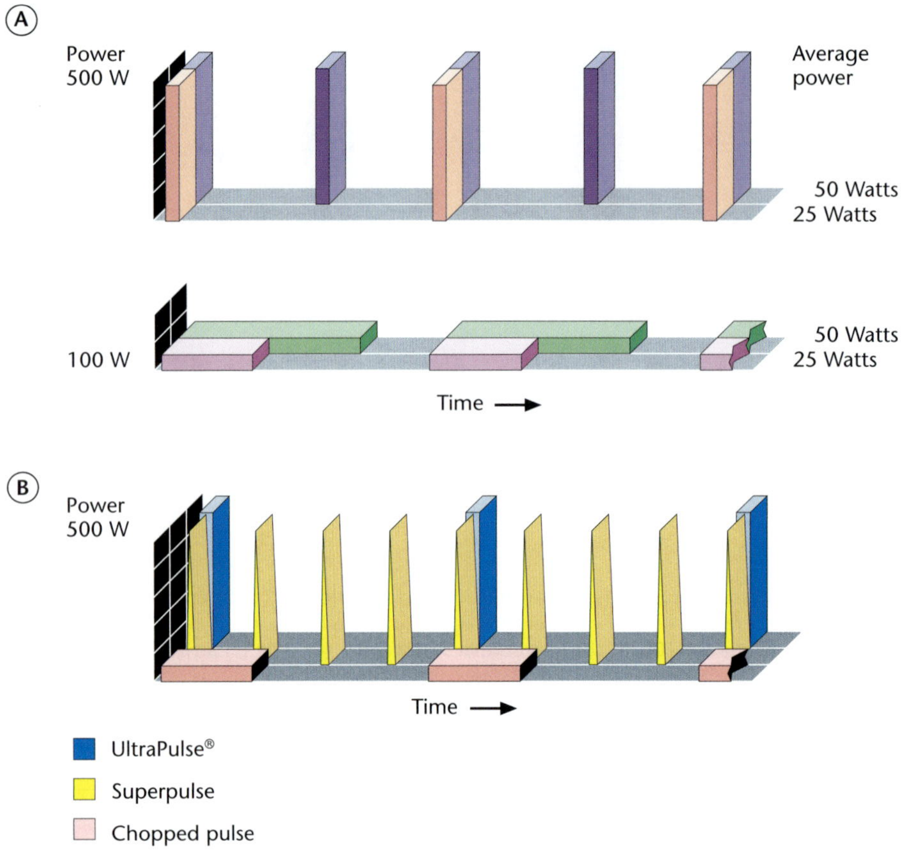

Figure 6.3 (A) To generate identical fluence at skin surface, a chopped pulse (continuous wave) must be maintained for a longer period than with ultrapulsed or superpulsed lasers, which generate a higher peak power over a shorter time. (B) Comparison of ultrapulse, superpulse, and chopped-pulse CO_2 laser fluence. At same average power, superpulsed laser must deliver 4 to 5 pulses for each ultrapulse. A chopped pulse is seven times longer than an ultrapulse for this same energy. (Courtesy Coherent Laser Corp., Palo Alto, CA.)

zone of thermal damage that no coagulation or hemostasis results when used in its purely ablative mode. The specific thermal effects in tissue will be discussed for each laser.

R. Rox Anderson and Parrish coined the term 'selective photothermolysis' in 1983 to describe the process by which a chromophore is heated by laser light absorption in a time period shorter than its thermal relaxation time.[9] The latter is the amount of time required for a material to lose 50% of its heat by conduction to its surroundings. Thus, when a chromophore is heated by selective photothermolysis, only the intended target is damaged and there is minimal diffusion of heat and no consequent injury to the surrounding structures. The mechanism of injury involves both thermal coagulation and/or photoacoustic injury in the form of supersonic high pressure shock waves. For both the CO_2 and Er:YAG lasers, the predominant mechanism is photothermal. The pulse fluence necessary to achieve vaporization and thus ablation of skin tissue with the CO_2 laser is $5\,J/cm^2$.[8] This can be calculated based on two factors: the latent heat of vaporization of water is $2500\,J/cm^3$, and the energy (E_v) absorbed per unit volume of tissue is E_v = fluence × μ_a. The depth of penetration of the 10,600 nm wavelength has been calculated to be 20 μm, or $1/\mu_a$, where μ_a is the absorption coefficient for water (equal to $500\,cm^{-1}$). Solving for fluence in the above equation, fluence = 2500/500 = $5\,J/cm^2$. The actual thickness of tissue ablation varies from 20 to 60 μm. For this thickness of tissue, the thermal relaxation time (τ_r) can be calculated to be ~800 μs. This is based on the equation $\tau_r = d^2/4\kappa$, where d = 20 μm (thickness of vaporized layer) and κ, the thermal diffusivity of skin tissue, is ~$1.3 \times 10^{-3}\,cm^2/s$.[8] Therefore, to achieve selective photothermolysis with the CO_2 laser, a pulse of energy of at least $5\,J/cm^2$ must be delivered in under 800 μs. For each 20 μm of tissue that is ablated, 3–4 times this amount is thermally damaged.[8] It is this latter effect that allows for hemostasis, collagen remodeling and wound healing. This 60–100 μm zone of coagulation is modest compared to the 300–1000 μm layer of damage that results from the use of continuous wave (CW) CO_2 lasers. Thus, the superficial penetration and high-powered, short-pulsed CO_2 laser allows precise layer by layer control of tissue ablation. Figure 6.2 depicts the zones of vaporization, irreversible thermal damage, and reversible damage. Although a lower-power, longer-duration laser will vaporize an equivalent volume of tissue as a high-power, short-pulsed laser, the former will do so with much more peripheral damage due to the longer time allowed for thermal diffusion. The volume of tissue vaporized depends on the amount of energy deposited per unit area (fluence). However, the width of the zone of adjacent tissue damage depends on the pulse duration, or time of laser exposure.[10–12]

Laser dwell time is the amount of time that the beam is on in one location. Low power densities require longer dwell times to achieve the same effect as high power densities. The longer the dwell time and the slower the heating, the more desiccation and charring of tissue that results. Further heating of charred tissue results in extremely high temperatures of 300–600°C. This is because carbonized and desiccated tissue acts as a heat sink for laser absorption. There is no buffer of water to absorb the heat and thus temperatures escalate rapidly. Continuous wave lasers must be rapidly scanned across the treated area in order to keep the dwell time less than the thermal relaxation time.

Superpulsed CO_2 lasers deliver pulse energies in the 30–50 mJ range. The peak power per pulse is 2–10 times higher than CW CO_2 lasers, but the average power over time is similar (see Fig. 6.3). We have seen that the 5 J/cm^2 minimum energy for vaporization can be achieved with a 250-mJ pulse and a 2.5-mm spot size. But for a single pulse of 40 mJ, one would need a 1-mm spot size to achieve 5 J/cm^2. This small spot size results in very uneven vaporization with the creation of ridges and grooves (unless the beam has a 'top-hat' energy design). To achieve the vaporization threshold with the larger 2.5-mm spot size, the 40 mJ pulses of a superpulsed laser must be layered in a sequence of 6–10 pulses (each with a pulse duration of 100–900 μs) such that interpulse cooling is not long enough to prevent the vaporization threshold from being reached. The rapid pulses are broken into short streams of pulses by mechanically shuttering and imposing a second duty on the superpulsed laser. Typically, the second duty cycle consists of a 50-ms burst of 6–10 pulses. Each burst is able to reach the vaporization threshold, and these bursts are safely repeated at a frequency of 2–10 Hz without creating unwanted thermal damage. One study showed that when conduction was the only mechanism for heat removal, the rate of delivery of these streams of pulses should be less than 5 Hz.[13] Experiments on guinea pig skin and confirmatory studies in human skin confirm that 50-ms pulses result in less thermal damage than longer shuttered pulses. The 'off' period protects tissue from excessive heat accumulation.[14–17] One must also consider the liquid phase that forms during laser–tissue interaction that is thought to act as a conduit for heat conduction from the impact crater to the surrounding tissues.[15,18] It has been shown that the thermal relaxation time for this phase is ~19 ms. However, it has not been shown that shuttered pulses less than 50 ms are clinically useful.

CO_2 Lasers

The Ultrapulse laser introduced by Coherent (now Lumenis) solved the problem of having to create second duty cycles (pulses of pulses) with the superpulsed lasers. This was the first laser capable of delivering very high fluence pulses (~200–500 mJ) with large spot sizes capable of tissue vaporization with a single pulse. A computer pattern generator allows the user to rapidly and precisely scan a series of spots within a predefined pattern shape (e.g. a parallelogram) and to select the degree of spot overlap. This facilitates even contouring of treated areas. The depth of vaporization with an ultrapulse laser was studied in pig skin using pulses of 250–450 mJ. The first pass caused complete vaporization of epidermis with <4 μm of dermal necrosis; subsequent passes caused thermal damage ranging in depth from 53–106 μm.[8,19] In human skin, the depth of thermal damage using the ultrapulse laser was 20 μm after one pass, 40 μm after two passes, and 70 μm after three passes.[8,20,21] It has been shown clinically that two to three passes of the CO_2 laser can smoothen deep rhytides that measure at least 1 mm in depth.[22–26]

A newer generation of superpulsed CO_2 laser, the NovaPulse, has been developed. Unlike the original superpulsed lasers, this device can generate 7 J/cm^2 of fluence by rapidly moving a small spot size through a computer pattern generator.

The TruPulse (Tissue Technologies) laser can produce peak powers up to 10,000 watts at very short pulse durations (~65–125 μs). The handpiece utilizes square spots available in 1, 3, and 5 mm. The fluence delivered is in the 5–7 J/cm^2 range, but it is delivered so fast (10 times less than the thermal relaxation time of skin) that very superficial ablation is accomplished per laser pass with little thermal injury. Only partial epidermal ablation may be achieved with a single pass. Less thermal injury and greater collagen production compared to the Novapulse and FeatherTouch were found in one study.[27]

Another laser system that can achieve results similar to those of the Ultrapulse is the Sharplan SilkLaser. This device offers two modes: the Feathertouch and Silktouch. This scanned laser uses a continuous wave CO_2 laser beam that is scanned over a defined pattern so rapidly that the tissue dwell time in any given spot is less than 1 ms. Thus the effect is essentially the same as that of a high-energy pulsed system. The SilkLaser flashscanner uses oscillating mirrors in the laser handpiece to rapidly scan a 0.1–0.25 mm focused beam in a spiral pattern across the tissue. The scanner covers areas ranging in size from 0.6 to 15 mm in patterns that can be circular, hexagonal, elliptical, or square. The beam profile is 'top-hat' or non-Gaussian so that even vaporization is achieved across the beam contact area. A difference between the SilkTouch and the FeatherTouch modes is that in the former, the beam is scanned twice with a dwell time of less than 1 ms, while in the latter the beam is scanned only once with a faster dwell time of less than 300 μs. The power in the FeatherTouch mode must be doubled to maintain the fluence above the vaporization threshold. For a given pass of the laser beam, more tissue is vaporized using the SilkTouch mode with resultant greater thermal coagulation. Unlike other CO_2 lasers, when power is increased with the SilkLaser, the thickness of tissue removed with each scan also increases. With the UltraPulse and TruPulse lasers increases in power result in increased rates of pulsing.

In 1997 a new scanner called the SureTouch was developed for use with most 20–30 W continuous wave CO_2 lasers. This device focuses the beam into a smaller spot size to provide irradiance sufficient to deliver 5 J/cm^2. The power requirement is roughly half that of the FeatherTouch system yet it provides equal zones of residual thermal damage. Rather than scanning in a spiral pattern, various geometric shapes can be used with the SureTouch.

To understand the thermal effects beyond vaporization of tissue with the CO_2 laser, we must understand the effect of heat on the individual structures within tissue. The rate of cell injury increases with temperature. Thus epidermal necrosis occurs after 5 seconds at 60°C and after 1 s at 70°C.[28,29] Vaporization occurs at 100°C to leave behind a layer of cellular and proteinaceous debris. Within the dermis, collagen I is the most temperature sensitive macromolecule and is the main structural component providing support. Reversible loss of tertiary structure occurs at temperatures less than 50°C, with irreversible denaturation of collagen I taking place at temperatures beyond this.[7] Elastin, on the other hand, is very stable, even at high temperatures.

For most nonresurfacing indications, the resurfacing CO_2 lasers are used to minimize residual thermal damage with its associated increase in residual scarring. Only when maximal hemostasis is needed such as when treating rhinophyma would one consider the use of a CW CO_2 laser.

Er:YAG Lasers

With the Er:YAG laser at 2940 nm, the energy is so efficiently absorbed by water (12–18 times that of the 10,600 nm wavelength) that its narrow depth of penetration (2–5 μm) results in a very superficial layer of tissue ablation with minimal surrounding thermal injury (20–50 μm compared to 60–100 μm for CO_2).[30–32] The absorbed heat is immediately dissipated as steam and smoke plume. The absorption coefficient μ_a of the 2940 nm wavelength for water is 12,800 cm^{-1}, compared to 500 cm^{-1} for the 10,600 nm wavelength, thus accounting for the superficial absorption and finer ablation. It is also able to do so at a lower fluence of 0.5–1.5 J/cm^2 compared to the CO_2 laser. Because of this high absorbance in tissue, the Er:YAG laser achieves ablation primarily through a photomechanical rather than a photothermal effect. That is, the immediate heating of water is so rapid that structures are literally exploded by high pressure shock waves. Bloodless ablation in the normal mode of use (pulse width ~200 μs) is achieved with up to two or three passes. However, the relative lack of thermal injury with Er:YAG lasers results in poor hemostasis after four or more passes and much less collagen shrinkage (1–2%) compared to the CO_2 laser. To address this problem, modulated systems have been developed that incorporate coagulation to effect hemostasis.

Three Er:YAG lasers now combine features of ablation and coagulation into their systems: The Derma-K (Lumenis), the dual-mode Contour (Sciton, Palo Alto, CA), and the CO_3 (Cynosure, MA). The Derma-K is a hybrid that combines a conventional ablative Er:YAG with a low-power CO_2 laser for coagulation. The dual mode Contour consists of two Er:YAG laser heads. One delivers short-pulsed ablative energy and the other provides long-pulsed subablative coagulative energy. The CO_3 laser is a variable pulse system that delivers both short ablative and long coagulative pulses from the same Er:YAG laser head.[33]

With this concept in mind, the modulated Er:YAG systems can provide results very similar to traditional CO_2 resurfacing lasers by providing controlled thermal desiccation of tissue.[33] The Derma-K laser delivers subablative, coagulative CO_2 pulses to tissue in between ablative Er:YAG pulses. The CO_2 pulse can fill from 50% to 100% of the 'off' period of the Er:YAG duty cycle. The power of the CO_2 pulse can also be varied to provide optimal tissue ablation and hemostasis.[34] The CO_3 laser is a pure Er:YAG laser that produces variable length pulses to effect ablation and hemostasis.

Finally, the Sciton Contour uses 'optical multiplexing' to stack individual Er:YAG pulses of high fluence and short ablative (microsecond) pulse-widths with subablative pulses of low-fluence and long (5–10 ms) pulse-widths (coagulative) to effect zones of vaporization and user-selected depths of coagulation similar to the CO_2 laser. It uses a rotating mirror to alternate pulses from both the ablative and coagulative lasers. The control panel of the Contour allows the surgeon to select the depth of both ablation (1 J/cm^2 is equal to ~2–4 μm of ablation) and coagulation in microns.[33] The system also adjusts the displayed fluence based on the degree of selected overlap of spots within the computer pattern generator. For example, if one increases the overlap of spots from 10% to 30%, the fluence increases by 65%.[33] The computer pattern generator used with the Contour places the laser pulses in a random pattern within the geometric shaped used, rather than placing them in sequential rows within the pattern. This avoids excessive heat accumulation and limits thermal damage.

Zachary and Goldman have used the Contour laser in particular with results similar to CO_2 laser resurfacing. The Contour Er:YAG laser can be used in one of three ways: purely ablative, dual-mode ablative-coagulative, or pure coagulative. With settings of 50% spot overlap, 84 μm of ablation (21 J/cm^2) and 50–100 μm of coagulation, significant tissue contraction and hemostasis were achieved. However, the technique was noted to be more challenging as a result of the lack of visual cues to which one may be accustomed with the CO_2 laser. The color changes observed with increasing depth using a CO_2 laser are not observed with the modulated Er:YAG lasers. Specifically, the typical chamois color that results from ablation of the papillary dermis, or the 'water-logged cotton thread' appearance upon reaching reticular dermis with the CO_2 laser, is not seen with Er:YAG resurfacing. Unlike the CO_2 laser, Er:YAG does not have the typical plateau response with ablation after three passes. Although vaporization does diminish as tissue becomes desiccated, the absorption at 2940 nm by desiccated tissue is still significant and estimated to be ~{2/3} that of hydrated tissue (i.e. 2–2.5 μm per 1 J/cm^2 of fluence compared to 2–4 μm per 1 J/cm^2 for hydrated tissue).[33,35–37]

Clinical Application

Patient Selection

Several factors should be taken into account when considering a patient for cutaneous laser surgery. Fitzpatrick skin type, sebaceous gland density, amount of photodamage, and history of tendency toward hypertrophic scarring or postinflammatory hypo- or hyperpigmentation are all important aspects of patient selection. For cutaneous laser ablation, the ideal patient has type I–II skin because the risk for postinflammatory hyperpigmentation will be minimal. The risk increases proportionately with Fitzpatrick skin type, especially types II–IV. Both hyper- and hypopigmentation are risks for types V–VI skin.

Laser ablation can remove several epidermal lesions associated with aging such as seborrheic keratoses, actinic keratoses, Bowen's disease, actinic cheilitis, and solar lentigines. Other lesions that can be treated include melasma, molluscum contagiosum, syringomas, epidermal nevi, warts, xanthelasma, sebaceous hyperplasia, angiofibromas, trichoepitheliomas, and rhinophyma.[22,30]

Patient expectations are of paramount importance in patient selection and satisfaction. 'Before and after' photographs of other patients may be helpful in educating individuals about the degree of improvement one can expect. It must be emphasized that not all lesions will be eliminated and that one must balance the degree of improvement desired with the effects of the postoperative recovery period. Traditionally, the major decision as to which laser to use was based on the severity of the lesions to be treated. The traditional Er:YAG lasers allow for a much faster recovery time with less posttreatment erythema. However, this occurs at the expense of less clinical improvement. Although the traditional single-mode low-powered Er:YAG laser required several passes to ablate the epidermis and had limited capacity to vaporize beyond papillary dermis due to lack of hemostasis, the introduction of the dual-mode Er:YAG lasers has led to depths of ablation and coagulation comparable to traditional CO_2 lasers. The attendant risks of scarring and prolonged posttreatment erythema that accompany CO_2 resurfacing procedures also apply to these newer Er:YAG systems. Delayed onset permanent hypopigmentation is a significant risk with CO_2 laser ablation. There seems to be a much lower incidence of hypopigmentation following Er:YAG procedures (~5% of treated patients).[38,39] However, when comparing equal depths of combined ablation and coagulation, the rate of hypopigmentation may be very similar with either CO_2 or Er:YAG lasers. Asian skin is prone to post-inflammatory hyperpigmentation with both the CO_2 and dual-mode Er:YAG lasers. With the latter, however, the hyperpigmentation is very responsive to amelioration by hydroquinone containing agents.[38,40]

One must counsel patients on the amount of time required for reepithelialization, the extensive wound care regimens that need to be employed, and the risk for significant prolonged redness for months after treatment. The degree of erythema corresponds to the depth of ablation. Although the traditional purely ablative Er:YAG lasers result in faster reepithelialization and less postoperative erythema, this is due to the superficial depth of ablation. When modified 'hot' Er:YAG lasers are used that achieve depths of ablation equivalent to CO_2 lasers, the time to healing and resolution of erythema can be just as long. Those patients who are unable to accept prolonged healing or who are not psychologically prepared for the physical appearance of deeper ablation might be better suited to superficial Er:YAG ablation. In this case it is important to explain that the results will also not be as impressive as with deeper ablative procedures.

Contraindications to ablative laser procedures include isotretinoin use within the past 12 months (due to risk for hypertrophic scarring), and impaired wound healing from a collagen vascular disease or immune disorder.[22,41–47] Prior resurfacing procedures may predispose to more fibrotic collagen that could be more difficult to vaporize effectively.[41,42] Also, lack of skin appendages from scarring, fibrotic skin disease (e.g. scleroderma), or prior radiation may retard reepithelialization.[23,48] Patients who smoke should be instructed to decrease or stop this as much as possible so that optimal wound healing will not be impaired. Written consent explaining risks and benefits as well as pre- and postoperative photographs are essential.

Pretreatment Regimen

Hyperpigmentation following laser ablation occurs in the majority of patients with Fitzpatrick skin type IV or greater.[49] For this reason, minimal sun-exposure in the perioperative period is helpful. The optimal time of year for ablative laser procedures is late autumn and winter. Since hydroquinone targets melanin production in basal layer melanocytes, and the basal layer is routinely ablated with laser resurfacing, it should not be expected that pretreatment with this bleaching agent will diminish postresurfacing hyperpigmentation. Reepithelialization occurs primarily from the adnexal structures where hydoquinone does not likely penetrate.[50,51] In her series of 100 consecutive patients, Alster reported that no effect on hyperpigmentation was observed when pre-treatment with tretinoin and AHA was compared to placebo.[52]

A history of bacterial, herpetic, or fungal infections should be noted so that proper antimicrobial prophylaxis can be instituted. If the lesion(s) to be treated are in the perioral area, regardless of a history of HSV infection, the patient is given anti-viral agents prophylactically. We use valacyclovir 500 mg PO b.i.d. for 10 days starting on the morning of the procedure.

The thermally coagulated dermal tissue that begins to slough after treatment provides a growth medium for bacteria. Consequently, initiation of anti-staphylococcal coverage with cephalexin, dicloxacillin, or azithromycin is generally recommended when treating large numbers of lesions or large areas commencing one day before or on the morning of ablative laser surgery and lasting for ~1 week.[53]

Anesthesia

Anesthesia used for ablative laser resurfacing consists of local lidocaine with epinephrine (adrenaline) or nerve blocks if treating larger facial areas, lesions on fingers, hands, toes, feet and penis. Conscious sedation and general anesthesia may be considered for children or when large areas are to be treated such as many genital warts.

Local infiltration of lidocaine 1% with epinephrine is useful for treatment of the periorbital region, but injections to block the supraorbital, supratrochlear, infraorbital, and mental nerves are more useful for anesthesia of the central face. The cheeks may be anesthetized using tumescent lidocaine infusion due to ineffective numbing with nerve blocks alone and the requirement for large amounts of concentrated local anesthetic with direct infiltration.[54] We have used a mixture of equal parts 2% lidocaine with 1:100,000 epinephrine, 0.5% bupivacaine, 1:10 sodium bicarbonate 8.4%, and 75 U hyaluronidase. The bicarbonate serves to neutralize the pH, providing less discomfort on injection, and the hyaluronidase increases the tissue diffusion.[21]

Finally, conscious sedation with midazolam, propofol and fentanyl and even general anesthesia are sometimes required for larger cases to maximize patient comfort.

Specific Applications

The most basic categorization of the CO_2 laser in terms of clinical application is whether it is used as an ablative instrument or as a surgical scalpel to cut tissue. Spot size and power alone will determine which effect is seen. With a focused spot of 0.2 mm and a power output of 5 W, the irradiance is $5/(p \cdot (0.01\,cm)^2) = 16{,}000\,W/cm^2$. With irradiance of such magnitude, tissue cutting is the result. The width of the cut is determined by the spot size and the depth of the incision is determined by the irradiance. The laser can be defocused by moving the handpiece away from the skin surface thus increasing the spot size. With larger spots of 2–4 mm, tissue ablation rather than cutting is the result. Again, using 5 W as the example and a spot size of 2 mm, the irradiance becomes $160\,W/cm^2$. Since irradiance determines speed of vaporization, low power-densities (larger spot size) effect ablation while high irradiance (small spot size) results in cutting. Thus it is important to realize that for a given laser power, irradiance varies inversely with the square of the beam radius. To effect cutting at a larger spot size, the laser would need to generate extremely high powers instead of the typical 5–25 W.

Nonablative implementation of the CO_2 laser through the use of low fluences ($3.7–4.4\,J/cm^2$) has been used to treat thin epidermal and superficial dermal lesions. This mode of use is that of nonlaser-specific thermal injury with a sequence of effects characterized first by redness, then whitening, then vaporization or charring. The therapeutic range for this method is very narrow; low fluences are ineffective and high fluences can lead to scarring.[55,56] Like the case of the superpulse laser, a repetition rate of <5 Hz is recommended to avoid heat accumulation and excessive thermal damage.

Continuous wave CO_2 lasers can be used for both excisional and ablative applications. The excisional mode has been used for blepharoplasty,[57–61] rhinophyma reduction,[57,62–64] (and see pp. 167, 168) scalp reduction,[65] keloid excision,[62,66,67] and the creation of recipient sites for hair transplantation. The advantage of this technique is the excellent hemostasis and decreased postoperative pain and edema.[68] A study comparing CW CO_2 laser to cold-steel surgery in 13 patients undergoing blepharoplasty found that the CO_2-laser-treated sides of these patients had reduced intraoperative time and bleeding, and less post-operative ecchymosis and edema.[69] However, another study showed comparable results between cold steel and laser surgery with no advantage using the CO_2 laser.[70] A third study in 1992 in ten patients with upper and lower blepharoplasties again found superior results with the CO_2 laser due to speed of surgery and visibility of the operative field as well as less post-operative pain and faster healing.[71] The amount of thermal damage produced along the incisional edges must be weighed against the advantage of hemostasis. Excessive thermal damage will produce delayed wound healing, dehiscence, or possible hypertrophic scarring. Use of the UltraPulse laser for excisional or incisional surgery utilizing a focused beam and an incisional handpiece can provide char-free incisions that will not interfere with wound healing. This incises with a pulsed beam whose frequency and energy can be varied independently to achieve the ideal blend of cutting and coagulation. Even the 'continuous' wave mode of the UltraPulse produces a pulsed beam with a frequency of 1000–3000 Hz. The zone of thermal injury surrounding incisions made by the UltraPulse laser was observed in one study to be only about 115 μm.[72]

The most common method of use in dermatologic surgery for both CO_2 and Er:YAG lasers is that of ablation for various indications, including epidermal nevi, actinic keratoses, seborrheic keratoses, Bowen's disease, actinic cheilitis, rhinophyma, verrucae, sebaceous hyperplasia, solar elastosis, acne scarring, rhytides, xanthelasma, melasma, dyschromia, and various other benign tumors. The various lesions that can be effectively treated with ablative CO_2 and Er:YAG lasers are discussed below.

Ablation Technique

CO_2

Extensive prepping of the skin prior to laser treatment is unnecessary because the heat of the laser sterilizes the treated areas. The treated areas should be wrapped with wet towels to decrease the risk of fire. If treatment of the periorbital area is planned, non-reflective sterile metal eyeshields should be placed under the eyelid(s) after application of anesthetic eyedrops such as tetracaine. When using one of the superpulsed (e.g. Novapulse, Lumenis), Ultrapulse (Lumenis), or scanned (Silktouch) CO_2 lasers, tissue is vaporized using minimal overlap of laser pulses to prevent excess thermal damage. After each pass of the laser, the desiccated white debris must be wiped away with saline soaked gauze before the next pass because this debris acts as a heat sink and CO_2 laser energy delivered to this layer will result in excessive thermal injury and possible scarring. The wet gauze also serves to rehydrate the desiccated tissue. Dry gauze should be used to remove any remaining water and exudates prior to another pass because this surface water would absorb the energy and prevent further tissue ablation. Additional laser passes are used until the desired depth of vaporization is reached or until the treated lesion(s) are removed. One should not continue ablation once the distinctive yellowish color of the desiccated reticular dermis has been reached. Bleeding is not usually encountered with CO_2 laser ablation except when treating very thick lesions such as rhinophyma or vascular lesions such as warts.

As opposed to Er:YAG resurfacing, treatment with the CO_2 laser allows an indication of the depth of vaporization. This is due to color changes that reflect the degree of thermal injury. The relative lack of thermal injury with Er:YAG treatment accounts for the lack of color changes with depth.[35] After epidermal ablation, the white, desiccated, proteinaceous debris is wiped away to reveal a pink (vascularized) layer of papillary dermis. Deeper ablation into the papillary dermis reveals a characteristic 'chamois' color while further passes will disclose coarse collagen bundles akin to 'wet cotton threads' in appearance upon reaching the reticular dermis. The latter should be considered the endpoint, beyond which ablation is generally unsafe due to destruction of the adnexal structures from which reepithelialization occurs and consequent risk of scarring. The desired treatment endpoint is visible removal of the target lesion and a smooth, even surface.

Risks associated with CO_2 laser ablation range from milia, prolonged posttreatment erythema, exacerbation of acne, transient hyperpigmentation, delayed onset permanent hypopigmentation, infection, and contact dermatitis to hypertrophic scarring, ectropion, and systemic infection.

Lumenis UltraPulse

This laser uses radio frequency-excited gas-slab technology to achieve a peak output power of 500 watts and can generate fluences of 5–7 J/cm^2. It can be used with a 3-mm collimated handpiece or with a computer pattern generator (CPG) that precisely places 2.25-mm spots within a given geometric pattern. With the exception of treating small areas or edging, it is generally recommended that the CPG be used in most ablative applications due to the precise control obtained, speed, and ease of operation. To treat large areas, the following CPG settings should be used:

- Pattern 2 (parallelogram) or pattern 3 (square)
- Pattern size: 9 (largest)
- Density: 5
- Energy: 300 mJ/pulse
- Power: 60 W
- Repetition rate: 1–1.5 Hz.

One sequentially lays down the patterns immediately adjacent to one another without skip or overlap. Wet gauze should be used to gently debride the tissue coagulum as vigorous rubbing could create additional injury that may prolong postoperative erythema. Subsequent passes in areas requiring deeper ablation are performed in a similar manner.

Shoulders or edges of the target lesion can be treated individually using the 2.25-mm spot with the CPG off or by using the 3-mm collimated handpiece at 350–500 mJ. The coagulum should be wiped away with saline-soaked gauze as with other areas prior to another pass.

Sharplan SilkLaser

This laser can generate fluences of 5–15 J/cm^2. It has 'start safe' default settings that serve as a reasonable first step for most ablative indications. One must select either the SilkTouch or FeatherTouch mode, the handpiece, scan size and scan shape. The software adjusts the scan time for the selected parameters and suggests a proper power setting. The time interval between scans is selected by the surgeon to allow enough time to move the handpiece in position for the next scan. The scan time varies from 0.2 to 0.5 s, depending on the size of the scan.

The number of passes delivered determines the depth of ablation. In the SilkTouch mode, one pass approximates the depth of a Jessner's solution/35% trichloroacetic acid (TCA) chemical peel. Two to three passes approximate the depth of dermabrasion, and four or more passes provide results similar to those of a deep Baker's phenol peel. The FeatherTouch mode, as its trade name implies, provides gentler resurfacing. Two passes in this mode are required for equivalent ablation to one pass with the SilkTouch mode. Increases in power in the FeatherTouch mode increases depth of vaporization without a significant concomitant increase in thermal damage. One can increase the power to decrease the number of passes required to achieve a desired endpoint.

In a fashion similar to the fine-tuning of edges or shoulders of lesions with the single beam of the UltraPulse, it may be beneficial to decrease the scan size of the SilkLaser after one to three passes and individually sculpt the shoulders of these lesions. The edges of the field of treatment typically receive only one laser pass to allow for feathering. A further technique to achieve this end is to angle the handpiece away from perpendicular to spread the spiral scan farther apart at the edges of the field.

Traditional Er:YAG

As with CO_2 ablation, the area to be treated should be wrapped with wet towels. Eye protection with intraocular anti-reflective metal eyeshield(s) should be used if treating the eyelid(s).[22] Wiping between laser passes is unnecessary because proteinaceous debris is ablated with each subsequent pass.

The fluence required for ablation using the Er:YAG laser is ~1J for every 4µm of tissue vaporized. One adjusts the fluence to an appropriate setting for the amount of ablation desired. A fluence of $10 J/cm^2$ will reliably vaporize 40µm of tissue, thus ablating epidermis in about two passes. The endpoint is visible effacement of the lesion(s) or until reticular dermis has been reached. With the traditional Er:YAG, bleeding may prevent deeper ablation. However, rapid pulse stacking can allow deeper ablation by ablating the accumulating blood along with additional tissue. Bleeding may be controlled with pressure or with soaks of 1% lidocaine and epinephrine.[22] In this case, the surface must be dried prior to the next pass to prevent surface water absorption by the laser. Because of the relative lack of visual cues as to the depth of ablation, one must keep track of how many passes have been delivered once the papillary dermis has been reached.

Various spot sizes can be used. Repetition frequencies of 1–10Hz with spot sizes of 3–7mm are typical. One should use ~50% overlap of spots either freehand or with a computer pattern generator. When using a feathering technique to blend the perimeters of treated lesion, the hand piece may be pulled away from the skin surface to a distance greater than ~12cm to cause some divergence in the beam and thus a decrease in fluence.

Long Pulse Er:YAG

The Cynosure CO_3 utilizes a variable pulse Er:YAG laser (0.5–10ms) to effect ablation and coagulation. The long pulse duration may be below the tissue vaporization threshold resulting in thermal coagulation effects approaching those of short-pulsed CO_2 lasers.[36] The endpoint is similar to CO_2 lasers with vaporization of epidermis and papillary dermis to leave behind coagulated collagen indicated visually by a visible yellow color. The color change is more subtle with the Er:YAG laser, even given the long pulses delivered for coagulation. The amount of thermal damage is intermediate between that obtained using purely short pulsed Er:YAG lasers and resurfacing CO_2 lasers. Also, wiping between passes rehydrates the tissue and can eliminate the yellow color. The Cynosure CO_3 laser has been shown to result in less thermal necrosis than both the Sciton optically multiplexed Er:YAG laser and the CO_2 laser but with approximately equivalent clinical efficacy.[36]

Settings used with long-pulsed Er:YAG lasers are generally similar to the short pulsed Er:YAG laser. Ablation at a setting of $10 J/cm^2$ fluence will vaporize 40µm per pass. Freehand technique or use of a scanner may be performed. When performing freehand ablation, 50% overlap of spots and pulsing at 5Hz or more efficiently removes tissue equivalent to two passes without overlap. The longer coagulative pulses should be set for a length of time commensurate with the desired effect.

Wound Care

During the initial postoperative period following laser ablation, there is significant exudation and sloughing of thermally denatured collagen and patients experience a burning sensation for 24–48 hours due to the partial thickness wound created. This wound heals by reepithelialization from cutaneous adnexal structures (predominantly the pilosebaceous units) over 5–10 days (longer with an increased number of passes or areas off the face, faster if ablated with Er:YAG laser).[51,73–75] Edema in the first 48 hours can be controlled with ice-packs, head elevation at bed-time, and oral corticosteroids. Two wound-care regimens, the open technique and the closed technique, can be used based on the well-known fact that a moist wound environment promotes wound healing. This is likely due to the creation of a medium favorable to keratinocyte migration from the wound edges and from cutaneous appendages, and also due to retention of various cytokines and growth factors in the immediate vicinity of the reepithelializing wound.[51,73–80]

The Closed Technique

Semiocclusive biosynthetic dressings such as hydrocolloids (Duoderm), composite foams (Flexzan, Revitaderm), hydrogels (Vigilon or Second Skin), polyurethane films (Silon TSR, Tegaderm, Op-site), calcium alginate (Sorbsan), and polymer mesh (N-terface) increase the rate of wound reepithelialization and significantly diminish postprocedural discomfort. Duoderm is especially useful for wound care after treatment of warts on the hands and feet. They serve to provide a moist wound environment while also removing exudates from the wound to prevent crusting.[81,82] These dressings are left on for 3–5 days and obviate the need for patient compliance during that time period. Many physicians have begun to favor the closed technique over the open technique,[83] although the former is not without its complications. Wound maceration and increased rate of infection have been reported.[84] An alternative is to combine an open and closed technique. This entails use of a semi-occlusive dressing for 48–96 hours followed by an open technique. Pain management using this technique may require only acetaminophen.[85]

The Open Technique

Fewer physicians tend to use the open technique as a sole postoperative regimen because it tends to be more painful, pruritic and uncomfortable for the patient. In addition, it depends on patient compliance with soaks and emollient application. The required frequency of these applications is difficult for patients during the exudative phase of healing, especially while sleeping, and crust is more likely to form with this technique.[81] The regimen consists dilute acetic acid soaks several times per day (a capful of white vinegar in a pint of warm water makes an approximately

0.25% acetic acid solution) to remove exudate and debris followed immediately by application of moisturizing ointments such as Aquaphor Healing ointment, Theraplex, Crisco, or Catrix-10. When only a few small lesion(s) have been treated the wound care regimen can be simplified by washing the area with tap water twice per day followed by ointment application. Antibiotic ointments such as Bacitracin and Polysporin have a significant risk of causing contact dermatitis, and are therefore not recommended.[22,53,86–89]

Excessive application of ointment may result in milia, folliculitis, acne, and increased risk of bacterial and candidal infections[88] while too little results in crusting, bleeding, and delayed reepithelialization. Patients using this technique need to be seen daily to ensure proper wound healing and to provide education. Pain management using this technique may require narcotic analgesia.

Postoperative erythema ranges from 1 to 4 months depending on the laser used and the depth of ablation. A green-tinted make-up can camouflage the erythema to normalize the appearance of skin tone. Topical corticosteroids are generally not used unless patients experience significant pruritus not related to yeast infection. Avoidance of ultraviolet light exposure is imperative during the entire period of postlaser erythema to minimize the risk of hyperpigmentation.

Practical Application of Laser Energy and Laser Safety

Table 6.1 *Ablative Laser Indications*

Ablative lasers as the potential treatment of choice	Ablative lasers offer distinct advantages	Ablative lasers where no specific advantage exists
Actinic cheilitis	Veruccae	Superficial BCC
Epidermal nevi	Condyloma accuminata	Bowen's disease
Rhinophyma	Various benign dermal tumors (e.g. adenoma sebaceum, trichoepitheliomas, syringomas)	Squamous cell carcinoma
Eyeliner tattoos	Erythroplasia of Queyrat Actinic keratoses Seborrheic keratoses Red tattoo reactions Xanthelasma Burn debridement Neurofibromas Other superficial lesions (balanitis xerotica obliterans, lichen sclerosus, Zoon's balanitis, etc.)	Cherry angiomas Solar lentigines Granuloma faciale Angiokeratomas

CO_2 Laser as the Treatment of Choice

Actinic Cheilitis

The video that accompanies this chapter demonstrates variable pulse Er:YAG laser vermilionectomy for the treatment of actinic cheilitis.

Actinic cheilitis is the term employed for lesions arising from epidermal dyplasia on the lip. This entity is analogous to actinic keratoses which arise on other areas of the body. The lower lip is most commonly involved. Many treatment options exist for actinic cheilitis, but unfortunately, regardless of the treatment option selected, recurrence is common.[90] Typical treatments include cryosurgery[91,92,280,281] topical agents such as 5-fluorouracil[90,93] or imiquimod,[94–98] chemical peels,[99] photodynamic therapy,[100–104] electrosurgery,[105] surgical vermilonectomy,[91,106–109] and ablative laser resurfacing (Fig. 6.4). Surgical vermilionectomy and mucosal advancement likely has the lowest recurrence rate, but perioperative morbidity can be significant and an unnatural

A

B

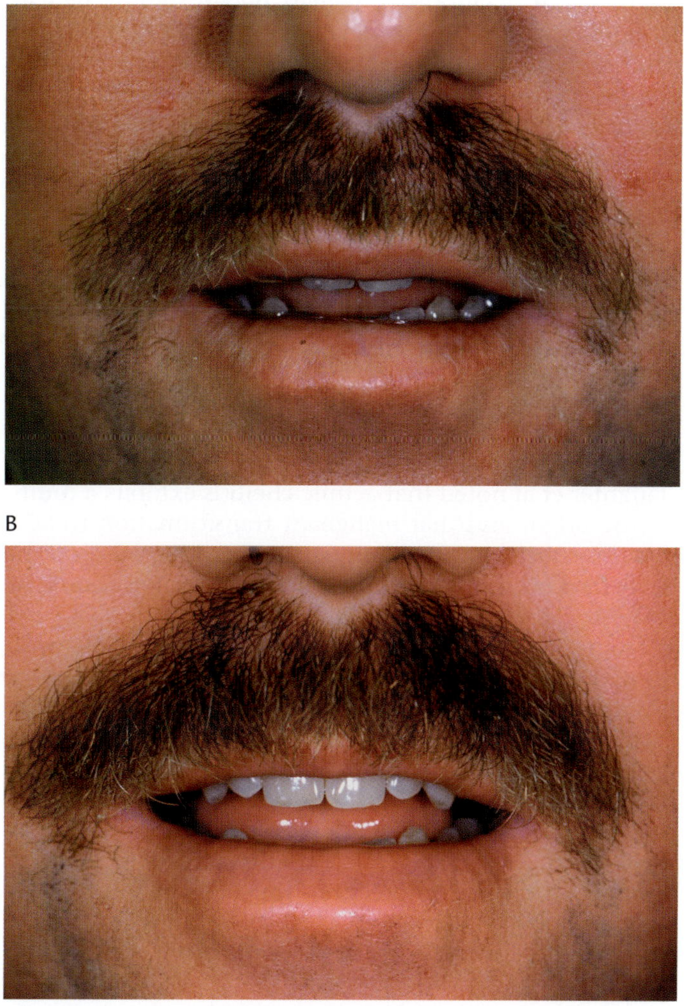

Figure 6.4 Lower lip actinic cheilitis (A) before and (B) 6 weeks after variable pulse Er:YAG laser (CO_3) vermilionectomy with complete reepithialization and normalization of mucosa.

appearance of the vermilion border can result.[90] In one study, 15.4% of patients exhibited labial scar tension, 25% experienced paresthesias, 71.7% had irritation from misaligned beard hairs, and 7.7% had visible scars.[108] For cryotherapy, unpredictable results have been reported.[110] Although 5-fluorouracil may be effective, patient compliance may be less than desirable due to the pain and discomfort associated with this treatment. The advantages of the CO_2 laser are a lower incidence of scarring, faster healing, and less pain compared to other modalities.

Actinic cheilitis is a premalignant condition that occurs more commonly on the lower lip and resembles chapping. The latter is a transient condition that resolves with constant moisturization. Actinic cheilitis, like actinic keratoses, does not resolve without specific treatment and carries the risk of evolving into squamous cell carcinoma (SCC). The appearance of this malignant change may initially be indistinguishable from that of actinic cheilitis. Clinically these lesions appear as red and white, atrophic, scaly, flat-topped papules or plaques with crusting and/or fissures (see Fig. 6.4A). The vermilion border may be ill-defined. In one study three out of six biopsies with a diagnosis of actinic cheilitis also showed histologic evidence of SCC.[111] Another study showed that five out of ten patients with clinical diagnoses of benign hyperkeratosis had lip biopsies consistent with well-differentiated SCC. Thirteen patients with clinical diagnosis of actinic cheilitis had biopsies performed that were serially sectioned at 1-mm intervals. Forty-two regions of dysplasia and 12 regions of SCC were identified.[112]

SCC may follow actinic cheilitis after a long latent period (20–30 years), although this interval is variable. Once there is clinical and histologic evidence of actinic cheilitis, a patient is at significant risk for development of a second lesion or SCC of the lip. This has been estimated to occur in 5–14% of patients.[113–115] Because SCC of the lower lip metastasizes in ~11% of patients, it is imperative to recognize and treat premalignant dysplasia. Multifocal lesions of actinic cheilitis suggest a field effect of actinic damage and carcinogenesis for the lower lip. Indeed, Slaughter et al noted that actinic cheilitis exhibits a multicentric origin and that malignant transformation to SCC may be subclinical and unpredictable.[116] Because of the field effect on the lower lip, the entire vermilion should be ablated.

From 1985 to 1992, the results of treatment with the CO_2 laser for actinic cheilitis have been reported for 123 patients. In follow-up periods ranging from 11 to 36 months only two patients experienced focal recurrences.[110,117–120]

Either the CO_2 laser or the variable pulsed Er:YAG laser can be utilized for lip epidermis vaporization.[121,122] Note that short pulsed Er:YAG lasers do not provide hemostasis and are therefore impractical for use on the highly vascular lip.

Technique for treating actinic cheilitis:

1. Patient receives prophylactic antiviral medication.
2. Local anesthetic is infiltrated into the lip commissures after achieving mental nerve block anesthesia of the rest of the lower lip or infraorbital nerve block for the upper lip. Infiltration of the vermilion region with local anesthetic or normal saline flattens the surface and hydrates the submucosa, which allows for more precise ablation of the epidermis and mucosa while preserving the underlying submucosa.
3. A single pass with the CW CO_2 laser using a 2- to 3-mm spot size and moving the handpiece at a rate of 1 cm/s will suffice to remove the epidermis. One will notice whitening, bubbling, and vesiculation of the epidermis. This should be wiped with saline-soaked gauze.
4. Two tissue morphologies should be evident after this first pass. Most of the ablated tissue should appear pink and pliable. A few areas will exhibit a fibrotic, gray spotty, or yellowish appearance and may represent deeper actinic damage.[110,118,123] These areas should be ablated with another pass with a desired end-point of a 'cotton-white' appearance. A more recent study suggests that these areas do not represent deeper actinic damage and states that ablation to the level of the papillary dermis is adequate.
5. Multiple passes (two or three) are needed with the variable pulsed Er:YAG or resurfacing CO_2 lasers.

Wound care consists of the repeated application of ointment. An initial bandage on the lip can be placed for the patient's trip home and first postoperative day. Prolonged use of bandages on the mucosal lip is impractical. Healing time ranges from 3 to 8 weeks. One study that closely monitored time to healing found that 98.5% of patients had reepithelialization by 4 weeks.[120] Complete healing takes roughly 2 weeks with the variable pulse Er:YAG laser. Healing has been reported to occur in 2.5 weeks with only 6% incidence of scarring when using a superpulsed CO_2 laser with a secondary 50 ms shuttered pulse.[124] When the Ultrapulse laser was used, average time to reepithelialization was 13 days with zero scarring.

One must take care not to create excessive thermal damage at the vermilion border as this can lead to scarring. Minimization of scarring also depends upon proper wound care, lack of infection, and superficial ablation. It should be kept in mind that actinic cheilitis is purely an epidermal process, and as such, vaporization need not extend beyond the papillary dermis.[120]

Eyeliner Tattoo

Although Q-switched lasers are used for most tattoo removal applications, CO_2 or Er:YAG ablation of eyeliner tattoos is still an effective and pragmatic treatment. The goal of tattoo removal in this location is avoidance of scarring or damage to eyelash follicles. Therefore excision is not the best option. With Q-switched lasers, multiple procedures are required. Because ablation may be accomplished precisely and effectively with the resurfacing lasers, the tattoo can be easily vaporized without eyelid or eyelash follicle damage.[125]

Rhinophyma

Rhinophyma is characterized by sebaceous gland hyperplasia, with the sebaceous ducts dilated and filled with

A

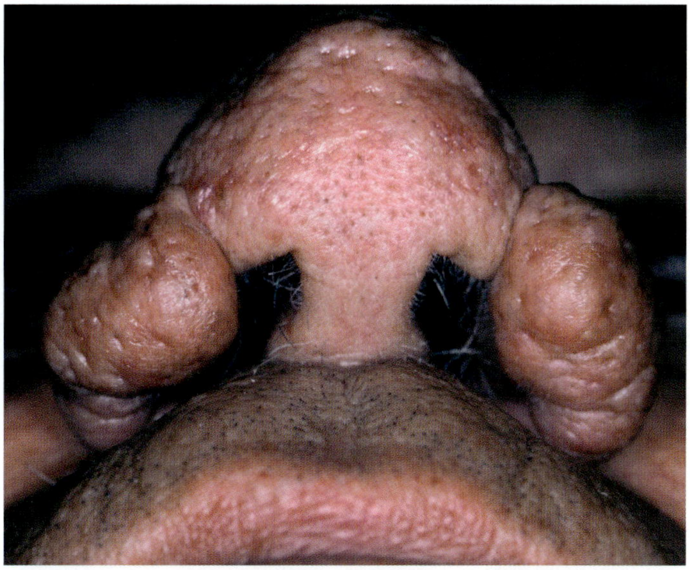

B

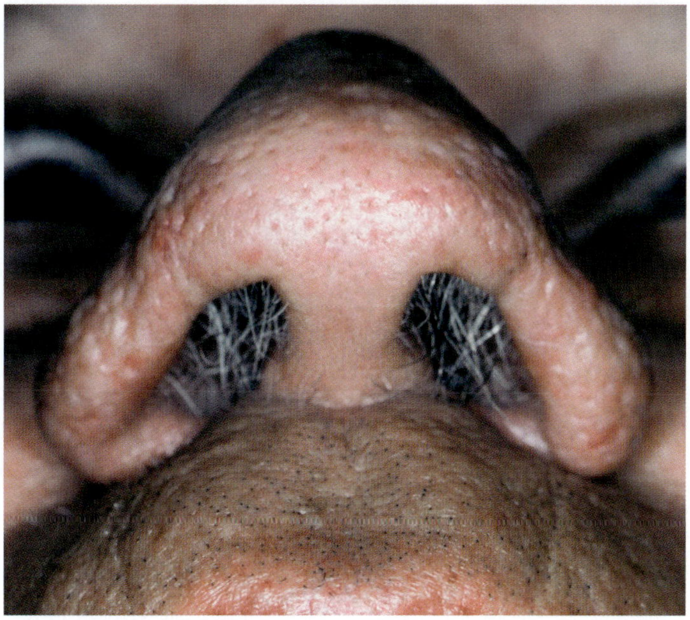

Figure 6.5 Rhinophyma (A) before scanned CO_2 laser (SilkTouch) vaporization and sculpting. (B) Nine months after vaporization with improved nasal ala contour and nostril patency.

sebum and keratinous debris. Variable amounts of dermal fibroplasia and connective tissue increase may also occur. The goal of surgical management of rhinophyma is to debulk the hypertrophied tissue and leave an adequate glandular reserve to allow scarless reepithelization. Many patients request treatment, not for cosmetic considerations, but to improve air movement (Fig. 6.5). After healing there is often greater nostril patency due to both fibrosis that stiffens the nasal alae as well as reduction of bulk that tends to push in on the nose opening.

Many techniques have been used to treat rhinophyma, including dermabrasion,[126–131] cold steel surgical sculpting,[130–134] cryosurgery,[135–139] electrosurgery[127,128,136,137,140–142] CO_2 laser ablation,[140–152] and Er:YAG laser ablation.[153,154] Dermabrasion may result in incomplete ablation of rhinophymatous tissue due to technical difficulties. Cryosurgery often results in uneven ablation because it is difficult to achieve a uniform depth of freezing. Scarring and hypopigmentation often occur. Electrosurgical sculpting allows easy tissue removal but heat conduction to deeper tissues may result in scarring. Lack of hemostasis with cold-steel surgery for rhinophyma makes this a suboptimal treatment modality.

CO_2 continuous wave laser ablation allows for precision in nasal shaping. Hemostasis during the procedure allows visualization of the treated areas and greater control over contouring.[155] The use of prerhinophymatous photographs helps to prevent oversculpting. Care must be taken, especially at the ala, not to overtreat, which can lead to scarring and nasal flaring. Consideration of the residual 1–2 mm of thermally denatured tissue with the CW CO_2 laser should be taken into account. There is a definite risk of scarring when ablating to a deep plane.[144] One must be aware of the extent of ablation by recognizing sebaceous gland structures as deeper layers of tissue are removed. During vaporization, the dermis contracts and sebum is visibly expressed from the sebaceous glands, indicating that scarring is unlikely at this depth. Reepithelialization occurs by approximately 3–4 weeks with CW CO_2 lasers (Fig. 6.6).

A resurfacing CO_2 laser or variable pulsed Er:YAG laser can be used to treat mild to moderate rhinophyma. Reepithelialization is complete in approximately 2–3 weeks. The risk of scarring with resurfacing lasers is very low.[121] Some hypopigmentation is often seen and a reduced number of more prominent pores can also occur. Frank scarring is seen more often when using CW lasers.

Technique:

1. Outline the entire nose with additional markings of the rhinophymatous tissue.
2. Perform a nasal 'ring' block by infiltrating local anesthetic along the nose cheek junction to anesthetize the infratrochlear, supratrochlear and infraorbital nerve branches. Infiltrate local anesthetic at the base of the collumella and finally inject anesthetic at the nasal bone and cartilage junction to the left and right of midline to anesthetize the anterior ethmoidal nerves. This should provide complete nasal skin anesthesia and obviate the need for extensive painful injections into the often stiff rhinophymatous tissue.
3. Wrap the nose with wet towels and cover the patient's eyes with wet eye patches.
4. Ablate the rhinophymatous tissue until the nose shape approximates that of its prerhinophymatous state (compare with the 'before' photographs). With resurfacing lasers, maximal energy fluences and pulse rates, along with pulse stacking, will be needed to achieve sufficient ablation. Although it has been advocated that, for severe rhinophyma, it may be advantageous to first use the CW CO_2 laser with a small spot size to excise and debulk large phymatous areas followed by the use of a larger spot size for vaporization and fine contour-

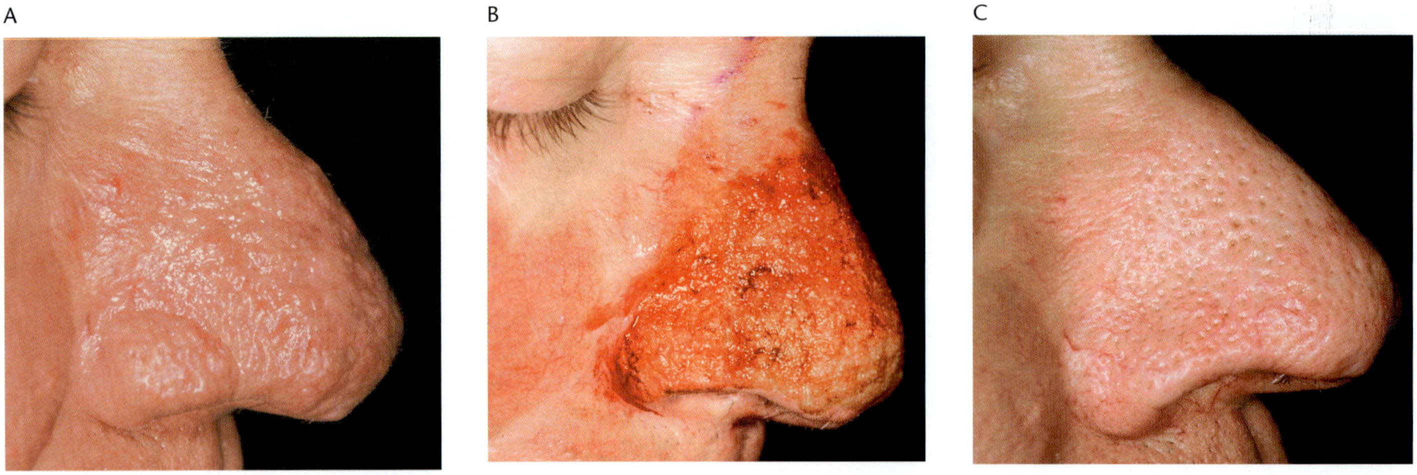

Figure 6.6 Rhinophyma (A) before, (B) immediately after and (C) 8 months after scanned CO_2 laser (SilkTouch) vaporization and sculpting.

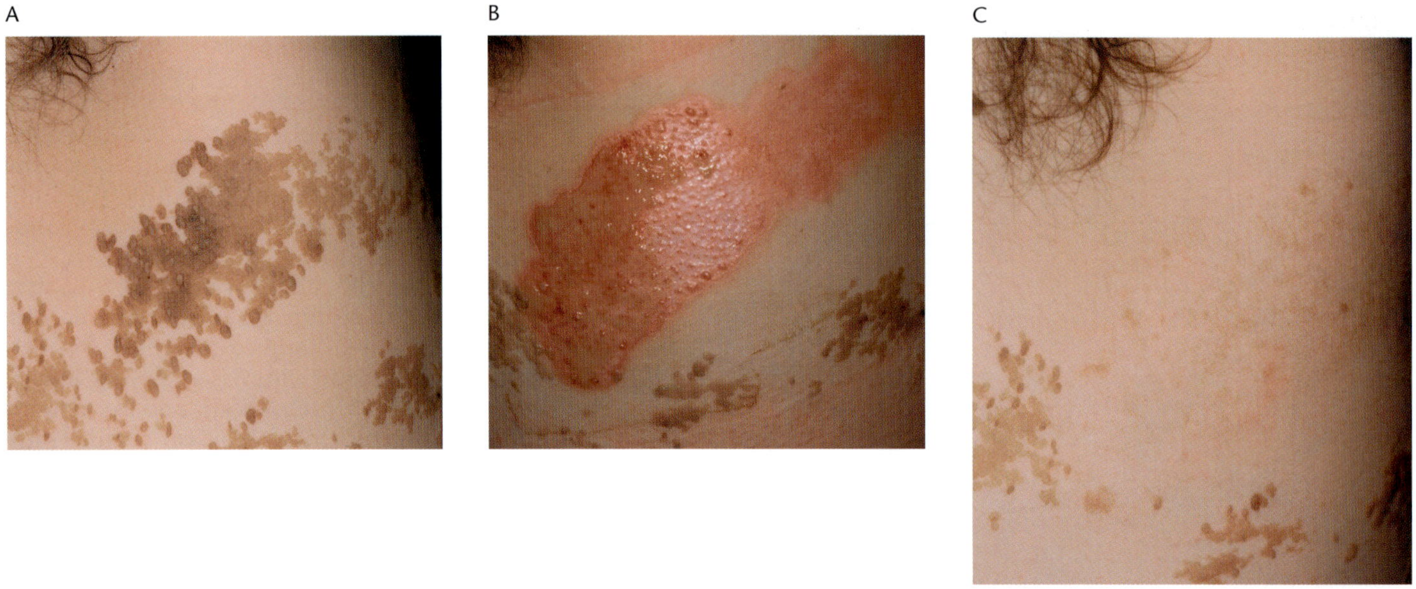

Figure 6.7 Widespread systematized epidermal nevus (A) before, (B) 1 week after and (C) 2 years after partial treatment with a scanned CO_2 laser (SilkTouch) showing effacement of the treated portion without recurrence, but, as anticipated, with residual hypopigmentation.

ing,[142,146,149,151,152,156] we rarely cut away rhinophyma nodules with the laser in the focused mode as we have found that areas so treated heal with scarring. Ablation should stop while still in the sebaceous tissue plane. Once large vessels have been encountered or there is no more sebaceous tissue noted ablation has proceeded too deeply and those areas will be at increased risk for scarring. It is better to err on the side of under-treatment rather than overtreatment. Consider the anticipated postlaser treatment coagulated tissue slough and tissue contraction due to posttreatment fibrosis. Special care should be taken at the nasal ala groove where too deep an ablation can result in unattractive nasal flaring.

5. Feather the treatment area by ablating into the papillary dermis the rest of the nose.
6. Hemostasis is achieved with lidocaine with epinephrine soaked gauze. Larger vessels that cannot be coagulated with the laser are sealed with spot electrocoagulation.
7. Acetic acid soaks several times per day are followed with Aquaphor Healing Ointment application.

Epidermal Nevi

Epidermal nevi are developmental abnormalities resulting in excess keratinocytes. Lesions usually manifest early in life and have a predilection for the neck, trunk and extremities.[157] While tumors, such as basal cell carcinoma and squamous cell carcinoma have been reported to arise within these lesions, this is a rare occurrence and removal is primarily of a cosmetic nature. Excision is usually not an option due to the large size of many epidermal nevi. Laser ablation with CO_2[155,158] or Er:YAG lasers[159] can successfully remove these lesions (Fig. 6.7). Care must be taken to balance efficacy versus scarring. Epidermal ablation only will allow for recurrence of the abnormal keratinization. Excessive ablation will lead to scarring. The ideal depth of ablation is to the papillary dermis below the inferior tips

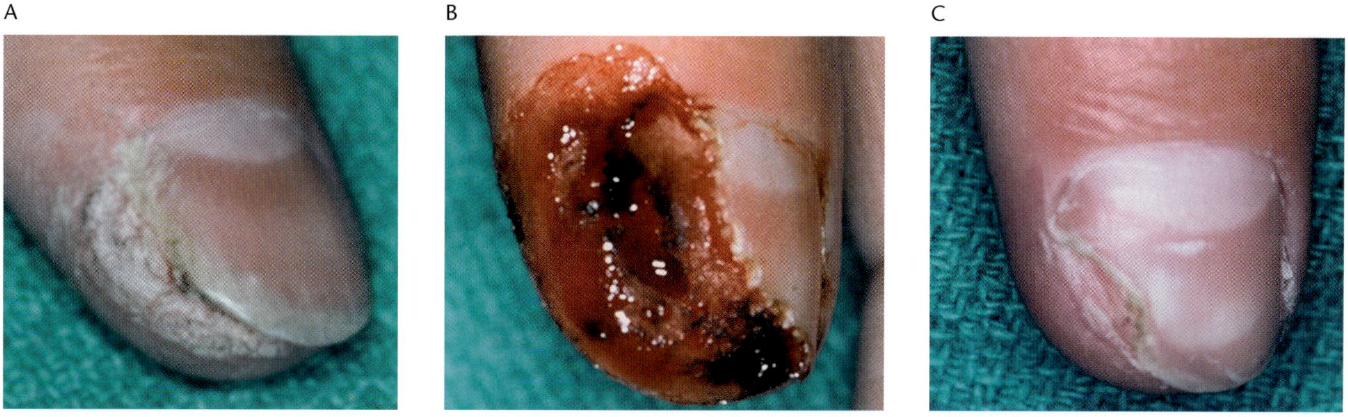

Figure 6.8 Subungual and periungual left index finger recalcitrant verruca vulgaris (A) before, (B) immediately after and (C) 2 months after traditional carbon dioxide laser vaporization including vaporization of the lateral nail plate. The normal nail is growing back proximally.

of the rete ridges. The patient can expect hypopigmentation from the procedure and occasional scarring or recurrence.[121,160,161] The Er:YAG laser was used to treat 20 patients with epidermal nevi in one study. After a single laser treatment, successful elimination of the verrucous epidermal nevi was observed in 15 of 20 patients. Five patients (25%) showed a relapse within 1 year after the treatment.[159]

The CO_2 laser may be combined with pigment targeting lasers to decrease the risk of scarring. The CO_2 laser is used to first ablate the clinically visible epidermal nevus followed by treatment with the frequency doubled Q-switched Nd:YAG laser at 3.5–4.0 J/cm^2.

Lesions For Which Ablative Lasers Offer Distinct Advantages

Verrucae

Development of human papilloma virus induced verrucae is a common cutaneous disease process. The use of continuous wave or pulsed lasers has been shown to have efficacy in the 56–81% range.[121,162,163] Studying the effects of any treatment for verrucae is extremely difficult. Given the high spontaneous resolution range of verrucae, a large number of patients is needed to demonstrate a statistically meaningful benefit. In general, we reserve ablative laser techniques for warts that have been refractory to less invasive and less costly measures.

In our experience, patients are referred for laser surgery after other measures have failed. Unfortunately, recurrent or refractory lesions respond less well to laser treatment than do primary lesions. Lim and Goh found that 80% of primary warts responded to laser therapy, whereas only 48% of refractory lesions responded.[164] Warts that are particularly difficult to eradicate include those occurring in a periungual location (Fig. 6.8). Cure rates using CO_2 laser ablation range from 32% to 71%.[165,166] Scarring[167] and dystrophic nail changes[165] have resulted due to the need for aggressive therapy with the CO_2 laser. The Er:YAG laser has been used successfully and has a better safety profile.[168,169] Of note, viral particles may be present up to 1 cm away from the clinically apparent wart, so laser therapy probably does not remove all virions.[170] Most likely, the laser, like other destructive techniques, reduces the viral load and allows for innate immunity to control the remainder. As most recurrences develop at the peripheral margin of a treated wart, laser ablation should incorporate a zone of 3–5 mm of clinically normal appearing tissue around the verruca. Because immunocompromised patients have very resistant warts, laser therapy should only be used to debulk painful verrucae or those that interfere with normal function. The patient should be informed that an immunocompromised state portends the development of recurrent and new warts.

When treating virally mediated diseases with ablation, special safety considerations are warranted. Viable viral particles have been demonstrated in the smoke plume generated from the treatment of verrucae.[171,172] Plantar warts (HPV type 1) are the richest in viral particles.[173–176] Because HPV 6 and 11 cause both respiratory papillomatosis and genital warts, a major risk of inhalational HPV infection exists when treating condyloma accuminata. Although viral transmission to the laser surgeon has not been convincingly demonstrated, personal safety precautions are recommended.[177] Intact and viable HIV particles have been identified in CO_2 laser plumes when HIV-infected tissue was treated.[121] No transmission of HIV through laser plumes has been reported to date.

Because of these factors, high efficacy smoke evacuators have to be employed and the evacuation tube opening should be within 1 cm of the laser plume. All personnel should don high-filtration laser masks with a particle filtration threshold of 0.1 micrometer.

Technique for treating verrucae:

1. Anesthetize the intended treatment area.
2. Manually remove thickened hyperkeratotic debris. This tissue has low water content and tends to act as a heat

sink with laser impact, creating excessive thermal diffusion and tissue injury.

3. Select laser and parameters: Continuous wave CO_2 lasers generally result in greater tissue damage and increased risk of scarring compared to pulsed CO_2 or Er:YAG lasers.
4. Sweep the laser over the verrucae 1–3 times. A cleavage plan at the dermoepidermal junction will be created allowing the keratotic epidermis to be curetted away. Vaporize any apparent wart tissue remaining. Lightly coagulate the papillary dermis to seal blood vessels. Visualization with magnification is helpful to observe tissue response upon laser impact. Wart tissue bubbles upon treatment whereas normal epidermis exhibits dermatoglyphs that appear to contract with laser contact. For periungual warts, vaporization of the nail plate to gain access to subungual extension of verrucae is not only helpful, but it eliminates the need for nail plate avulsion (Fig. 6.8B).
5. Apply a biocclusive dressing such as Duoderm. As a large amount of exudate may form early in the wound healing process, daily dressing changes are required. Once the exudative phase diminishes, less frequent dressing changes can be done.

Condyloma Accuminatum

Human papilloma virus is also responsible for anogenital warts. The physician who treats anogenital warts should be aware of the psychosocial aspects of this disease. Sexual partners require screening and treatment. We refer all female patients and female partners of male patients to their gynecologist for cervical examination. As with verrucae, HPV can be isolated as far as 1.5 cm away from clinically apparent lesions.[170] It is unlikely that the laser alone will eradicate the virus.[178]

Patients with perianal lesions may benefit from anoscopic examination to evaluate for the presence of internal lesions. Additionally, after ablation of the clinically apparent lesions, adjuvant therapy to eradicate residual virus should be considered. Interferon-α has been shown to improve clearance when used after laser. Studies utilizing adjuvant interferon were performed prior to the introduction of imiquimod for the treatment of genital warts. While not specifically studied for adjuvant treatment after laser ablation of external condyloma, the use of imiquimod is rational, and much simpler than intralesional interferon. Imiquimod is a topically applied immune modulation agent that induces the local production of cytokines, including interferon. One small study of anal canal condyloma suggested that adjuvant imiquimod decreases recurrence after ablative therapy.[179]

Technique for treating condyloma:

1. Consider acetowhitening with 5% acetic acid to help delineate clinically subtle lesions.
2. Anesthetize the intended treatment area.
3. Insert moistened cotton gauze into the anal sphincter.
4. Using a pulsed laser, treat each lesion and a 3–5-mm margin of normal appearing skin.
5. Wound care: reepitheliazation takes 3–4 weeks.
   a. Sitz baths with saltwater solution should be performed three or four times daily
   b. use a hair dryer instead of wiping
   c. consider the use of stool softeners
   d. refrain from sexual intercourse, douching or the application of topical creams.

Evidence suggests that the risk of viral transmission during laser ablation of condyloma is greater than of verrucae. Of particular concern is the development of mucosal or respiratory tract papilloma. Special attention to mask usage and laser plume evacuation is warranted.[171,180]

Actinic Keratoses

Similar to actinic cheilitis, there are many treatment modalities available for actinic keratoses (AKs). The options listed for actinic cheilitis are also viable choices for AKs. Laser ablation with either a pulsed CO_2 or Er:YAG laser[181] can be employed. Note that CW CO_2 laser treatment of AKs can leave hypopigmentation and scarring.

Laser ablation of AKs is generally performed in a regional manner (Fig. 6.9). An entire anatomic unit or subunit is typically treated, rather than focusing on individual lesions. Ablation to the papillary dermis is essential. Treatment may be combined with trichloroacetic acid to peel surrounding fields of actinic keratoses. When lesions develop in previously treated areas, the surgeon should be suspicious that they represent squamous cell carcinomas that were not completely vaporized. However, AKs can develop from actinically damaged follicles. It may be prudent to biopsy larger or thicker lesions prior to laser ablation to rule out squamous cell carcinoma. Reepithelization takes place over 10–14 days. A bio-occlusive dressing speeds healing.

Seborrheic Keratoses

Seborrheic keratoses are benign hyperplastic neoplasms of the epidermis. Current treatment modalities are primarily destructive in nature. Ablative laser treatment can effectively vaporize these lesions with little risk of scarring or pigmentary alteration. It is debatable if the laser offers benefit over less costly alternatives such as liquid nitrogen cryotherapy. The clinician who endeavors to destroy these

A

B

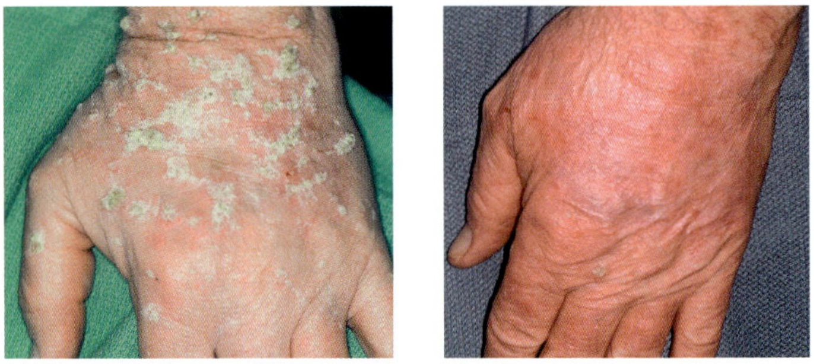

Figure 6.9 Extensive left dorsal hand hypertrophic actinic keratoses (A) before and (B) 5 years after continuous wave CO_2 laser vaporization of the entire dorsal hand area.

lesions (and thus foregoes histologic analysis of the lesion) should be cognizant of the fact that a number of malignancies, including squamous cell carcinoma, basal cell carcinoma and melanoma have been reported to arise within and associated with seborrheic keratoses.[182]

Miscellaneous Conditions

Various lesions in difficult surgical locations may be addressed advantageously using ablative lasers. A number of inflammatory conditions have been reported to respond to ablation with the CO_2 laser. Note that experience with treating these conditions is limited to small numbers and large scale clinical trial data are not available. For this reason, lasers should not be considered the primary treatment. Some of these conditions include: balanitis xerotica obliterans,[183] Zoon's balanitis, kraurosis vulvae, lichen sclerosis et atrophicus, porokeratosis,[184] keratoderma, chondrodermatitis nodularis helices,[185] granuloma faciale,[186] genital lichen planus,[187] oral florid papillomatosis,[188] psoriasis, [189] and Hailey–Hailey disease.[177,190] Because some of these lesions occur primarily on the genitalia, eyelids, or in intertriginous areas, they are particularly well-suited for treatment with ablative lasers due to surgical challenges associated with these anatomic locations. Psoriasis is the exception in that surgical treatment is not usually used for this condition. However, ablation of chronic psoriatic plaques with CO_2 laser treatment has been reported to achieve long-term results.[191] CO_2 lasers can be employed to treat a number of dermal growths. Adenoma sebaceum of tuberous sclerosis,[192] trichoepitheliomas,[193,194] syringomas,[195] hidrocystomas,[196] neurofibromas,[197] myxoid cysts,[198] tricholemmomas of Cowden's disease,[199] sebaceous hyperplasia,[200] syringocystadenoma papilliferum,[201] and xanthelasma[202] have all been treated with laser ablation.

The Er:YAG laser has been used to effect nail ablation,[203,204] in the generation of recipient holes for hair transplantation in cicatricial alopecia,[205] and in the treatment of post-burn scars.[206] It has also been used to treat Zoon's balanitis,[207] xanthelasma,[208] syringomas,[209] multiple eruptive hair cysts,[210] colloid milium (Fig. 6.10),[211] milia, hidradenomas, acrochordons, melasma and solar lentigines.[212]

Of these conditions, the benign dermal growths have been treated with other surgical methods such as excision and repair, shave excision, dermabrasion, cryosurgery, electrosurgery, KTP and Nd:YAG laser treatment, and with various acids and tretinoin. There are one or more disadvantages with these techniques, including scarring or surface texture change, difficult or awkward surgical technique, lesion recurrence, or incomplete lesion removal.

We favor resurfacing lasers over continuous wave lasers for these applications. This is especially true when multiple lesions are present. In such cases entire cosmetic subunits should be deepithelialized with a large spot size before addressing the dermal tumors. For individual lesions, the growth is vaporized by using relatively low-power settings in the 3- to 5-W range with a spot size that matches the size of the lesion. Depending upon the depth of the lesion being treated, the entire lesion may not be destroyed. Ablation should be carried out to the level of the dermis, but since residual thermal damage will extend 0.5 to 1 mm beyond the level of ablation, one should not try to remove the entire lesion if there is deep extension. A useful endpoint is a smooth cutaneous contour. Patients

A

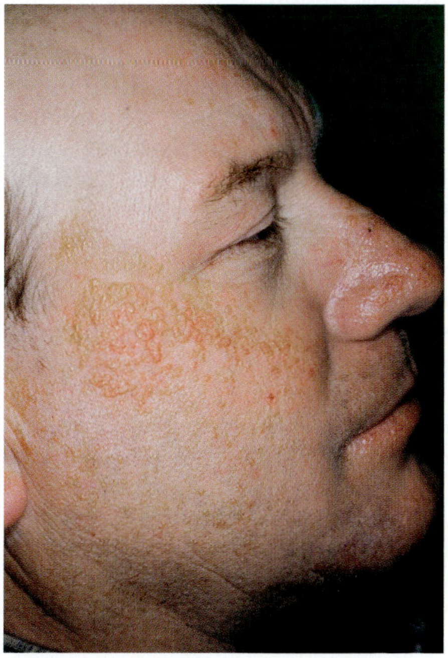

B

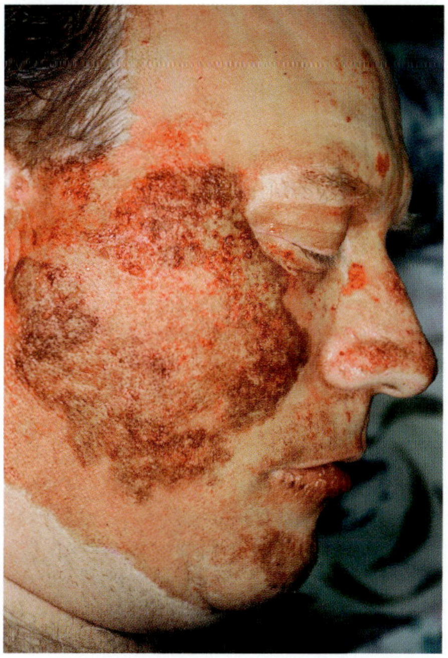

C

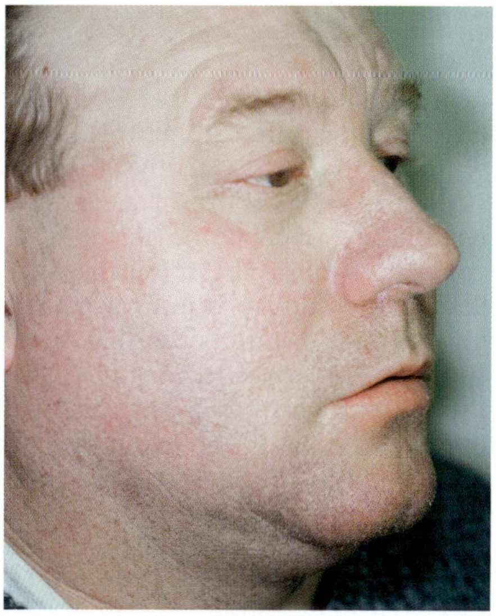

Figure 6.10 Extensive colloid millium (A) before, (B) immediately after and (C) 4 months after variable pulse Er:YAG laser (CO_3) aggressive full-face ablation with residual erythema.

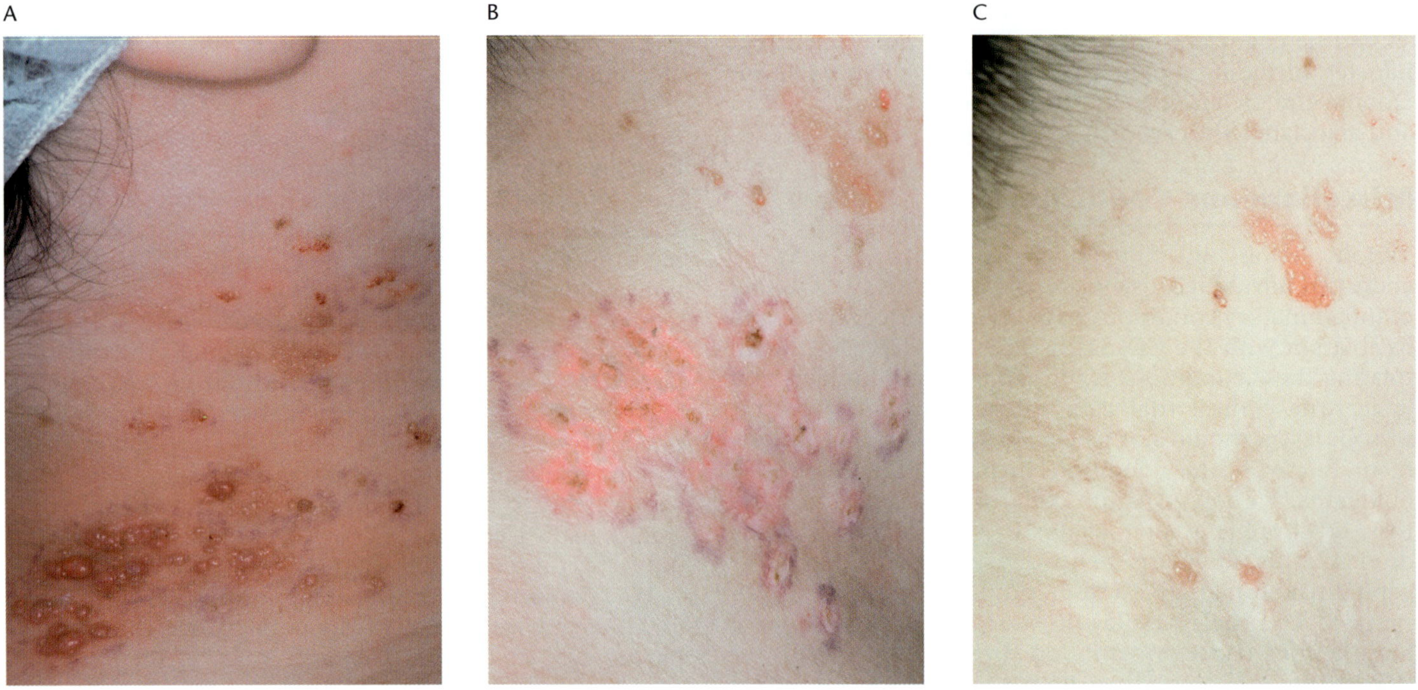

Figure 6.11 Right neck lymphangioma circumscriptum (A) before, (B) immediately after and (C) 7 months after continuous wave CO_2 laser vaporization with 90% lesion effacement in the treated area along with the expected residual hypopigmentation and textural alteration.

should be cautioned that some lesions may recur with time and new lesions may develop in the treated areas. Re-epithelialization is complete in approximately 2 weeks. While residual hypopigmentation may occur, scarring is rare.

Laser tattoo removal has primarily fallen within the domain of Q-switched lasers. However, in selected circumstances, CO_2 or Er:YAG laser ablation can be considered. In patients with allergic reactions to tattoo ink, the use of a Q-switched laser can lead to systemic reactions.[213] In these cases, ablation of the tattoo can be considered. Additionally, patients who desire tattoo removal without the multiple treatment sessions required with Q-switched lasers may benefit from laser ablation, which can usually achieve tattoo removal in a single treatment session. To diminish scarring, the entire depth of the tattoo is not ablated. Approximately 30–50% of the ink is removed via laser. The remainder of the tattoo ink is leached out through the application of 40 to 50% urea paste for 10 to 14 days.[214] Some patients may require a second 'touch-up' treatment to remove any residual visible tattoo ink 6 months after the initial ablative treatment. Another option is to ablate the epidermis overlying the tattoo to gain better access to the pigment for Q-switched laser therapy in the same treatment session. Epidermal ablation results in less beam scattering for the Q-switched laser. This technique may reduce the number of treatment sessions with a Q-switched laser by 50% without significantly increasing the risk of scarring. We have found the short-pulse Er:YAG laser to be particularly useful for tattoo ablation as there is no need for thermal tissue coagulation. The ultimate cosmetic outcome is superior if the entire region of the tattoo is ablated, rather than simply tracing the outline of the tattoo. The latter approach can lead to a ghost of the tattoo remaining. Ultimately, the treated area resembles a superficial burn scar.

For tattoos that have been treated with Q-switched lasers, certain pigments (skin-colored, white, brown, some red pigments) that contain iron or titanium oxides undergo a reduction reaction that converts the treated pigment into a black color. Additional Q-switched laser therapy is not an option for this black pigment, but it can be efficiently ablated with a resurfacing laser.

Lymphangioma circumscriptum can be approached with the CO_2 laser (Fig. 6.11). In many cases, the patient's chief concern is the drainage of lymphatic fluid from the lesions. The CO_2 laser can be employed to ablate the superficial lesions into the middermis (Fig. 6.11B). Reepithelialization occurs after a highly exudative phase with excessive lymphatic drainage lasting a couple of weeks. This is followed by a layer of fibrosis that can prevent drainage from the area. If the proliferation is superficial, laser ablation may result in permanent resolution. However, these lesions often have deeper components, and complete ablation may not be possible without excessive scarring. In these cases, recurrences are frequently seen after several years.

Postsurgical wounds that are allowed to heal by second intention can be improved by immediate postoperative laser resurfacing, which involves sculpting the wound edges and feathering the ablation across the cosmetic subunit (Fig. 6.12). It is primarily useful for nasal defects in which a full-thickness skin graft or second intention healing are contemplated. In a study of post-Mohs micrographic surgery defects of the nose, the edge of the wound was contoured with a resurfacing laser. The sites, once healed, had excellent cosmetic results.[215]

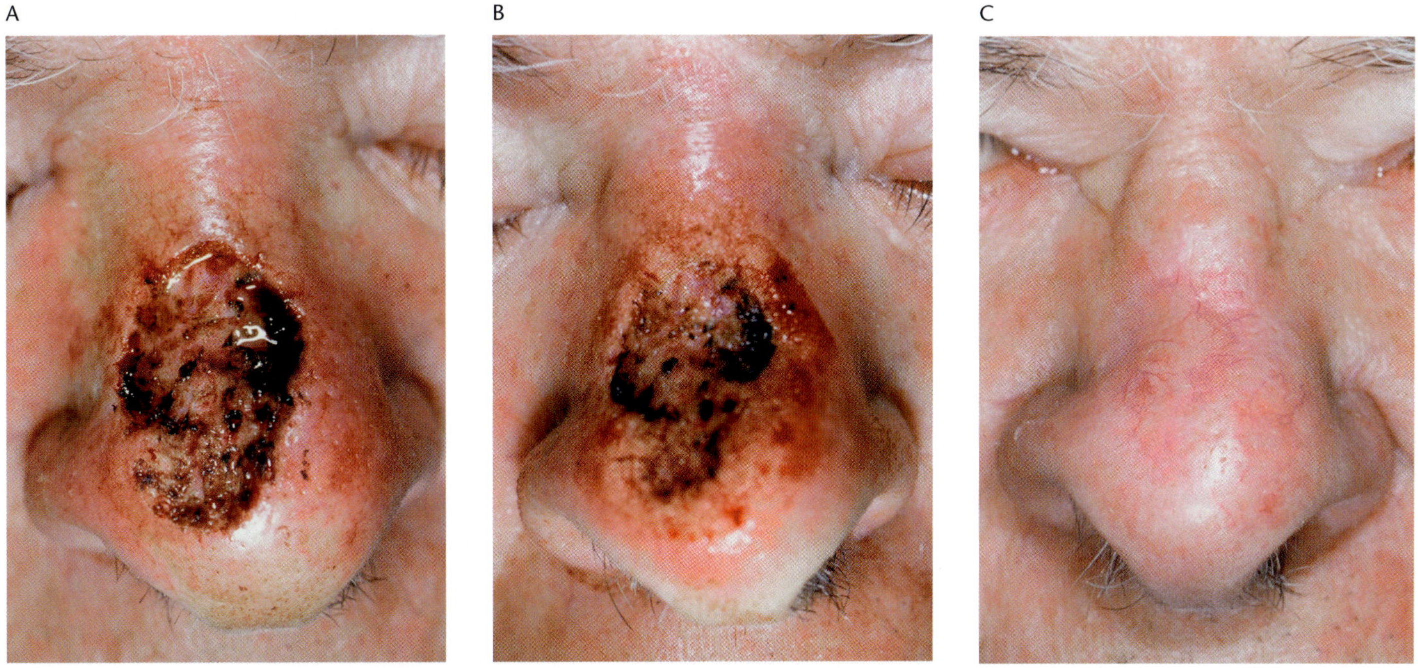

Figure 6.12 Dorsal nose Mohs surgery defect (A) before, (B) immediately after and (C) 6 months after wound edge vaporization, sculpting and peripheral feathering with a variable pulse Er:YAG laser (CO_3).

Surgical wounds repaired with grafts or flaps may heal with uneven wound edges, texture mismatch and/or color mismatch. These scars have been traditionally improved with spot dermabrasion 6–8 weeks after surgery. Laser contouring with a resurfacing CO_2 or Er:YAG laser can achieve similar improvement by flattening the scar irregularity and blending the skin texture and color mismatch (Fig. 6.13). The ablation is carried out until a flattening of the scar has been achieved and the entire cosmetic subunit is ablated into the papillary dermis. Reepithelialization is usually complete within 10 days.

Excisions performed on infected issue may best be performed using a CO_2 laser as the heat that is generated sterilizes the surgical field. Debridement of decubitus ulcers, exuberant granulation tissue, and various cutaneous infections such as botryomycosis and cutaneous leishmaniasis as well as ablation of dermatophyte-infected nails have been effectively carried out with a CO_2 laser.[216] Treatment of hidradenitis suppurativa,[217–219] acne keloidalis nuchae,[220] and dissecting folliculitis of the scalp[221] have also been reported.

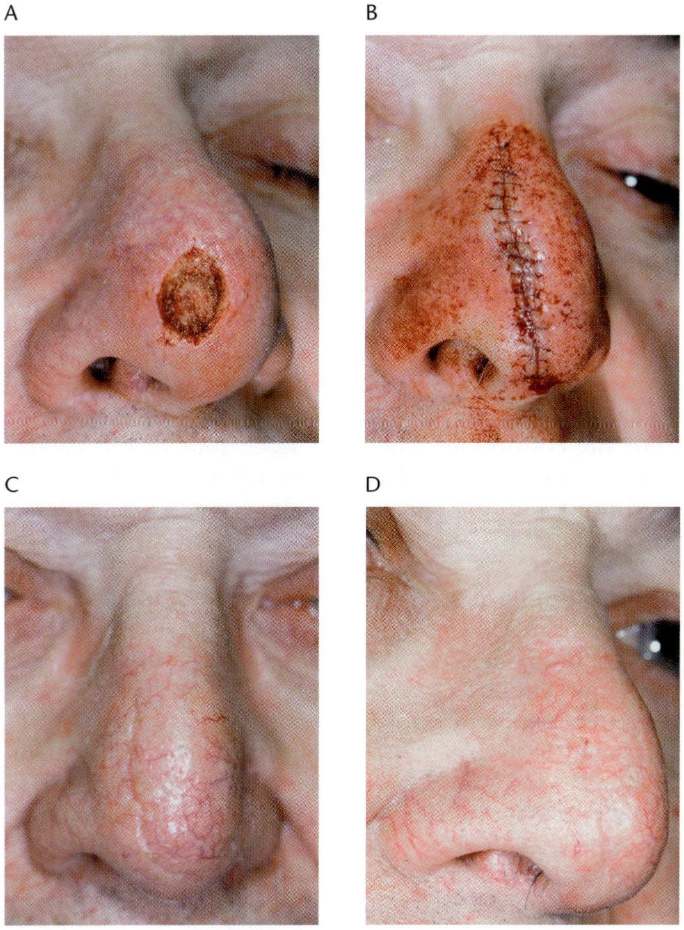

Figure 6.13 (A) Right dorsal nose Mohs surgery defect; (B) immediately after linear defect repair; (C) 6 weeks after surgery with prominent and depressed suture line; (D) 6 weeks after variable pulse Er:YAG laser (CO_3) aggressive full-face ablation with smoothing of the suture line irregularity.

Lesions For Which Laser Ablation Offers No Distinct Advantages

Skin Cancer

Ablative laser therapy currently plays little role in the management of cutaneous malignancy. No well-designed, large clinical trials with a sufficient follow-up period have validated the use of ablative lasers in the management of basal cell carcinoma (BCC).[222] One small study showed that superficial BCCs could be completely vaporized if tissue ablation occurred to the level of the mid-dermis or deeper.[223] Wheeland et al showed that CO_2 laser ablation of 370 superficial BCCs in 52 patients resulted in no recurrences after a mean follow-up of 20 months.[224] In a recent case report, CO_2 laser ablation was used to treat approximately 45 facial basal cell carcinomas after curettage in a patient with Gorlin's syndrome.[225] Full face resurfacing was performed after individual lesion ablations. In a 10-month follow-up period, six basal cell carcinomas were identified. The importance of an adequate depth of ablation was also demonstrated by the fact that in one study, complete tumor vaporization was not achieved in five of eight superficial BCCs treated with one to two resurfacing CO_2 laser passes. In the same study, the authors found no residual tumor when three CO_2 laser passes were performed.[226] Fitzpatrick[227] reported the treatment of 15 patients with Bowen's disease and 12 patients with large multifocal BCCs using the Ultrapulse CO_2 laser. With a mean follow-up of 6 to 18 months, all lesions were clinically clear. However, until more supportive data are available, the routine use of ablative laser therapy for basal cell carcinoma cannot be recommended.

Superficial malignancies such as squamous cell carcinoma in situ (Bowen's disease) or lentigo maligna may seem suitable for laser ablation. However, our experience from Mohs surgery is that these malignancies frequently have atypical cells within the hair follicles. These cells serve as a reservoir of abnormal cells and multifocal recurrences can occur. The Er:YAG laser has been used to enhance the delivery of 5-fluorouracil. In one study, lesions of Bowen's disease pretreated with the Er:YAG laser showed more rapid clinical and histologic responses to topical 5-FU than those treated with 5-FU alone.[228]

An exception to the lack of distinct advantage of lasers in the treatment of skin cancer is erythroplasia of Queyrat (squamous cell carcinoma in situ on the glans penis). This condition appears to be more amenable to laser ablation[229–232] as there are no follicular units down which atypical cells can extend; however the treatment is not universally successful. In one of the largest series published to date, van Bezooijen and colleagues treated 12 patients with the continuous wave CO_2 laser; four of the 12 had disease recurrence.[229] The authors advocate ablation of 5 to 8 mm of normal-appearing skin around the clinically apparent lesion. Combination therapy with CO_2 laser ablation and Nd:YAG laser treatment has been used for more invasive penile lesions.[233–236] When compared to partial penectomy, recurrence rates with laser ablation are approximately the same (16% versus 17.6%) but without the surgical mutilation. In one study of 30 patients with various degrees of penile intraepithelial neoplasia or invasive SCC, treatment with CO_2, Nd:YAG, KTP (one patient), or combination CO_2 and Nd:YAG lasers resulted in 22 of 23 patients remaining free of malignancy for up to 2 years' follow-up.[237]

Vulvar intraepithelial neoplasia (VIN) has been treated effectively with the CO_2 laser. CW CO_2 laser therapy was used in the 1980s in two trials that achieved cure rates of 91% and 94%.[238,239] Repeated treatment sessions were necessary due to recurrences at the untreated borders of the lesions. A recent study using a pulsed CO_2 laser for excision, vaporization, or both yield cure rates of 76.9% for a single session of patients treated with laser vaporization and 78.4% for those treated with laser excision.[240] A second laser procedure was carried out in all cases of relapsed VIN, with an overall cure rate of 96.8% after two treatments.

Conservative excision remains the treatment of choice for lentigo maligna. However, certain lesions in precarious anatomic locations may lead to significant deformity after surgical excision. Lesions of lentigo maligna on the ear, temple, nose, and cheek were treated with a CO_2 laser in four patients.[241] These individuals were found to be lesion free at 15 months' mean follow-up. No long term studies on the use of lasers for lentigo maligna are available.

Vascular Lesions

With the advent of specific vascular lasers such as the 585 and 595 nm pulsed dye lasers, and the 532 nm KTP laser, the use of ablative lasers to treat vascular lesions is rarely necessary. The only potentially useful application of an ablative laser today is in the treatment of thick, hypertrophic, nodular components of mature port wine stains and hemangiomas.[242–248] Full ablation should not be performed due to the inevitable scarring that would result. Rather, superficial vaporization of the nodular components with a pulsed CO_2 or Er:YAG laser should be performed followed by treatment of the remaining vascular component with a pulsed dye laser.

Epidermal Pigmented Lesions

As with vascular lesions, there are more specific lasers that target pigmented lesions thereby making treatment of lentigines, ephelides, and labial melanotic macules with ablative lasers less desirable due to the risk of scarring.

Continuous Wave (CW) CO_2 Laser Excision

The CW CO_2 laser is primarily utilized as a surgical tool. In a focused mode, the device can provide precise tissue cutting. When defocused, the laser provides excellent hemostasis.

Laser Blepharoplasty

The CW CO_2 laser has been used in blepharoplasty surgery. Benefits of the laser include hemostatic cutting of tissue. The surgeon can thus open the orbital septum, remove fat pads and achieve hemostasis simultaneously. However, limited studies directly comparing laser blepharoplasty with other modalities fail to show any long-term benefits solely attributable to the use of the CO_2 laser. A shortcoming of CW CO_2 laser incisional surgery is the lack of tactile feedback that the surgeon obtains with other modalities such as a steel scalpel or electrosurgical needle. Additionally, the surgeon must be aware of and take precautions against the risk of ocular injury from the laser.[249]

Laser Excision of Keloids

As CO_2 laser surgery gained increased clinical application, there was initial enthusiasm that laser excisional surgery would be particularly useful for keloid excision (Fig. 6.14). Keloids are characterized by unregulated collagen deposition and tend to occur in certain body locations, most

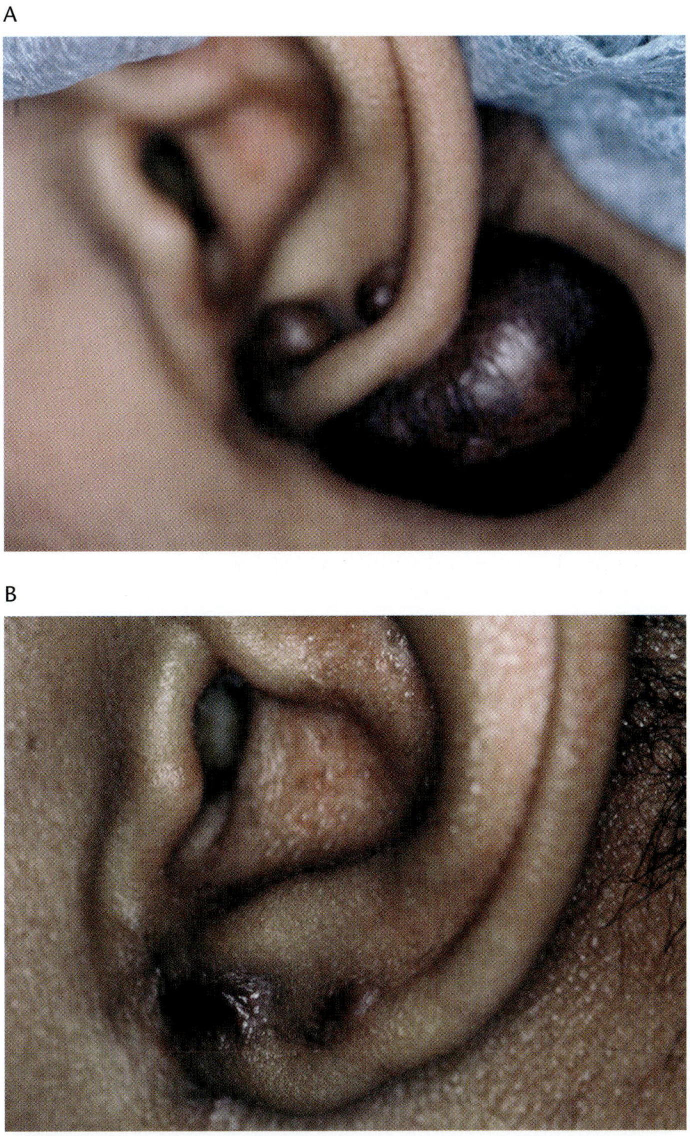

Figure 6.14 Left earlobe 'dumbbell' keloid (A) immediately before and (B) 5 months after continuous wave CO_2 laser excision. The wound was allowed to heal by second intention except for the defect through the full-thickness of the ear-lobe, which was sutured closed. Intralesional 40 mg/mL triamcinolone acetonide was injected immediately after laser surgery.

notably the ears, chest and upper back/shoulders. In prone individuals, a traumatic event, even a slight injury, may incite keloid formation. Surgical excision of keloids with the CO_2 laser was postulated to be less traumatic than excision via scalpel. Unfortunately, the keloid recurrence rate with CO_2 laser surgery alone was unacceptably high, in the order of 50–70%. Additional studies have demonstrated similar recurrence rates between laser excision and standard surgical excision.[250,251]

The CO_2 laser has utility as a surgical device as it provides excellent hemostasis as it cuts. Recently, the role of blood thinners in dermatologic surgery as an area of concern has been called into question. Published data have suggested that, for cutaneous surgery, blood thinners may not lead to an increased rate of serious bleeding complications as compared with patients with normal coagulation. From a practical standpoint, the surgeon can achieve similar cutting capacity with hemostasis from most standard electrosurgical units. [252]

Complications of Er:YAG and CO_2 Ablative Surgery

The complications that result from Er:YAG and CO_2 laser ablation of epidermal and dermal lesions are essentially the same potential complications that can result from any wound. The surgeon must monitor for appropriate wound healing in the postoperative course and intervene if there should be signs of infection (bacterial, fungal or viral) or hypertrophic scarring. The surgeon must be cognizant of site specific sequela, such as nail abnormalities after periungal surgery or herpes labialis reactivation after actinic cheilitis treatment. Fortunately, dermatologic surgeons are well-versed in wound healing and the creation of wounds from laser, dermabrasion or chemical peeling.

Complications can be divided into six categories: immediate predictable effects, infectious, eczematous, follicular; scarring; and pigmentary changes.

Immediate Predictable Effects

Erythema of treated areas lasts 6–12 weeks on average (shorter with Er:YAG, longer with CO_2 laser ablation). This is considered a normal part of the healing process. For up to 12 months after laser surgery, erythema and flushing can occur at the treated sites upon emotional upset or exertion. Depending on the depth of ablation, there may even be persistent erythema for up to 12 months following CO_2 laser ablation procedures.[24,87,253,254]

Pigmentary Changes

Postinflammatory hyperpigmentation is the most common adverse effect following laser ablation procedures and occurs more commonly in Fitzpatrick skin types III–VI. Transient hyperpigmentation has been reported in up to 36% of patients.[255] Sun avoidance, even through window glass, is imperative as there is a direct relationship between the degree of sun exposure postoperatively and frequency of hyperpigmentation. Pretreatment with tretinoin and hydroquinone may reduce the incidence of hyperpigmentation following laser surgery.[256] These topical products should be restarted at the very earliest sign of hyperpigmention postoperatively. If started early enough, hyperpigmentation usually resolves within months after initiation of topical bleaching creams and tretinoin.

Another major pigmentary complication is permanent hypopigmentation, which can develop up to 1 year following ablative laser surgery. This adverse effect has been reported in up to 16% of patients and appears to be less frequent following laser ablation than after dermabrasion or deep chemical peels.[256] It is more frequent if a patient has previously been treated by dermabrasion.[86,255] The degree of hypopigmentation can range from pale new 'sun-protected' skin to depigmented skin. Mismatches in color between treated and untreated areas can be avoided by treating the entire face or at least entire cosmetic units with feathering into surrounding areas.

Follicular

During the postoperative healing period, ointments are used to facilitate reepithelialization. However, follicular occlusion during the reepithelialization process may result in the development of milia and acne. These adverse effects usually occur during the first few weeks after laser ablation and generally respond to standard acne treatments.

Eczematous

Contact dermatitis may result from the use of topical anesthetic preparations.[87,257] Postoperative erythema and hyperpigmentation may occur with greater frequency in patients who experience contact dermatitis in the perioperative period.[53] These eczematous reactions generally respond well to mid-potency topical steroid applications and bland emollients. When ablative laser procedures are performed in the perioral region, perioral dermatitis may develop. This usually responds to standard therapy with tetracyclines.

Infectious

Infection is a concern with any ablative procedure, including dermabrasion, ablative laser surgery, and chemical peeling. As discussed earlier, pretreatment with antiviral prophylaxis is imperative. Manuskiatti et al showed that ciprofloxacin is effective in preventing infection with both Gram-positive and Gram-negative bacteria prior to CO_2 laser resurfacing.[258] One study showed that fluconazole administered between days 3 and 8 postoperatively significantly promoted reepithelialization in patients undergoing full-face CO_2 laser skin resurfacing.[259]

Scarring

Fortunately, CO_2 and Er:YAG laser ablation rarely results in hypertrophic scarring. One must treat conservatively and err on the side of under-treatment rather than risk the development of scarring. Limiting the number of laser passes and ensuring proper post-operative wound care will minimize the chance of scarring.[86,256,257] When pulse stacking is used with a CO_2 laser or a greater number of passes is delivered, excessive thermal damage may result in unwanted scarring. One can always perform further ablation at a future follow-up visit, and therefore avoidance of deep ablation in the initial procedure would be prudent. Topical and intralesional steroids, silicone gel sheeting, or pulsed dye laser photocoagulation should be used to treat any areas that are developing early scarring.

Summary

Despite recent advances in non-ablative and Q-switched laser technologies, the ablative CO_2 and Er:YAG lasers play an important role in the management of a diverse number of cutaneous lesions.

References

1. Goldman L. Laser treatment of melanoma. In: Goldman L, ed. Laser cancer research. New York: Springer-Verlag; 1966.
2. Stellar S, Polanyi TG. Lasers in neurosurgery: a historical overview. J Clin Laser Med Surg 1992 Dec; 10(6):399–411.
3. Polanyi TG, Bredemeier HC, Davis TJ Jr. CO_2 laser for surgical research and medical and biological engineering. New York: Pergamon; 1970.
4. Aschler P, Ingolitsch E, Walter G et al. Ultrastructural findings in CNS tissue with CO_2 laser. In: Kaplan I, ed. Laser surgery II. Jerusalem: Academic Press; 1976.
5. Ben-Bassat M, Ben-Bassat J, Kaplan I. An ultrastructural study of the cut edges of skin and mucous membrane specimens excised by carbon dioxide laser. In: Kaplan I, ed. Laser surgery. Jerusalem: Academic Press; 1976.
6. Absten GT. Laser biophysics for the physician. In: Ratz JL, ed. Lasers in cutaneous medicine and surgery. St Louis: Mosby; 1986.
7. Olbricht SM. The CO_2 laser: use as an ablative instrument. In: Ardnt KA, Dover JS, Olbricht SM, eds. Lasers in cutaneous and aesthetic surgery. Philadelphia: Lippincott-Raven; 1997.
8. Anderson RR. Laser–tissue interactions in dermatology. In: Ardnt KA, Dover JS, Olbricht SM, eds. Lasers in cutaneous and aesthetic surgery. Philadelphia: Lippincott-Raven; 1997.
9. Anderson RR, Parrish JA. Selective photothermolysis: precise microsurgery by selective absorption of pulsed radiation. Science 1983; 220(4596):524–7.
10. McKenzie AL. How far does thermal damage extend beneath the surface of CO_2 laser incisions? Phys Med Biol 1983; 28(8):905–12.
11. Green HA, Burd E, Nishioka NS et al. Mid-dermal wound healing. A comparison between dermatomal excision and pulsed carbon dioxide laser ablation. Arch Dermatol 1992; 128(5):639–45.
12. Hall RR. The healing of tissues incised by a carbon-dioxide laser. Br J Surg 1971; 58(3):222–5.
13. Brugmans MJ, Kemper J, Gijsbers GH et al. Response of biological materials to pulsed non-ablative CO_2 laser irradiation. Lasers Surg Med 1991; 11(6):587–94.
14. Lanzafame RJ, Naim JO, Rogers DW et al. Comparison of continuous-wave, chop-wave, and super pulse laser wounds. Lasers Surg Med 1988; 8(2):119–24.
15. Schomacker KT, Walsh JT Jr, Flotte TJ et al. Thermal damage produced by high-irradiance continuous wave CO_2 laser cutting of tissue. Lasers Surg Med 1990; 10(1):74–84.
16. Fitzpatrick RE, Ruiz-Esparza J, Goldman MP. The depth of thermal necrosis using the CO_2 laser: a comparison of the superpulsed mode and conventional mode. J Dermatol Surg Oncol 1991; 17(4):340–4.
17. Fitzpatrick RE, Goldman MP, Ruiz-Esparza J. Clinical advantage of the CO_2 laser superpulsed mode. Treatment of verruca vulgaris, seborrheic keratoses, lentigines, and actinic cheilitis. J Dermatol Surg Oncol 1994; 20(7):449–56.
18. Zweig AD, Meierhofer B, Muller OM et al. Lateral thermal damage along pulsed laser incisions. Lasers Surg Med 1990; 10(3):262–74.
19. Fitzpatrick RE, Tope WD, Goldman MP et al. Pulsed carbon dioxide laser, trichloroacetic acid, Baker–Gordon phenol, and dermabrasion: a comparative clinical and histologic study of cutaneous resurfacing in a porcine model. Arch Dermatol 1996; 132(4):469–71.

20. Kauvar AN, Waldorf HA, Geronemus RG. A histopathological comparison of 'char-free' carbon dioxide lasers. Dermatol Surg 1996; 22(4):343–8.
21. Dover JS, Hruza G. Lasers in skin resurfacing. Australas J Dermatol 2000; 41(2):72–85.
22. Ratner D, Tse Y, Marchell N et al. Cutaneous laser resurfacing. J Am Acad Dermatol 1999; 41(3 Pt 1):365–89.
23. Weinstein C. Carbon dioxide laser resurfacing. Long-term follow-up in 2123 patients. Clin Plast Surg 1998; 25(1): 109–30.
24. Lask G, Keller G, Lowe N. Laser skin resurfacing with the SilkTouch flashscanner for facial rhytides. Dermatol Surg 1995; 21(12):1021–4.
25. Fitzpatrick RE. Laser resurfacing of rhytides. Dermatol Clin 1997; 15:431–447.
26. Ross EV, Grossman MC, Duke D et al. Long-term results after CO_2 laser skin resurfacing: a comparison of scanned and pulsed systems. J Am Acad Dermatol 1997; 37(5 Pt 1):709–18.
27. Alster TS, Nanni CA, Williams CM. Comparison of four carbon dioxide resurfacing lasers. A clinical and histopathologic evaluation. Dermatol Surg 1999; 25(3):153–8.
28. Henriques FC, Moritz AR. Studies of thermal injury. I. The conduction of heat to and through skin and the temperatures attained therein: a theoretical and experimental investigation. Am J Pathol 1947; 23:531.
29. Moritz AR, Henriques FC. Studies of thermal injury. II. The relative importance of time and surface temperatures in the causation of cutaneous burns. Am J Pathol 1947; 23:695.
30. Alster TS. Cutaneous resurfacing with CO_2 and erbium: YAG lasers: preoperative, intraoperative, and postoperative considerations. Plast Reconstr Surg 1999; 103(2):619–32.
31. Walsh JT Jr, Flotte TJ, Deutsch TF. Er:YAG laser ablation of tissue: effect of pulse duration and tissue type on thermal damage. Lasers Surg Med 1989; 9(4):314–26.
32. Hohenleutner U, Hohenleutner S, Baumler W et al. Fast and effective skin ablation with an Er:YAG laser: determination of ablation rates and thermal damage zones. Lasers Surg Med 1997; 20(3):242–7.
33. Zachary CB. Modulating the Er:YAG laser. Lasers Surg Med 2000; 26(2):223–6.
34. Goldman MP, Marchell N, Fitzpatrick RE, Tse Y. Laser resurfacing of the face with the combined CO_2/Er:YAG laser. Dermatol Surg 2000; 26:102–4.
35. Zachary CB, Grekin RC. Dual mode Er:YAG laser systems for skin resurfacing. Lasernews.net, LLC; 1999.
36. Rostan ER, Fitzpatrick RE, Goldman MP. Laser resurfacing with a long pulse Erbium:YAG laser compared to the 950msec pulsed CO_2 laser. Laser Surg Med 2001; 29:136–41.
37. Rostan EF, Goldman MP, Fitzpatrick RE. Laser resurfacing with a dual mode long pulse Erbium:YAG laser compared to the 950msec pulsed CO_2 laser. Am J Cosmetic Surg 2000; 17(4).
38. Bass LS. Erbium:YAG laser skin resurfacing: preliminary clinical evaluation. Ann Plast Surg 1998; 40(4):328–34.
39. Weinstein C. Erbium laser resurfacing: current concepts. Plast Reconstr Surg 1999; 103(2):602–16.
40. Goldman, MP. The use of hydroquinone with facial laser resurfacing. J Cutaneous Laser Therapy 2000; 2:73–7.
41. Brody HJ. Chemical peeling. In: Baxter S, Brody HJ, eds. Chemical peeling and resurfacing, 2nd edn. St Louis: Mosby; 1997:1–256.
42. Alster TS. Laser resurfacing of rhytides: manual of cutaneous laser techniques. Philadelphia: Lippincott-Raven; 1997:104–21.
43. Roenigk HH Jr, Pinski JB, Robinson JK. Acne, retinoids, and dermabrasion. J Dermatol Surg Oncol 1985; 11(4):396–8.
44. Rubenstein R, Roenigk HH Jr, Stegman SJ. Atypical keloids after dermabrasion of patients taking isotretinoin. J Am Acad Dermatol 1986; 15(2 Pt 1):280–5.
45. Katz BE, MacFarlane DF. Atypical facial scarring after isotretinoin therapy in a patient with previous dermabrasion. J Am Acad Dermatol 1994; 30(5 Pt 2):852–3.
46. Zachariae H. Delayed wound healing and keloid formation following argon laser treatment or dermabrasion during isotretinoin treatment. Br J Dermatol 1988; 118(5):703–6.
47. Brody HJ. Update on chemical peels. Adv Dermatol 1992; 7:275–88; discussion 289.
48. Apfelberg DB, Varga J, Greenbaum SS. Carbon dioxide laser resurfacing of peri-oral rhytids in scleroderma patients. Dermatol Surg 1998; 24(5):517–19.
49. Yang CC, Chai CY. Animal study of skin resurfacing using the ultrapulse carbon dioxide laser. Ann Plast Surg 1995; 35(2):154–8.
50. Martinet N, Harne LA, Grotendorst GR. Identification and characterization of chemoattractants for epidermal cells. J Invest Dermatol 1988; 90(2):122–6.
51. Krawczyk WS. The pattern of epidermal cell migration during wound healing. J Cell Biol 1971; 49:247–63.
52. West TB, Alster TS. Effect of pretreatment on the incidence of hyperpigmentation following cutaneous CO_2 laser resurfacing. Dermatol Surg 1999; 25(1):15–17.
53. Lowe NJ, Lask G, Griffin ME. Laser skin resurfacing. Pre- and posttreatment guidelines. Dermatol Surg 1995; 21(12):1017–19.
54. Weinstein C. Carbon dioxide laser resurfacing. In: Coleman WP, Hanke CW, Alt TH, Asken S, eds. Cosmetic surgery of the skin. St Louis: Mosby; 1998.
55. Dover JS, Smoller BR, Stern RS. Low-fluence carbon dioxide laser irradiation of lentigines. Arch Dermatol 1988; 124(8): 1219–24.
56. Kamat BR, Tang SV, Arndt KA. Low-fluence CO_2 laser irradiation: selective epidermal damage to human skin. J Invest Dermatol 1985; 85(3):274–8.
57. Bissacia E, Scarborough DA. Laser surgery. In: Bissacia E, Scarborough DA, eds. The Columbia manual of dermatologic cosmetic surgery. New York: McGraw Hill; 2002.
58. Seckel BR, Kovanda CJ, Cetrulo CL et al. Laser blepharoplasty with transconjunctival orbicularis muscle/septum tightening and periocular skin resurfacing: a safe and advantageous technique. Plast Reconstr Surg 2000; 106(5):1127–41.
59. Lessner AM, Fagien S. Laser blepharoplasty. Semin Ophthalmol 1998; 13(3):90–102.
60. Glassberg E, Babapour R, Lask G. Current trends in laser blepharoplasty. Results of a survey. Dermatol Surg 1995; 21(12):1060–3.
61. Baker SS, Muenzler WS, Small RG et al. Carbon dioxide laser blepharoplasty. Ophthalmology 1984; 91(3):238–44.
62. Wheeland RG. Cosmetic use of lasers. Dermatol Clin 1995; 13(2):447–59.
63. Karim Ali M, Streitmann MJ. Excision of rhinophyma with the carbon dioxide laser: a ten-year experience. Ann Otol Rhinol Laryngol 1997; 106(11):952–5.
64. Vidimos AT. Treatment of rhinophyma with the carbon dioxide laser. J Oral Maxillofac Surg 1991; 49(9):1032.
65. Wheeland RG, Bailin PL. Scalp reduction surgery with the carbon dioxide laser. J Dermatol Surg Oncol 1984; 10(7): 565–9.
66. Lim TC, Tan WT. Carbon dioxide laser for keloids. Plast Reconstr Surg 1991; 88(6):1111.

67. Norris JE. The effect of carbon dioxide laser surgery on the recurrence of keloids. Plast Reconstr Surg 1991; 87(1):44–9.
68. Kaplan I. The CO_2 laser in plastic surgery. Lasers Surg Med 1986; 6(4):385–6.
69. David LM, Sanders G. CO_2 laser blepharoplasty: a comparison to cold steel and electrocautery. J Dermatol Surg Oncol 1987; 13(2):110–14.
70. Mittelman H, Apfelberg DB. Carbon dioxide laser blepharoplasty – advantages and disadvantages. Ann Plast Surg 1990; 24(1):1–6.
71. Morrow DM, Morrow LB. CO_2 laser blepharoplasty. A comparison with cold-steel surgery. J Dermatol Surg Oncol 1992; 18(4):307–13.
72. Biesman BS. Blepharoplasty: laser or cold steel? Skin Therapy Lett 2003; 8(7):5–7.
73. Clark RA. Cutaneous tissue repair: basic biologic considerations. I. J Am Acad Dermatol 1985; 13(5 Pt 1):701–25.
74. Geronemus RG, Mertz PM, Eaglstein WH. Wound healing. The effects of topical antimicrobial agents. Arch Dermatol 1979; 115(11):1311–14.
75. Fazio MJ, Zitelli JA, Goslen JB. Wound healing after cosmetic surgery. In: Coleman WP, Hanke CW, Alt TH, Asken S, eds. Cosmetic surgery of the skin. St Louis: Mosby; 1998;18–38.
76. Brown CD, Zitelli JA. Choice of wound dressings and ointments. Otolaryngol Clin North Am 1995; 28(5):1081–91.
77. Chen WY, Rogers AA, Lydon MJ. Characterization of biologic properties of wound fluid collected during early stages of wound healing. J Invest Dermatol 1992; 99(5):559–64.
78. Eaglestein WH. Experiences with biosynthetic dressings. J Am Acad Dermatol 1985; 12(2 Pt 2):434–40.
79. Demling RH. Burns. N Engl J Med 1985; 313(22):1389–98.
80. Kannon GA, Garrett AB. Moist wound healing with occlusive dressings. A clinical review. Dermatol Surg 1995; 21(7): 583–90.
81. Newman JP, Fitzgerald P, Koch RJ. Review of closed dressings after laser resurfacing. Dermatol Surg 2000; 26(6):562–71.
82. Weiss RA, Goldman MP. Interpenetrating polymer network wound dressing vs. petrolatum and polyethylene oxide hydrogel following facial CO_2 laser resurfacing or dermabrasion. Dermatol Surg 2001; 27:449–51.
83. Apfelberg DB. Summary of the 1997 ASAPS/ASPRS Laser Task Force Survey on laser resurfacing and laser blepharoplasty. American Society for Aesthetic Plastic Surgery. American Society of Plastic and Reconstructive Surgeons. Plast Reconstr Surg 1998; 101(2):511–18.
84. Sriprachya-Anunt S, Fitzpatrick RE, Goldman MP. Infections complicating pulsed carbon dioxide laser resurfacing for photoaged facial skin. Dermatol Surg 1997; 23(7):527–35; discussion 535–6.
85. Goldman MP, Skover G, Roberts TL, Fitzpatrick RE, Lettieri JT. Optimizing wound healing in the post-laser abrasion face. J Am Acad Dermatol 2002; 46:399–407.
86. Weinstein C. Ultrapulse carbon dioxide laser removal of periocular wrinkles in association with laser blepharoplasty. J Clin Laser Med Surg 1994; 12(4):205–9.
87. Waldorf HA, Kauvar AN, Geronemus RG. Skin resurfacing of fine to deep rhytides using a char-free carbon dioxide laser in 47 patients. Dermatol Surg 1995; 21(11):940–6.
88. Weinstein C, Ramirez O, Pozner J. Postoperative care following carbon dioxide laser resurfacing. Avoiding pitfalls. Dermatol Surg 1998; 24(1):51–6.
89. Fisher AA. Lasers and allergic contact dermatitis to topical antibiotics, with particular reference to bacitracin. Cutis 1996; 58(4):252–4.
90. Robinson JK. Actinic cheilitis. A prospective study comparing four treatment methods. Arch Otolaryngol Head Neck Surg 1989; 115:848–52.
91. Cataldo E, Doku HC. Solar cheilitis. J Dermatol Surg Oncol 1981; 7(12):989–95.
92. Lubritz RR, Smolewski SA. Cryosurgery cure rate of premalignant leukoplakia of the lower lip. J Dermatol Surg Oncol 1983; 9(3):235–7.
93. Epstein E. Treatment of lip keratoses (actinic cheilitis) with topical fluorouracil. Arch Dermatol 1977; 113(7):906–8.
94. Burns CA, Brown MD. Imiquimod for the treatment of skin cancer. Dermatol Clin 2005; 23(1):151–64.
95. Stockfleth E, Christophers E, Benninghoff B et al. Low incidence of new actinic keratoses after topical 5% imiquimod cream treatment: a long-term follow-up study. Arch Dermatol 2004; 140(12):1542.
96. Szeimies RM, Gerritsen MJ, Gupta G et al. Imiquimod 5% cream for the treatment of actinic keratosis: results from a phase III, randomized, double-blind, vehicle-controlled, clinical trial with histology. J Am Acad Dermatol 2004; 51(4):547–55.
97. Lebwohl M, Dinehart S, Whiting D et al. Imiquimod 5% cream for the treatment of actinic keratosis: results from two phase III, randomized, double-blind, parallel group, vehicle-controlled trials. J Am Acad Dermatol 2004; 50(5):714–21.
98. Navi D, Huntley A. Imiquimod 5 percent cream and the treatment of cutaneous malignancy. Dermatol Online J 2004; 10(1):4.
99. Witheiler DD, Lawrence N, Cox SE et al. Long-term efficacy and safety of Jessner's solution and 35% trichloroacetic acid vs 5% fluorouracil in the treatment of widespread facial actinic keratoses. Dermatol Surg 1997; 23(3):191–6.
100. Kim HS, Yoo JY, Cho KH et al. Topical photodynamic therapy using intense pulsed light for treatment of actinic keratosis: clinical and histopathologic evaluation. Dermatol Surg 2005; 31(1):33–6; discussion 36–7.
101. Gilbert DJ. Treatment of actinic keratoses with sequential combination of 5-fluorouracil and photodynamic therapy. J Drugs Dermatol 2005; 4(2):161–3.
102. Gold MH, Goldman MP. 5-aminolevulinic acid photodynamic therapy: where we have been and where we are going. Dermatol Surg 2004; 30(8):1077–83.
103. Dragieva G, Prinz BM, Hafner J. A randomized controlled clinical trial of topical photodynamic therapy with methyl aminolaevulinate in the treatment of actinic keratoses in transplant recipients. Br J Dermatol 2004; 151(1):196200.
104. Piacquadio DJ, Chen DM, Farber HF et al. Photodynamic therapy with aminolevulinic acid topical solution and visible blue light in the treatment of multiple actinic keratoses of the face and scalp: investigator-blinded, phase 3, multicenter trials. Arch Dermatol 2004; 140(1):41–6.
105. Laws RA, Wilde JL, Grabski WJ. Comparison of electrodessication with CO_2 laser for the treatment of actinic cheilitis. Dermatol Surg 2000; 26(4):349–53.
106. Grotting JK. Chronic lower lip lesions; treatment by the lip-shave operation. Minn Med 1956; 39(8):527–8.
107. Spira M, Hardy B. Vermilionectomy. Review of cases with variations in technique. Plast Reconstr Surg 1964; 33:39–46.
108. Sanchez-Conejo-Mir J, Perez Bernal AM, Moreno-Gimenez JC. Follow-up of vermilionectomies: evaluation of the technique. J Dermatol Surg Oncol 1986; 12(2):180–4.
109. Birt BD. The 'lip shave' operation for pre-malignant conditions and micro-invasive carcinoma of the lower lip. J Otolaryngol 1977; 6(5):407–11.

110. Dufresne RG Jr, Garrett AB, Bailin PL. Carbon dioxide laser treatment of chronic actinic cheilitis. J Am Acad Dermatol 1988; 19(5 Pt 1):876–8.
111. LaRiviere W, Pickett AB. Clinical criteria in diagnosis of early squamous cell carcinoma of the lower lip. J Am Dent Assoc 1979; 99(6):972–7.
112. Schmitt CK, Folsom TC. Histologic evaluation of degenerative changes of the lower lip. J Oral Surg 1968; 26(1):51–6.
113. Wurman LH, Adams GL, Meyerhoff WL. Carcinoma of the lip. Am J Surg 1975; 130(4):470–4.
114. Booth F, Coldwater K, Paletta FX. The treatment of leukoplakia and carcinoma in situ of the lower lip. Ann Surg 1957; 145(1):74–80.
115. Moller R, Reymann F, Hou-Jensen K. Metastases in dermatological patients with squamous cell carcinoma. Arch Dermatol 1979; 115(6):703–5.
116. Slaughter DP, Southwick HW, Smejkal W. Field cancerization in oral stratified squamous epithelium; clinical implications of multicentric origin. Cancer 1953; 6(5):963–8.
117. Whitaker DC. Microscopically proven cure of actinic cheilitis by CO_2 laser. Lasers Surg Med 1987; 7(6):520–3.
118. Stanley RJ, Roenigk RK. Actinic cheilitis: treatment with the carbon dioxide laser. Mayo Clin Proc 1988; 63(3):230–5.
119. Zelickson BD, Roenigk RK. Actinic cheilitis. Treatment with the carbon dioxide laser. Cancer 1990; 15;65(6):1307–11.
120. Johnson TM, Sebastien TS, Lowe L et al. Carbon dioxide laser treatment of actinic cheilitis. Clinicohistopathologic correlation to determine the optimal depth of destruction. J Am Acad Dermatol 1992; 27(5 Pt 1):737–40.
121. Hruza GJ. Skin resurfacing with lasers. Fitzpatrick's J Clin Dermatol 1995; 3:38–41.
122. Hruza GJ, Dover JS. Laser skin resurfacing. Arch Dermatol 1996; 132:451–5.
123. David LM. Laser vermilion ablation for actinic cheilitis. J Dermatol Surg Oncol 1985; 11(6):605–8.
124. Fitzpatrick RE, Ruiz-Esparza J. The superpulsed CO_2 laser. In Roenigk RK, Roenigk H, eds. New trends in dermatologic surgery. London: Martin Dunitz; 1993.
125. Fitzpatrick RE, Goldman MP, Dierickx C. Laser ablation of facial cosmetic tattoos. Aesthetic Plast Surg 1994; 18(1):91–8.
126. Albom M. Surgical gems: electrosurgical treatment of rhinophyma. J Dermatol Surg 1976; 2(3):189–91.
127. Staindl O. Surgical management of rhinophyma. Acta Otolaryngol 1981; 92(1–2):137–40.
128. Cheney ML, Graves TA, Blair PA. Rhinophyma: a surgical management. J La State Med Soc 1987; 139(2):13–14, 17–18.
129. Kemble JV. Correction of deformities of the nose. Practitioner 1980; 224(1342):399–404.
130. Fulton JE. Modern dermabrasion techniques: a personal appraisal. J Dermatol Surg Oncol 1987; 13(7):780–9.
131. Fisher WJ. Rhinophyma: its surgical treatment. Plast Reconstr Surg 1970; 45(5):466–70.
132. Anderson R, Dykes ER. Surgical treatment of rhinophyma. Plast Reconstr Surg 1962; 30:397–402.
133. Freeman BS. Surgical treatment of rhinophyma. Plast Reconstr Surg 1962; 30:397–402.
134. Karge HJ, Konz B. Surgical methods in the treatment of rhinophyma. J Dermatol Surg 1975; 1(3):31–2.
135. Strempel H. A new dermatome for surgical treatment of rhinophyma. J Dermatol Surg Oncol 1981; 7(2):153–6.
136. Linehan JW, Goode RL, Fajardo LF. Surgery vs electrosurgery for rhinophyma. Arch Otolaryngol 1970; 91(5):444–8.
137. Verde SF, Oliveira Ada S, Picoto Ada S. How we treat rhinophyma. J Dermatol Surg Oncol 1980; 6(7):560–1.
138. Nolan JO. Cryosurgical treatment of rhinophyma. Case report. Plast Reconstr Surg 1973; 52(4):437–8.
139. Sonnex TS, Dawber RP. Rhinophyma-treatment by liquid nitrogen spray cryosurgery. Clin Exp Dermatol 1986; 11(3):284–8.
140. Greenbaum SS, Krull EA, Watnick K. Comparison of CO_2 laser and electrosurgery in the treatment of rhinophyma. J Am Acad Dermatol 1988; 18(2 Pt 1):363–8.
141. Eisen RF, Katz AE, Bohigian RK et al. Surgical treatment of rhinophyma with the Shaw scalpel. Arch Dermatol 1986; 122(3):307–9.
142. Farina R. Rhinophyma; plastic correction. Plast Reconstr Surg 1950; 6(6):461–6.
143. Ali MK, Callari RH, Mobley DL. Resection of rhinophyma with CO_2 laser. Laryngoscope 1989; 99(4):453–5.
144. Bohigian RK, Shapshay SM, Hybels RL. Management of rhinophyma with carbon dioxide laser: Lahey Clinic experience. Lasers Surg Med 1988; 8(4):397–401.
145. Roenigk RK. CO_2 laser vaporization for treatment of rhinophyma. Mayo Clin Proc 1987; 62(8):676–80.
146. Wheeland RG, Bailin PL, Ratz JL. Combined carbon dioxide laser excision and vaporization in the treatment of rhinophyma. J Dermatol Surg Oncol 1987; 13(2):172–7.
147. Shapshay SM, Strong MS, Anastasi GW et al. Removal of rhinophyma with the carbon dioxide laser: a preliminary report. Arch Otolaryngol 1980; 106(5):257–9.
148. Amedee RG, Routman MH. Methods and complications of rhinophyma excision. Laryngoscope 1987; 97(11):1316–18.
149. Hassard AD. Carbon dioxide laser treatment of acne rosacea and rhinophyma: how I do it. J Otolaryngol 1988; 17(6):336–7.
150. Hallock GG. Laser treatment of rhinophyma. Aesthetic Plast Surg 1988; 12(3):171–4.
151. Haas A, Wheeland RG. Treatment of massive rhinophyma with the carbon dioxide laser. J Dermatol Surg Oncol 1990; 16(7):645–9.
152. el-Azhary RA, Roenigk RK, Wang TD. Spectrum of results after treatment of rhinophyma with the carbon dioxide laser. Mayo Clin Proc 1991; 66(9):899–905.
153. Fincher EF, Gladstone HB. Use of a dual-mode erbium:YAG laser for the surgical correction of rhinophyma. Arch Facial Plast Surg 2004; 6(4):267–71.
154. Orenstein A. Treatment of rhinophyma with Er:YAG laser. Lasers Surg Med 2001; 29(3):230–5.
155. Simo R, Sharma VL. Treatment of rhinophyma with carbon dioxide laser. J Laryngol Otol 1996; 110(9):841–6.
156. Goldman L, Perry E, Stefanovsky D. A flexible sealed tube transverse radio frequency excited carbon dioxide laser for dermatologic surgery. Lasers Surg Med 1983; 2(4):317–22.
157. McKee PH. Tumors of the epidermal appendages. In: Pathology of the skin, 2nd ed. Chicago: Mosby-Wolfe; 1996.
158. Garden JM, Geronemus RG. Dermatologic laser surgery. J Dermatol Surg Oncol 1990; 16(2):156–68.
159. Park JH, Hwang ES, Kim SN et al. Er:YAG laser treatment of verrucous epidermal nevi. Dermatol Surg 2004; 30(3):378–81.
160. Hohenleutner U, Wlotzke U, Konz B et al. Carbon dioxide laser therapy of a widespread epidermal nevus. Lasers Surg Med 1995; 16:288–291.
161. Ratz JL, Bailin PL, Wheeland RG. Carbon dioxide laser treatment of epidermal nevi. J Dermatol Surg Oncol 1986; 12:567–570.
162. Logan RA, Zachary CB. Outcome of carbon dioxide laser therapy for persistent cutaneous viral warts. Br J Dermatol 1989; 121:99–105.

163. McBurney EI, Rosen DA. Carbon dioxide laser treatment of verrucae vulgaris. J Dermatol Surg Oncol 1984; 10:45–48.
164. Lim JT, Goh CL. Carbon dioxide laser treatment of periungual and subungual viral warts. Aust J Dermatol 1992; 33:87.
165. Street ML, Roenigk RK. Recalcitrant periungual verrucae: the role of carbon dioxide laser vaporization. J Am Acad Dermatol 1990; 23(1):115–20.
166. Apfelberg DB, Druker D, Maser MR et al. Benefits of the CO_2 laser for verruca resistant to other modalities of treatment. J Dermatol Surg Oncol 1989; 15(4):371–5.
167. McBurney EI, Rosen DA. Carbon dioxide laser treatment of verrucae vulgares. J Dermatol Surg Oncol 1984; 10(1):45–8.
168. Tosti A, Piraccini BM. Warts of the nail unit: surgical and nonsurgical approaches. Dermatol Surg 2001; 27(3):235–9.
169. Wollina U, Konrad H, Karamfilov T. Treatment of common warts and actinic keratoses by Er:YAG laser. J Cutan Laser Ther 2001; 3(2):63–6.
170. Ferenczy A, Mitao M, Nagai N et al. Latent papillomavirus and recurring genital warts. N Engl J Med 1985; 313:784–8.
171. Bergbrant IM, Samuelsson L, Olofsson S et al. Polymerase chain reaction for monitoring human papillomavirus contamination of medical personnel during treatment of genital warts with CO_2 laser and electrocoagulation. Acta Derm Venereol 1994; 74:393–395.
172. Carden JM, O'Banion K, Shelnitz LS et al. Papillomavirus in the vapor of carbon dioxide laser-treated verrucae. JAMA 1988; 259:1199–1202.
173. Abramson AL, DiLorenzo TP, Steinberg BM. Is papillomavirus detectable in the plume of laser-treated laryngeal papilloma? Arch Otolaryngol Head Neck Surg 1990; 116(5):604–7.
174. Ferenczy A, Bergeron C, Richart RM. Human papillomavirus DNA in CO_2 laser-generated plume of smoke and its consequences to the surgeon. Obstet Gynecol 1990; 75(1):114–18.
175. Jenson AB, Sommer S, Payling-Wright C et al. Human papillomavirus. Frequency and distribution in plantar and common warts. Lab Invest 1982; 47(5):491–7.
176. Laurent R, Kienzler JL, Croissant O et al. Two anatomoclinical types of warts with plantar localization: specific cytopathogenic effects of papillomavirus. Type I (HPV-1) and type 2 (HPV-2). Arch Dermatol Res 1982; 274(1–2):101–11.
177. Don PC, Carney PS, Lynch WS et al. Carbon dioxide laserabrasion: A new approach to management of familial benign chronic pemphigus (Hailey–Hailey disease). J Dermatol Surg Oncol 1987; 13:1187–94.
178. Sood S, Hruza GJ. Treatment of verrucae vulgaris and condyloma acuminatum with lasers. Dermatol Ther 2000; 90:101.
179. Kaspari M, Gutzmer R, Kaspari T, Kapp A, Brodersen JP. Application of imiquimod by suppositories (anal tampons) efficiently prevents recurrences after ablation of anal condyloma. Br J Dermatol 2002; 63:757–759.
180. Gloster HM, Roenigk RK. Risk of acquiring human papillomavirus from the plume produced by the carbon dioxide laser in the treatment of warts. J Am Acad Dermatol 1995; 32:436.
181. Jiang SB, Levine VJ, Nehal KS et al. The effect of carbon dioxide laser surgery on the recurrence of keloids. Plast Reconstr Surg 1991; 87(1):44–9.
182. Thomas I, Kihiczak NI, Rothenberg J, Ahmed S, Schwartz RA. Melanoma within the seborrheic keratosis. Dermatol Surg 2004; 30:559–61.
183. Ratz JL. Carbon dioxide laser treatment of balanitis xerotica obliterans. J Am Acad Dermatol 1984; 10:925–8.
184. Merkle T, Hohenleutner U, Braun FO et al. Reticulate porokeratosis-successful treatment with CO_2 laser vaporization. Clin Exp Dermatol 1992; 17:178–81.
185. Taylor MB. Chondrodermatitis nodularis helicis: Successful treatment with the carbon dioxide laser. J Dermatol Surg Oncol 1991; 17:862–4.
186. Wheeland RG, Ashley JR, Smith DA et al. Carbon dioxide laser treatment of granuloma faciale. J Dermatol Surg Oncol 1984; 10(9):730–3.
187. Bain L, Geronemus R. The association of lichen planus of the penis with squamous cell carcinoma in situ and with verrucous squamous carcinoma. J Dermatol Surg Oncol 1989; 15(4):413–17.
188. Persky MS. Carbon dioxide laser treatment of oral florid papillomatosis. J Dermatol Surg Oncol 1984; 10(1):64–6.
189. Alora MB, Anderson RR, Quinn TR et al. CO_2 laser resurfacing of psoriatic plaques: a pilot study. Lasers Surg Med 1998; 22(3):165–70.
190. McElroy JA, Mehregan DA, Roenigk RK. Carbon dioxide laser vaporization of recalcitrant symptomatic plaques of Hailey–Hailey disease and Darier's disease. J Am Acad Dermatol 1990; 23:893–7.
191. Bekassy Z, Astedt B. Carbon dioxide laser vaporization of plaque psoriasis. Br J Dermatol 1986; 114(4):489–92.
192. Wheeland RG, Bailin PL, Kantor GR et al. Treatment of adenoma sebaceum with carbon dioxide laser vaporization. J Dermatol Surg Oncol 1985; 11:861–4.
193. Rosenbach A, Alster TS. Multiple trichoepitheliomas treated with a high-energy, pulsed carbon dioxide laser. Dermatol Surg 1997; 23:708–10.
194. Wheeland RG, Bailin PL, Kronberg E. Carbon dioxide (CO_2) laser vaporization for the treatment of multiple trichoepithelioma. J Dermatol Surg Oncol 1984; 10:470–5.
195. Apfelberg DB, Maser MR, Lash H et al. Superpulse CO_2 laser treatment of facial syringomata. Lasers Surg Med 1987; 7:533–7.
196. Bickley LK, Goldberg DJ, Imaeda S et al. Treatment of multiple apocrine hidrocystomas with the carbon dioxide (CO_2) laser. J Dermatol Surg Oncol 1989; 15:599–602.
197. Roenigk RK, Ratz JL. CO_2 laser treatment of cutaneous neurofibromas. J Dermatol Surg Oncol 1987; 13(2):187–90.
198. Huerter CJ, Wheeland RG, Bailin PL et al. Treatment of digital myxoid cysts with carbon dioxide laser vaporization. J Dermatol Surg Oncol 1987; 13(7):723–7.
199. Wheeland RG, McGillis ST. Cowden's disease – treatment of cutaneous lesions using carbon dioxide laser vaporization: a comparison of conventional and superpulsed techniques. J Dermatol Surg Oncol 1989; 15(10):1055–9.
200. Walther T, Hohenleutner U, Landthaler M. Sebaceous gland hyperplasia as a side effect of cyclosporin A. Treatment with the CO_2 laser. Dtsch Med Wochenschr 1998; 123(25–26): 798–800.
201. Jordan JA, Brown OE, Biavati MJ et al. Congenital syringocystadenoma papilliferum of the ear and neck treated with the CO_2 laser. Int J Pediatr Otorhinolaryngol 1996; 38(1): 81–7.
202. Alster TS, West TB. Ultrapulse CO_2 laser ablation of xanthelasma. J Am Acad Dermatol 1996; 34:848–9.
203. Neev J, Nelson JS, Critelli M et al. Ablation of human nail by pulsed lasers. Lasers Surg Med 1997; 21(2):186–92.
204. Leshin B, Whitaker DC. Carbon dioxide laser matricectomy. J Dermatol Surg Oncol 1988; 14(6):608–11.
205. Podda M, Spieth K, Kaufmann R. Er:YAG laser-assisted hair transplantation in cicatricial alopecia. Dermatol Surg 2000; 26(11):1010–14.
206. Eberlein A, Schepler H, Spilker G et al. Erbium:YAG laser treatment of post-burn scars: potentials and limitations. Burns 2005; 31(1):15–24.

207. Albertini JG, Holck DE, Farley MF. Zoon's balanitis treated with Erbium:YAG laser ablation. Lasers Surg Med 2002; 30(2):123–6.
208. Borelli C, Kaudewitz P. Xanthelasma palpebrarum: treatment with the erbium:YAG laser. Lasers Surg Med 2001; 29(3): 260–4.
209. Riedel F, Windberger J, Stein E. Treatment of peri-ocular skin lesions with the erbium:YAG laser. Ophthalmologe 1998; 95(11):771–5.
210. Kageyama N, Tope WD. Treatment of multiple eruptive hair cysts with erbium:YAG laser. Dermatol Surg 1999; 25(10): 819–22.
211. Ammirati CT, Giancola JM, Hruza GJ. Adult-onset facial colloid milium successfully treated with the long-pulsed Er:YAG laser. Dermatol Surg 2002; 28(3):215–19.
212. Dmovsek-Olup B, Vedlin B. Use of Er:YAG laser for benign skin disorders. Lasers Surg Med 1997; 21(1):13–19.
213. Ashinoff R, Levine VJ, Soter NA. Allergic reactions to tattoo pigment after laser treatment. Dermatol Surg 1995; 21: 291–4.
214. Chernoff G, Slatkine M, Zair E et al. Silk Touch. A new technology for skin resurfacing in aesthetic surgery. J Clin Laser Med Surg 1995; 13:97–100.
215. Ammirati CT, Cottingham TJ, Hruza GJ. Immediate postoperative laser resurfacing improves second intention healing on the nose. 5-year experience. Dermatol Surg 2001; 27:147–52.
216. Olbricht SM. Use of the carbon dioxide laser in dermatologic surgery. A clinically relevant update for 1993. J Dermatol Surg Oncol 1993; 19(4):364–9.
217. Lapins J, Marcusson JA, Emtestam L. Surgical treatment of chronic hidradenitis suppurativa: CO_2 laser stripping-secondary intention technique. Br J Dermatol 1994; 131(4):551–6.
218. Finley EM, Ratz JL. Treatment of hidradenitis suppurativa with carbon dioxide laser excision and second-intention healing. J Am Acad Dermatol 1996; 34(3):465–9.
219. Dalrymple JC, Monaghan JM. Treatment of hidradenitis suppurativa with the carbon dioxide laser. Br J Surg 1987; 74(5):420.
220. Kantor GR, Ratz JL, Wheeland RG. Treatment of acne keloidalis nuchae with carbon dioxide laser. J Am Acad Dermatol 1986; 14(2 Pt 1):263–7.
221. Glass LF, Berman B, Laub D. Treatment of perifolliculitis capitis abscedens et suffodiens with the carbon dioxide laser. J Dermatol Surg Oncol 1989; 15(6):673–6.
222. Hruza GJ. Laser treatment of epidermal and dermal lesions. Dermatol Clin 2002; 20:147–64.
223. Horlock N, Grobbelaar AO, Gault DT. Can the carbon dioxide laser completely ablate basal cell carcinomas? A histological study. Br J Plas Surg 2000; 53:286–293.
224. Wheeland RG, Bailin PL, Ratz JL et al. Carbon dioxide laser vaporization and curettage in the treatment of large or multiple superficial basal cell carcinomas. J Dermatol Surg Oncol 1987; 13(2):119–25.
225. Doctoroff A, Oberlender SA, Purcell SM. Full-face carbon dioxide laser resurfacing in the management of a patient with the nevoid basal cell carcinoma syndrome. Dermatol Surg 2003; 29(12):1236–40.
226. Humphreys TR, Malhotra R, Scharf MJ, Marcus SM, Starkus L, Calegari K. Treatment of superficial basal cell carcinoma and squamous cell carcinoma in situ with a high-energy pulsed carbon dioxide laser. Arch Dermatol 1998; 134:1247–52.
227. Fitzpatrick RE. The ultrapulse CO_2 laser: selective photothermolysis of epidermal tumors. Lasers Surg Med 1993; Suppl 5:56.
228. Wang KH, Fang JY, Hu CH. Erbium:YAG laser pretreatment accelerates the response of Bowen's disease treated by topical 5-fluorouracil. Dermatol Surg 2004; 30(3):441–5.
229. Van Bezooijen BPJ, Horenblas S, Meinhardt W, Newling DWW. Laser therapy for carcinoma in situ of the penis. J Urol 2001; 166:1670–71.
230. Greenbaum SS, Glogau R, Stegman SJ et al. Carbon dioxide laser treatment of erythroplasia of Queyrat. J Dermatol Surg Oncol 1989; 15(7):747–50.
231. Rosemberg SK. Carbon dioxide laser treatment of external genital lesions. Urology 1985; 25(6):555–8.
232. Rosemberg SK, Fuller TA. Carbon dioxide rapid superpulsed laser treatment of erythroplasia of Queyrat. Urology 1980; 16(2):181–2.
233. Blatstein LM, Finkelstein LH. Laser surgery for the treatment of squamous cell carcinoma of the penis. J Am Osteopath Assoc 1990; 90(4):338–44.
234. Rosemberg SK. Lasers and squamous cell carcinoma of external genitalia. Urology 1986; 27(5):430–3.
235. Boon TA. Sapphire probe laser surgery for localized carcinoma of the penis. Eur J Surg Oncol 1988; 14(2):193–5.
236. Malloy TR, Wein AJ, Carpiniello VL. Carcinoma of penis treated with neodymium YAG laser. Urology 1988; 31(1): 26–9.
237. Malek RS. Laser treatment of premalignant and malignant squamous cell lesions of the penis. Lasers Surg Med 1992; 12(3):246–53.
238. Baggish MS, Dorsey JH. CO_2 laser for the treatment of vulvar carcinoma in situ. Obstet Gynecol 1981; 57(3):371–5.
239. Townsend DE, Levine RU, Richart RM. Management of vulvar intraepithelial neoplasia by carbon dioxide laser. Obstet Gynecol 1982; 60(1):49–52.
240. Penna C, Fallani MG, Fambrini M et al. CO_2 laser surgery for vulvar intraepithelial neoplasia. Excisional, destructive and combined techniques. J Reprod Med 2002; 47(11):913–18.
241. Kopera D. Treatment of lentigo maligna with the carbon dioxide laser. Arch Dermatol 1995; 131(6):735–6.
242. Slutzki S, Shafir R, Bornstein LA. Use of the carbon dioxide laser for large excisions with minimal blood loss. Plast Reconstr Surg 1977; 60(2):250–5.
243. Kaplan I, Sharon U, Ger R. The carbon dioxide laser in clinical surgery. In Wolbarsht M, ed. Laser applications in medicine and biology, vol 2. New York: Plenum; 1974.
244. Apfelberg DB, Maser MR, Lash H et al. Benefits of the CO_2 laser in oral hemangioma excision. Plast Reconstr Surg 1985; 75(1):46–50.
245. Marsili M, Cockerell CJ, Lyde CB. Hemangioma-associated rhinophyma. Report of a case with successful treatment using carbon dioxide laser surgery. J Dermatol Surg Oncol 1993; 19(3):206–12.
246. Shafir R, Slutzki S, Bornstein LA. Excision of buccal hemangioma by carbon dioxide laser beam. Oral Surg 1977; 44(3):347–50.
247. Ohshiro T. The CO_2 laser in the treatment of cavernous haemangioma of the lower lip: a case report. Lasers Surg Med 1981; 1(4):337–45.
248. Aronoff BL. The use of lasers in hemangiomas. Lasers Surg Med 1981; 1(4):323–35.
249. Biesman B. Laser blepharoplasty. In: Dover JS, Arndt KA, Geronemus RG, Alora MBT, eds. Illustrated cutaneous and aesthetic laser surgery, 2nd edn. Stamford, CT: Appleton & Lange; 2000.

250. Hom DB. Treating the elusive keloid. Arch Otolaryngol Head Neck Surg 2001; 127(9):1140–3.
251. Stern JC, Lucente FE. Carbon dioxide laser excision of earlobe keloids. A prospective study and critical analysis of existing data. Arch Otolaryngol Head Neck Surg 1989; 115(9): 1107–11.
252. Alcalay, J. Cutaneous surgery in patients receiving warfarin therapy. Dermatol Surg 2001; 27(8):756–8.
253. Lowe NJ, Lask G, Griffin ME et al. Skin resurfacing with the Ultrapulse carbon dioxide laser. Observations on 100 patients. Dermatol Surg 1995; 21(12):1025–9.
254. Alster TS, Garg S. Treatment of facial rhytides with a high-energy pulsed carbon dioxide laser. Plast Reconstr Surg 1996; 98(5):791–4.
255. Alster TS, West TB. Resurfacing of atrophic facial acne scars with a high-energy, pulsed carbon dioxide laser. Dermatol Surg 1996; 22(2):151–4.
256. Bernstein LJ, Kauvar AN, Grossman MC et al. The short- and long-term side effects of carbon dioxide laser resurfacing. Dermatol Surg 1997; 23(7):519–25.
257. Fitzpatrick RE, Goldman MP, Satur NM et al. Pulsed carbon dioxide laser resurfacing of photo-aged facial skin. Arch Dermatol 1996; 132(4):395–402.
258. Manuskiatti W, Fitzpatrick RE, Goldman MP et al. Prophylactic antibiotics in patients undergoing laser resurfacing of the skin. J Am Acad Dermatol 1999; 40(1):77–84.
259. Conn H, Nanda VS. Prophylactic fluconazole promotes reepithelialization in full-face carbon dioxide laser skin resurfacing. Lasers Surg Med 2000; 26(2):201–7.

Chapter 7

Skin Resurfacing with Ablative Lasers

Alex S. Carcamo and Mitchel P. Goldman

Introduction

Interest has surrounded facial rejuvenation for centuries. The use of topical agents such as soured milk, vegetable extracts, and mud packs has been documented in ancient civilizations. However, only in the last decade has rejuvenation been approached from a scientific basis. With the aging of the American population, particularly those 76 million individuals referred to as the 'baby boomers' turning age 50, much attention has been focused on 'anti-aging' therapies. In particular, the use of retinoic acid, alpha-hydroxy acids, and antioxidants in conjunction with sunscreens and sunblocks has been investigated to prevent or reverse the photoaging process. Although these agents may have significant benefit, they generally fall short of the clinical expectations of those using them as a primary rejuvenation treatment.

To achieve a more dramatic clinical endpoint, a variety of chemical agents have been used to induce a layer of necrosis of variable depths, effectively peeling away the outermost layer of sun-damaged skin, with subsequent dermal healing and reepithelialization resulting in a more youthful appearance. Similar results have been achieved by mechanically removing these outer layers with dermabrasion.

Ablative laser resurfacing of photodamaged skin has rapidly become the treatment of choice for rejuvenation of photoaging facial skin. This chapter details the use of the carbon dioxide (CO_2) and the erbium:yttrium-aluminum-garnet (Er:YAG) lasers to rejuvenate the skin.

Overview of the Clinical Literature on Skin Resurfacing with Ablative Lasers

Over a decade of clinical literature has established the ablative resurfacing lasers as effective, safe and versatile tools for rejuvenation of photodamaged skin. The CO_2 laser, which produces infrared light with a 10,600 nm wavelength, was the first resurfacing laser to be utilized for cutaneous resurfacing. Given that water represents 70% of the total volume of the skin and the CO_2 laser's wavelength is strongly absorbed by water, this laser was initially considered an ideal tool for superficial ablation of the skin. However, early on the CO_2 laser was used in a continuous wave mode with a tissue-dwell time that was well above the thermal relaxation time of the superficial skin (1 ms). This resulted in the generation of excessive nonspecific thermal damage, which clinically translated into high rates of scarring and pigmentary disturbances.[1] The disappointing experience with the continuous wave (CW) CO_2 laser in the 1980s resulted in a subsequent loss of interest in laser technology for cutaneous resurfacing.

However, important research over the following 10 years led to increased knowledge of the laser–tissue interaction and the mechanisms of rhytid ablation culminating in the development of a new generation of improved resurfacing lasers. The early 1990s marked the arrival of a new generation of CO_2 lasers that more closely implemented the principles of selective photothermolysis[2] by delivering peak fluences above the ablation threshold of cutaneous tissue (5 J/cm^2) with tissue-dwell times that were shorter than the 1-ms thermal relaxation time of the epidermis. These new-generation CO_2 lasers limited tissue-dwell time either by shortening the pulse duration, e.g. UltraPulse (Coherent – now Lumenis, Inc., – Santa Clara, CA) or by using scanning technology to rapidly sweep a continuous wave CO_2 laser beam over the tissue such that the laser beam did not remain in contact with any particular spot on the tissue for longer than 1 ms, e.g. SilkTouch (Sharplan Laser Corporation – now Lumenis Inc., – Santa Clara, CA). These high-peak-power, short pulsed and rapidly scanned CO_2 laser systems made it possible for laser surgeons to precisely and effectively ablate 20–30 µm of skin per pass, leaving behind a considerably smaller residual zone of thermal damage (up to 150 µm) than left behind by the previous generation of continuous wave CO_2 lasers (up to 600 µm).[2] Clinically, this technological advancement translated into superior clinical results and a much more favorable safety profile than seen previously with the continuous wave CO_2 lasers.

Given the impressive clinical results achieved with the high-peak-power, short pulsed and rapidly scanned focused-beam CO_2 lasers, they quickly replaced chemical peels and dermabrasion as the treatment of choice for cutaneous resurfacing. However, the impressive results achieved with these new-generation CO_2 lasers were not without drawbacks. Adverse sequelae such as delayed hypopigmentation and prolonged erythema occurred.[3–5] These side effects, as well as the significant 'downtime' typically associated with CO_2 laser resurfacing, were not acceptable to many patients and significantly dampened the initial enthusiasm associated with their use.

As the CO_2 laser typically operates near its tissue ablation threshold (5 J/cm^2) in most resurfacing applications, a large fraction of its energy is invested in heating rather than ablating tissue.[6] Consequently, the CO_2 laser produces relatively large residual thermal damage zones and causes significant dessication of the target tissue after only a few passes. With each subsequent pass the amount of vaporized tissue decreases while thermal damage increases and a 'plateau' of ablation is typically reached after the fourth pass. Nonspecific thermal damage has a negative impact not only on the CO_2 laser's ablative capacity, but also on its side effect profile. Our research suggests that the relatively large thermally induced residual zone of necrosis (up to 150 µm) left behind by the CO_2 laser is one of the main factors contributing to its adverse sequelae including prolonged erythema, postoperative pain, delayed healing, infection and scarring.

Given the complications encountered with CO_2 laser resurfacing, clinicians began looking for an alternative resurfacing laser. Ideally, this would be a laser system capable of carrying out considerably greater ablation with a significantly reduced residual zone of nonspecific thermal damage. The arrival of the erbium:yttrium-aluminum-garnet (Er:YAG) laser in the mid 1990s made available to clinicians a laser system which successfully met both of these 'ideal' criteria.

With a wavelength of 2940 nm (near-infrared light) and a coefficient of absorption for water that is 16 times greater than that of the CO_2 laser,[7] the energy absorbed by the Er:YAG laser is in a much thinner layer of tissue (1 µm) than the CO_2 laser's irradiation. Its greater affinity for water (16 times greater than that of the CO_2 laser) allows the Er:YAG laser to carry out precise and efficient ablation of tissue with very little scattering of the laser beam and minimal residual thermal damage. Short pulsed (350 µs) Er:YAG lasers reliably ablate 5 to 15 µm of tissue per pass at a fluence of 5 J/cm^2, producing a residual zone of thermal damage not exceeding 15 µm.[5,8] In contrast, the CO_2 laser produces 20 to 60 µm of tissue ablation and up to 150 µm of residual thermal damage per pass.[9] Moreover, given the limited zone of residual thermal damage produced by the Er:YAG laser, tissue desiccation does not significantly increase with each subsequent pass and the ablation 'plateau' characteristic of CO_2 laser resurfacing is not reached.[10] Its minimal optical penetration depth and limited zone of residual thermal damage endow the Er:YAG laser with superior capacity for efficient, precise and controlled tissue ablation. This has translated clinically into faster recovery times and a significantly more favorable side effect profile than seen after CO_2 laser skin resurfacing.[2,6,11–13] Additionally, the Er:YAG laser's capacity to confine ablation superficially, has significantly reduced anesthesia requirements and anesthesia-related complications associated with laser skin resurfacing.

Because of its greater safety margin, the Er:YAG laser has proven advantageous for resurfacing of nonfacial skin (i.e. neck, forearms, hands) that, given its relative lack of adnexae and its tendency toward slower healing, is considered by most experts to be 'off-limits' to CO_2 laser treatment.[14,15] Additionally, patients with darker Fitzpatrick skin phototypes (III and above) who experience a high rate of pigmentary alteration following CO_2 laser resurfacing,[5,16–18] have been effectively treated with the Er:YAG laser with a considerably lower incidence of postoperative pigmentary alterations.[2]

Given its advantages, it was initially postulated that the short pulsed Er:YAG would completely replace the CO_2 laser as a resurfacing tool. However, this initial enthusiasm was tempered by the realization that resurfacing with the Er:YAG laser was hindered by poor intraoperative hemostasis, which limited ablation depth, and by the Er:YAG's limited ability to effect significant tissue shrinkage, both of which translated into clinical results that were considerably less impressive than those previously achieved with the CO_2 laser.[11,19–24]

Many experts believed that the comparatively superior results achieved with the CO_2 laser were due to thermally induced tissue changes. A number of studies showed that treatment with the CO_2 laser led to heating of dermal collagen, collagen contraction and reactive dermal neocollagen synthesis. Immediate tissue contraction of 25%–40% was reported during CO_2 laser resurfacing.[25] In contrast, early studies failed to show significant tissue contraction with short pulsed Er:YAG laser skin resurfacing.

With the thought that thermally induced tissue contraction was important for long-term laser resurfacing results, 'modulated' Er:YAG lasers combining the precise ablation capability of the short pulsed Er:YAG laser with a 'CO_2-like' coagulative effect were introduced.[21] Modulated Er:YAG lasers have demonstrated clinical efficacy comparable to that of the short pulse CO_2 laser in a number of studies.[21,26,27] Moreover, studies have demonstrated faster reepithelialization and recovery times and significantly lower incidence of postoperative complications after modulated Er:YAG laser skin resurfacing as compared to CO_2 laser skin resurfacing. Modulated Er:YAG lasers have achieved good to excellent improvement of class III and above rhytides with a side effect profile and convalescence time that is somewhere between that of the CO_2 and short pulse Er:YAG lasers.[28–30] The modulated Er:YAG lasers have given cosmetic surgeons a true alternative to CO_2 laser resurfacing.

Modifications of technical protocols have continued to improve clinical outcomes. Combination therapy with the CO_2 and Er:YAG lasers allows cosmetic surgeons to capitalize on the unique benefits of each laser system and to minimize their disadvantages. Erbium:YAG laser treatment can be used to bypass the ablation 'plateau' characteristic of CO_2 resurfacing. Improved postoperative healing can be attained when the short pulsed Er:YAG laser is used to remove the residual zone of thermal necrosis left behind after CO_2 resurfacing.[31,32] A similar benefit on healing can be derived with the modulated Er:YAG lasers if resurfacing with their 'CO_2-like' long pulse is followed by treatment with their short pulse Er:YAG mode.

Additionally, the ablative lasers have turned out to be extremely versatile therapeutic tools. Cosmetic surgeons now regularly combine ablative laser resurfacing with other problem-specific nonablative technologies to address multiple cosmetic concerns for the patient in a single treatment session. The efficacy of Q-switched lasers in the treatment of pigmented lesions is enhanced when these lasers are utilized after ablative resurfacing. Treatment of vascular lesions with the pulsed dye laser or other vascular lasers has been shown to be extremely successful when performed prior to skin resurfacing with an ablative laser.[33] Despite early reports advising against it,[34–36] full-face laser resurfacing is now safely being combined with rhytidectomy to achieve a more comprehensive approach to facial rejuvenation. Large series of patients treated with the combination of rhytidectomy and laser skin resurfacing have reported complication rates that are no greater than those typically seen with either treatment modality alone.[37–39]

Given its capability to produce precise depths of ablation with minimal residual thermal damage, the Er:YAG laser has proven particularly advantageous in cutaneous resurfacing of face-lift flaps with potentially compromised vascular supply. Combination therapy is helping cosmetic surgeons achieve results that are superior to those attainable with either treatment modality alone. Additionally, by reducing cost and convalescence time, combination therapy is making cosmetic surgery more appealing to a number of patients.

Pretreatment and posttreatment protocols have improved as well. Although some controversy remains surrounding the topic of antibiotic prophylaxis, a number of studies in the last decade have provided relevant information on common pathogens, effective antibiotic prophylaxis regimens and clinical situations at increased risk for infection after cutaneous laser resurfacing.[40–45] Improved laser wound care regimens have reduced recovery time and decrease morbidity after laser skin resurfacing. The benefits of occlusive dressings in accelerating laser wound healing have been well established in a number of studies.[40,42,46–50] Timely institution of medications in the postoperative period is now allowing surgeons to effectively address a number of expected postoperative symptoms and complications including postoperative erythema and edema, pruritus and postinflammatory hyperpigmentation.[51,52]

In the last decade, considerable progress has also been made in the treatment of the adverse sequelae of laser skin resurfacing. Topical photochemotherapy and excimer laser therapy are now available options for the treatment of delayed onset hypopigmentation.[53,54]

A decade of improved clinical outcomes and lower rates of complications have resulted in a considerable increase in the utilization of resurfacing lasers by dermatologic, cosmetic and plastic surgeons alike. Moreover, patient satisfaction with laser skin resurfacing remains high. A recent prospective study surveyed patients 30 months after laser skin resurfacing and found that 88% of these patients felt their appearance had improved, 75% of them would recommend the procedure and 71% of them would undergo laser skin resurfacing again.[55]

Given its wide acceptance among cosmetic surgeons and its high patient satisfaction ratings, laser skin resurfacing is likely here to stay. Newer technologies which may further enhance results, minimize downtime and make laser skin resurfacing a viable treatment option for a greater number of patients are already on the horizon. One of these new technologies, the FRAXEL laser (Reliant Technologies, Palo Alto, CA), implements the concepts of fractional photothermolysis allowing increased collagen production with a decrease in epidermal damage and faster healing.[56] This chapter will summarize our 15+ years experience with laser resurfacing.

The CO_2 Laser

Although physicians showed considerable interest in development of resurfacing parameters with the CO_2 laser in the early to middle 1980s, the safety profile for use of the CW CO_2 laser prohibited its use in this manner. Successful low-fluence CW CO_2 laser removal of the epidermis was reported[57,58] as well as revision of skin grafts[59] and treatment of acne scars[60] in 1985–1991. However, this technique was found to be too risky to use over large surface areas because it has too high a risk of scarring. These treatment techniques can be traced back to Leon Goldman's report of treatment of actinic cheilitis with the CO_2 laser in 1968.[61] This treatment technique, however, was not widely used for this condition until popularized by David's report of a series of patients in 1985.[62]

The more limited use of the CO_2 laser in combination with trichloroacetic acid (TCA) peeling was reported first by Brauner and Schliftman[63] in 1987 and by David et al[64] in 1989 for the treatment of wrinkling.

CO_2 Laser Development

The development of superpulsed CO_2 lasers, in conjunction with Anderson and Parrish's development of the theory of selective photothermolysis[65] and work being done on burn debridement, allowed the potential for defining the necessary laser parameters for skin resurfacing. Work done by our group[66–71] plus critical information obtained by Green et al[72–74] led to the realization that cutaneous resurfacing could be accomplished with a high-energy, pulsed CO_2 laser. From 1988 to 1991, however, no laser manufacturer showed interest in developing such a CO_2 laser for this purpose. Fortunately, however, Coherent had developed such a laser for ear–nose–throat and gynecologic use. This laser was poorly received in these fields and was about to be withdrawn from production when we approached Coherent with our proposal.[75]

Working with Dale Koop of Coherent, Richard Fitzpatrick modified this laser for resurfacing by developing a collimated handpiece, increasing the pulse energy to 500 mJ, enlarging the spot size to 3 mm, and developing a computer pattern generator (CPG) to standardize the placement of laser impacts on the skin surface. A protocol involving treatment with single-pulse vaporization was developed and involved single-impact passes with approximately 10%–20% spot overlap of a gaussian beam and wiping away desiccated tissue debris between passes.

Initially the laser was used in treatment of various cutaneous lesions, as traditionally performed with CW or superpulsed CO_2 lasers, to understand the potential limitations or complications of the laser. At the same time, a histologic study was performed on a porcine model to explore the wound depths and healing characteristics in comparison to commonly used resurfacing modalities.[76] Relatively predictable depths of injury, ranging from intraepidermal to 350 μm, could be produced by varying the pulse energy and the number of laser passes (Fig. 7.1).

Weinstein[3] reported the first series of patients treated with the high-energy, pulsed CO_2 laser for cosmetic benefit. She reported 36 patients who had upper and lower lid laser blepharoplasty in conjunction with periorbital resurfacing. Excellent results (complete eradication of static periocular lines) were seen in 81%; reepithelialization required 8.4 days on average and erythema took 4.7 weeks to fade. One patient had transient scarring, one had transient ectropion, and three had mild hypopigmentation. Lowe et al[4] reported that 100 patients had been successfully treated and that gradual improvement was seen over the first 6 months postoperatively, with average improvement being 4.17 on a scale of 6.0 (maximum). The initial use of the laser was confined to the perioral and periorbital regions, because these areas were most difficult to treat by traditional methods. Improvement in pretreatment photodamage by approximately 50% or more was reported by our group[77] (Fig. 7.2). It became apparent that full-face resurfacing was possible and resulted in even better cosmetic improvement.

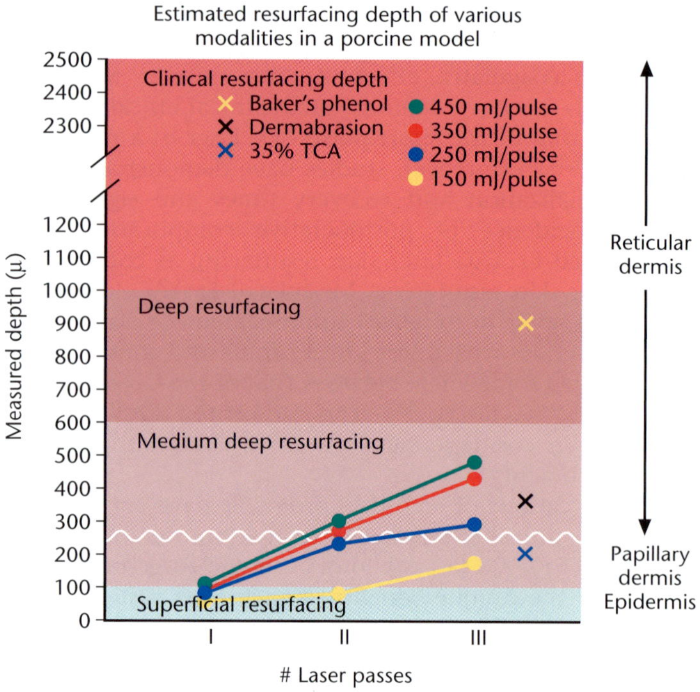

Figure 7.1 Varying pulse energies and passes of UltraPulse CO_2 laser resulted in resurfacing depths comparable to those of trichloroacetic acid (TCA) peels or dermabrasion, but not those of phenol peels.

The SilkTouch scanning system (Sharplan Laser Corp., Allendale, NJ) was developed around the same time and used for ablative rectal surgery,[78] laser uvuloplasty[79] in the management of obstructive sleep apnea, and hair transplantation.[80] This laser system was also being evaluated in a single pass for laser cutaneous resurfacing.[81] Our protocol of multiple single passes with wiping between passes was adapted for this system as well. The first clinical series reports appeared in 1995.[82,83]

The first reports of 47 patients and 40 patients showed an average improvement of greater than 50% and 3.5 on a scale of 6.0.[82,83] Erythema was seen to last 1 to 4 months[82] or averaged 6 weeks.[83] Persistent erythema was seen to correlate with depth of ablation. Postinflammatory hyperpigmentation was the most common complication, occurring in 17%, exclusively in patients with skin types III or IV. Bacterial infections occurred in 6%, with herpes simplex disseminating in one patient.[82]

A third laser, the SurgiPulse XJ150 (Sharplan) uses two paried 200-mJ energy peaks rather than a single 500-mJ peak as seen with the Coherent UltraPulse CO_2 laser. With a peak energy of 200 mJ, very little energy actually exceeds the critical irradiance required for tissue vaporization. Because of this, an increased number of laser passes was found to be necessary for treatment, and a 63% mean average improvement was seen, compared with 82% mean improvement after UltraPulse laser treatment.[84]

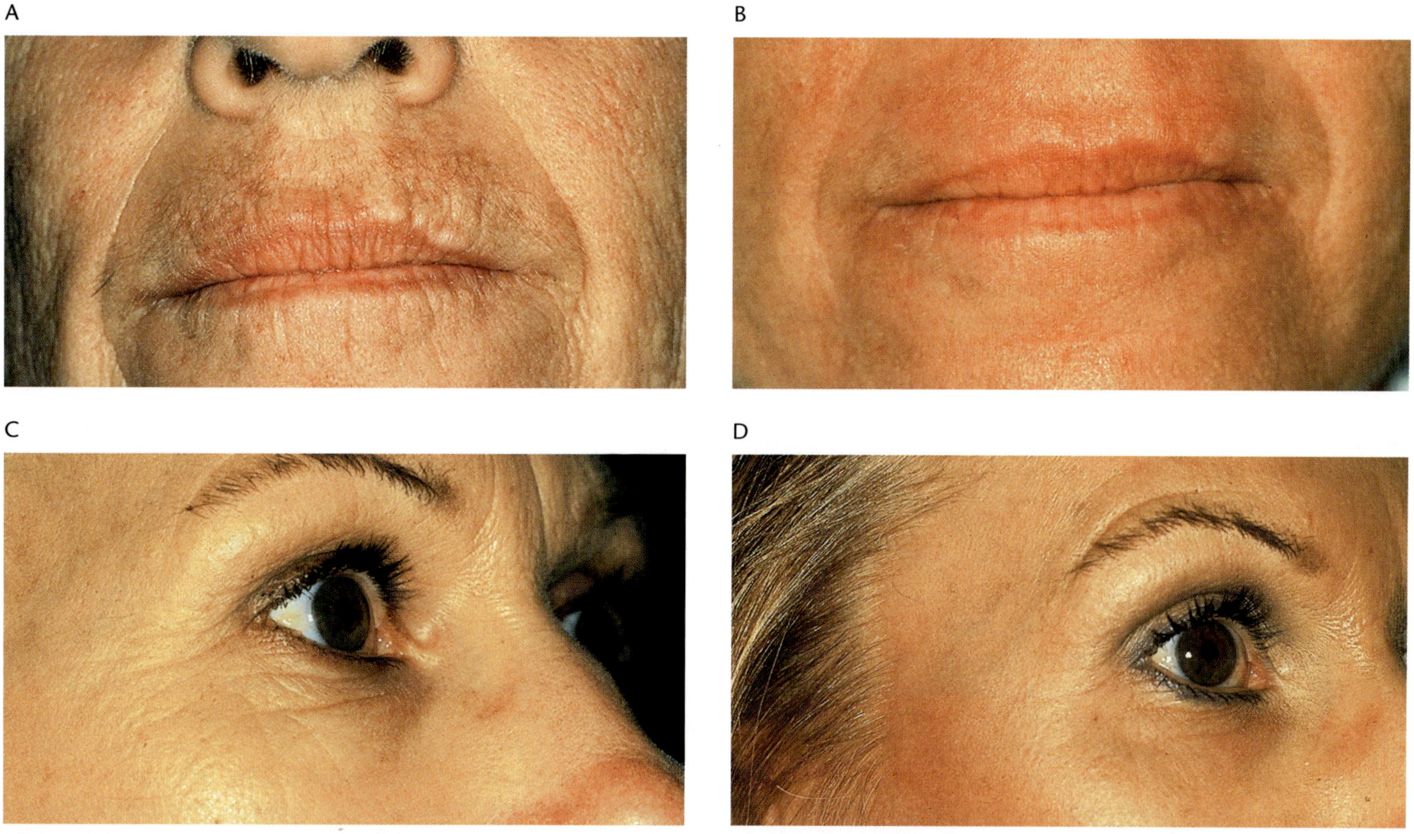

Figure 7.2 Significant perioral photodamage (class III, level 7) (A) before treatment; (B) 6 months postoperatively, dramatic improvement, with photodamage now rated class I, level 2; (C) periorbital photodamage (class II, level 6) before treatment; (D) 9 months postoperatively, significant improvement, with photodamage now rated class I, level 3.

These recent advances in high-energy, pulsed CO_2 lasers, combined with the development of safe and effective treatment protocols, have resulted in an explosion of interest, promotion, and use of these lasers for rejuvenation of facial photodamage.[3,4,77,81–94]

Advantages of the Pulsed CO_2 Laser

The potential advantages of pulsed-laser cutaneous resurfacing relate to the precise control of tissue vaporization, minimization of residual thermal damage, and achievement of hemostasis. These advantages are achieved by single-pulse vaporization of tissue using a high-energy, submillisecond, pulsed CO_2 laser. The CO_2 wavelength (10,600 nm) is efficiently absorbed in water, resulting in an optical penetration depth of 20 to 30 μm.[73,74,95] The absorption coefficient (μ_a) of water at 10.6 μm is approximately 790 cm − 1 and in tissue 553 cm − 1 (790 cm − 1 × 70%, assuming water content of tissue to be 70%).[95] Each pulse exposure should remove about one optical penetration depth (20–30 μm) of tissue and leave two to four times that (40–120 μm) of residual thermal damage. In cutaneous applications, intracellular water is the laser's target, and on absorption, heat transfer results in instantaneous tissue heating to greater than 100°C boiling of water and its vaporization and cellular ablation. If this energy is delivered with a continuous beam, the tissue becomes progressively desiccated, and because of loss of its water target, heat accumulates in tissue, reaching temperatures of up to 600°C. This results in diffusion of heat to several hundred micrometers below the level of vaporization.

A layer of thermal necrosis greater than 100 μm interferes with wound healing and may result in significant scarring when it extends deeper into the dermis.[70,96,97] To avoid this, the laser energy must be delivered rapidly, in less time than it takes the tissue to cool (estimated to be 1 ms or less).[65,70,73,74,76,98–114]

If the individual pulses do not deliver adequate energy to vaporize tissue, multiple pulses become necessary and complicate the situation because of heat diffusion between pulses.[70] Ideally, the tissue should be vaporized in a single pulse because this dissipates heat away from the treated tissue and does not allow significant heat diffusion to occur below the level of vaporization.

Delivery Systems and CO_2 Laser–Tissue Interactions

A study regarding the effects of pulse duration on the ablation threshold and residual thermal damage[102] revealed a number of significant findings regarding the laser–tissue interaction. These findings included the following: (1) that when tissue ablation occurs, the pulse duration is not critical because a rapid temperature drop occurs just below the ablation front;[103,106] (2) that residual thermal damage in this situation approaches a theoretic minimum of 50 µm;[103,105–108] and (3) that increases in pulse width cause increased thermal damage at the edges of craters resulting from a Gaussian beam. Also, an increase in the ablation threshold at longer pulse durations is related to thermal diffusion during the pulse. To confine thermal damage, the velocity of ablation is critical and requires a value of 0.65 cm or greater to achieve minimal thermal damage.

The ablation depth per pulse at 7.5 J/cm^2 was found to be 35 µm, too small to account for the clinical improvement seen in two or three passes of the CO_2 laser in treating wrinkles measuring 300 µm in depth. This aspect is discussed in greater detail later.

As an alternative to pulsed delivery, a CW CO_2 laser may be used with a scanning system that sweeps the beam across tissue rapidly enough that the tissue dwell time is less than the thermal relaxation time of the tissue, simulating the tissue effects of a pulsed delivery system.[4,82]

The laser beam may be delivered using a focused system, in which the beam is focused with lenses to a point having maximal fluence or irradiance. The distance from that focal point is a major determinant of tissue reaction, resulting in decreasing energies with increased handpiece-to-tissue distances. Alternatively, the beam may be delivered in a collimated manner, in which the beam is parallel and nondivergent, having the same fluence or irradiance independent of handpiece-to-tissue distances.

Although several new pulsed lasers were introduced in the mid-1990s, two laser systems have been used to pioneer this field and have generated virtually all the published data available: the UltraPulse laser (Coherent) and the SilkTouch scanner (Sharplan). The UltraPulse laser can deliver up to 500 mJ in a single pulse with a duration of less than 1 ms. This energy is delivered with a 3-mm collimated beam, generally used with 3 to 5 W resulting in a repetition rate of 6 to 10 Hz. Rapid, precise placement of these high-energy pulses ensuring single-pulse tissue interaction is achieved with a computer pattern generator (CPG),[109–112] using a 2.25-mm beam, 300 mJ per pulse, and a power of 60 W resulting in a placement of 81 pulses in one of six patterns at a rate of 220 Hz and with pulse densities varying from no overlap to 60% overlap (Fig. 7.3).

The Sharplan system uses a standard CW CO_2 beam focused to a 200-µm spot that is manipulated through rotating mirrors to scan tissue rapidly, resulting in a tissue dwell time of less than 1 ms. Scanning patterns of 4, 6, or 9 mm may be chosen.

In clinical use, two passes with the Sharplan SilkTouch systems appear to be approximately equal to three passes with the UltraPulse laser in terms of the amount of tissue removed and the depth of residual thermal necrosis.[113]

Experimental data and theoretic calculations reveal the necessary pulse fluence to vaporize epidermal tissue to be approximately 5 J/cm^2.[95] To utilize a large spot size and deliver a pulse less than 1 ms in achieving this threshold fluence, a very high irradiance is necessary. When a spot size of 2.5 mm is used, 250 mJ must be delivered in less than 1 ms.[70] This is generally delivered with a Gaussian beam, so a peripheral ring of about 10% may exist in which this threshold may not be reached. This suprathreshold energy will immediately vaporize intracellular water, leaving behind cellular proteinaceous debris. The depth of vaporization is proportional to the pulse energy. However, when the laser is interacting with the dermis, a new situation exists. Water is now primarily extracellular, in the dermal matrix, which is dominated by the structural proteins collagen and elastin. Type I collagen will melt at temperatures greater than 60°C but requires fluences much greater than 5 J/cm^2 for vaporization. Nonvaporization heating of the dermis will have little adverse effect as long as the pulse width is less than 1 ms and pulses are delivered to the same tissue spot at rates less than 5 Hz. If the delivery rate is greater than this, heat will accumulate between pulses, and thermal damage by diffusion may occur. This can result in poor wound healing or scarring.

CPG settings

	Face				Eyelids			
	Pulse energy	Pattern	Size	Density	Pulse energy	Pattern	Size	Density
1st pass	300 mJ	3	9	6	200 mJ	5	9	5
2nd pass	300 mJ	3	9	5	200 mJ	5	8	4
3rd pass	300 mJ	3	8	4	None			

Figure 7.3 Computer pattern generator (CPG) settings should not use densities greater than 6 if cumulative thermal damage from excessive pulse overlap is to be avoided.

Histologic studies have revealed a relationship between depth of ablation and pulse energy as well as the number of passes.[76,95,98–103,114] A comparision between the CO_2 laser used with various pulse energies and numbers of passes and TCA peeling, dermabrasion, and Baker's phenol peel on a porcine model showed that typical pulse energies at one to three passes produced a wound depth intermediate between a 35% TCA peel and dermabrasion, but much more superficial than a phenol peel.[76] Most histologic studies have shown the first CO_2 laser pass to result in epidermal ablation and subsequent passes to result in variable depths of dermal ablation and necrosis. The amount of residual thermal necrosis has also been shown to correlate with both pulse energy and number of passes, with each pass delivering the same amount of energy with less vaporization and more extensive heat absorption because of the layer of desiccated tissue at the treatment surface (Table 7.1 and Fig. 7.4).[76,98–101,103]

Published reports have correlated clinical signs with anatomic depths of ablation.[115] A pink color of tissue was found to correlate with superficial papillary dermis, chamois-cloth appearance for deeper papillary dermis, and waterlogged cotton-thread appearance for reticular dermis. We have found this to be true, but only in deep ablation, such as with treatment of plantar warts or basal cell carci-

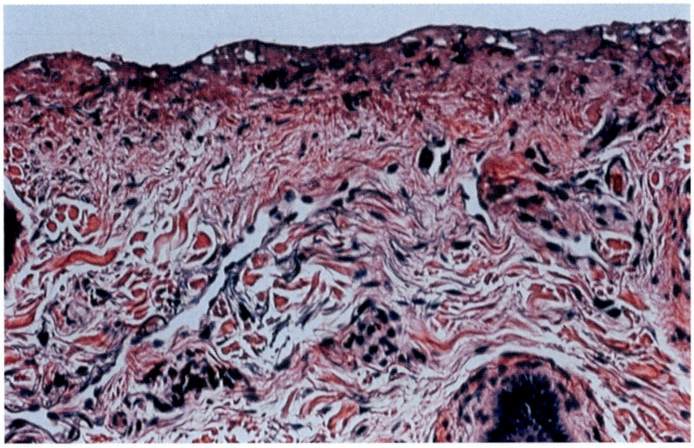

Figure 7.4 Residual thermal damage after two or three passes of UltraPulse CO_2 laser averages approximately 70 µm.

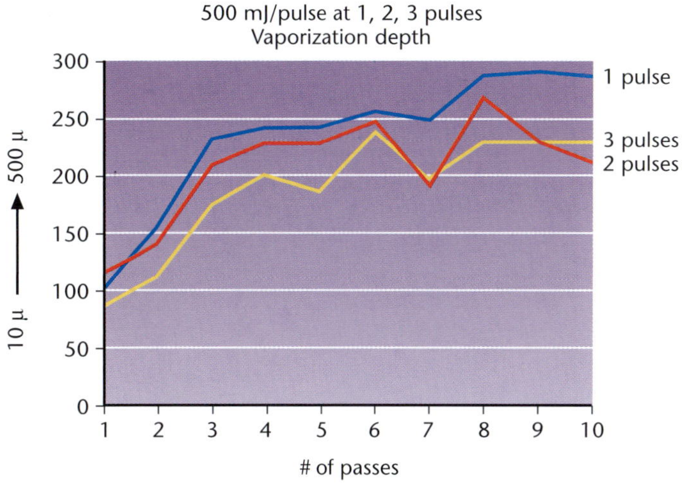

Figure 7.5 With pulsed CO_2 laser ablation, using one, two, or three pulses per impact site at 10 Hz, ablation plateau is reached in three to four passes, limiting ablation depth to approximately 250 µm.

Table 7.1 *Residual Thermal Necrosis with CO_2 Laser Treatment**

Laser passes	Area of necrosis (µm)
One	15.5 ± 7.0
Two	53.0 ± 21.2
Three	40.0 ± 21.7
Four	50.2 ± 26.4

Data from E. Bernstein, UltraPulse CO_2 Multicenter Clinical Trial.
*Pulse width less than 1 msec, fluence 7.1 J/cm^2.

noma (BCC) of the back. When thinner layers of ablation are used, as in resurfacing, these subtle clinical signs are not seen. Unfortunately, a second report that has received a tremendous amount of attention stated that color was an indication of depth of ablation: pink indicating epidermis, gray indicating papillary dermis, and chamois yellow indicating reticular dermis.[88] These color changes are actually a misinterpretation of anatomic changes and not a reliable indicator of tissue depth. If little residual thermal necrosis (less than 30 µm) exists, thermal reaction will not be sufficient to coagulate fine papillary vessels, and the tissue will be pink because of the visible capillary blood flow. This is typical of the appearance of the tissue after a single laser pass removing the epidermis. After a second or third laser pass, the laser is reacting with the dermis and leaves 70–100 µm of thermal necrosis, adequate for hemostasis and resulting in whitish gray tissue. Further laser passes tend to leave more thermal injury, resulting in progressive yellow-brown discoloration, which is a sign of thermal injury, not an indication of penetration into the reticular dermis.

These color changes probably do correlate to some degree with depth of injury, but many inexperienced physicians have interpreted this report too literally and spend much wasted time attempting to recognize subtle color changes, when attention to the laser–tissue interaction with better comprehension would be much more informative.

One study used posttreatment biopsies to compare three pulsed CO_2 lasers with a CW CO_2 laser. After one, two, and three passes, the depth of residual thermal damage measured 30, 80, and 150 µm, respectively, with the SilkTouch laser; 30, 100, and 150 µm with the SurgiPulse laser; and 20, 50, and 70 µm with the UltraPulse laser.[98] The CW CO_2 laser left a 400-µm layer of thermal necrosis.

Although early studies appeared to show a relatively constant amount of tissue to be ablated per pass[76] (approximately 75 µm), it became clear in clinical use that a decreasing amount of tissue was ablated per pass. To investigate this hypothesis, as well as the effects of single-pulse vaporization versus multipulse vaporization, or ‘pulse stacking’, and its possible relationship to scarring, a study on excised tissue was done.[116] Skin excised for ‘face-lift’ surgery was treated with one through ten passes, wiping with saline between passes and using single-pulse, double-pulse, and triple-pulse impacts at 10 Hz on the same impact site. Biopsies were done to study the depth of ablation as well as residual thermal necrosis. Whether single, double, or triple pulses were used at either 250 mJ or 500 mJ per pulse, a similar curve was generated showing that an ablation plateau was reached after three or four passes at 225 to 250 µm in the dermis (Fig. 7.5).

Residual thermal necrosis showed a linear relationship to both pulse energy and number of passes, with single-pulse vaporization gradually increasing to a maximum of 100 µm at pass number seven. However, pulse stacking had a marked impact on residual thermal necrosis, because double pulses added significantly more thermal injury per pass and triple pulses even more per pass, about 30 µm (Fig. 7.6). This additional thermal injury may significantly affect wound healing and result in a much deeper wound than intended. Pulse stacking may occur intentionally by concentrating repeated laser impacts on the same tissue site or

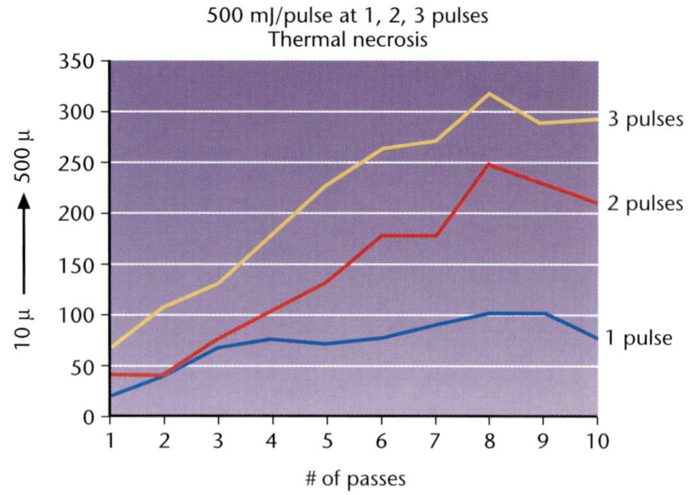

Figure 7.6 When multiple pulses impact same site at 10 Hz (double or triple sets), a cumulative thermal effect occurs resulting in increasing loss of control of residual thermal necrosis. Single tissue impacts, however, result in excellent control of residual thermal damage, even after 10 laser passes.

Average fluence

Density	Overlap	Average fluence (J/cm^2)					
1	–10%	2.4	3.3	4.1	4.9	6.5	8.2
2	0%	3.0	4.0	4.9	5.9	7.9	9.9
3	10%	3.7	4.9	6.1	7.3	9.8	12.2
4	20%	4.6	6.2	7.7	9.3	12.3	15.4
5	30%	6.0	8.1	10.1	12.1	16.1	20.2
6	35%	7.0	9.4	11.7	14.0	18.7	23.4
7	40%	8.2	11.0	13.7	16.5	21.9	27.4
8	50%	11.9	15.8	19.8	23.7	31.6	39.5
9	60%	18.5	24.7	30.9	37.0	49.4	61.7
Pulse energy		150 mJ	200 mJ	250 mJ	300 mJ	400 mJ	500 mJ

Figure 7.7 Most effective fluences for treatment are 5 to 18 J/cm^2, corresponding to green and yellow zones of this chart. CPG settings of 9 can result in a fluence as high as 60 J/cm^2.

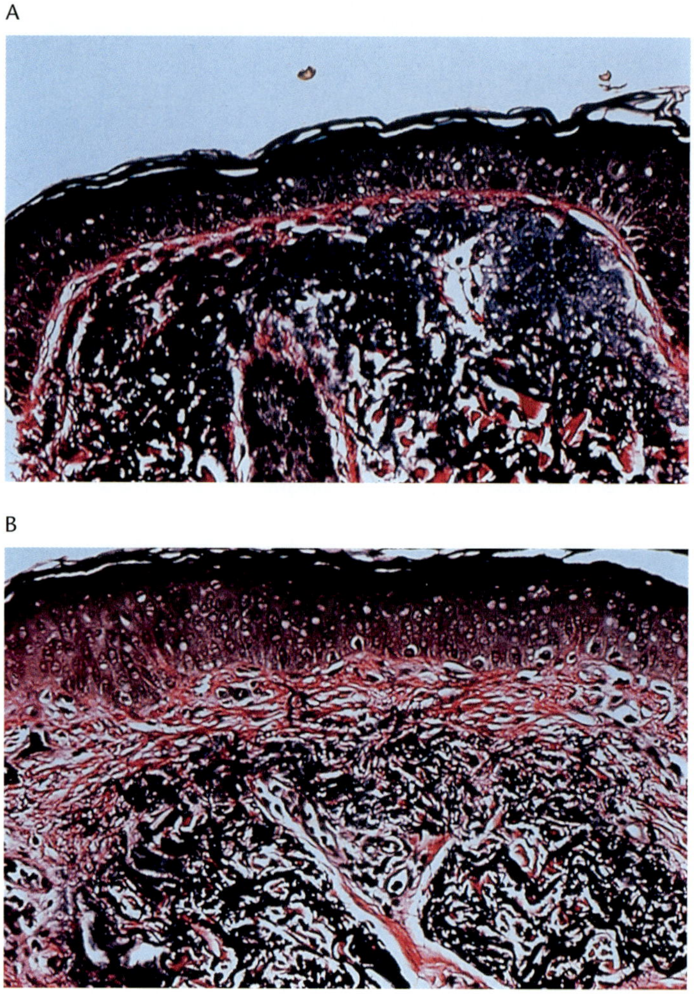

Figure 7.8 (A) Before treatment. (B) Using elastic tissue stains, a 600% increase in Grenz zone is noted 90 days after resurfacing, indicating new collagen formation. In addition, layer of solar elastosis is reduced.

unintentionally by moving the handpiece at too slow a pace or by using a CPG density that results in too much pulse overlap (densities 7, 8, and 9) corresponding to 40%, 50%, and 60% overlap. This may be a significant factor in causing scarring, hypopigmentation, or poor wound healing (Fig. 7.7).

Another finding from this study is that in using single-pulse vaporization with a fluence of 3–7 J/cm^2 and a pulse width of less than 1 ms, CO_2 laser resurfacing is a self-limiting procedure, plateauing at a depth of 250–300 μm in the dermis, too superficial a wound to result in scarring because of depth alone. Therefore adherence to proper treatment techniques is critical in avoiding excessive thermal injury.

Previous histologic studies of dermabraded skin revealed a new, orderly epidermis overlying an upper papillary dermal band of new collagen or 'scar'. Similar results (increased collagen I formation in the papillary dermis) have been reported after 10 months of treatment with topical tretinoin for photoaged skin. Biopsy specimens obtained at baseline and 3 and 12 weeks after dermabrasion were analyzed and correlated with clinical assessment.[117] Clinical reduction in wrinkling correlated significantly with an increase in fibroblast procollagen-1 in RNA and an increase in procollagen-1 protein, suggesting that clinical improvement may be a result of increased collagen synthesis. Similar increases in Grenz zone collagen have been reported after laser resurfacing,[99,100,104] which we have found as well.[118] This new collagen production and remodeling may be a significant factor in achieving rejuvenation of facial photodamage, as well as in improvement in atrophic acne scars (Fig. 7.8). Continued improvement in facial wrinkling has been noted to occur for as long as 6 months postoperatively and in acne scars for 12 months or more. Long-term biopsies (up to 4 years postoperatively) have shown reversal of epidermal dysplasia, maintenance and continued thickening of the Grenz zone, and marked improvement in the layer of solar elastosis underlying the Grenz zone, with reduction in overall depth and development of a more fibrillar character (Figs 7.9 and 7.10).

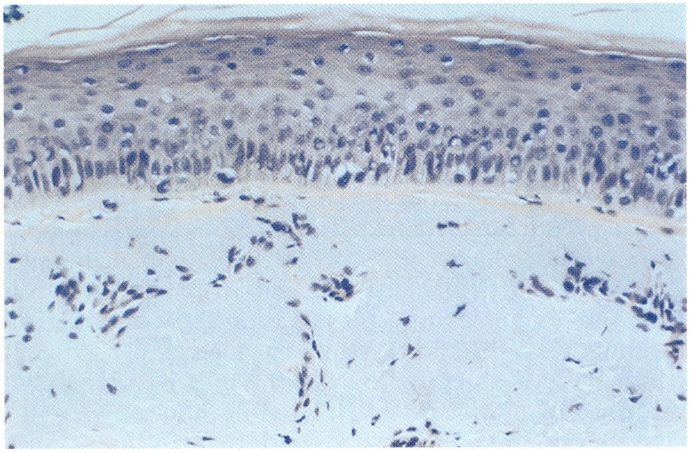

Figure 7.9 Ultraviolet (UV) light damage to skin results in epidermal atrophy and flattening of rete ridges with development of precancerous and cancerous epidermal cells. Amorphous elastotic material (solar elastosis) replaces normal collagen and elastin. Capillaries become reduced in number with thin fragile walls.

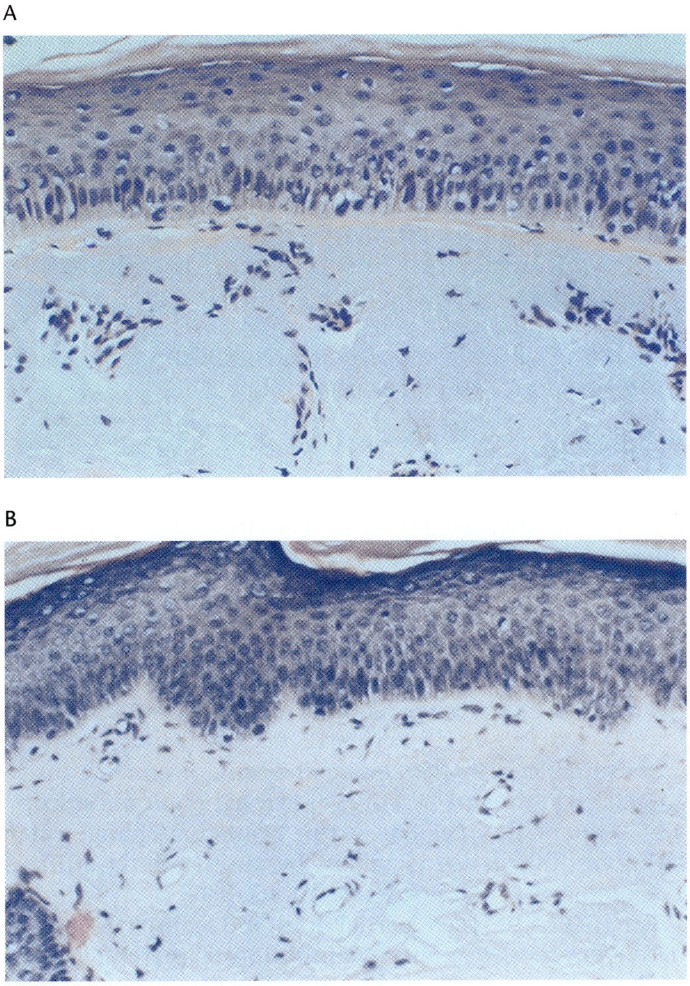

Figure 7.10 Long-term biopsies (2 years or more postoperatively) have demonstrated normalization of epidermis, continued gradual thickening of Grenz zone, and reduction of solar elastosis. In addition, solar elastosis was found to become progressively less homogenous and amorphous with much greater fibrillar content (see also Figure 7.9).

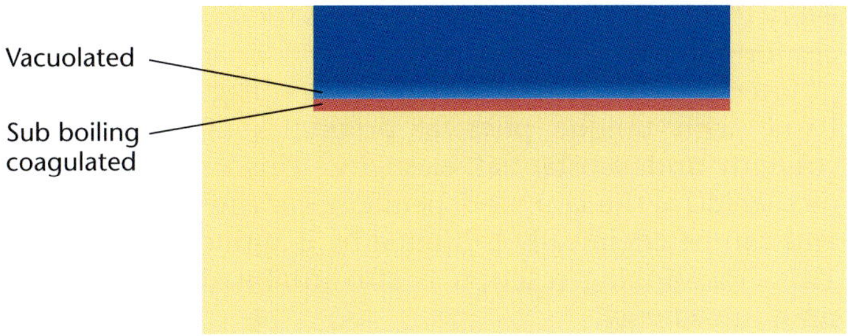

Figure 7.11 Zones of thermal damage in tissue instantaneously heated above 70°C but below 100°C. Normal tissue has a temperature of 37°C. Between this 70°C layer and normal 37°C tissue is a gradient of temperature in which collagen shinkage occurs, ideally at 63°C.

A further consideration is that consecutive passes with the laser result in the laser encountering desiccated, thermally denatured collagen with little water to act as a target for the laser. This results in a progressively decreased depth of vaporization per pulse. When less of the pulse energy goes into vaporization, progressively more energy is deposited into the tissue, potentially causing thermal necrosis by diffusion. In this situation the pulse width and repetition rate become critical.

In addition to the vaporization and coagulation effects of these lasers removing up to 250 to 300 μm of tissue in the dermis, with decreasing tissue ablation with each sequential pass, a second mechanism of laser–tissue interaction appears to be important in achieving the desired clinical results. A discernible shrinkage of the skin is visible as the laser reacts with the dermis, tightening loose folds of skin. This is thought to be a result of heat-induced collagen shrinkage.[77]

When the CO_2 laser interacts with tissue, three distinct zones of tissue alteration correlate to the degree of tissue heating. The zone of direct impact results in vaporization of intracellular water and tissue ablation. Underlying this is a zone of irreversible thermal damage and denaturation resulting in tissue necrosis. Below this layer is a zone of reversible, nonlethal thermal damage (Fig. 7.11), in which collagen shrinkage is thought to occur, accounting for the visible tissue tightening observable as the CO_2 laser interacts with the dermis.

Collagen Shrinkage

Collagen fibers provide the framework and mechanical strength of skin. The microscopically visible fiber is composed of a bundle of fibrils that are readily distinguishable by electron microscopy. These fibrils are made up of a unit filament, the protofibril, which has the same chemical and configurational structure as the collagen molecule.

The collagen molecule is a highly unique and unusual protein containing three polypeptide chains in a helical conformation with the presence of hydroxyproline and hydroxylysine. The repetitive positioning of glycine at every third amino acid locus accounts for its unique helical conformation.

Intermolecular cross-links provide collagen connective tissue with unique physical properties of high tensile strength and substantial elasticity. This cross-linking is mediated by the copper-dependent enzyme lysyl oxidase and can be chemically inhibited by β-aminopropionitrile. This cross-linking reaction is also inhibited by heat and photonic energy.

Thermal Effects

The knowledge regarding collagen shrinkage and tightening comes from a variety of sources, including biochemistry and thermokinetics,[119–139] tissue studies,[143–152] thermokeratoplasty,[153–195] orthopedics,[196–201] and tissue-welding studies.[117,202–235] The group having the closest clinical correlation to tissue shrinkage during resurfacing is found in tissue-welding studies, but clinical studies in orthopedics and ophthalmology have involved the thermal effects of type I collagen and are directly translatable to cutaneous work. The changes in collagen that occur in resurfacing mirror the collagen changes seen in all these areas of collagen research.

The response of collagen to heat is different than that of other body tissues. The hydrothermal shrinkage of collagen fibers has long been recognized as a characteristic of collagen.[156] The mechanism of this thermal contraction is proposed to be a molecular structure transition between the triple helix and a random coil.[110–112,129] Temperature elevation ruptures the ultrastructural cross-links that stabilize the collagen helix and results in immediate contraction in the fibers to about one-third their original length, with a corresponding increase in the caliber of individual fibers without alteration in the structural integrity of the tissue. Although the application of heat dissociates the interpeptide bonds, the cross-linkage between tropocollagen molecules remains intact, and the contraction of these linked molecules leads to shortening of the collagen fiber.[160]

The thermal stability of collagen is also species dependent as well as related to its hydroxylation. As new collagen is formed, it becomes progressively more cross-linked with time, so younger, newer collagen is less heat stabile than mature collagen and contracts at a lower temperature. The shrinkage temperature for collagen lies within a very narrow range within which collagen fibers will shrink without destroying collagen fibrils. The higher the amino acid content, the more stable is the helix. The temperature at which half the helical structure of molecular strands is lost is called the melting temperature (Tm). For intact collagen fibers, the comparable index is the shrinkage temperature (Ts). For calf skin, the Tm of tropocollagen has been shown to be 39°C (only 2°C above body temperature), whereas the collagen Ts is 65°C.[112] The relationship between denaturation of collagen in the solid state and in the dissolved state has possible physiologic significance. It has been proposed that denaturation of extractable collagen in vivo at physiologic temperatures is a necessary state in the catabolism of collagen, preparing it for proteolytic digestion.[113,114]

The viscosity of a tropocollagen solution drops sharply at 39°C as the helical structure is disrupted to random coils and a disrupted structure called gelatin results. This same type of reaction with intact collagen results in visible shrinkage along the long axis of collagen fibers and occurs at a very specific temperature. Rabbit cornea has been shown to shrink 40%–50% at 65°C.[156] Mammalian collagen, including human scleral and skin tissue, shrinks at 61°C–63°C, whereas human cornea shrinks at a lower temperature, 55°C–58°C.[158] However, the thermal properties of collagen vary with both the age of the animal and the environmental conditions.[115,140,141] Hyalinization of collagen, a characteristic microscopic finding of thermal injury, indicates merger of unraveled, swollen collagen fibers and has been reported to occur at temperatures greater than 58°C. Changes in birefringence (double refraction), indicating thermally coagulated collagen with unraveling of collagen fibrils and loss of unique striations, reportedly occurs at 70°C–75°C.[142]

In a well-organized discussion of photothermal effects induced by laser irradiation of tissue, Thomsen[142] separates these biologic thermal effects into three different thermodynamic processes based on observations by Pearce,[143] as follows:

1. Lower-temperature (about 43°C–150°C) damage by heat accumulation processes, which may be lethal or nonlethal depending on times of heat exposure.
2. Higher-temperature (100°C+) effects, dominated by water vaporization and effects of water vapor release.
3. High-temperature ablation (about 300°C–1000°C), resulting in tissue vaporization, combustion, molecular dissociation, and plasma formation.

Thermal Coagulation

The visible thermal changes seen in collagen on light microscopy represent thermally induced, irreversible alterations of proteins and other biologic molecules, organelles, membranes, and cells, referred to as thermal coagulation. These alterations are caused primarily by thermal denaturation of structural proteins, are seen immediately after heating, and are always lethal. This differs from the low-temperature tissue injury that occurs, which may be demonstrable with electron microscopy or enzyme histochemistry in the first 24 hours or through light microscopy 48–72 hours after cellular death. Nonlethal changes may be more difficult to document because staining artifacts can mimic the pathologic alterations.

Thermally induced partial loss and complete loss of native birefringence and hyalinization of thermally coagulated collagen are easily recognizable. The normally seen birefringence is related to the regular arrangement of molecules forming the collagen fibrils. Thermally coagulated collagen examined by electron microscopy reveals unraveling of collagen fibrils with loss of the unique striations of collagen and an increase in fibrillar diameters.[141] The unraveled strands merge, and the individual fibers become less distinct, forming the swollen, hyalinized (glassy) collagen fibers seen with light microscopy. Birefringence changes induced by thermal reaction in collagen include a gradual loss of bright image intensity as well as color shifts of histologic stains. The loss of bright image intensity in thermally coagulated collagen may result from thermal disruption of the intramolecular and intermolecular bonds of collagen, leading to destruction of the regular arrangement among collagen molecules. The unraveling of collagen fibrils may expose new dye-binding sites and thus result in the color shifts seen. Normal fibers have been found to be intermixed with altered fibers in examination of tissue-welding sites induced by thermal changes from laser irradiation.[126,202,203]

The easily recognizable changes of thermal necrosis of collagen reflect the effects of higher temperatures (70°C–75°C) that result in cellular death and therefore are not necessarily desirable in resurfacing procedures, at least not greater than 200 to 300 μm in depth. Whether more subtle alterations in birefringence and color shifts can be definitively correlated with corresponding electron microscopy changes and shown to represent a layer of nonlethal thermal injury, but irreversible structure change has not been demonstrated. Our hypothesis is that such a layer exists just below the layer of visibly altered thermal changes. However, the only, or primary, collagen shrinkage may occur in the area of tissue necrosis. If this is true, maintenance of tissue shrinkage seen would depend on efficient collagen replacement of this necrotic layer while maintaining this shortened tissue matrix. This would be difficult to achieve, because this layer sloughs within 1 week in normal wound healing, much faster than the synthesis and cross-linking of new collagen occur.

In general, however, researchers agree that the thermal profile of laser–tissue interaction must be controlled to prevent excessive tissue heating and thermal necrosis when performing laser resurfacing. If, in addition, a tissue layer of collagen can be heated in the range of 60°C–70°C to achieve the desired shrinkage without completely denaturing collagen or changing the skin's structural integrity, and if this thermally altered collagen persists in this state, then maintenance of this shortened, tightened condition would be achieved. Replacement of this altered collagen in the healing process might cause regression of the collagen contraction achieved.[192] Indeed, in the absence of trauma, the half-life of type I collagen has been shown to be consistent with the life span of the experimental animal.[144] Some authors assume this to be true of human collagen as well, but the stability and longevity of collagen and its normal homeostatic replacement are for the most part unknown. It is known to be an ongoing process controlled by fibroblasts and dependent on collagenase secretion. The half-life of corneal collagen is reported to be 10 years or more; however, this is a unique location because it has no direct vascular supply.[145]

Collagen Structure

Collagen is a protein that undergoes self-assembly into macromolecular structures. Collagen solutions will readily polymerize into collagen fibrils that are indistinguishable from those found in vivo. Reactive carbonyl moieties generate intermolecular cross-links (collagen aldehydes reacting with other collagen amino acids), uniting the collagen molecules into a continuous polymeric network.[127] Thus collagen molecules, which contain carbonyl groups, self-assemble into fibers, which then become cross-linked because of reactions between the carbonyl groups and other amino acids of adjoining molecules. This structure is maintained by hydrogen bonds.[128]

Collagen protofibrils are composed of laterally aggregated, staggered molecules, which when cross-linked, form a strong, macroscopic three-dimensional network. The molecular stagger results from interactions between the amino acid side chains and consequently has the requisite precision to bring the lysyl side chains into proximity to form intermolecular cross-links.[130] This occurs in a spontaneous, progressive manner. As previously mentioned, this precise intermolecular cross-linking is species specific, because the relative abundance of different cross-links varies greatly depending on the tissue of origin of the collagen.[127]

Flexibility in side-chain interactions suggest that rather than a unique reaction being involved, a myriad of conformations occur at the molecular surfaces.[130] The fluidity of the surface domains would allow collagen molecules in soft tissues to slip relative to one another when stress is applied.[131]

Denaturation

The loss of the specific structure of a macromolecule without chemical degradation is considered to be denaturation. Collagen in solution undergoes denaturation at about 30°C. Reconstitution of collagen fibrils from these heated solutions is no longer possible, so its biologic function is destroyed as well. However, this process tends to be reversible. The polypeptide strands making up the original collagen molecule have a considerable but incomplete capacity to resume the intrachain characteristics of the native state.[131] Therefore the denaturation temperature involves a considerable range that is both time and temperature dependent. The shrinkage process also has been described as a rate phenomenon; in general a 2°C rise in temperature reduces the time for shrinkage by half.[132]

A similarity exists between the denaturation of soluble collagen and the thermal shrinkage of collagen. A study of the shrinkage temperature of normal human skin versus that of various pathologic states revealed a range of 57°C–65°C, with normal skin having an average shrinkage temperature of 62.9°C and abnormal skin averaging 61.9°C.[146] A transient lengthening was observed just before the instantaneous shrinkage. An energy of activation near 140 kcal is found for tendon collagen. From thermodynamic considerations, it is concluded that the only bonds involved in thermal shrinkage are the hydrogen bonds between chains. The cooperative nature of the 'melting' of hydrogen bonds remains as the common feature of both the denaturation of soluble collagen and the hydrothermal contraction of collagenous tissue.[128]

Mammalian collagen, either skin or tendon, contracts sharply at 60°C–70°C (Ts) to about one-third to one-quarter its initial length. The tensile strength of the fiber is greatly lowered and shows 'rubber-like elasticity'.[132] Completely shrunken collagen loses its orderly structure. This structural alteration is an irreversible process once it is completed. The disoriented collagen formed is in a low state of entropy and consequently tends to fold into a more random configuration, thereby gaining in entropy.

The change from an oriented structure to a random state of configuration of the protein units is a natural consequence of the structure's tendency to increase its entropy. Instantaneous shrinkage of collagen takes place at temperatures at which the free energy of activation is about 25 kcal per mole, and the heat of the activation process has been determined to be 25 cal per gram.[132]

At about 60°C the process is initiated in tendon collagen by the appearance of tiny nodules. As the temperature is raised, more energy is available to rupture additional cross-links, which increases the thermal movement of the chains. A point will be reached at which the structure is weakened to the extent that it will assume a more stable configuration by chain folding. The nodules visibly enlarge and coalesce, and shrinkage of the tendon takes place. Further heating results in loss of structure and relaxation of collagen strands. This threshold for relaxation was found to be 78°C, but it rises with increasing age because of an increase in the number of thermally stable bonds.[140] In one study, human tendons were shown to contract sharply to 70% of their original length at about 70°C but to fall apart physically at temperatures higher than 80°C.[147]

Studies of thermokeratoplasty, in which corneal flattening is achieved through application of heat, have shown that in the corneal stroma the highest temperatures do not achieve additional shrinkage, but rather result in thermal injury and necrosis.[156,190] White et al[217,232] and Kopchok et al[233] have shown in tissue-welding studies that collagen bonding occurs if tissue apposition is precise and the temperature is controlled to prevent denaturation of the tissue elements. Higher energies and higher temperatures have also been shown to disrupt the laser seal when tissue-welding vessels.[231–234] Furthermore, kinetic modeling of the laser–tissue fusion process was done with guidelines such that excessive heating desiccates collagen fibers to a brittle state unsuitable for fusion.[133] Clearly, overheating collagen is counterproductive.

On the other hand, a number of studies have demonstrated that the percent shrinkage of collagen is directly proportional to the heat applied to tissue while remaining within a narrow range and without exceeding the excessive heating threshold.[104,147–149,192,212] However, when evaluating percent shrinkage of various tissues, the clinician must keep in mind that the degree of shrinkage of tissue will depend not only on the collagen contraction, but also on the mechanical properties of the surrounding tissue.

Clinical Developments

Thermally induced changes in collagen were first investigated in refractive surgery 100 years ago by Lans,[153] who applied electrocautery to the peripheral cornea of rabbit eyes and achieved correction of astigmatic changes of up to 6.00 diopters. However, he found variability in the predictability of the curvature changes induced. In 1914 Wray[154] successfully used cautery clinically to treat a patient with hyperoptic astigmatism, and O'Connor[155] confirmed its benefit in selected cases in 1933 and reported persistence of refractive correction for 10 years postoperatively.

The determination of corneal collagen shrinkage temperatures in 1964[158] resulted in greater interest in thermokeratoplasty, and in the mid-1970s several investigators explored this as a treatment option for keratoconus.[156,157,161–173] Because of reports of a high incidence of regression[163] and various complications,[164–166] this procedure was never widely used, although Itoi[167] advocated its use because only 7% of his 750 patients treated subsequently required corneal transplantation.

In the 1980s, radiofrequency devices[168,169] and a retractable thermal probe (Michrome wire)[170–172] were used in an attempt to deliver heat in a more controlled manner but were abandoned because of poor predictability and regression of effects.[173,174]

Since then, lasers have been investigated as devices to deliver heat more precisely with selective targeting,[175] based primarily on a theoretic model developed by Mainstern.[176] At least five different lasers have been studied: CO_2[177–180] yttrium-erbium-glass (Y-Er-glass),[181] cobalt:magnesium fluoride,[159] hydrogen fluoride,[179–182] and holmium:YAG (Ho:YAG).[175,183–195] Only the Ho:YAG has been evaluated in clinical trials. In general, long-term follow-up (up to 2 years) has shown treatment with the Ho:YAG laser to induce moderate curvature changes with no significant complications. However, a small percentage (27% in one study)[57] of patients had continuous regression of the retractive changes throughout the first year. Some of this regression may be related to the treatment parameters used, and many unanswered questions remain at this time. Evidence indicates that persistent local contraction of collagen is present in treated rabbit eyes and that new collagen formation occurs as well. The significance of this new collagen formation and its effects on regression of the refractive benefits is controversial. Inhibition of new collagen formation by corticosteroids has been suggested as a potential method of preserving postoperative refractive stability.[190]

Collagen remodeling and new collagen formation are thought to be possibly counterproductive, because the brisk stromal wound healing may result in replacement of the thermally altered collagen by newly synthesized molecules not maintaining the new, shortened profile. In addition, the new collagen may adversely affect the refraction by having a different ultrastructure, as would a scar, or by altering curvature through filling in interstices, thickening the stroma, or counteracting the curvature changes.

Mechanical tissue factors such as the elasticity (or loss of it) of adjacent tissues may contribute to regression even though the collagen contraction is maintained. Epithelial hyperplasia resulting from laser injury also is thought to be a secondary event that may alter refraction.

Studies have shown that keratocyte injury occurs when stromal collagen is heated to 79°C.[180,195] Avoiding injury to the epithelium and keratocytes by development of a better delivery system and maintaining corneal temperature in the narrow range of 60°C–75°C would be optimum: above the shrinkage temperature of corneal collagen and below that lethal to keratocytes.

A natural transition from the use of collagen shrinkage as a therapeutic modality in ophthalmology to its use in orthopedics was reported by Fing et al,[196] who used heat not on the eye itself, but on extraocular muscle tendon. They reported the successful treatment of strabismus by shrinking the muscle tendon. Indeed, much of the basic knowledge regarding collagen shrinkage secondary to heating has been obtained through laboratory studies using excised tendons as the collagen source, so these clinical results are not surprising.

An in vitro study using a rabbit model was performed to investigate the potential of using laser energy (Ho:YAG laser) to the joint capsule of the shoulder to decrease capsular redundancy in patients with shoulder instability.[197] This study showed a significant and strong correlation between energy density applied and percent shrinkage of capsular tissue. Up to 40% shrinkage was seen without loss of normal relaxation properties of the tissue, indicating normal stability in response to stress. However, the higher energies resulted in a decrease in stiffness, indicating more compliant tissue. Once again, as seen in other tissue studies, this indicates that overheating may cause adverse tissue effects and disruption of collagen bonds.

In a multicenter clinical trial, patients with glenohumeral instability were shown to have dramatic improvement 6 months postoperatively after nonablative reduction of their joint capsule using the Ho:YAG laser.[200]

A further study using tissue baths heated to a designated temperature was performed on cadaver shoulders to determine the specific tissue effects of a range of temperatures.[201] This study revealed significant tissue shrinkage to occur at temperatures at or above 65°C. The percent shrinkage correlated with the temperature applied and ranged from 11% ± 15% at 65°C to 59% ± 5.4% at 80°C. Histologic and electron microscopy (EM) studies revealed progressive alterations in collagen, with hyalinization on light microscopy and loss of distinct edges of fibers visible with EM at 65°C, but complete homogenization with light microscopy and loss of fibrillar structure with EM seen at 80°C. This study revealed that distinct fibrillar structure was lost at or above 70°C, indicating transition of fibrillar collagen to an amorphous state. A previous EM study using the Ho:YAG laser to shrink the joint capsule, however, revealed that fibril diameters increased dramatically with less distinct edges, but with preservation of individual fibers. The difference may be secondary to the methods of heating or other factors. The authors point out, however, that wound healing factors must be considered and postulate that after adequate healing, the tissue may have normal architectural properties with maintenance of its shortened length.

After laser resurfacing, EM studies have revealed three distinct zones of collagen morphology.[150] In the most superficial tissue at the base of tissue vaporization is a zone of homogeneous, completely denatured collagen without discrete fibrillar components. This corresponds with the layer of thermal necrosis visible on light microscopy. An intact tertiary structure is necessary for diffraction of polarized light (birefringence). Loss of this structural integrity is associated with loss of birefringence and with tinctorial changes resulting from exposure of stain-binding sites within the unraveled collagen fiber.[150] These changes result in the area of thermal necrosis that is visible on light microscopy. The exact correlation of the EM zones to this visible zone is not known at this time. However, below the first homogeneous zone is a zone of significant population of less structurally defined collagen fibers of increased diameter interspersed among normal collagen fibers. Below this is a zone of normal collagen fibers.

Skin Rejuvenation

Clinical observations have confirmed the value of collagen shrinkage in rejuvenation of photodamaged skin. This is a significant component of the clinical improvement seen in laser resurfacing. Its exact mechanism and relative importance have been debated. We have hypothesized that the shortened collagen fibers result in a shrunken matrix on which collagen remodeling occurs, resulting in preservation of this tightened skin. That the tightened skin does persist to variable degrees is confirmed by study of photographs over time, as well as by the occurrence of laser-induced ectropion, a condition of excessive tissue tightening.

Tissue contraction is grossly visible on impact of the pulsed CO_2 laser with skin during resurfacing being most profound on the first and second dermal passes after removal of the epidermis. Although some component of this tissue contraction is undoubtedly secondary to tissue volume loss as a consequence of vaporization of tissue water, a large portion is thought to be from collagen contraction. Gardner et al[104] found a positive linear correlation between the number of passes and the degree of skin shrinkage. A linear regression model showed a 6% size reduction per pass with the SilkTouch laser and a 5% reduction per pass with the UltraPulse laser. Rehydrating the tissue between passes resulted in only slight correction of the shrinkage (Fig. 7.12). Analysis of a single specimen treated with the SilkTouch laser for five consecutive passes with rehydration between passes revealed about 15% reduction on the first pass and a plateau at about 31% reduction after three to five passes. Temperature elevation in the tissue was approximately 20°C and unchanged with each pass. Ross et al[149] observed a positive correlation between contraction of the treated area and both fluence and the number of laser passes in their studies on pig skin.

CO_2 Laser Skin Resurfacing

The most important factor in performing CO_2 laser resurfacing is single-pulse laser–tissue interaction (Fig. 7.13). If vaporization is accomplished in a single pulse, the heat of

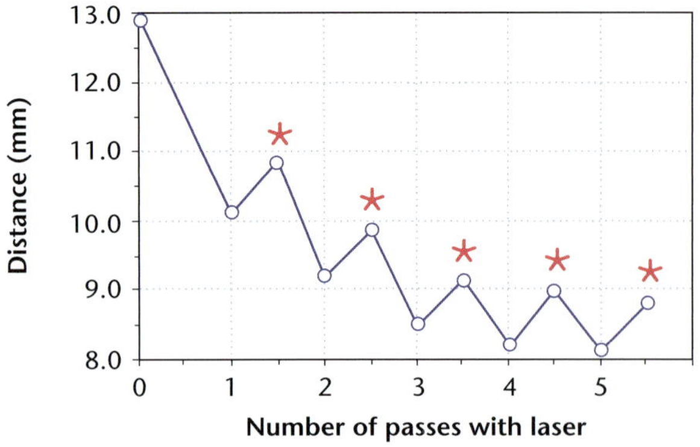

Figure 7.12 Collagen shrinkage as seen per pass with UltraPulse CO_2 laser. Asterisks represent rehydration between passes. (From Gardner ES, Reinisch L, Stricklin GP et al. Lasers in Surgery and Medicine. 19:379, © 1996. Reprinted with permission from Wiley-Liss, Inc., a subsidiary of John Wiley & Sons, Inc.)

A

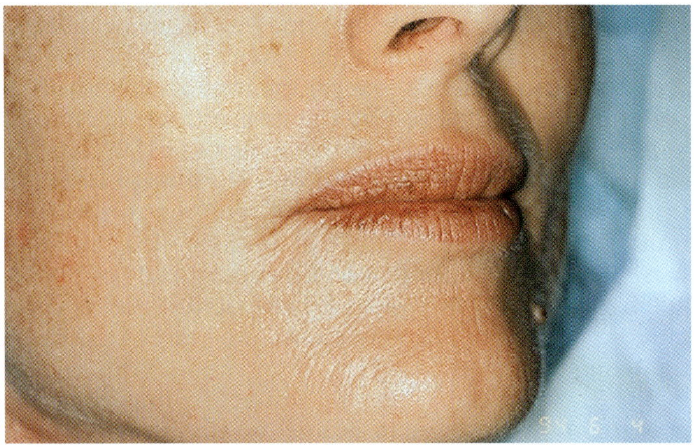

B

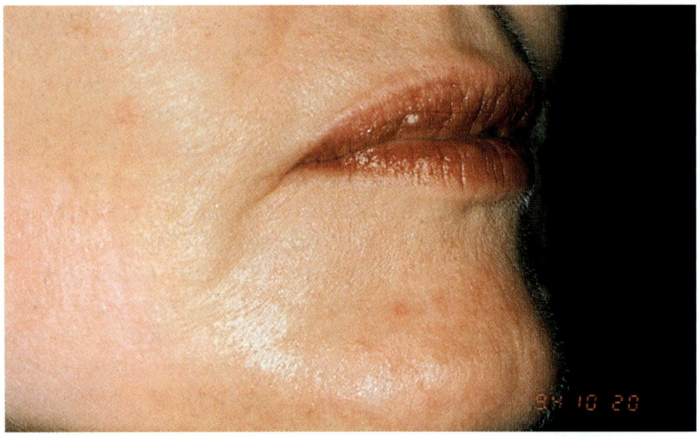

Figure 7.13 (A) Relatively superficial lines may be completely removed by ablating to depth of wrinkle line. (B) Improvement depends on ablation of solar elastosis and wound healing. Collagen shrinkage and new collagen formation are not necessary for this improvement to occur.

the laser–tissue interaction is released in the vapor created, and thermal diffusion deep into the treated tissue will not occur. If the tissue cannot be vaporized (i.e. the threshold for vaporization is not reached), it is critical that the pulse duration be less than the thermal diffusion time. In this

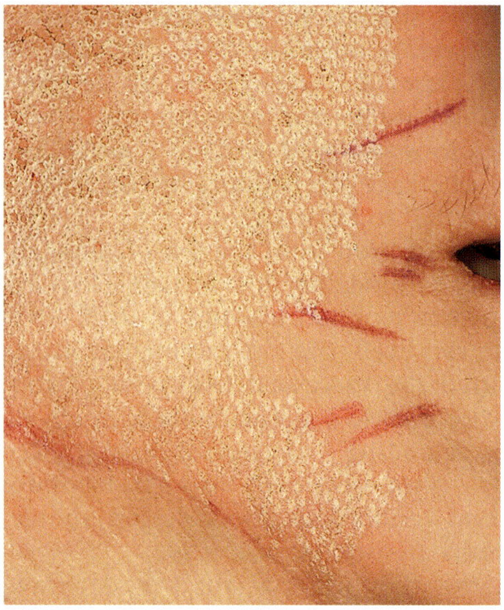

Figure 7.14 Initial CO_2 laser pass effectively removes epidermis by vaporizing a 40- to 50-µm layer and causing a subepidermal vesicle to form. Surface is covered with white, desiccated, proteinaceous debris from epidermis immediately after first pass. This needs to be wiped away with saline-soaked gauze.

situation the laser–tissue interaction site will cool off before there is time for thermal diffusion to occur. If laser pulses are stacked one on top of another, additive thermal effects will occur because of heat retention. For the CO_2 laser, the pulse repetition rate must be less than an estimated 5 Hz to allow tissue cooling between pulses and to avoid cumulative thermal effects.[151]

The technique used with the Coherent UltraPulse 5000 is described here. Similar techniques with appropriate modifications specific to individual systems to achieve the same laser–tissue interaction may be used for other systems as well.

UltraPulse Technique

When performing resurfacing procedures by hand with a 3-mm collimated beam, it is critical to move the handpiece at a rate that allows single-pulse laser–tissue interaction, with minimal overlapping (generally a rate of 4 to 10 Hz). When using the CPG, the patterns should not be overlapped, and the individual laser impacts within the pattern should have minimal overlap (generally densities of 3 to 6).

The surface is covered with a single pass of laser impacts, resulting in white, desiccated debris composed of proteinaceous epidermal tissue remaining after intracellular tissue water vaporization (Fig. 7.14). This tissue debris should be wiped away with saline-moistened gauze to remove the remaining epidermis. The first pass generally removes the epidermis and leaves only minimal residual thermal damage (10–30 µm) depending on epidermal thickness, with more thermal damage in thin epidermis, such as eyelid or neck skin. This same procedure is repeated over the entire surface to be treated for the second pass. The only difference is that during this pass, the CPG is

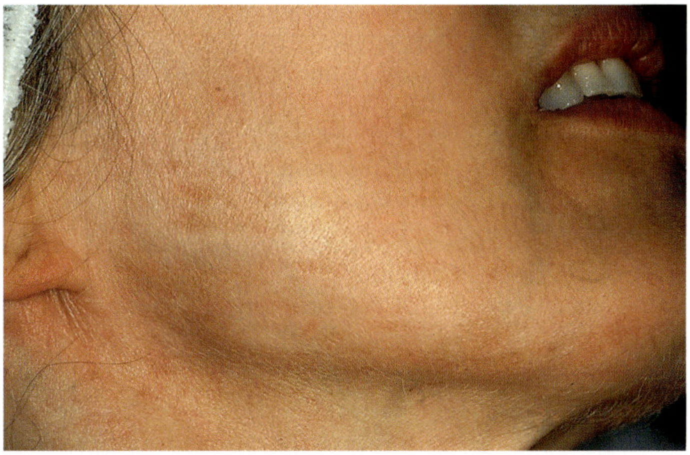

Figure 7.15 Single pass of CPG may result in linear streaks of hyperpigmentation, resulting from differential thermal effects leaving a mixture of non-sun-damaged cells and sun-damaged cells. To prevent this, a second pass is performed at 90 degrees to first pass.

oriented at 90 degrees to the direction used for the first pass. The reason for this is to avoid the appearance of linear pigment streaks that may be associated with the pattern of the CPG (Fig. 7.15).

Generally, the third pass is applied more selectively to areas of more significant photodamage and wrinkling. If photodamage remains visible over the entire treatment area, the entire area is treated again. In general, however, the third pass is confined to the glabellar area, upper lip, nasolabial folds, and lateral cheeks. A fourth pass with the Coherent CPG is only rarely needed except in cases of advanced, severe photodamage and is therefore not recommended (see Fig. 7.3).

Generally, after the third pass with the Coherent CPG, treatment with the 3-mm beam is used in selective areas to flatten high tissue points by vaporization and to tighten loose skin or ablate wrinkles by pulling the base of wrinkle lines up and achieving as smooth a surface as possible to act as a base for new collagen formation.

In performing resurfacing, clinicians should keep in mind the following:

1. Always 'feather' the peripheral areas by decreasing the density of pulse application as well as the pulse energy (decrease to 200–250mJ), or angle the beam at 45 degrees to spread the fluence over a larger surface area.
2. Feather into the hairline a distance of 5–15mm and well under the jawline (3–5cm) (Fig. 7.16).
3. Use feathering parameters to treat the eyelid surfaces, and use no more than two passes in the immediate periorbital area, except isolated spot application to persisting folds of tissue.
4. Carefully observe the laser–tissue interaction of the eyelids to avoid excessive tightening of tissue and possible scleral show or ectropion, especially in patients with a prior blepharoplasty.
5. Use the 3-mm beam to make a single pass along the vermilion borders of the upper and lower lips, because this is the most common area of persistence of wrinkle lines. This also helps to emphasize the vermilion border.

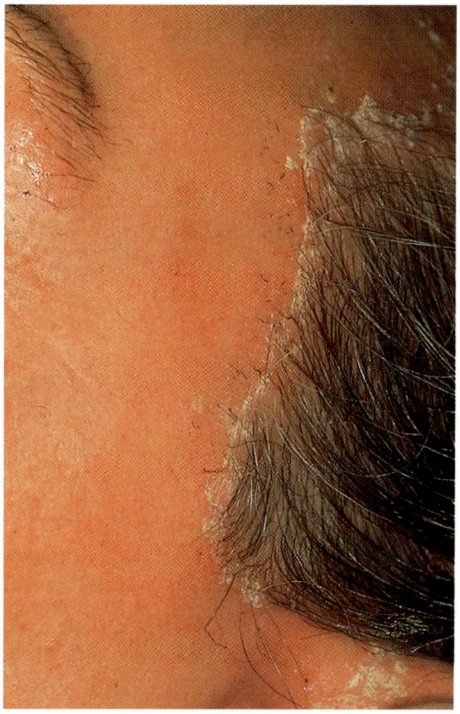

Figure 7.16 'Feathering' into hairline 5 to 15mm to avoid leaving a line of contrast anterior to hairline. Hair will regrow normally in this feathered zone, but it is not possible to treat inside scalp without coagulating shaft of hairs.

6. Do not routinely cross the vermilion border. Treat up to the border, because this will make the lips appear fuller and emphasize the vermilion border as a result of the collagen tightening of the lip.
7. Treat lines that cross the vermilion border individually by tracing over the line with the laser once all the other areas have been treated, rather than treating the entire vermilion surface.
8. After completion of treatment with the CPG, carefully search the treatment surface for signs of residual seborrheic keratoses, actinic keratoses, or SCC in situ and for thickened scars, and vaporize these to a flat surface using the 3-mm beam with pulse-stacking treatment technique or with the Er:YAG laser.
9. Always carefully observe the immediate tissue response regarding contraction or yellow-brown discoloration. If this discoloration persists after wiping with saline, this is a sign of thermal necrosis (Fig. 7.17).
10. Use the 3-mm spot in placing impact sites at 3- to 5-mm intervals to achieve tightening of the skin without significant thermal risk (concentric lines of these treatment spots moving away from a site to be tightened is effective). This is particularly useful on the eyelids and midcheeks.

The endpoint of treatment is when one of the following conditions is seen:

1. The wrinkle or scar is removed.
2. A yellow–brown discoloration indicating thermal damage is seen.
3. No further skin tightening is observed.

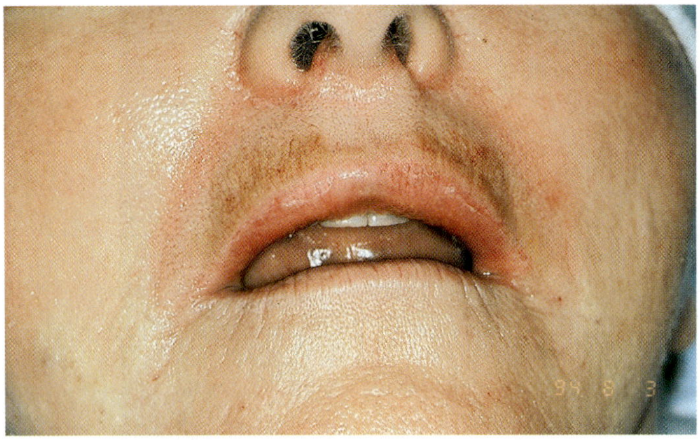

Figure 7.17 Persistent yellow-brown discoloration of dermis after wiping with saline is a sign of thermal injury that may be extending deeper into dermis.

No reason exists to continue treating an area when any of these signs is observed. Leave that area untreated from that point on and concentrate on other tissue sites.

SilkTouch Technique

The treatment technique using the Sharplan SilkTouch embodies the same basic principles, but with modifications specific to the system. Because the beam is not collimated, one must be careful to hold the handpiece at the proper distance from the skin at all times and to avoid movement during the scan of each 'pulse'. Also, the beam is not Gaussian in its energy distribution, so no built-in compensation exists for overlap of patterns. However, the scan pattern is a circle, which necessitates either having skip spaces with nonoverlapping pattern placement or overlapping each pattern on four sides to create a square. Caution must be observed in monitoring these pattern overlaps for signs of excessive thermal injury to the treated tissue. A square-pattern scan has recently been added to the capabilities of the scanner, as well as 'light-touch' capabilities, with a scanning system similar to Coherent's CPG, using a small spot size but a true pulse of laser energy with less than 1-ms duration.

Either a 3.7-mm scan using 5–8W or a 6.5- or 9.0-mm scan with 15–20W is chosen. With the Sharplan system, increasing the power results in an increased depth of vaporization: 18W vaporizes deeper than 16W. Typical settings are 18W for the 6.5- and 9.0-mm scan and 7W for the 3.7-mm scan. Scan duration is 0.2s 'on' and 0.3 to 0.4s 'off' in the repetitive mode.

Generally, two passes of one of the larger patterns are used, then the 3.7-mm scan and spot is used in the same manner as with the Coherent 3-mm collimated beam at the vermilion border and along 'shoulders' of persistent lines. Feathering is accomplished by decreasing the power and angling the handpiece to less than 90 degrees. The eyelids are treated with decreased wattage as well and generally only a single pass.

With the newer FeatherTouch-SilkTouch system, it is easier to obtain superficial resurfacing using the FeatherTouch mode, scanning circles or squares 3–15mm in diameter.

Weinstein[236] reports the histologic findings using a 10-mm square at 36W, corresponding to a fluence of $10 J/cm^2$, as follows:

1. Single pass: epidermal vaporization with dermal coagulation necrosis of 10μm
2. Two passes: epidermal vaporization with dermal coagulation necrosis of 30μm
3. Three passes: epidermal vaporization with dermal coagulation of 50μm

The depth of vaporization into the dermis is not given.

When the same settings are used on the SilkTouch mode, the pattern is scanned twice: once inward, then outward. The total time on tissue is longer, the fluence is higher ($28 J/cm^2$), and the thermal injury is greater, as follows:

1. Single pass: epidermal vaporization with dermal coagulation necrosis of 70μm
2. Two passes: epidermal vaporization with dermal coagulation necrosis of 100μm

The depth of vaporization into the dermis is not reported.

To accomplish excellent results, it is necessary to have an understanding of the basic mechanisms of action of laser resurfacing. Basically, four mechanisms are involved: (1) single-pulse vaporization; (2) collagen shrinkage and skin tightening; (3) new collagen formation and remodeling of collagen; and (4) multipulse coagulation of collagen.

Collagen Shrinkage and Skin Tightening

It was not initially anticipated that collagen shrinkage would be a component of the laser–tissue interaction. However, unexpected improvement in redundant folds of the eyelids, loose skin of the cheeks, nasolabial folds, and the other deep wrinkle lines, coupled with the visible skin tightening observable with the laser–tissue interaction, has led to use of heat-induced collagen shrinkage for clinical benefit (Box 7.1).

This skin-tightening effect allows achievement of comparable clinical results at a more superficial level of tissue removal than is necessary with other resurfacing modalities, such as dermabrasion and chemical peels. The amount of tightening observed depends on the number of passes delivered, unknown specific tissue factors (possibly the numbers and health of intact collagen fibers), tissue thickness, and anatomic location. Thin tissue such as eyelid and neck skin tightens very readily and often profoundly, even to the point of causing ectropion in eyelid skin. Temporal skin is generally thinner compared with other facial skin and also tightens more significantly. Tightening of cheek skin may be important in reducing nasolabial fold prominence and 'jowls' under the jaw line. Tightening may be used very selectively to achieve desired clinical effects

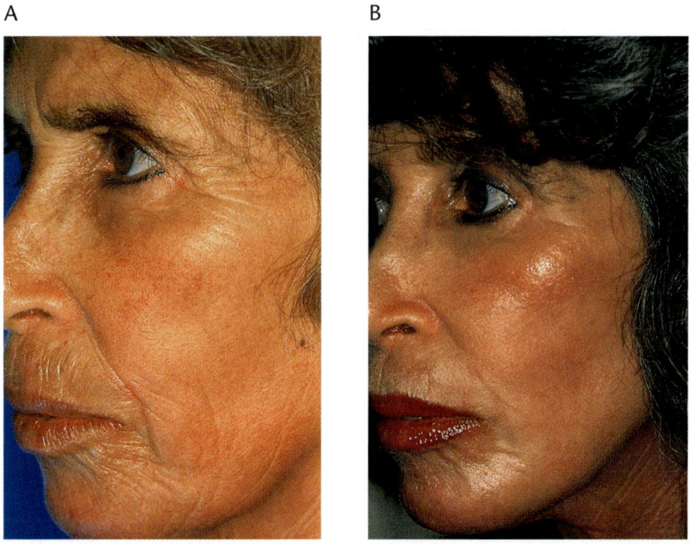

Figure 7.18 Skin tightening and collagen shrinkage result in clinical improvement in nasolabial folds and cheeks. (A) Before treatment; (B) 1 year after full-face CO_2 laser resurfacing.

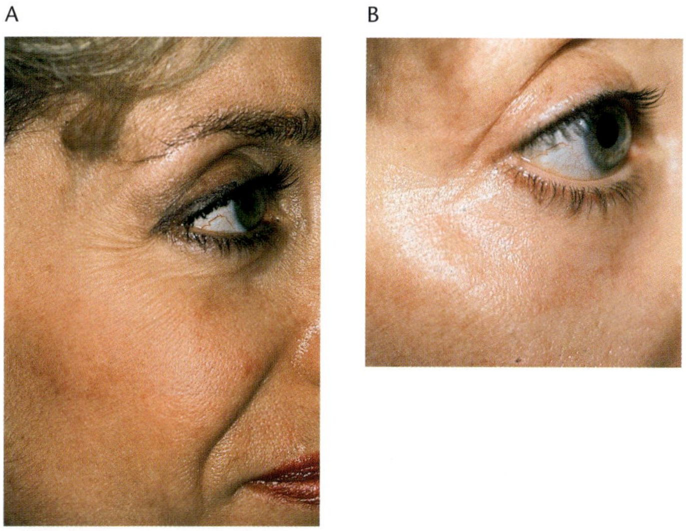

Figure 7.19 Improvement in loose, folded tissue of photodamaged lower-eyelid skin usually occurs primarily from collagen tightening. (A) Before therapy; (B) 4 months after CO_2 laser resurfacing.

Box 7.1 *Collagen Shrinkage with CO_2 Laser*

Collagen Molecule

- Three polypeptide chains in helical conformation result from repetitive positioning of glycine at every third amino acid locus.
- Intermolecular cross-links provide tensile strength and are inhibited by heat.
- Heat dissociates interpeptide bond; molecules remain intact.
- Hydrothermal shrinkage occurs through molecular structure transition from a triple helix to a random coil.
- Immediate contraction of fibers occurs to about one-third their original length.
- Collagen is progressively more cross-linked with time, so new collagen is less stable and contracts at lower temperature.

Collagen-heat Reaction

- Polypeptide strands of heated tissue have capacity to resume the original intrachain characteristics.
- Collagen readily self-assembles into fibrils, which cross-link in a spontaneous, progressive manner.
- A myriad of molecular conformations are possible.
- Denaturation process is both time and temperature dependent; in general a 2°C rise in temperature reduces shrinkage time by 50%.
- Very narrow temperature range exists for shrinkage without destroying fibrils.
- Instantaneous shrinkage temperature of human collagen was found to be 62.9°C, with range of 57°C–65°C.
- As temperature rises, more and more cross-link bonds are broken until loss of structure and denaturation occur.
- Percent shrinkage is directly proportional to heat applied, while not exceeding threshold for denaturation.

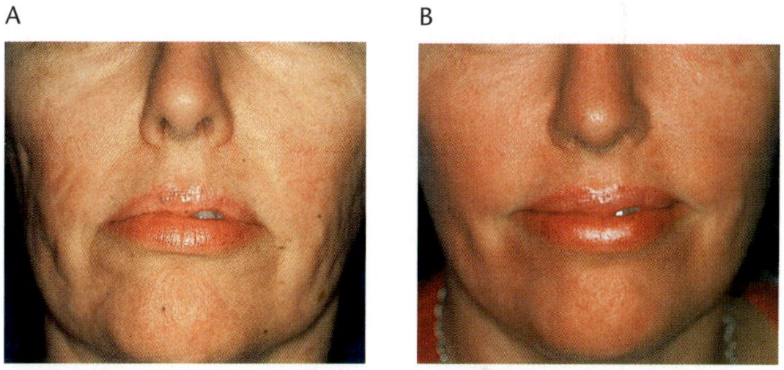

Figure 7.20 Atrophic acne scars may respond dramatically to a single treatment with CO_2 laser by using collagen tightening selectively and artfully to elevate scars. (A) Before treatment; (B) 4 months after CO_2 laser resurfacing.

(Fig. 7.18). Precise tightening of folds of loose eyelid tissue (Fig. 7.19) or atrophic scars (Fig. 7.20) can dramatically improve clinical results without significant risk if careful clinical observation is used.

By targeting high points of glabellar and forehead lines, better smoothing of these areas may be achieved. This type of tissue change has been shown to persist 4 years or more and is thought to be a permanent structural change in the skin once the new collagen formation has occurred.

New Collagen Formation and Collagen Remodeling

To avoid excessive thermal injury, it is recommended that the laser resurfacing procedure be discontinued when signs of thermal injury are seen, that is, yellow-brown discoloration of the skin. Often, when treatment is discontinued because of visible thermal effects, visible wrinkle

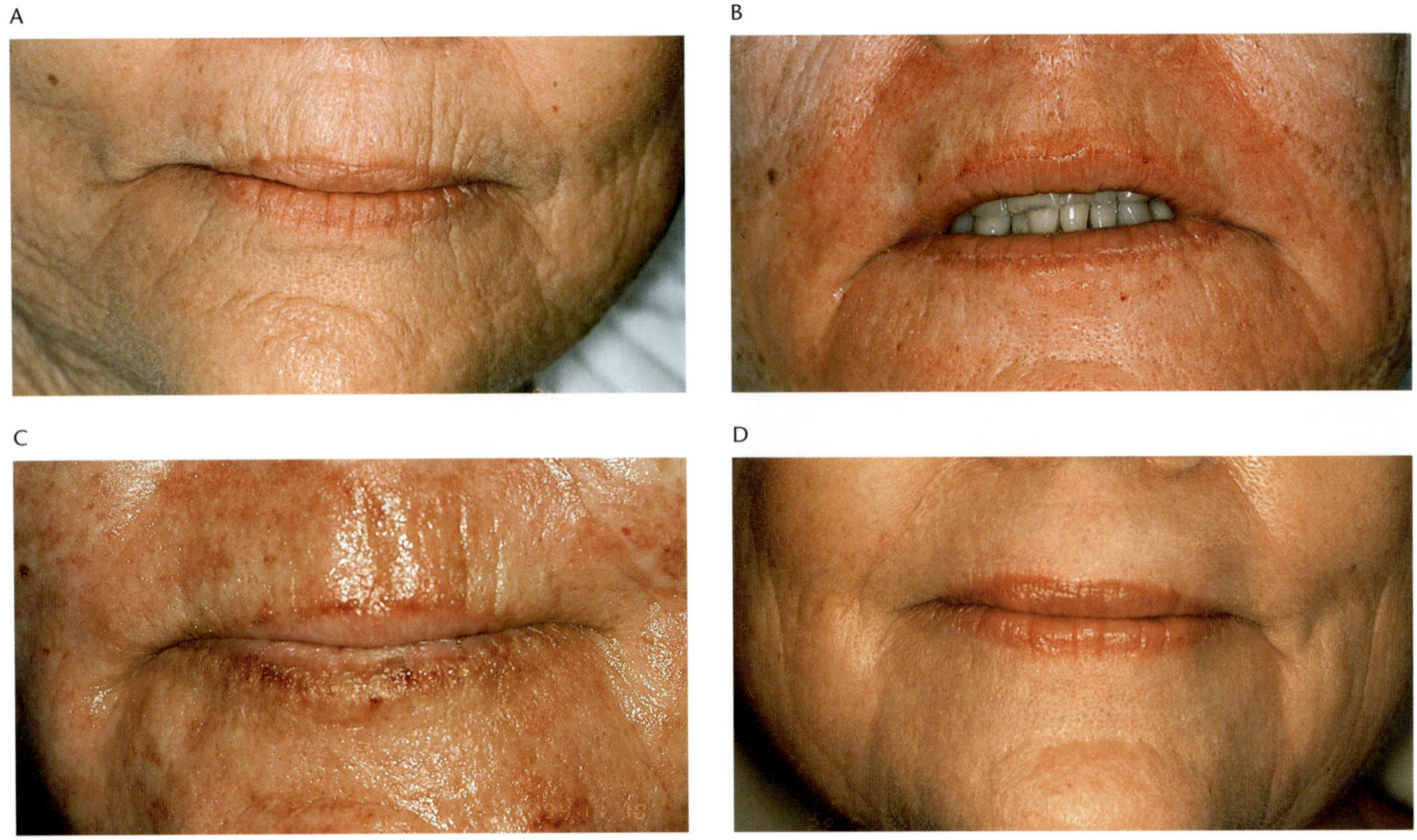

Figure 7.21 Clinical improvement often occurs in a delayed manner secondary to new collagen formation and collagen remodeling. (A) Deep upper-lip lines before treatment. (B) Immediately after treatment, these lines remain very visible. (C) 3 days after treatment, swelling intensifies visibility of some lines. (D) 6 months later, lines are gone.

lines are still present, particularly on the glabella and forehead and upper lip (Fig. 7.21A,B). These lines may gradually improve during the healing process and may gradually subside over 6 to 12 weeks (Fig. 7.21C,D). This occurs as a consequence of new collagen formation and collagen remodeling.

A multicenter study demonstrated that UltraPulse laser resurfacing results in up to a 600% increase in the Grenz zone layer. A new layer of healthy, fine collagen fibrils is laid down parallel to the epidermis and measures 100 to 400 μm in depth, replacing the layer of solar elastosis vaporized by the laser.

Multipulse Coagulation

The most efficient fluences for vaporizing the epidermis have been shown to be in the range of 5–19 J/cm^2. Single-pulse vaporization generally uses fluences of about 7 J/cm^2. However, when one pulse is stacked on top of another without sufficient tissue cooling time, additive thermal effects occur. When using the CPG with the UltraPulse laser, a density of 9 results in as high an energy density as 60 J/cm^2 to be delivered to the tissue. It has been clinically observed that after making three or four passes with the UltraPulse laser using CPG densities of 4 to 6, nothing visible appears to occur to the tissue. Neither the depth of vaporization nor the thermal injury appears to be increasing. Biopsy studies confirm this impression, as long as single-pulse vaporization is being used.[116]

However, these same tissue studies have shown that with stacking pulses on top of one another, the zone of thermal necrosis gradually increases and may increase to greater than 300 μm, even though the depth of vaporization remains basically unchanged. The procedure of vaporization appears to level off because the tissue target (i.e. water) changes as the procedure progresses. In the first pass the laser is interacting with intracellular water. Once the epidermis has been stripped away, however, the laser is acting primarily with extracellular water in the dermis. In addition, the water content of the epidermis is closer to 80%, whereas in the dermis the water content is closer to 60%. The dermis is made up primarily of protein fibrils of collagen and elastic tissue. These fibers have a much higher threshold of vaporization than water. Therefore the amount of tissue vaporized with each pass becomes less and less.

Complicating the situation even further is the layer of thermal necrosis, which measures generally between 50 and 100 μm, is desiccated and has very little water. Therefore it is difficult to vaporize deeper than 200 to 300 μm using single-pulse vaporization with a collimated

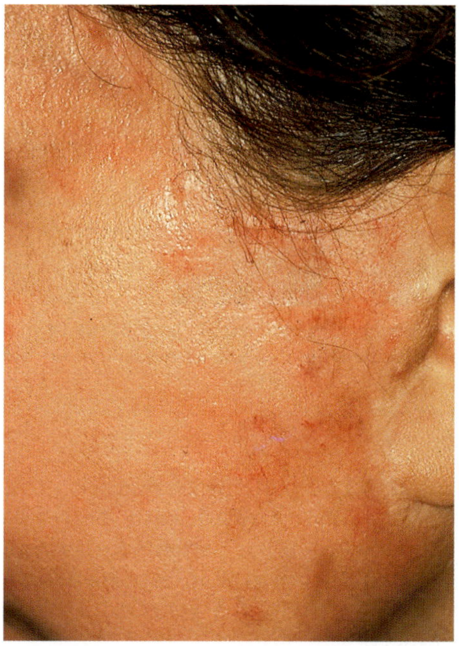

Figure 7.22 Failure to adhere carefully to single-pulse vaporization may result in inadvertently stacking pulses and extending thermal necrosis deeply into dermis. This may result in delayed wound healing and scarring.

beam. However, stacking pulses results in cumulative thermal effects and may allow deeper vaporization because of the higher fluence that results from rapid pulse succession.

This is a hazardous procedure because the residual thermal damage is greater with pulse stacking and may progress to the point of interfering with wound healing, which may cause scarring. This occurs without obvious clinical signs of potential problems, but subtle signs may be distinguished by experienced observation. When stacking pulses on top of each other, a yellow-brown discoloration of the tissue is observed clinically. This is initially subtle and clears with saline wiping. As further passes are performed, the yellow color gradually deepens to brown and will not wipe away. When this yellow–brown discoloration is seen, the physician can be certain that this area will be the last to heal and that this tissue will slough. Although this pulse-stacking technique can be used to resurface deeper because of the resultant tissue slough, it is a potentially dangerous technique that can result in poor wound healing and scarring (Fig. 7.22).

If a decision is made to use this technique clinically, it is imperative to learn the signs of depth of injury by observation of tissue healing with variable levels of treatment on repeated occasions. As mentioned earlier, the three endpoints of treatment are elimination of the wrinkle or scar, a yellow-brown discoloration indicating thermal damage, and no further collagen shrinkage or tightening. When any one of these is reached, the laser procedure should be terminated in that area of the face. It is much safer to retreat residual lines after an adequate healing time of 6 months or longer.

Table 7.2 *Facial Wrinkling: Clinical Classifications*

Class	Wrinkling	Score	Degree of elastosis
I	Fine wrinkles	1–3	Mild: fine textural changes with subtly accentuated skin lines
II	Fine to moderate-depth wrinkles	4–6	Moderate: distinct papular elastosis (individual papules with yellow translucency under direct lighting) and dyschromia; moderate number of lines
III	Fine to deep wrinkles; numerous	7–9	Severe: multipapular and confluent elastosis (thickened, yellow, and pallid) lines; with or without redundant skin folds approaching or consistent with cutis rhomboidalis

Facial Wrinkling

To evaluate the severity of wrinkling and photodamage present and therefore achieve some degree of predictability of response to resurfacing, a clinical classification and numeric scoring system has been adapted from other photodamage assessment systems. Although other wrinkling and photodamage assessment scales exist, the need for a system related purely to visible wrinkling and visible textural changes secondary to solar elastosis was thought to be more relevant to the topic of wrinkle eradication.[77]

Use of this scoring system allows broad classification into mild, moderate, and severe categories as well as a subjective numeric severity score (Table 7.2). Assessing patients both before and after treatment in a study with an average follow-up of about 90 days revealed that the average patient's preoperative score decreased approximately 50% as a consequence of resurfacing.[84] This means that mild wrinkles generally resolve completely, moderate wrinkles become mild, and severe wrinkles become moderate. Other studies[3,4,82] using different assessment systems have come to basically the same conclusion: wrinkles generally improve 50%–70%, with superficial lines eliminated, deeper lines softened, skin texture normalized, precancerous lesions eliminated, and lentigines and seborrheic keratoses eliminated. These are realistic expectations for the patient, although occasionally even severe wrinkles may completely resolve. The treated area may continue to improve for several months after laser resurfacing as collagen remodeling takes place.

Our studies of patients with an average follow-up of 2 years postoperatively (range 1–4 years) have revealed an excellent preservation of these results. Generally, as anticipated, the lines first to recur are those caused by muscle motion ('crow's feet', glabellar, forehead). Excellent preservation of results was seen, however, because 3-month versus 25-month scores revealed an average improvement

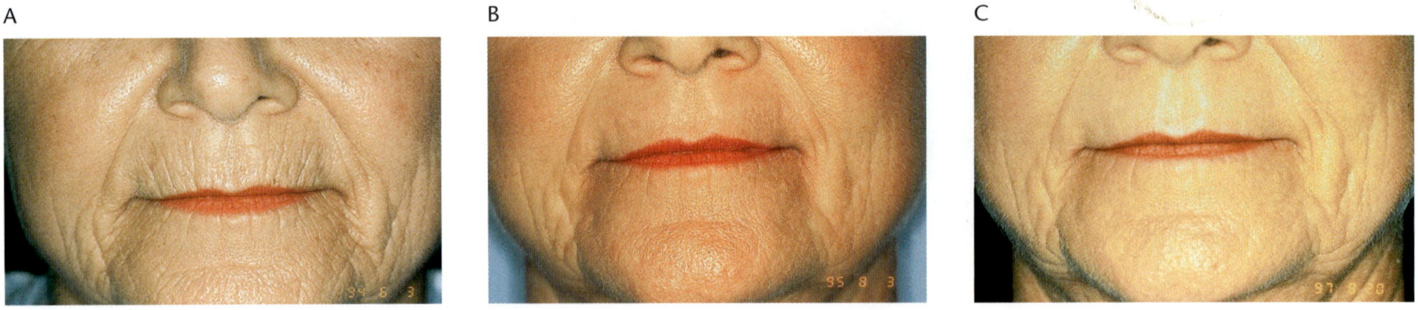

Figure 7.23 Excellent long-term results after CO_2 laser resurfacing of facial wrinkles. (A) Before surgery: class III, level 8. (B) 14 months postoperatively: class II, level 4. (C) 39 months postoperatively: class II, level 4. Note progression of photoaging of medial cheeks, which were not treated.

Table 7.3 *The Average Decrease in Photodamage at 90 days and 1 year after Full-Face Resurfacing*

Area	90 Days (%)	1 Year (%)
Perioral	69	64
Cheeks	89	72
Forehead	80	48
Periorbital	79	52

in preoperative photodamage scores periorally of 49% versus 38%, respectively, while periorbital scores were 46% versus 31% improved (Fig. 7.23). Interestingly, patient satisfaction for these two areas was 55% for the perioral area and 80% for the periorbital area. Overall, 94 of 104 patients (90%) considered laser resurfacing to be a beneficial procedure that they would recommend to others.[237] This may be true because the laser removes the textural and pigmentary abnormalities (the 'weathered' look) even though the muscles may still be able to fold the skin into wrinkles.

Other investigators have found similar results. Burns (personal communication) had independent observers grade 95 consecutive full-face resurfacing procedures at 90 days and 1 year postoperatively using a scale of 1 to 8 and found an average decrease in photodamage scores (Table 7.3). No difference was seen in outcome whether patients were treated with the Coherent system or the Sharplan system.

Ross et al[238] reported the long-term results of 28 patients treated with either the SilkTouch or the UltraPulse laser and found that their pretreatment photodamage scores continued to improve from 60 days to the reassessment point at 1 year. Scores improved 43% in the SilkTouch group and 34% in the UltraPulse group, but no statistical difference was seen between the two groups. The immediate thermal damage was found to be about 30% greater in the SilkTouch group, with a wider zone of fibroplasia (220 μm vs. 150 μm in the UltraPulse group) at 1 year postoperatively. No statistical difference was seen in adverse effects for the two groups, although focal hypopigmentation was noted in two patients treated with the SilkTouch laser and one patient treated with both. Weinstein[236] reports that follow-up of her patients for as long as 5 years after resurfacing has shown that improvement visible at 6 months was still present at 5 years and that the overall results are indeed long-lasting.

In addition, 24 subjects were treated with the SilkTouch laser on one side of the face and 35% TCA on the opposite, for correction of periorbital wrinkling. Using a scoring system of 1 to 5, pretreatment scores were found to diminish 56% with laser treatment versus 20% with chemical peeling at 6 months. The outcome difference was statistically significant. Posttreatment erythema, however, lasted 4.5 months versus 2.5 months for the respective groups.[239]

Long-term follow-up of 12 patients having photodamage treated with dermabrasion and followed for 6 months to 8 years showed that not only did cosmetic improvement persist over these time periods, but the need for continued treatment of premalignant and malignant lesions was virtually eliminated. All patients were noted to have maintenance of smooth, supple skin with pigmentation slightly lighter than adjacent nondermabraded skin. The problem of course is that even though this laser resurfacing can improve the appearance of wrinkling by over 50%, the patient continues to age. We typically are seeing our patients back after 10 years asking for a second laser resurfacing procedure.

Other Indications of the CO_2 Laser

Acne

Laser resurfacing can achieve significant improvement in acne scarring. The procedure can be made very precise by sculpting the edges of the scars and vaporizing more tissue away only in the areas of scar tissue while doing only superficial resurfacing in the rest of the cosmetic unit being treated. The tissue-tightening effects can achieve dramatic improvement in soft atrophic scars with sloping walls (see Fig. 7.20). Some 'ice pick' and bound-down scars should first be removed with punch excision, punch elevation, or punch grafting, with laser resurfacing performed 6 to 12 weeks later if maximum improvement is desired[240] (Fig. 7.24). Those not treated first with excision will improve, but the degree of improvement achieved will depend on the scar's depth and the operator's skill. In general, a 30% to 50% improvement is the treatment goal. However, a study using the Coherent UltraPulse CO_2 laser to treat moderate to severe atrophic acne scars in 50 patients revealed an average clinical improvement of 81% at 6 months after treatment, with progressive improvement occurring during that period.[18]

We always treat acne scars with the Er:YAG laser after resurfacing with the CO_2 laser. The use of the Er:YAG allows for continued sculpting of the acne scar without an increase in nonspecific thermal damage.

Patients should be advised that acne scars are always difficult to treat by any method, and the patient rarely reaches the level of satisfaction desired in a single surgical procedure. The same is true for laser resurfacing, but additional laser procedures add significant degrees of improvement.

A

B

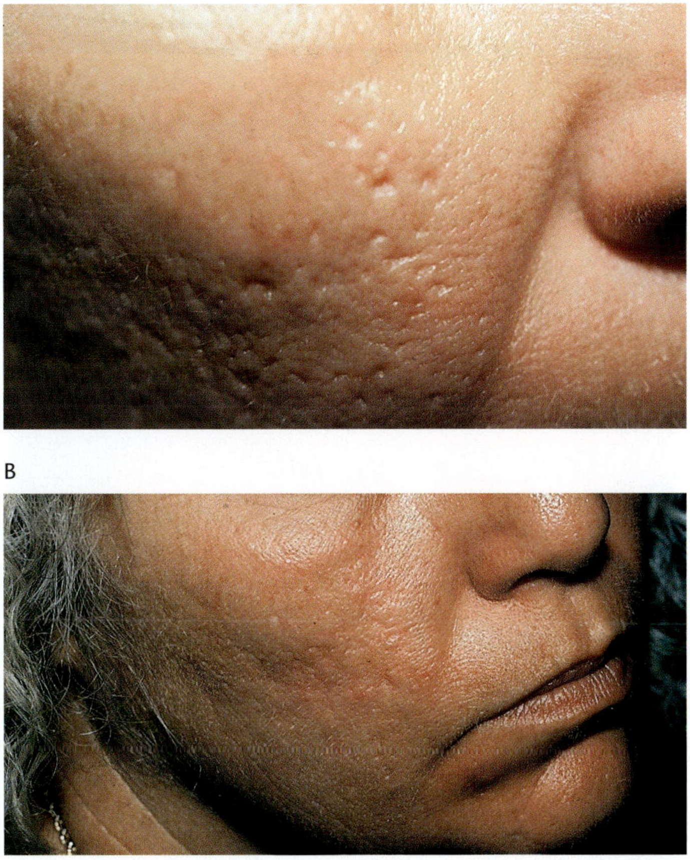

Figure 7.24 'Ice pick' or bound-down scars will improve greatly if scar excisions are performed before CO_2 laser resurfacing. (A) Before excision; (B) 1 year after laser resurfacing.

Scars

Crateriform varicella scars and isolated acne scars can be improved with spot laser resurfacing. The area around and over the scar is vaporized with one laser pass. Additional passes with the Er:YAG laser are concentrated along the edge of the scar crater until it has been completely effaced.

Postsurgical (Fig. 7.25) and traumatic scars and skin grafts (Fig. 7.26) can be dramatically improved if resurfaced.[59,60,241] It is best to wait until the scar has completely healed (3 to 6 months) (Fig. 7.27). This is an artistic endeavor and involves the vaporization of elevated tissue high points as well as skin tightening to elevate loose atrophic tissue. This is often a process of trial and error, attempting various maneuvers in small selective areas with observation of tissue effects before deciding to use an approach in a larger surface area.

Actinic Cheilitis

Actinic cheilitis has proved to be a condition for which CO_2 laser therapy is considered the treatment of choice.[62,242–251] It can be successfully treated by performing a laser vermilionectomy using any of the resurfacing lasers.[240] This procedure usually requires only one pass with the laser over the vermilion surface and then spot treatment of persistently visible actinic damage. This has significantly reduced postoperative healing to approximately 10 days, in contrast to the 4 weeks required when the conventional CO_2 laser was used in the past.[62,242–251]

A B C

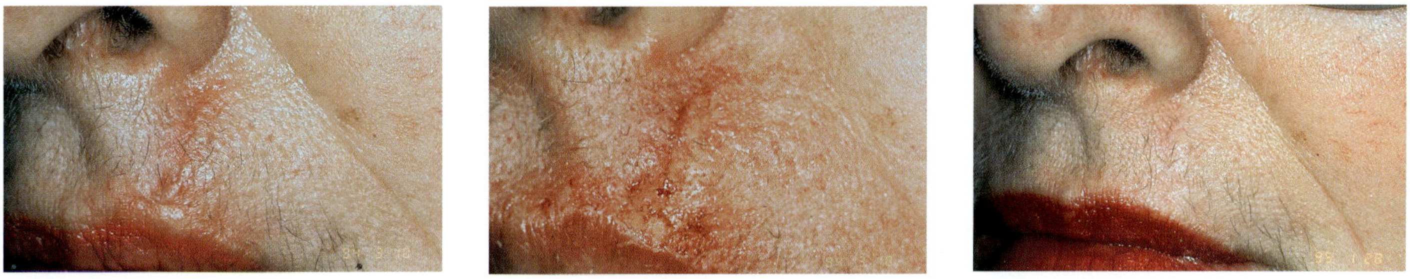

Figure 7.25 (A) Linear scar 6 weeks after repair of Mohs surgical defect. (B) Immediately after resurfacing with UltraPulse CO_2 laser at 500 mJ, 3-mm-diameter spot size, with three passes given to vaporize scar. (C) 9 months after resurfacing, virtual disappearance of scar.

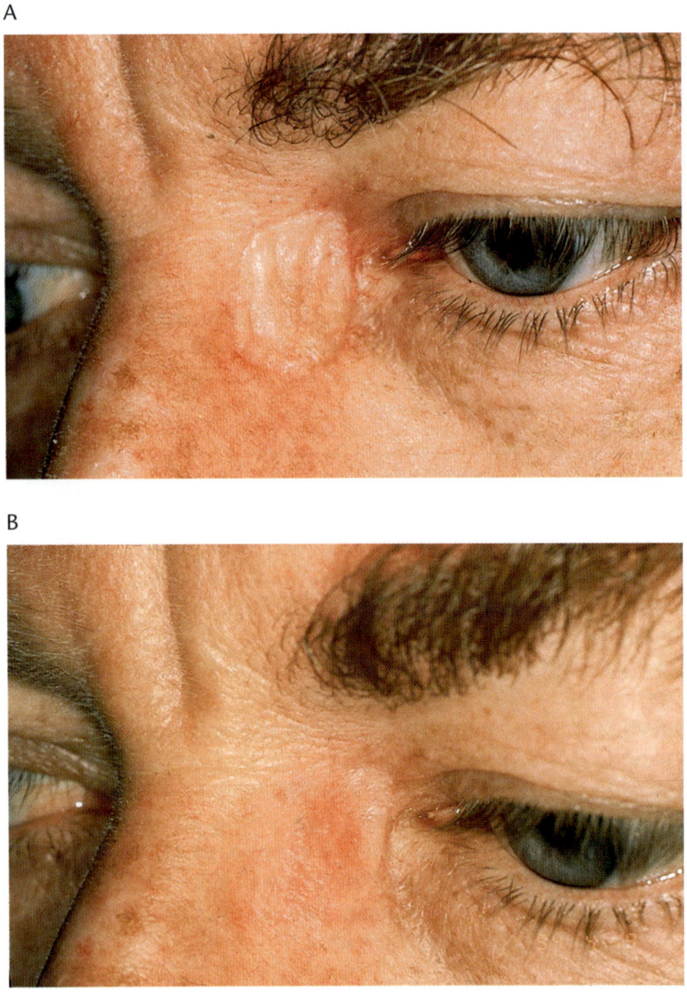

Figure 7.26 (A) 6 weeks after full-thickness skin graft repair of Mohs surgical defect. (B) 4 months after laser resurfacing of skin graft with laser parameters identical to those in Fig. 7.27.

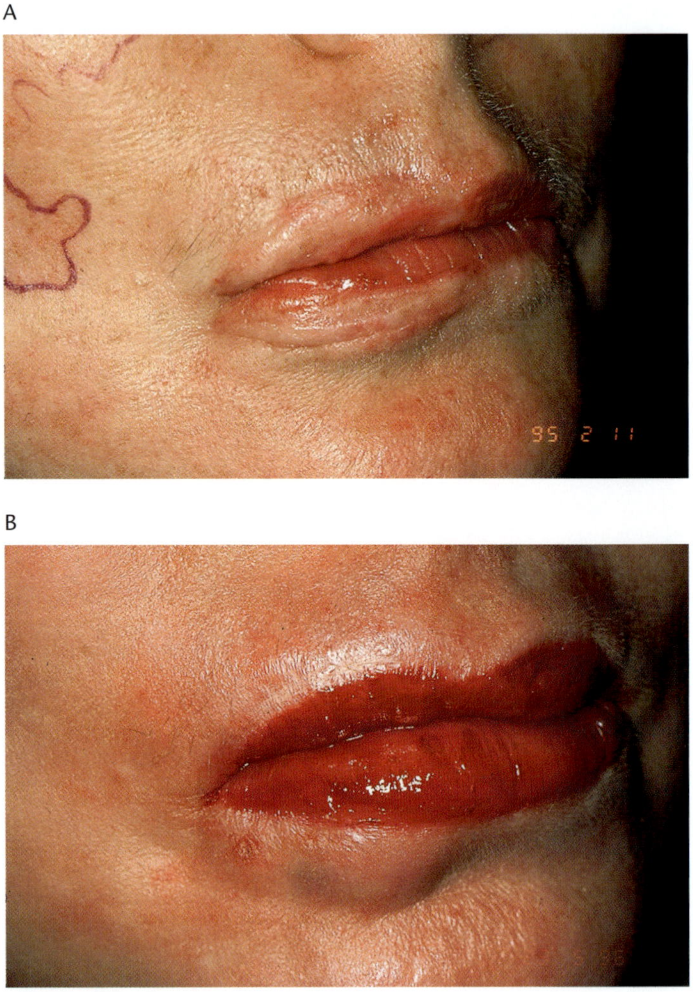

Figure 7.27 (A) Obvious deformity of scarred lips after full-thickness tissue loss and reconstructive surgery. (B) UltraPulse CO_2 laser was used to sculpt scar tissue and normalize lip contours.

Also, the risk of scarring is greatly reduced because the extent of thermal damage is much less.

Actinic keratoses unresponsive to conventional treatment with liquid nitrogen and topical 5-fluorouracil can be treated by removing the epidermis with one pass and then concentrating treatment on visible dermal extensions using one of the resurfacing lasers. This is especially useful on the dorsal hands and scalp but may be a primary or sole indication for laser resurfacing.

In our experience, treatment of these lesions in large surface areas results in much greater efficacy of treatment, with significantly decreased numbers of lesions occurring and their interval of recurrence greatly lengthened (see Chapter 6).

Pigmentation

Pigmentation irregularities such as postinflammatory hyperpigmentation or melasma can sometimes be improved with laser resurfacing. It is very important to use tretinoin (Retin-A) and hydroquinones for an extended period before and after the procedure.[252,253] Other lasers more specific for melanin or medium-depth chemical peels are often preferable because they do not require anesthesia and recovery time is much shorter.[254–258] Melasma responds variably, in a similar manner to its response to other modalities.[259] Usually these pigment abnormalities are a secondary component of treatment and not the primary treatment objective. If they are the primary reason for treatment, care must be taken to ensure that other, more pigment-specific therapies are not desirable for whatever reason.

Rhinophyma and Benign Growths

Rhinophyma[260,261] and various small benign growths such as syringoma,[262] trichoepithelioma,[263] dermatosis papulosa nigra, xanthelasma,[264] adenoma sebaceum,[265] sebaceous hyperplasia, and epidermal nevi[266,267] have traditionally been treated with the conventional CO_2 laser and respond in an even more excellent manner to the resurfacing CO_2 lasers (see Chapter 6).

CO_2 Laser Resurfacing: Surgical Considerations

Regional Versus Full-Face Resurfacing

The two areas of photodamage and wrinkling that have been shown to respond dramatically well to laser resurfacing are the perioral and periorbital regions.[77] These areas are not improved by face-lifting procedures and although blepharoplasty may improve the skin laxity, it does not smooth away the wrinkle lines and textural changes of the periorbital region. Chemical peels and dermabrasion have given disappointing results in both these regions after treatment by the average practitioner. Treatment success in these regions has given laser resurfacing its popularity. Either of these areas may be successfully treated as an isolated region, but if both areas are to be treated, it is far better to treat the entire face.

In general, full-face resurfacing will give a better clinical result in all patients, because treatment of the full cheeks results in better tightening of the nasolabial lines, lateral 'crow's feet', and midcheek creases. The same is true of treating the entire forehead and its effects on glabellar lines, lateral temporal lines, and upper aspects of crow's feet. In addition, the even pigmentation and smoothing of the skin results in a much more pleasant cosmetic appearance than blending new, smooth skin to photodamaged skin and creating a patchwork pattern. From a practical standpoint, it is also much easier for the patient to deal with postoperative erythema that is uniform over the full face rather than patchy erythema with multiple borders to blend. We rarely treat only a single anatomic unit, almost never treat an isolated wrinkle or scar, and never treat two isolated anatomic units simultaneously without treating the intervening skin. In our office, 90%–95% of patients receive full-face treatment.

Timing of Treatment

Whether to treat early or later is an issue that frequently arises. The potential advantages of treating early, rather fine, subtle wrinkle lines is that the procedure can be done more superficially and with less risk of prolonged erythema, pigment changes, or scarring. Also, greater potential exists for removing all the photodamaged tissue, achieving a more long-lasting result, and providing a preventive benefit regarding future wrinkling. However, these early changes are usually relatively subtle clinically and, even when fully removed, result in only modest cosmetic benefits. The primary benefit may be in halting progression of photodamage. The pros and cons of performing a relatively aggressive procedure for a relatively minor cosmetic problem need to be discussed in detail with the patient and a decision made with realistic expectations (Table 7.4).

Table 7.4 *Early Versus Later CO_2 Laser Treatment of Wrinkles**

Pros	Cons
Treatment of early wrinkling	
More superficial resurfacing necessary	Use of relatively aggressive treatment for relatively minor cosmetic problem
Less risks of scarring, prolonged erythema, and pigment loss	Must weigh risk/benefit ratio
Complete elimination of wrinkles typically achieved	Patients often very demanding and critical of less-than-perfect results
Long-lasting results achieved with good maintenance program	Deeper resurfacing procedure and more aggressive therapy necessary
Dramatic improvement often achieved	Greater risks of scarring, prolonged erythema, and pigment loss
	Improvement might be subtle
Treatment of late wrinkling	
Medical benefit (e.g. removal of actinic keratoses, squamous cell carcinoma in situ) common	More than one procedure necessary for complete elimination of wrinkles
Significant psychologic benefit	Persistence of benefits variable, depending on depth of preexisting damage as well as maintenance program
Patient satisfied with improvement, with no expectation of complete eradication of wrinkles	

*Both are successful. Both patient and physician must have realistic expectations. In general, earlier treatment preferable to later treatment because of decreased risks and enhanced ability to achieve excellent results.

Degree of Photodamage and Pigmentation

When dealing with more advanced photodamage, full-face resurfacing is almost always necessary. Complete removal of deep lines in a single procedure may not be possible, as previously discussed. The anticipated improvement is 50% to 70%[3,4,77,82–84] (Fig. 7.28). If further improvement is desired, a second treatment may be done after 6 to 12 months to allow new collagen formation and collagen remodeling. Patients with more advanced photodamage are usually very pleased with their clinical improvement even though it may not be complete eradication of wrinkle lines. Complete elimination of wrinkle lines usually is not the patient's goal, and overaggressive treatments may result in prolonged healing or hypopigmentation from deep levels of tissue ablation and deep resurfacing. The physician must effectively communicate to the patient that some degree of decreased pigmentation is a consequence of treatment.

Sun-damaged skin, with a history of decades of sun exposure, has a different pigmentation than non-sun-damaged skin that is related to the depth of resurfacing. Removal of the epidermis alone may result in healing with a population of melanocytes derived from the most superficial aspect of the follicular epithelium. These melanocytes have a significant history of prior sun damage and may produce persistent dyspigmentation. Deeper resurfacing results in progressive elimination of this sun-exposed subset of follicular epithelial melanocytes, yielding a more uniform pigmentation. An effective means of communicating this to patients is to have them compare the pigment of a non-sun-exposed area, such as the skin of the medial upper arms, to that of their face. This is likely to be the color of their newly healed skin, with non-sun-exposed epithelium and papillary dermis having developed during the healing process. If a strong color contrast is seen, a decision must be made regarding: (1) selection of epidermal resurfacing only, which can be accomplished with a 20% TCA peel or Er:YAG laser resurfacing; and (2) consideration of forming the transition zone from treated to non-treated skin.

The natural shadowing under the jaw line makes this area a good transition area. For some patients the contrast will be too great if they do not wear makeup. It may be preferable, however, to have this contrast occur at the jaw line rather than at midneck (chosen by some physicians because the upper neck heals better than the lower neck and can be treated more aggressively), the clavicular level, or the V of the neck or upper chest. Resurfacing of the neck to the clavicles or down to the middle anterior chest has not been recommended with the CO_2 laser because the risk of side effects is too high. The erbium laser may be used successfully in this regard with proper technique. Some physicians use 20% to 25% TCA applied in a light coat, with only spotty frosting occurring. The latter two choices may be appropriate for a woman who always wears a collared shirt and rarely or never has her entire upper chest and shoulder area visually exposed. When these areas are more visible from the clothing worn, especially in those frequently involved in athletics, women may prefer more superficial resurfacing and a transition zone at the jaw line.

To preserve normal pigmentation, even though it may be reduced in contrast to sun-damaged skin, it is necessary to avoid deep, midreticular dermal tissue removal. This type of pigment loss is considered a complication and is usually associated with prolonged erythema (Fig. 7.29). It should be avoidable by adhering to our recommended techniques.

Lines of Expression

Lines of expression – forehead lines, glabellar lines, and particularly 'crow's feet' lateral canthal lines – are caused by muscle contraction and will always recur, even if completely erased after the procedure. As long as the muscles

A B

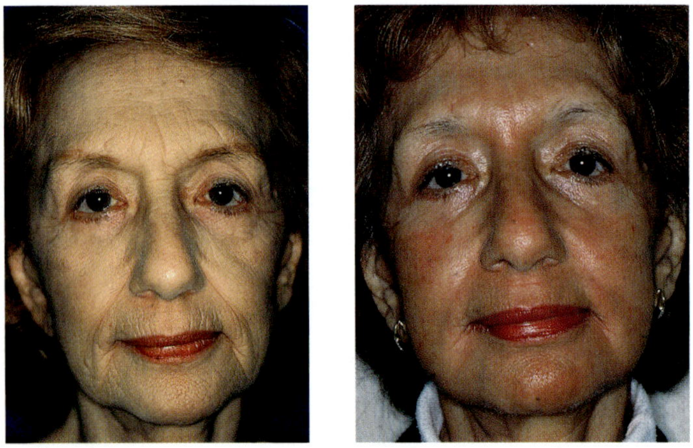

Figure 7.28 Anticipated improvement results for full-face resurfacing are 50% to 70%. Complete elimination of some wrinkle lines definitely will occur, but other lines may only soften. (A) Before surgery; (B) 3 months postoperatively.

A B C

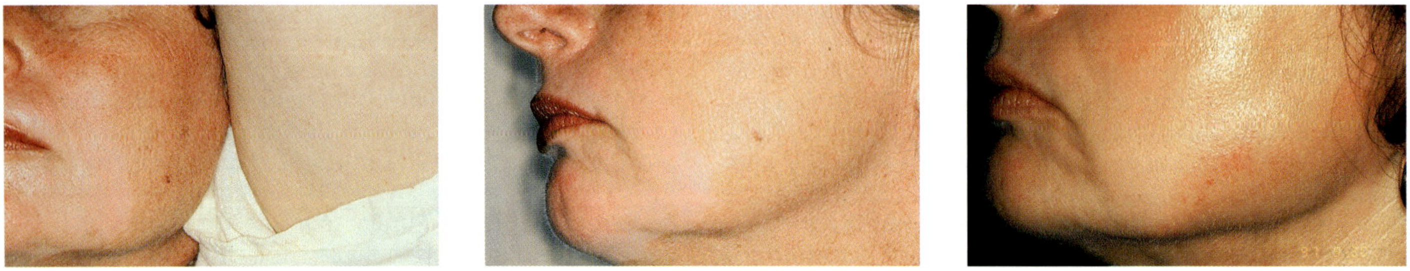

Figure 7.29 (A) True hypopigmentation occurs with loss of melanocytes and results in pigment loss that is usually more significant than that of non-sun-exposed skin. (B) This type of pigment loss contrasts sharply with photodamaged skin. (C) Treatment of this condition is oriented toward removal of contrasting photodamaged skin.

A

B

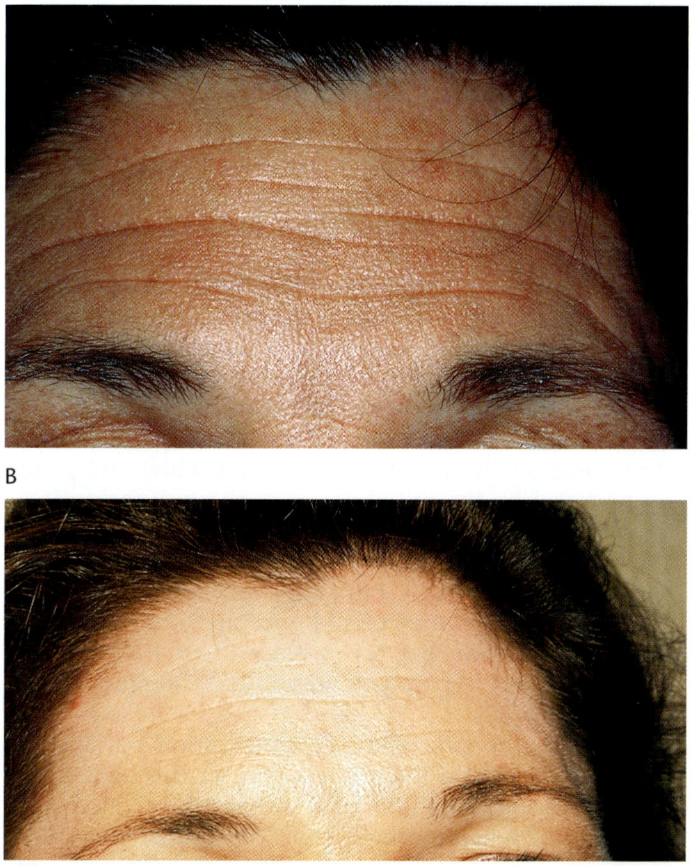

Figure 7.30 (A) Deep lines of forehead, glabella, and lateral canthi caused by muscle movement frequently recur after laser resurfacing. (B) Pretreatment with Botox results in more significant, longer-lasting improvement.

involved continue to fold the skin, a crease is formed. Several surgical procedures may be used to denervate or demuscle some of these areas. However, a very useful adjunctive procedure is the injection of botulin toxin type A (Botox) to block nerve transmission to these muscle groups.[268–271] These injections should be performed 1 to 2 weeks preoperatively to block these muscle groups and prevent motion in these areas for 3–4 months during the time of new collagen formation and remodeling. Enhanced results are seen and should give a more lasting clinical improvement (Fig. 7.30). We recommend continuing with Botox injections every 3–4 months for 1 year to achieve longer-lasting results.

Contraindications

Box 7.2 lists possible contraindications to resurfacing.

Box 7.2 *Relative Contraindications to Skin Resurfacing*

Possible Abnormal Wound Healing
- Prior isotretinoin (Accutane) treatment within 1 to 2 years
- Keloids/hypertrophic scars
- Scleroderma/collagen vascular diseases
- Immunosuppressive drugs

Decreased Adnexal Structures of Skin
- Prior radiation therapy
- Prior deep phenol peel
- Burn scars

Infectious Diseases
- Human immunodeficiency virus/acquired immunodeficiency syndrome
- Hepatitis C
- Active herpes simplex
- History of recurrent infections/anergy

Koebnerizing (Isomorphic) Diseases
- Labile psoriasis
- Severe eczema
- Vitiligo

Medical Conditions
- Significant diabetes
- Problematic hypertension
- Significant cardiovascular/pulmonary disease

Preoperative Care

Currently, there is no consensus on what the most appropriate preoperative skin care regimen to prepare the skin for cutaneous laser resurfacing is.[40,252,253] In fact, many recent studies have questioned the need for a preoperative skin care regimen at all.

Topical tretinoin has been shown by a number of studies to stimulate epithelial proliferation and regeneration and to decrease epidermal melanin content.[271,272] Additionally, topical tretinoin acid has been shown in a number of studies to speed reepithelialization and improve clinical outcome when used to prime the skin before dermabrasion and chemical peels.

Extrapolation from the literature reporting the benefits of tretinoin acid when used prior to dermabrasion and chemical peels led to its widespread use by cosmetic surgeons prior to laser skin resurfacing. In a 1998 survey of physician members of the American Society of Laser Medicine and Surgery, 80% of the 116 responders reported that they pretreated cutaneous laser resurfacing patients with topical tretinoin.[2]

However, the widespread use of tretinoin preoperatively was not based on well-controlled clinical studies. Recent investigations have questioned the benefit of pretreatment with topical tretinoin prior to cutaneous laser resurfacing. In a randomized, side-by-side comparative study, Orringer et al pretreated patients who underwent CO_2 laser skin resurfacing of the forearms with topical tretinoin (0.05%) for 3 weeks. Biopsy specimens were obtained at baseline and at various times (1 day to 6 months) posttreatment. They found no evidence of enhanced collagen formation, accelerated reepithelialization or quicker resolution of postoperative erythema with tretinoin pretreatment before CO_2 laser resurfacing.[274]

Moreover, adverse side effects secondary to tretinoin pretreatment have been reported. Some authors believe that topical application of tretinoin before cutaneous laser resurfacing may contribute to prolonged erythema postoperatively.[275] Skin irritation and exacerbation of facial telangiectasias are also potential hazards of tretinoin therapy according to other authors.[276,277] Given the lack of well-controlled clinical trials showing a benefit, and the risk, albeit small, of adverse side effects, it seems judicious to reexamine the current widespread use of tretinoin as a pretreatment medication for the laser resurfacing patient.

Up to one-third of patients experience postinflammatory hyperpigmentation after laser resurfacing.[16] The risk of hyperpigmentation after laser resurfacing parallels the degree of a patient's natural skin pigmentation and it is most prevalent in patients with Fitzpatrick skin phototypes greater than III.[5] To reduce the incidence of postinflammatory hyperpigmentation, many laser surgeons routinely pretreat patients with skin phototypes III–VI with a combination of topical skin lightening agents including tretinoin, hydroquinone, kojic acid, azelaic acid and alpha-hydroxy acids for 4 to 8 weeks prior to cutaneous laser resurfacing.[253]

The widespread use of these skin lightening agents before cutaneous laser resurfacing was highlighted by a 1998 survey of physician members of the American Society of Laser Medicine and Surgery; 80% of the 116 responders reported that they routinely pretreated their patients with topical tretinoin, 69% pretreated with hydroquinone and 10% pretreated with glycolic acid cream.

Hydroquinone inhibits tyrosinase, a key enzyme in the melanin synthesis pathway, and is directly toxic to melanocytes. Tretinoin promotes melanosome transfer and keratinocyte turnover and decreases epidermal melanin content. Azelaic acid, kojic acid, and glucosamine also inhibit tyrosinase and pigment synthesis. Reported benefits of alpha hydroxyl acids (i.e. glycolic acid) include increased epidermal thickness, decreased stratum corneum thickness and reversal of basal cell layer atypia.

Despite their widespread use, currently there is a great debate over whether pretreatment with these skin bleaching agents helps prevent hyperpigmentation after cutaneous laser resurfacing (Table 7.5). Data from several recent studies suggests that these agents are ineffective in the prophylaxis of hyperpigmentation after cutaneous laser resurfacing. West et al randomized 100 consecutive CO_2 laser skin resurfacing patients (skin phototypes I–III) to receive pretreatment with 10% glycolic acid cream b.i.d. or a combination of tretinoin 0.025% cream b.i.d. and hydroquinone 4% q.h.s. or no pretreatment at all. The overall incidence of postinflammatory hyperpigmentation was 11.1%, 32.3% and 50% in patients with skin phototypes I, II and III, respectively. Most importantly, they observed no significant difference in the incidence of postinflammatory hyperpigmentation between those patients that received pretreatment and those who did not.[52]

Postinflammatory hyperpigmentation is largely caused by the migration of melanocytes from deep within the adnexal epithelium or from cutaneous wound edges after resurfacing. Because of their limited penetration depths, topical bleaching agents may not exert any effect on these deeply situated melanocytes. Instead, they most likely affect superficially located melanocytes which are generally removed by the initial passes of the resurfacing laser. Topical bleaching agents like tretinoin and hydroquinone may be most effective, not as prophylactic agents during the preoperative period, but rather as therapeutic agents during the postoperative period once melanocyte and keratinocyte migration has taken place (3 to 4 weeks postoperatively) and hyperpigmentation has manifested itself clinically.[52,53]

To reduce the risk of hyperpigmentation patients are encouraged to avoid having a suntan at the time of the laser resurfacing procedure. Daily application of a full-spectrum sunscreen containing Parsol 1789 and/or micronized zinc is an important, noncontroversial, aspect of the pre and post operative care of the cutaneous resurfacing patient.

Table 7.5 *Agents to Treat Hyperpigmentation*

Agent	Mechanism of action
Hydroquinone	Cytotoxic to melanocytes
Azelaic acid	Inhibits tyrosinase and pigment synthesis
Kojic acid	Inhibits tyrosinase and pigment synthesis
Glucosamine	Inhibits tyrosinase and pigment synthesis
Tretinoin	Promotes melanosome transfer and keratinocyte turnover
Alpha-hydroxy acids	Promotes keratinocyte turnover

Antibiotic Prophylaxis

The use of antibiotic prophylaxis for cutaneous laser resurfacing remains a controversial issue. A number of studies have found antibiotics to be effective in prevention of infection after cutaneous laser resurfacing.

Bernstein et al observed no infections in a series of 50 patients who underwent full-face resurfacing and were treated with 250 mg of dicloxacillin q.i.d., starting the day before resurfacing and continuing for 1 week.[279] Nanni et al reported no bacterial infections in 500 consecutive cases of full-face cutaneous laser resurfacing, using 1 g intravenous (IV) cefazolin intraoperatively followed by 500 mg of azithromycin on postoperative day 1 and 250 mg for at least 4 days.[280] Waldorf et al found three instances of clinical infection in a series of 47 patients undergoing facial laser resurfacing that were prescribed 250 mg of dicloxacillin q.d. or 333 mg of erythromycin b.i.d. for 1 week throughout the reepithelialization period. The patients who developed infection were not taking antibiotics nor receiving aggressive wound care.[281] Ross et al reported that two of four patients without antibiotic prophylaxis undergoing full-face laser resurfacing developed *Staphylococcus aureus* infection, whereas none of four patients with Gram-positive antibiotic prophylaxis developed infection. Notably, they also reported a Gram-negative infection in a patient who had received Gram-positive antibiotic prophylaxis.[44]

Gaspar et al performed a randomized prospective study of 31 patients undergoing full-face CO_2 laser resurfacing and found four culture-positive clinical infections in the group of patients not receiving antibiotic prophylaxis (n = 14) and no cases of infection in the group of patients (n = 17) treated with cephalexin 500 mg PO b.i.d. started the day before surgery and continued for 5–10 days. The most common pathogen found in this study was *Staphylococcus aureus*. An occlusive dressing was used postoperatively in their patients.[282] Sriprachya-Anunt et al retrospectively found a 4.3% rate of culture-positive infection in a series of 395 patients undergoing facial skin laser resurfacing. However, the rate of infection increased seven-fold (from 1.35% to 9.82%) with a change from oral antibiotic prophylaxis (azithromycin 250 mg q.d. or a similar antibiotic for 7 days) to intranasal mupirocin and gentamicin otic solution, and the use of occlusive dressings rather than an open wound care technique postoperatively. The most common organism found was *Pseudomonas aeruginosa*, followed by *Staphylococcus aureus* and *Staphylococcus epidermidis*. Several combinations of Gram-positive and Gram-negative organisms were found in their study. Prophylactic ciprofloxacin (500–750 mg) b.i.d. for 5 to 7 days, starting the morning of surgery was recommended by these authors, especially when an occlusive dressing technique is used.[41] Manuskiatti et al reported on the infection rates of a large series of 356 patients that underwent facial skin resurfacing with the CO_2 laser. They observed an 8.2% bacterial infection rate when antibiotic prophylaxis was not given and a closed wound care technique was utilized. The infection rate decreased to 4.3% in the group of patients that received antibiotic prophylaxis with ciprofloxacin. Of note, infections in the group of patients that received prophylaxis occurred almost exclusively after discontinuation of ciprofloxacin.[43]

The 'pseudo-tissue-culture' environment maintained by occlusive dressings is an ideal growth medium not only for host cells that will carry out reepithelialization, but also for pathogenetic bacteria that can cause infection. As the studies described above suggest, antibiotic prophylaxis can help reduce the rate of infection after ablative laser skin resurfacing, especially when a closed wound care technique is utilized postoperatively. Furthermore, many authors believe that both Gram-positive and Gram-negative antibiotic coverage should be instituted when occlusive dressings are utilized for wound care after cutaneous laser skin resurfacing.[41,278]

There are some authors, however, that have not found antibiotic prophylaxis effective in reducing rates of infection after cutaneous laser resurfacing. In a retrospective study of 133 consecutive patients undergoing CO_2 laser resurfacing, Walia et al found a significantly higher rate of infection in patients receiving intraoperative (cephalexin 1 g IV) or postoperative (azithromycin 1.5 g PO for 5 days) antibiotics. The most common pathogens found were *Pseudomonas* and *Enterobacter* species. The authors concluded that prophylactic antibiotics are not necessary, especially if good postoperative care is followed.[283,284]

The literature shows that staphylococcal infection may be prevented by the prophylactic use of systemic antibiotics such as dicloxacillin, azithromycin, or ciprofloxacin.[16,43,253] The use of intranasal mupirocin (Bactroban),[285] however, has not proved to be advantageous and may even worsen the situation. All staphylococcal infections occurred in the group of patients using intranasal Bactroban in a study of patients randomly assigned to use or not to use Bactroban for 3 days preoperatively and 7 days postoperatively.[116]

Given that we use an occlusive dressing postoperatively, we begin antibiotic prophylaxis for both Gram-positive and Gram-negative bacteria (Omnicef 300 mg PO b.i.d.) the night before surgery and continue it for a total of 10 days. Utilizing this regimen we have observed no instances of infection after cutaneous laser resurfacing in our practice in the past 7 years.

The prevention of bacterial infections should not be taken lightly, because toxic shock syndrome (TSS) has been reported after a benign cutaneous infection with *Staphylococcus aureus* after laser resurfacing in three patients to date. Also, scarring secondary to disruption of wound healing has resulted from *Staphylococcus aureus* and *Pseudomonas* infection.

Another postoperative infection that may result from the moist wound environment is cutaneous candidiasis. This has been found to correlate with a prior history of vaginal yeast infection.[41] Prophylaxis with a single dose of fluconazole (400 mg) on the day of surgery is recommended. To date, we have not seen a yeast infection occur in a patient who received this prophylactic treatment preoperatively. The presentation of this infection postoperatively may include typical signs and symptoms of cutaneous candidiasis, but also may be atypical and present only as slow wound healing, itching, and erythema. It should always be suspected in a patient with unexplained poor wound healing. A potassium hydroxide preparation from a scraping of a suspicious area or a culture usually confirms the diagnosis.

In contrast to the controversial nature of antibacterial prophylaxis, most authors today advocate antiviral prophylaxis for herpes simplex virus for all patients undergoing full-face or perioral skin laser resurfacing.[40,42,45] Resurfacing laser-induced epidermal trauma and thermal injury can reactivate latent labial herpes simplex virus. The deepithelialized surface left behind after cutaneous laser resurfacing is highly susceptible to rapid dissemination of the herpes simplex virus. The incidence of herpetic outbreak in the postoperative period has been reported in the range of 2% to 7%.[2,16] All patients should be administered prophylaxis for herpes simplex virus, because patients with no known prior history of herpes simplex infection have been noted to develop an acute episode in the immediate postoperative period.[77] Dissemination over the treatment area with resultant scarring has been observed to occur in these patients (Fig. 7.31).

Patients should be treated with an antiviral agent such as valacyclovir (Valtrex) or famcyclovir (Famvir) starting a day or two preoperatively if they have a prior history of herpes simplex infection or starting on the day of the

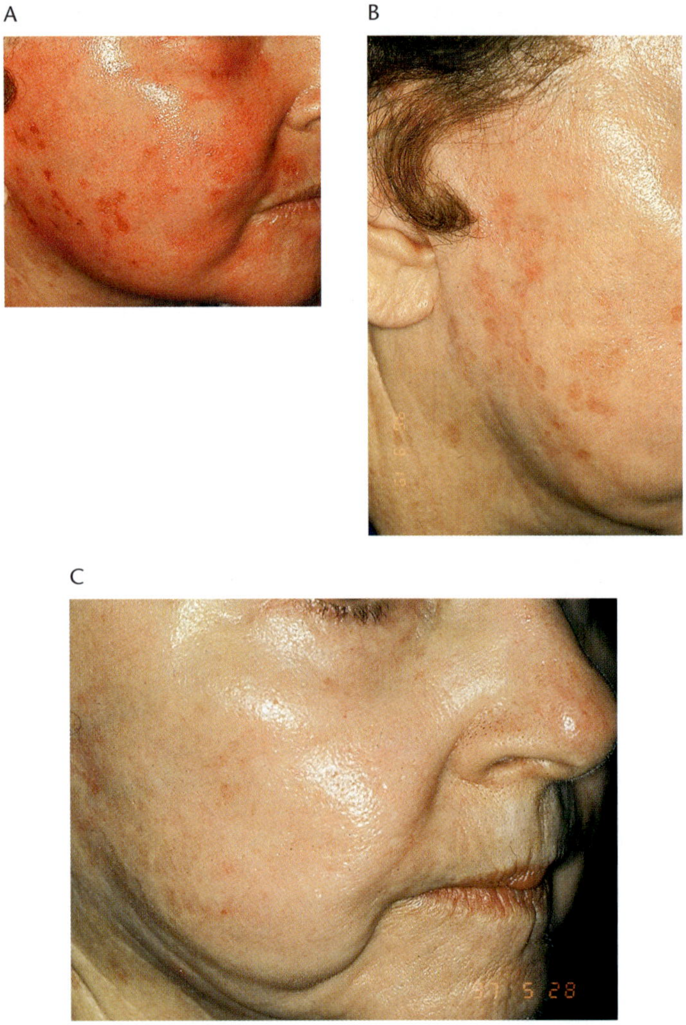

Figure 7.31 (A) Dissemination of herpes simplex occurred on day 4 postoperatively in patient with no prior history of herpes simplex infection, despite pretreatment with acyclovir (Zovirax). Valacyclovir (Valtrex) has been found to be superior as a preventive medication because much higher drug blood levels are achieved. (B) 10 months postoperatively, scarring from infection is apparent. (C) 8 months later, marked improvement has been achieved with pulsed dye laser treatment of scars.

procedure if no prior history. This treatment should be continued at least through the reepithelialization phase of wound healing (an additional 10 days). An acute treatment dose rather than a suppressive dose should be used. Valtrex (500 mg twice daily) and Famvir (250 mg twice daily) provide higher and longer-lasting blood drug levels than does acyclovir (Zovirax, 400 mg four times daily).

Immediate Preoperative Measures

The skin should be prepped with Techni-Care, a broad-spectrum, nontoxic microbicide that is antiviral, antifungal, and effective against both Gram-positive and Gram-negative bacteria; 30-s contact use has been shown to result in 99.99% bacterial reduction. Flammable agents such as chlorhexidine gluconate (Hibiclens) and isopropyl alcohol should not be used in the immediate preoperative stage unless thoroughly washed off with water preoperatively. Hibiclens and alcohol also have ocular toxicities, especially in a sedated patient (Table 7.6).

Metal eye shields should be inserted to protect the eyes.[286] Tetracaine (Tetcaine HCl Ophthalmic 0.5%) or a similar ophthalmic anesthetic solution is first placed in the eyes. Metallic eye shields with an external etching coated with sterile ophthalmic petrolatum should be used. Cox laser eye shields (Delasco, Council Bluffs, IO), which are available in three sizes, are inserted with a rubber vacuum plunger and have proved to be the most effective of those available because of ease of insertion and the ability to close the lids over them without distorting the overlying skin. When the eye shields are removed at the end of the procedure, the eyes should be flushed with sterile saline to wash out the petrolatum remaining on the conjunctival surface. This minimizes blurry vision postoperatively. If the periorbital area is not to be treated, the eyes may be protected with moistened gauze pads rather than eye shields.

The periphery of the patient's face should be draped with wet cloths before the procedure so that errant laser impacts do not contact a flammable surface or skin unintended for treatment. Some physicians advocate the use of aluminum foil, but we find this to be impracticable. If the glossy surface is the outer surface, reflection of an errant beam can occur; if the duller surface is exterior, reflection may still occur. Perhaps even more significantly, it is difficult to keep these foil sheets in place during the movement that necessarily occurs during the procedure. They are constantly falling off the surgical field, requiring replacement. A moist towel is easy to apply, is pliable, stays in place, and absorbs any errant laser beam that happens to hit it. The teeth may be protected by placement of wet gauze under the lips and over the teeth, but we have not found this to be necessary, except in patients with extensive porcelain crowns.

Anesthesia

For CO_2 laser resurfacing of the face, as for any surgical procedure, the goals of anesthesia are to provide optimal conditions for the surgeon while ensuring the patient's safety and comfort. Facial resurfacing is a highly stimulating and painful procedure requiring significant analgesia and alteration of consciousness level for optimal results. Muscle relaxation and loss of all reflexes are unnecessary and may be undesirable.

The sensory innervation of the face is complex and in some areas overlapping, making it difficult to attain adequate anesthesia using only nerve blocks. For complete and bilateral anesthesia, one must block the forehead; periocular, nasal, medial, and lateral face and cheeks; anterior areas of the ears; perioral region; and jaw lines. The medial forehead is blocked through the supraorbital and supratrochlear nerves. Sensory blockage of the entire face is difficult to achieve because a variety of nerves innervate this

Table 7.6 *Antimicrobials and Microbicides as Prophylaxis Before Skin Resurfacing*

	Chlorhexidine gluconate (Hibiclens)	Povidone iodine (Betadine)	Linear alcohol	Techni-Care
Substantivity (hours)	>6	3	None	>6
Occular irritation	Yes	Yes	Yes	Minimal
Scrub time (minutes)	8	3.5	11	0.5
Dermatitis potential	30%	30%	High	<1%
Formulation dependent	Yes	Yes	Variable	Yes
Amount needed (ml)	10	10	–	2.5
Tissue contraindications	Yes	Yes	Yes	None
Toxicity/chemical burns	Eyes, ears	Skin, genitalia	Eyes	Nontoxic*
Denatured by organic material	Minimal	Yes	No data	Minimal
Transdermal penetration/absorption	No	Yes	No	Yes
pH measurement	5.86	4.0	6.8	7.2

Data from a variety of sources.
*Safe for mucous membranes.

area and some of the blocks are very difficult to perform. The upper half of the ear is innervated through the mandibular nerve. The medial cheek, upper lip, and part of the skin overlying the nose are innervated through the infraorbital nerve. The lower lip and chin are innervated via the mental nerve. The upper outer cheek and lateral forehead are innervated through the maxillary nerve and the far lateral cheek and jaw line through the cervical plexus on each side.

Even with perfect technique, the 14 separate nerve blocks required for facial anesthesia may leave areas around the ear and lateral temporal region without adequate anesthesia.[287] Supplementation of the nerve blocks that are easily performed (infraorbital, mental, supraorbital, and supratrochlear) with local infiltration is painful and only partially effective.

Some physicians treat with only the use of topical anesthetic creams, such as lidocaine-prilocaine (EMLA cream). We have found this to be ineffective, because achievement of anesthesia results in maceration of tissue from the occlusive process, which then alters the laser–tissue interaction because of the excessive tissue water content. When this is not done, anesthesia is generally not achieved, and the procedure may be too painful to complete.

Another alternative now being popularized is tumescent anesthesia: using very dilute infiltration of 0.1% to 0.2% lidocaine (Xylocaine) in saline to distend the tissue subcutaneously, as is done with liposuction. This undoubtedly may produce adequate anesthesia but also may cause tissue distortion and alterations of the skin's mechanical properties. This interferes with identification of tissue laxity and its elimination through collagen shrinkage and skin tightening. Skin tightening depends not only on the pliability and ease of movement of the collagen, but also that of immediately adjacent tissue.

Some compromise in results would be anticipated with use of these local anesthetic techniques, either from inability to treat adequately because of incomplete anesthesia or alterations in the laser–tissue interaction. Local anesthesia techniques are generally supplemented with sedatives such as diazepam (Valium), midazolam (Versed), or lorazepam (Ativan) and analgesics such as meperidine (Demerol) or hydromorphine (Dilaudid), generally given orally or intramuscularly (IM). Possible side effects from these drugs must be considered as well in the choice of anesthesia. We prefer IV propofol sedation as our anesthesia, if feasible.

General anesthesia with endotracheal (ET) intubation for full-face laser resurfacing is an acceptable technique and has certain advantages. It ensures airway control, is safe and quickly administered, and allows the administration of adequate narcotic analgesia without concern for respiratory depression. However, not all facilities are equipped to provide general anesthesia. Also, patients or physicians may be reluctant to use general anesthesia for this procedure. A method of deep IV sedation combined with the use of the laryngeal mask airway (LMA) allows the procedure to be accomplished without ET intubation or an anesthesia machine.

Propofol is the primary agent used and provides rapidly induced, easily maintained, and quickly terminated loss of consciousness. IV midazolam is used to provide initial sedation and amnesia, while analgesia is provided by fentanyl (Sublimaze) supplemented intermittently with ketamine (Ketalar). To counteract potentially troublesome side effects of ketamine, all patients receive glycopyrrolate (Robinul) as a drying agent and midazolam and propofol before receiving ketamine. By using this regimen and limiting the total ketamine dose to about 1 mg/kg, patients have had no problems with 'bad dreams' or adverse psychic experiences.[287]

The requisite equipment for this technique consists of an electrocardiogram (ECG), blood pressure monitor, pulse oximeter, supplemental oxygen source, LMA, and an IV infusion pump, as well as an anesthesiologist to administer the anesthesia. Capnohepatography, while optional, is desirable to monitor adequacy of ventilation. Prudence dictates that any facility administering narcotics or sedatives have appropriately trained medical personnel, a fully stocked resuscitation cart, intubation equipment (laryngoscope, blades, ET tubes), a method for delivering positive-pressure ventilation (Ambubag or Jackson-Rees circuit), and a charged and functional defibrillator. A recovery area staffed with qualified nursing personnel should have the capacity to monitor ECG, blood pressure, and pulse oximetry.

Concern over the safety of laser energy in proximity to oxygen and the patient's face is understandable. All modern inhaled anesthetics are nonflammable, and although oxygen and nitrous oxide support combustion, neither is itself flammable. It is imperative that flammable liquids not be used in the facial preparation. The patient must be instructed not to use hairspray or other topical skin and hair products before surgery to avoid the introduction of unknown chemicals into the surgical field.

The oxygen delivery system consists of the LMA and the tubing from a green oxygen mask connecting the oxygen cylinder and the LMA, which includes a small pilot tube used to inflate the pharyngeal cuff. The LMA is very resistant to damage from the laser. An informal study performed in our facility revealed it to be resistant to penetration or inflammation despite 60 consecutive laser impacts while oxygen was flowing to enrich the immediate open-air vicinity. The pilot tube also is very resistant to laser damage, requiring 22 impacts before it was cut through, but never ignited. The green oxygen tubing, on the other hand, is easily damaged, and a few pulses will melt it. However, the oxygen flowing through the tube will not ignite, although any flammable object present in the field (e.g., dry gauze, dry hair) will ignite. ET tubes and LMA tubes can be fully protected by wrapping them with saline-soaked gauze or towels. With proper procedures and caution that no combustible liquids or other products are used near surgical areas, laser resurfacing in the presence of oxygen and an anesthetic delivery system such as an ET tube or LMA is safe.

Anesthesia for Erbium:YAG Laser Resurfacing

While a topical anesthesia approach has been found impractical for CO_2 laser skin resurfacing, topical ancsthetics such as LMX-5 (Ferndale Laboratories, Ferndale, MI) have been able to provide an effective level of anesthesia for superficial resurfacing with the Er:YAG laser. For deeper resurfacing with the short pulse Er:YAG laser, regional nerve blocks (supraorbital, supratrochlear, infraorbital, mental nerve blocks can be easily performed) and/or local infiltration with 1–2% lidocaine with 1:100,000 epinephrine can be used. However, for ablation into the dermis or full-face resurfacing with the Er:YAG laser, intravenous sedation performed by an anesthesiologist as described above under careful monitoring is generally required.

Wound Healing

Observations in animal models and clinical studies suggest a general sequence of events that occur in wound healing, largely controlled by fibroblasts.[288–294] This has been divided into three phases: inflammatory, proliferation, and maturation.

Inflammatory Phase

The inflammatory phase lasts 3 to 10 days.[291,294] After dermal trauma, blood vessels constrict, and leakage of plasma proteins (fibrinogen, fibronectin, plasminogen) and platelets occurs. Plasma and blood clot when exposed to tissue factors[295] and form a gel-like fibrin-fibronectin matrix. Inflammatory cells, new capillaries, and fibroblasts derived from the wound edges migrate into this matrix. Activated macrophages are probably the most important cells in this phase of healing, particularly for wound debridement.[296–299]

The fibrin–fibronectin matrix is degraded by inflammatory cells. Fibroblasts synthesize fibronectin, interstitial collagens, and GAGs to form a new fibrovascular connective tissue, or granulation tissue, within 2 to 4 days of injury.[289,300,301] Fetal wound healing has been found to proceed without scar formation and, unlike adult wounds, in which hyaluronic acid is present transiently, high levels of hyaluronic acid persist in fetal wounds until repair is completed. The fetal extracellular matrix contains abundant hyaluronic acid rather than collagen.[302,303] This may be the result of decreased degradation,[304] and other studies suggest that hyaluronic acid may have a regulatory effect on scarless fetal wound healing.[305,306] Topical treatment of wounds with hyaluronic acid was found to reduce scarring of tympanic membrane perforations.[307] Normal mature scars, hypertrophic scars, and keloids were found with distinctively different distributions of hyaluronic acid, possibly contributing to their different clinical appearances.[308]

Beneficial effects of topical hyaluronic acid have been demonstrated both clinically and histologically in cutaneous ulcer healing studies,[309–314] animal wound studies,[315–317] and in vitro and in vivo studies.[318–321]

Proliferation Phase

The prominent collagen formed during the inflammatory phase is type III collagen, which has a gel-like consistency.[322] Its synthesis is maximal between 5 and 7 days. The proliferation phase occurs over the next 10 to 14 days and is dominated by the proliferation of fibroblasts and synthesis of collagen as well as regeneration of the epidermis and neoangiogenesis. Reepithelialization is heralded by mitoses at wound edges and at appendages within 24 hours.[292] Epidermal proliferation is maximal at 24 to 72 hours.[293] Direct contact with fibronectin and type I collagen guides and stimulates epithelial cell migration in culture.[294] Soluble substances such as growth factors derived from platelets, macrophages, dermal parenchymal cells, and keratinocytes stimulate reepithelialization in animal models.[301] Continued collagen synthesis proceeds, stimulated by macrophage-derived and platelet-derived factors,[323] followed by capillary resorption and disappearance of fibroblasts.[324]

Lymphokines, complement, native collagens of types I to V, fibronectin, and platelet-derived growth factor may be potent mitogens and chemotactants for fibroblasts.[288,325] In addition, macrophages may be activated by blood and may play a key role in inducing a fibroproliferative response when there is significant blood within the healing wound.[288,297,326]

In the biosynthesis of collagen, procollagen is formed intracellularly by fibroblasts and secreted into the extracellular space.[324] It is then biochemically transformed into tropocollagen by proteases.[327–329] The tropocollagen molecules aggregate into immature soluble collagen fibrils, which are then cross-linked by the action of lysyl oxidase to form mature, stronger collagen fibers.[330]

Maturation Phase

The total amount of collagen in a wound reaches a maximum at 2 to 3 weeks, but collagen remodeling continues over months to years.[331] This characterizes the third phase of wound healing, the maturation phase. The earliest collagen fibers are thin and unorganized, becoming thicker, cross-linked, and parallel to skin tension lines with time. As new collagen is formed, abnormal or damaged collagen is broken down by collagenases and proteases produced by fibroblasts, macrophages, and inflammatory cells. Proteoglycans, responsible for water storage in the healing wound, decrease, and water is reabsorbed as the wound heals.[332,333]

Remodeling of the collagen matrix results in gradual shrinkage, thinning, and paling of the scar. Once the collagen bed is established as a stable matrix, collagen production and resorption continue in a steady, balanced state in a normally healed scar. Tensile strength increases from 5% of original strength at 2 weeks to 80% in a mature scar.[334] Contraction of a scar, which begins 1 week after wounding, is not caused by excessive deposition of collagen, but rather by the effects of transformation of fibroblasts to myofibroblasts.[335,336] These cells produce contractile proteins with characteristics of smooth muscle cells. Granulation tissue has been shown to contain as much actomyosin as an equivalent weight of smooth muscle.[337] Furthermore, it has been demonstrated that contraction of myofibroblasts can be inhibited by smooth muscle relaxants.[291,335] It has been proposed that migrating fibroblasts interact with their surrounding matrix components to reorganize connective tissue fibers to induce shrinkage.[338] These factors can result in as much as a 45% reduction in wound surface area.[291]

Effects of Treatment

The magnitude and timing of each phase of wound healing may vary significantly depending on the wounding procedures and modalities. A study was designed to characterize differential responses to cutaneous injuries of equal depth created by a dermatome, laser ablation, or standard thermal metal template.[339] When skin is wounded with a dermatome, the wound bed is immediately flooded with growth-factor-laden platelets and blood constituents. By contrast, the other thermal wounds are deficient in immediate blood-borne cytokines. At day 5, dermatome wounds showed an average reepithelialization of 54%, almost two times higher than that of laser injuries and four times higher than standard thermal burns. This difference had disappeared by day 10. At day 5, laser wounds contained the highest number of proliferating fibroblasts, which were significantly depressed in thermal burns. At day 10, this order was reversed, with thermal burns having the highest proliferative profile and laser wounds the lowest. Laser wounds showed the earliest peak in matrix metalloproteinase (MMP) expression, whereas burns showed the least expression at day 5. An assessment of angiogenesis showed peak values at day 5 in both excisional and laser wounds, with burns not peaking until day 10. Laser injuries appeared to mature the earliest. The amount of new granulation tissue in laser injuries was modest compared with excisional or burn injuries. Standard burns exhibited the highest degree of disorganization, a feature of immature wounds.

In summary, laser injuries showed early accelerated levels of angiogenesis, dermal fibroblast proliferation, and MMP expression but were dramatically slower to resurface. This delay in reepithelialization may be related to damage to keratinocytes that reside in the upper aspects of hair follicles and sweat ducts. More likely, the difference in laser wounds relate to the layer of necrotic tissue that needs to be digested before reepithelialization can proceed in non-laser-induced wounds. The differences in the MMP expression patterns of the three types of wound raise questions regarding proteolytic enzymes within the wound clearing and activating precursor of cytokines beneficial to wound healing. The data suggest that the function of MMPs within these wounds is not the proteolysis of devitalized tissues but rather the active remodeling of the wound environment.

Postoperative Care

If the patient develops noticeable intraoperative swelling, usually detected in the periorbital area, dexamethasone (Decadron, 10–12 mg by IV push) may be administered. Although some physicians routinely use a Decadron Dospak, oral prednisone (20 mg every day for 7 days), or triamcinolone (Kenalog, 40 mg IM) postoperatively, the effects on suppression of fibroblast activity and infection surveillance must be considered. Single-dose IV Decadron is rapidly cleared and thus should not interfere with wound healing. Because postoperative swelling generally clears rapidly (2 to 5 days), the choice of the shorter-acting corticosteroids is preferable.

Minimal thermal damage which results in poor coagulation of dermal blood vessels and poor hemostasis characterize treatment with the short pulsed Er:YAG laser. Application of wet gauze compression is useful to deal with the bleeding that is typically seen after resurfacing with the short pulsed Er:YAG laser.[12] Patients are told to expect a mild burning sensation for the first 1 to 3 days and significant swelling for the first 2 to 5 days postoperatively. The edema that develops in the first 48 hours postoperatively can be controlled with icepacks, head elevation at night and in severe cases, with oral corticosteroids.

During the first 3 to 5 days, significant serous exudate is present as well, related to the swelling and absence of an epithelial barrier. Use of topical antibiotics and other topical drugs should be particularly avoided during this phase, because the incidence of contact irritant and allergic dermatitis is enhanced by the absence of epithelium.[124] We have found the incidence to increase from about 3% to 4% when topical agents are used in nonlaser-treated skin to 20% or higher when they are used after laser skin resurfacing. Bacitracin is a frequent sensitizer, with a five-fold increase in dermatitis reported from 1990 to 1994.[340] In addition, a compound such as petrolatum, which usually does not cause contact sensitivity, has a greater potential to sensitize in this situation.[116,341]

Wound Care

The benefits of wound occlusion have been well documented.[50,342,343] Wound occlusion creates a moist environment that protects the wound from exogenous bacteria, inhibits crust formation, enhances reepithelialization and reduces patient discomfort. Occlusion can be achieved by either open or closed wound care techniques.

Open wound care techniques facilitate surveillance of the laser wound for clinical signs of infections or other complications. Additionally, they are relatively inexpensive and do not elicit the feeling of claustrophobia that some patients can experience with occlusive dressings. However, to achieve the healing benefits of occlusion, open wound care techniques demand around-the-clock wound care by the patient and thus are largely dependent on patient compliance.

Open-wound care generally consists of frequent soaking with cool distilled water containing a small amount of white vinegar. One teaspoon per cup is generally the starting concentration (0.25% acetic acid). The mildly acidic pH has an antibacterial effect, which is especially important in suppressing *Pseudomonas* species. The skin should be soaked for 20 minutes every 1 to 2 hours. The objective is to soak away the serous exudate and any necrotic tissue on the skin surface. Just patting the skin with a moist gauze pad is not adequate. Between soakings, the skin should be liberally and continuously coated with petrolatum (Vaseline), Aquaphor (Beiersdorf, Charlotte, NC) or Theraplex. This coating may be gently removed with gauze or facial tissue before the next soaking. Ice packs or frozen peas may be applied during this period for symptomatic pain relief.

The application of petrolatum to the wound surface results in a semiocclusive, moist environment. Studies have shown that wounds treated with petrolatum compared with those treated with a topical antibiotic have no increased incidence of infection and heal at the same rate.[334] In contrast, in a study of accidental burns treated with either petrolatum mesh gauze or nitrofurazone, 75% of the petrolatum group had bacteria reported as 'too numerous to count' compared with only 10% of the nitrofurazone group.[345]

The composition of a bland emollient apparently may have an effect on wound healing. A U.S.P. petrolatum ointment decreased wound healing by 17%, a white petrolatum cream increased wound healing by 24%, and a lotion with propylene glycol without petrolatum increased wound healing by 15%.[346]

Wound-healing studies have shown that vehicles with the proper combination of fatty acids result in faster healing than do petrolatum or Aquaphor.[347] Fatty acids that reflect the composition of fatty acids in human membranes are required for the proliferation of epithelial cells.[348,349] This mixture of fatty acids also significantly enhances the ability of pyruvate and vitamin E to inhibit reactive oxygen production and improve membrane function and cellular viability. These three components – vitamin E, pyruvate, and essential fatty acids – have been shown to be synergistic in reducing oxidative stress to keratinocytes and enhancing wound healing.[347]

Patients treated with an open wound care regimen are seen on the first and third days postoperatively, and any excess crust is gently removed with saline. The frequency of soaks and ointment application is tapered off as reepithelialization progresses. Once reepithelialization is complete, a mild facial cleanser (i.e. Neutrogena fresh foaming cleanser or Cetaphil facial cleanser) and a daily moisturizer-sunscreen are introduced.

The benefit of occlusive dressings in accelerating wound healing was first demonstrated in 1962[350] and confirmed in numerous studies.[342,351–361] Reepithelialization was shown to occur 30% to 45% more quickly, with decreased pain and inflammation and more cosmetically acceptable scar formation. In addition, new collagen formation has been shown to begin 3 days earlier than in open wounds,[362] with an increased rate of collagen synthesis.[363] The increased rate of reepithelialization produced by occlusive dressings is generally attributed to the moist wound environment and the absence of a crust that may impede cellular movement. In addition, occlusive dressings provide an environment that maximizes exposure to various endogenous growth factors. Continued exposure to epidermal growth factor has been shown to quicken epidermal resurfacing.[364]

Studies of varying the time of application or removal of an occlusive dressing have shown that for optimal healing, dressings need to be applied within 2 hours after wounding and should be left in place for at least 24 hours.[365] Waiting 24 hours before application almost precludes the occlusive dressing's effect on wound healing, but it still may have benefit in pain reduction. Early removal of the dressing greatly reduces the occlusive effects, but not if 24 or 48 hours has passed.

More recently, several studies have demonstrated that closed wound care techniques utilizing occlusive dressings for the first 48 to 72 hours after laser skin resurfacing reduce crusting, erythema, and edema (Fig. 7.32). Moreover, occlusive dressings have been reported to significantly decrease postoperative pain and patient discomfort and simplify wound care for patients when compared to open wound care techniques.[40,46–50]

The most popular commercially available closed-occlusive dressings for laser skin resurfacing wounds belong to one of the following categories: composite foams, polymer films, polymer meshes, hydrogels, hydrocolloids and alginates. These closed-occlusive dressing categories are reviewed below.

Occlusive Dressings for Laser Resurfacing Wounds (Table 7.7)

Composite Foam Dressings

These dressings have adhesive and absorptive properties and thus are useful in the care of the exudative wound that results after laser skin resurfacing. Flexzan (Dow Hickam

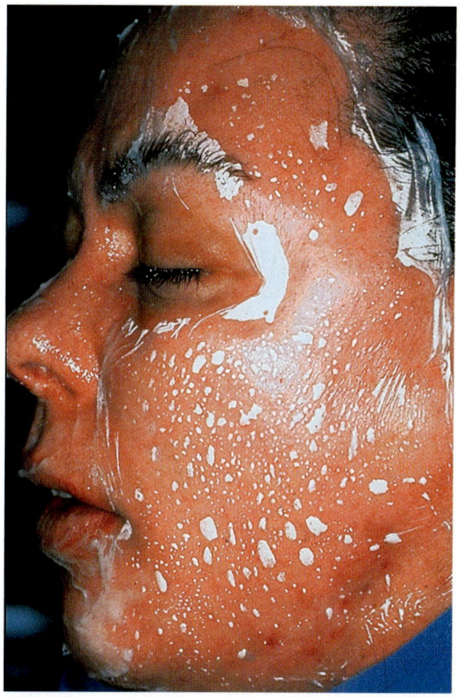

Figure 7.32 Silon II, a polyurethane film with multiple small slits, allows soaking directly through film and enhances wound healing during first 72 hours.

Table 7.7 *Biosynthetic Dressings*

Classification	Composition	Examples	Transmits oxygen
Polyurethane films	Polyurethane *or* co-polyester with adhesive backing	Op-Site Bioclusive, Opraflex, Uniflex, Blisterfilm, Visulin, Ensure, Clingfilm, Viofilm, Acuderm, Omniderm, Dermafilm, Silon II, Tegaderm	Fluid retention may be problem Difficult to handle Omniderm or Silon II better suited for exudative wounds
Hydrocolloids	Hydrophilic colloidal particles bound to polyurethane foam	DuoDerm, Actiderm, Tegasorb, Cutinova Hydro, Ultec, Comfeel Ulcus, Restore, Hydrapad, Granulfex E, Intrasite, Intact, Flexzan	
Hydrogels	60%–99% water cross-linked polymer, such as polyethylene or polyvinyl	Vigilon, Second Skin, Biofilm, Geliperm, Cutinova Gel, Elasto-Gel, Intrasite Gel, Span Gel, ClearSite	Gel formed by dressing often purulent in appearance and acrid in odor If wound very exudative, gel will leak beyond dressing
Calcium alginate	Composite of fibers from calcium alginate	Sorbsan	Capable of significant fluid absorption
Foams	Hydrophillic or hydrophobic polyurethane or gel film	Kaltostat	Require frequent dressing change Significant hemostatic properties
Others			
Biobrane	Silicone rubber with nylon and porcine collagen bilaminate	Cutinova Plus Ulcer Care, Lyofoam, Sythaderm Allevin, Epigard	Very high absorbency Similar to hydrogels
N-Terface	Monofilament plastic		Can become incorporated in wound if wound dries May delay reepithelialization
Cellophane wrap (contains 65% glycerin)	Cellulose with glycerin	Saran Wrap	Excessive fluid accumulation occurs Wick effect transfers fluids to outer membrane Oxygen transmission increases 1000-fold when material is wet

Pharmaceuticals) is the most popular commercially available dressing of this type.

Flexzan is composed of a polyurethane foam with open cells of graduated sizes that allows absorption of moisture at the skin surface and gas exchange but no entry of exogenous moisture or bacteria at its outer surface. Flexzan comes in white-colored sheets from which customized templates can be cut out to fit the resurfaced areas. Flexzan has a patterned adhesive coating. Individual strips of Flexzan stick to dry skin and should be overlapped to stabilize it over the face. Flexzan does not require additional gauze padding for absorption. It is opaque, and thus it must be removed in order to examine the patient's skin. Removal of the dressing does not harm the healing epithelium if done during the first 48 hours postoperatively while the wound is still in its exudative phase.[366]

Polymer Film Dressings

Silon TSR (Bio Med Sciences, Inc, Bethlehem, PA) is a thin (0.005 inch), transparent film of silicone polymer with a pattern of 2-mm slits spaced at 12-mm intervals, which allows for escape of wound exudate. Silon TSR comes designed as a face mask that is placed over the face after slits for the eyes, nose and mouth are cut out. The face mask maintains its adherence via surface tension forces from the wound's exudate and is secured with drawstrings that are tied posteriorly over the scalp. To provide absorption, a layer of gauze padding is laid down over the mask and is held in place with a band net dressing. Given its transparency, the skin can easily be inspected with the Silon TSR dressing in place. Omniderm is a water-vapor-permeable, wound-fluid-impermeable polyurethane film dressing that is bonded to acrylamide, a hydrophilic monomer. Omniderm is relatively inexpensive and has been found effective for wound care after CO_2 laser resurfacing[367] and dermabrasion.[368] Additionally, a new dual-silicone membrane dressing (DiamondSeal, Genzyme Biosurgery, Cambridge, MA) had a higher patient satisfaction rating (71% versus 54%) when compared to a popular occlusive tape dressing (Flexzan) in a series of patients that underwent full-face laser resurfacing and/or rhytidectomy.[366]

Polymer Mesh Dressings

Polymer sheets with numerous pores forming a mesh pattern characterize dressings in this category. Mepitel (Molnlycke Health Care, Molnlycke, Sweden) and N-Terface (Winfield Laboratories, Dallas, TX) are two commercially available representatives of this category.

N-Terface is a thin polyethylene mesh that comes in a face mask design which is applied to the face with an ointment that aids in its adherence to the wound. Gauze pads over the mesh are necessary for absorption and are secured with a band net dressing. Slippage can be a problem and an additional elastic face mask design wrap has been designed to stabilize the dressing. N-Terface is partially transparent and thus does not need to be removed for wound inspection.

Mepitel is a silicon polymer mesh with 1-mm pores that allow drainage of wound exudates to an overlying layer of gauze pads secured by a band net dressing. Mepitel adheres only to dry skin or nonresurfaced areas. When removed for inspection of the skin, it can be reapplied without any loss of its adherent properties.

Hydrogel Dressings

The dressings in this category are composed primarily of water. Vigilon (Bard Medical Division, Covington, GA) and 2nd Skin (Bionet, Little Rock, AR) are two commercially available hydrogels. They are soft, porous gels composed of a lattice of water molecules (96% water content) and 4% polyethylene oxide. The 2nd Skin hydrogel comes as precut rectangles that can be custom sized. There is a plastic film on either surface of the gel. The outer plastic film can be removed or left in place depending on how much occlusion is desired. The primary disadvantage of hydrogel dressings is that they lack adhesion. They are held in place with paper tape followed by placement of gauze pads over the dressing for absorption and a band net dressing to secure the assembly in place. These dressings are capable of marked fluid absorption, so they are well suited for exudative laser wounds. Dressing changes vary with the amount of exudate and are recommended every 6 to 8 hours for the 2nd Skin dressing.

Hydrocolloid Dressings

Hydrocolloid dressings use a water-impermeable polyurethane outer covering that is separated from the wound by a hydrocolloid material, usually carboxymethyl cellulose. This hydrocolloid interacts with the wound exudate to form a gel that does not adhere to the wound surface; however, these dressings do adhere to normal skin. Within the gel are endogenous enzymes that autolytically debride the wound.[361,369,370] Liu et al found that the hydrocolloid dressing Duoderm (ConvaTec, Princeton, NJ) effectively promoted wound healing following CO_2 laser resurfacing.[371]

Alginate Dressings

The alginate dressings are very absorptive and because they are nonadherent, require a secondary dressing. The dressing is easily removed with saline irrigation because it is soluble in solutions containing sodium ions.[372] Alginates have been used in the food and pharmaceutical industries since 1881 and are salts of alginic acid, derived from brown seaweeds. They are unique as dressings because of their action as hemostatic agents[373,374] and have not been shown to induce adverse tissue changes.[375] They may be ideal dressings for resurfacing, especially erbium laser therapy, in regard to the capillary oozing that occurs postoperatively. Liu et al. found that the popular alginate dressing Kaltostat (ConvaTec, Princeton, NJ) left behind difficult-to-remove fibers on the laser wound surface.[371] Other popular, commercially available alginate dressings for laser resurfacing wound care include Sorbsan (Bertek Pharmaceuticals), Restore Calcicare (Hollister), Tegagen HG (high gelling) and Tegagen HI (high integrity) (3M Health Care) and Comfeel Plus (Alginate-hydrocolloid dressing) (Coloplast).

Other Dressings

Biobrane (Dow Hickman, Sugar Land, TX) is a synthetic wound dressing composed of an ultra-thin, semi-permeable silicone membrane and a flexible nylon fabric. Both layers are covalently bonded to porcine collagen peptides to increase wound adherence and maintain a hydrophilic biocompatible surface. Levy et al treated 85 patients who underwent CO_2 laser resurfacing with a wound care regimen that included Biobrane dressing left on for the first 6 days postoperatively followed by application of cartilage extract ointment. These investigators found this wound care protocol effective in decreasing postoperative erythema and patient discomfort. Of note, they observed no cases of infection but reported three cases of contact dermatitis.[376]

In a study by Newman et al, comparing dressings from four different categories, Mepitel was found to be the most stable dressing (lowest incidence of slippage).[48] The Flexzan dressing showed good stability, good absorptive capacity and was liked by patients for its ease of care. Flexzan, however, was found significantly more time-consuming to change than other dressings because of its tendency to adhere to newly reepithelialized skin. Silon TSR and N-Terface, the easiest dressings to apply and change, had some problems with slippage. Silon TSR was rated by patients as a very comfortable dressing with the most natural feel. The 2nd Skin hydrogel dressing, remarkable for its pain-reducing effect and low incidence of pruritus, had the most problems with slippage.

In another study, Batra et al found that Silon TSR significantly reduced the severity and duration of erythema, swelling and crusting when compared to an open-wound care regimen after laser skin resurfacing.[46]

Pseudomonas aeruginosa favors a moist environment and readily colonizes burn wounds. A wound dressing that would provide the benefits of occlusion without encouraging the growth of *P. aeruginosa* in burn wounds might result in a more favorable prognosis for burn patients. Such a dressing would be beneficial in facial resurfacing as well.

A study evaluated three dressings regarding their ability to suppress *P. aeruginosa* inoculated on burn wounds of specific pathogen-free (SPF) pigs.[377] The three dressings evaluated were: (1) a hydrogel containing 22% polyvinyl pyrrolidone, 18% propylene glycol, and 60% water (Clear-Site: Conmed Corp.); (2) a hydrogel containing 65% glycerin, 17.5% water, and 17.5% polymeric matrix of acrylamide (Elasto-Gel: Southwest Technologies); and (3) a hydrocolloid made of pectin and sodium carboxymethylcellulose (DuoDerm: Conva Tec). All the wounds were clinically infected. However, wounds covered with the hydrogel containing glycerin had a significantly lower number of *P. aeruginosa* than the other wounds at all points in time. An in vitro study also showed that the hydrogel with glycerin caused a significant reduction in *P. aeruginosa*, as well as in *Escherichia coli* and *S. aureus*. Glycerin has been reported to have an antimicrobial effect that is attributed to dehydration,[378] and a 10% solution of glycerin and ichthammol showed particular activity against *P. aeruginosa*.[379]

These results suggest that the hydrogel with glycerin may be advantageous in promoting wound healing while providing an environment that does not support bacterial proliferation; however, this has not been tried clinically. K-Y Jelly, which has 17% glycerin content, has often been found to be too irritating to use on freshly resurfaced skin. Whether the glycerin hydrogel would be less irritating is unknown at this time.

Biocclusive dressings should be applied for only 48 to 72 hours postoperatively. Longer applications may increase the risk of bacterial or fungal colonization and infection with subsequent scarring. Sriprachya-Anunt et al found a 4.3% cumulative infection rate in patients who had closed dressings in place for 5 to 7 consecutive days or longer after facial skin resurfacing. The infection rate increased to 20% for those patients in their study who underwent full-face resurfacing followed by the Silon II semipermeable occlusive dressing. *P. aeruginosa* was the most common causative agent, followed by *S. aureus*, *S. epidermidis* and *Candida* species.[41]

Biocclusive dressings may encourage the development of infection because of the combination of moisture, necrotic tissue, and occlusion. However, the question of potentially increasing the risk of infection with occlusive dressings is not easy to answer. The literature on the effects of an occlusive dressing on the bacterial population is contradictory.

Some studies have shown that bacterial colonization under occlusion does not impair wound healing,[380–383] and that wound fluid and exudate collecting under an occlusive dressing have bactericidal activity.[384,385] Oliveria-Gandia et al demonstrated that occlusive dressings can act as barriers to invading wound organisms and that dressing composition can influence the growth of various pathogens.[377] Moreover, several studies found that wounds covered with occlusive dressings had reduced infection rates when compared to nonocclusive dressings.[346,359,361,385–390] Christian et al recently reported four cases of culture positive infections among 354 patients who underwent full-face CO_2 laser resurfacing (1.13% rate of infection) and were treated with occlusive dressings and empiric oral cephalexin. Three of the four infections developed 3 to 5 weeks after the laser resurfacing.[391] Newman et al evaluated the efficacy and safety of four different types of closed dressings following full-face laser resurfacing in 40 patients and observed no cases of infection.[48]

However, a study comparing semiocclusive dressings exposed to open air showed not only an increased number of microorganisms, but also a shift toward Gram-negative organisms.[380] Other investigators have shown a similar pattern on normal skin occluded with a plastic film.[383,389] Moreover, an increased incidence of infection after laser skin resurfacing has been reported in some studies when antibiotics have not been used.[41,116]

An increased susceptibility to Gram-negative infections in resurfacing patients would reflect our clinical experience as well. If semiocclusive dressings are to be used postoperatively, most physicians now would advise that: (1) antibiotic coverage should include Gram-negative organisms; (2) dressings should be changed frequently, if not daily; and

(3) occlusive dressings should be used for no more than 72 hours.

A semiclosed wound care technique that combines the advantages of both open and closed techniques is recommended by the authors who use Silon TSR dressing for wound occlusion during the first 72 hours followed by open wound care consisting of frequent 0.25% acetic acid soaks and application of moisturizers. Additionally, antibiotic prophylaxis for both Gram-negative and Gram-positive bacteria is started the evening before the procedure and continued for a total of 10 days.

After reepithelialization, the next phase of wound healing lasts another 7 to 10 days. During this phase, no further weeping occurs and swelling has usually resolved. Maturation of the epithelium still requires a moist environment. Of note, continued use of occlusive ointments such as petrolatum beyond complete reepithelialization has been associated with the occurrence of folliculitis in some patients.[253] Lighter preparations such as Theraplex emollient, Cetaphil moisturizer (Galderma Laboratories, Inc., Fort Worth, TX), Norwegian Formula emulsion (Neutrogena), and Curel (Bausch and Lomb, Inc., Rochester, NY) are preferred during this phase. Biologic agents such as vitamin C, essential fatty acids, hyaluronic acid, aloe vera, and topical photoprotective antioxidants such as green tea extract, idebenone, or ferulic acid may be beneficial in this phase. After the second week a lighter, high-moisture cream containing these biologic agents can be used and continued. Preoperative topical agents are restarted at 2 to 3 weeks postoperatively.

To minimize postoperative erythema we use 0.1% flurocinalone ointment (Synalar, Medicis, Scottsdale, AZ) applied to the face at night from postoperative day 5–21. We have not noted any decrease in wound healing or allergic reactions since this topical steroid ointment does not contain any preservatives or stabilizers. In addition, the addition of a topical steroid decreases postoperatuve pruritus and edema. Aquanil HC lotion (Person & Covey, Glendale, CA) is recommended for daytime use during the same period. This mild topical steroid is in a light, moisturizing, nonsensitizing base.

Close surveillance of patients during the postoperative period is important to provide emotional support and to detect abnormalities in the healing process at the earliest manifestation. Ideally, patients are seen 1 day, 3 days, 1 week, 3 weeks, 6 weeks, 3 months, 6 months, and 1 year postoperatively.

Complications of CO_2 Laser Resurfacing

As with all resurfacing procedures, the incidence of complications is related to both the depth of resurfacing and the patient's preexisting skin pigment type. Complications include infection, pigmentary changes, acne and milia, scarring, and ectropion. Swelling, erythema, petechiae, and itching are normal postoperative sequelae that may be more prominent in some patients.[252]

Postoperative Swelling

Postoperative swelling is generally mild to moderate, peaking on day 2 to 3 and most often resolving by day 5 to 7. At times, however, dramatic swelling may occur that is frightening and uncomfortable for the patient. Although we do not routinely use steroids in the postoperative course, in this situation of excessive swelling, IM Celestone (6–9 mg) or oral prednisone (40–60 mg daily for 3–5 days) may be valuable. Patients are also advised to soak their face frequently and to use ice packs or frozen peas as frequently as needed.

Erythema

Erythema occurs to some degree in all patients and reflects the increased blood flow and angiogenesis associated with dermal healing. The degree and persistence of erythema relate to the depth of resurfacing performed and the amount of nonspecific thermal injury produced, as well as to unidentified individual variables and possibly to preoperative and postoperative regimens. The regimens outlined previously appear to enhance wound healing and decrease erythema. In addition, the inflammatory reaction related to slough of thermal necrotic tissue may be a factor in prolonging erythema. Removal of this layer with the Er:YAG laser has been shown to be effective both in reducing erythema and infection and in enhancing the healing process and speeding its conclusion.

Itching

Itching is a common postoperative complaint, particularly during the second postoperative week. It can indicate infection, particularly candidiasis, but is then often accompanied by other signs, such as poor wound healing, beefy erythema in patches, and exudate. Contact dermatitis must be considered as well when pruritus occurs, particularly if any topical medications are being used. If these conditions are excluded, generally the itching will respond well to an antihistamine such as diphenhydramine (Benadryl, 10 or 25 mg) or loratadine (Claritin, 10 mg) or a topical steroid such as Synalar, as described above.

Infection

The combined incidence of bacterial, viral, and candidal infection has been found to be 4.7% in a multicenter study[392] and 4.3% in a retrospective study,[41] 12% in Burns' study (personal communication), 7.6% in our most recent study,[393] and 8.4% in the study of Waldorf et al.[82] Multiple organisms are typically found, and the microorganisms identified (*Staphylococcus* and *Pseudomonas* species) are similar to those found in burn injuries.[394–396]

The moist wound care and the layer of thermal necrosis provide an environment conducive to bacterial and candidal growth. The absence of the protective epidermal barrier further invites infection and allows dissemination of the infection across the surface of the treatment area. Biocclusive dressings further complicate the situation by trapping bacteria and increasing the incidence of infection.[41]

Infection should be suspected in the following situations:

1. Patient complains of persistent or new onset of pain.
2. Burning or intense itching is reported after day 2 or 3.
3. Patient has patchy, intense erythema, yellow exudate or crust, papules, pustules, or erosions.
4. 'Reversal of healing' is seen; that is, previously re-epithelialized areas become eroded.

Eighty percent of infections become symptomatic within 7 days and pain is the most common complaint, reported by 50% of patients. However, as previously mentioned, the use of antibiotics may alter this pattern, and antibiotics used for 10 to 14 days may eliminate postoperative bacterial infections. A sensation of burning and itching is the second most common symptom, reported by a third of patients.

When an infection is suspected, direct smears and cultures for bacteria, yeast, and herpesvirus should be taken, because the physical findings of infection may be atypical, with the absence of the epithelium and presence of a necrotic layer and edema. Correct diagnosis requires proper identification of the infectious agent.

All patients should be given appropriate antiviral medication at surgery, because the laser resurfacing procedure may be a potent factor in herpetic reactivation.[42] Should this occur despite antiherpetic prophylaxis, it is best to switch from valacyclovir to famciclovir, or vice versa, and to increase the dosage.

When candidal infections are encountered, a 400-mg dose of fluconazole should be given and occlusive topical regimens discontinued.

Bacterial infections should be treated according to culture and sensitivity results. Serious consideration should be given to prophylactic use of ciprofloxacin (500 mg twice daily) starting the evening before surgery and continuing for 10 to 14 days postoperatively.

Acne and Milia

Many physicians report an unusually high incidence of milia formation after laser resurfacing as well as increased or exacerbation of acne. Although the use of petrolatum-based ointments may be an exacerbating factor in many patients, particularly those with a prior history of acne, the incidence of this complication appears to parallel the degree of thermal injury to the tissue. Thermal injury may lead to a shock effect on sebaceous glands, causing their disruption and dedifferentiation of adnexal structures and producing an aberrant re-formation of the canal.[397] Dermabrasion, by contrast, generally results in improvement in acne; some physicians believe this is an invariable consequence of dermabrasion, although degree of improvement may vary.

Treatment of acne and milia is that traditionally used for acne: minimize occlusive ointments, reinstitute tretinoin and AHAs, and administer systemic tetracycline or minocycline. Gentle acne surgery performed at 2- to 4-week intervals may be beneficial as well. Isotretinoin (Accutane) may be started if the acne fails to respond to more conservative measures.

Hyperpigmentation

Hyperpigmentation is generally related to the degree of natural pigmentation and occurs in 20% to 30% of those with Fitzpatrick type III skin and nearly 100% of patients with type IV skin if treatment is performed without preoperative preparation.[84] Almost all episodes will resolve within 2 to 4 months if aggressively treated. Strict sun avoidance is a fundamental aspect of treatment and is enhanced by daily use of full-spectrum sunscreens containing titanium dioxide or Parsol 1789. Hydroquinone is cytotoxic to melanocytes and is the mainstay of treatment. Tretinoin promotes melanosome transfer and keratinocyte turnover and is almost always beneficial as well. Azelaic acid, kojic acid, and glucosamine inhibit tyrosinase and pigment synthesis and may be added to the regimen when patients are responding slowly. Topical vitamins C and E function as free-radical scavengers and help prevent further stimulation of melanocytes by UV radiation. Pretreatment with these agents will minimize the occurrence of hyperpigmentation, as well as its degree of severity and its favorable response to therapy.

Hypopigmentation

Hypopigmentation is a delayed phenomenon, generally not apparent for 6 to 12 months. True hypopigmentation must be differentiated from pseudohypopigmentation, a situation in which the resurfaced area has normal pigmentation reflective of non-sun-exposed skin, but contrasts distinctively with the more darkly pigmented sun-damaged skin. True hypopigmentation reflects a diminished melanocyte content of the skin and correlates with both the depth of resurfacing and the degree of thermal injury. These patients generally have long-lasting erythema, often have had problems with milia and acne as well, and may have areas of scarring. These patients typically have been treated with free-hand techniques allowing pulse stacking or with CPG patterns having greater than 50% overlap. These patients often have received more than three laser passes as well.

Treatment of hypopigmentation has been difficult, including the use of PUVA, eximer laser or UVB flashlamps (Relume, Lumenis). When segmental hypopigmentation or pseudohypopigmentation is present, resurfacing the remainder of the face will blend the area and decrease its visibility (see Fig. 7.29). An incidence of about 20% has been reported for hypopigmentation, but this must be examined carefully and pseudohypopigmentation separated as a different phenomenon, because it may not be preventable. In a review of 104 patients 1 to 4 years postoperatively, we found hypopigmentation in 19.2% (20 of 104). Pseudohypopigmentation was present in 65% of these patients and true hypopigmentation in 35%. Hypopigmentation was classified as mild in 85% of these patients. When examined more closely, these 20 patients

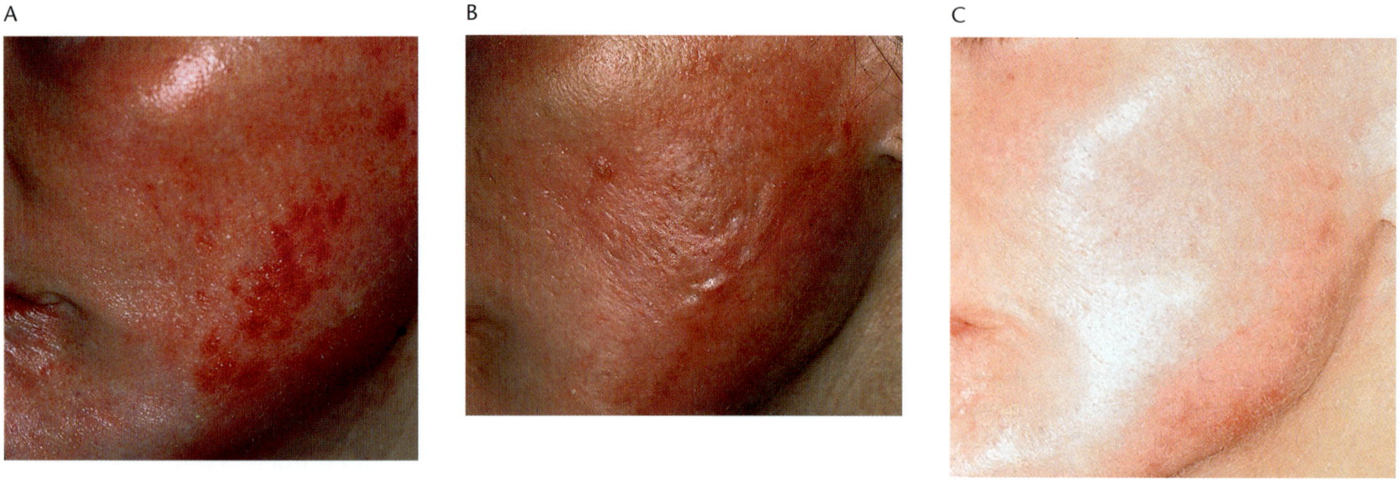

Figure 7.33 (A) *Pseudomonas* infection developed on day 8 after single-pass laser resurfacing, resulting in nonhealing erosions on lower cheek. (B) Although this area initially healed very well, at 4 months an obvious hypertrophic scar was developing, corresponding to site of infection. (C) Intensive treatment with intralesional 5-fluorouracil (45 mg/mL) and triamcinolone (Kenalog, 1 mg/mL) followed by pulsed dye laser (6 J/cm^2) resulted in scar resolution after approximately 1 year.

with hypopigmentation were also the patients having the worst photodamage preoperatively, those with the most significant clinical improvement, and those who were most pleased with their results. Pseudohypopigmentation should be viewed as a consequence of resurfacing in significantly photodamaged skin rather than a complication. However, patients should be forewarned of this aspect of the procedure.

Petechiae

Although of almost no long-term significance, the appearance of small petechiae is often a source of much concern to the patient. They appear just as reepithelialization is complete, conflicting with the patient's desire to return to public view. Small subepithelial hemorrhages from the immature basement membrane and undeveloped rete appear to be the cause. These factors render the skin more fragile and easily damaged with minor trauma from rubbing or scratching. Petechiae may continue for several weeks after the procedure but clear quickly without treatment.

Scarring

Erythematous and hypertrophic scars often result from excessive depth of tissue injury. This is usually caused by excess tissue heating and residual thermal damage well beyond the depth of tissue vaporized by the laser. Incorrect 'off' times, high scanner densities (greater than 40%), and failure to keep the handpiece moving during resurfacing are some of the treatment methods that lead to inadvertent overlap or 'stacking' of pulses, with the resultant accumulation of heat and residual thermal damage.

Scarring is also seen more frequently in patients who develop a postoperative infection, particularly in those who have had multiple prior surgical procedures, altering the anatomy of the region. In addition, patients treated more aggressively, resulting in a thicker layer of thermal necrosis, may be more prone to infection. Careful preoperative history taking to rule out predisposing factors and immediate treatment of postoperative infections are mandatory.

Scarring is much more frequently seen in treatment of nonfacial areas, such as the neck. Decreased adnexal structures, thinner dermis, and increased tissue tension and traction secondary to motion are predisposing factors. In a trial of 10 patients receiving a single laser pass of 300 mJ with CPG density of 6, we encountered scarring of the lower one third of the neck in three patients and patchy hypopigmentation in four patients (Fig. 7.33).

The earliest evidence for the development of a scar is usually erythema and pruritus. At this point the affected area should be cultured to rule out infection, and topical high-potency corticosteroids should be applied two or three times daily. If the affected area begins to thicken, intralesional injection of triamcinolone (10 mg/mL) with 5-fluorouracil (50 mg/mL) in a 1:9 dilution (1-mg triamcinolone with 45-mg 5-fluorouracil) should begin every 2 to 3 days. Topical silicone dressings should also be applied. If further progression occurs, we advise using the 585-nm flashlamp pumped pulse dye laser (PDL) or other vascular lasers or intense pulsed light (IPL) every 4 weeks. With these techniques, permanent scarring has been avoided (Fig. 7.34).

Ectropion

Contraction of previously scarred tissue of the lower eyelid leads to excessive tightening and exposure of the conjunctiva. This avoidable complication usually occurs in patients who have undergone resurfacing after a lower-lid blepharoplasty without stabilizing the lateral canthal tendon. It may also occur if laser resurfacing is performed too aggressively in this region without attention to the laser–tissue interaction.

A

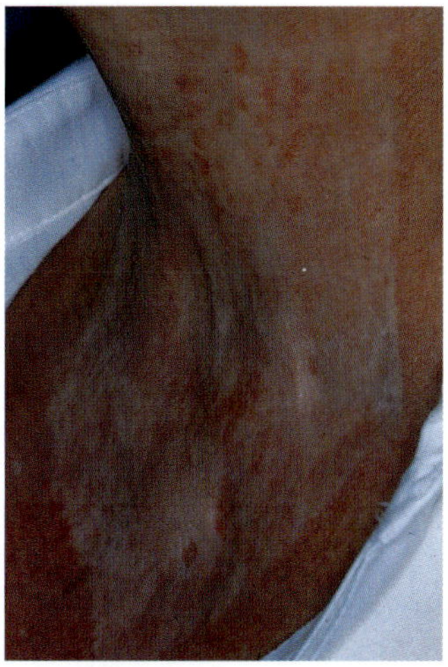

B

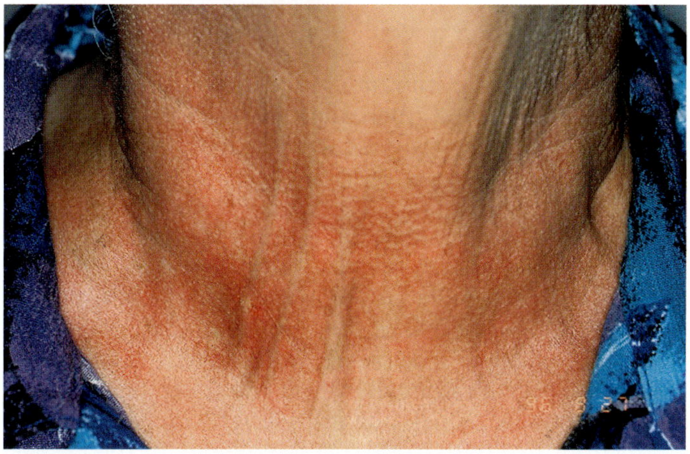

Figure 7.34 (A) Treatment of the neck in same manner as the face may result in severe scarring. (B) Treatment goals must be much more conservative, but even a single pass with the same laser parameters used for the face may result in scarring of the lower neck.

To minimize the occurrence of ectropion, we recommend that the patient's skin elastic recoil be tested, the so-called snap test, with close observation for loose tissue folds and the effect on the lid margin when tightened. If the lid margin moves easily, close observation during the procedure is essential to avoid excessive tightening of the lid. In addition, laser density should not exceed 20% to 30% in this region to limit nonspecific thermal damage of dermal tissue, and only one or two passes should be performed with careful attention to the tightening effect. The cheeks should be treated before the periorbital area so that the additive tightening effects of this area are known before periorbital resurfacing. Scleral show was found in 3% of patients less than 4 months postoperatively and in 2% more than 4 months postoperatively in a report of 1000 procedures.[398] Ectropion occurred in 0.3% of patients in this series.

Synechiae

Synechiae are adhesions that occur when two adjacent areas of deepithelialized skin are in contact with each other in a fold and a bridge of epithelium develops over the top of the fold. This occurs primarily on the lower eyelid and has the appearance of an unusual crease or faint white line 1 to 2 weeks postoperatively. Treatment consists of cutting the epidermal bridge with a fine-tipped scissors, lancet, or scalpel. The patient then must carefully roll a moist cotton-tipped applicator over the area frequently to avoid recurrence. Synechiae almost always resolve without problems.[398]

Erbium:YAG Laser

Erbium:YAG Laser–Tissue Interaction

The short pulsed Er:YAG laser is a flashlamp-pumped yttrium-aluminum-garnet (YAG) crystal laser system doped with atoms of the element erbium. Laser energy is generated within a cavity containing the flashlamp-excited YAG crystal rod, mirrors at each end, and a cooling system. On exiting the cavity, the laser light is focused into a beam delivery system that typically incorporates an articulated arm which allows the use of hand pieces capable of producing highly collimated beams. Erbium:YAG lasers used in cutaneous resurfacing typically have a bell-shaped Gaussian laser beam profile.[399]

The erbium:yttrium-aluminum-garnet (Er:YAG) laser produces light in the near-infrared (IR) portion of the electromagnetic spectrum at 2.94 μm. This wavelength was discovered by Soviet researchers in 1975[7] and its clinical use developed in Europe.[23,400–404] The broad water-absorption band extends from just under 2 μm to beyond 10 μm, ensuring superficial absorption of near-IR light. The Q-switched Er:YAG laser ablates approximately 15 to 20 μm of skin and leaves such a thin layer of thermal damage (5 μm) that it is not hemostatic. The Er:YAG laser has been investigated using a Q-switched pulse of 90 μs, but pulse-to-pulse instability and a low-intensity tail of a gaussian beam have made this beam profile undesirable. Instead, the laser is used in its normal-spiking mode, emitting a macropulse of approximately 250 μs, made up by a train of 1-μs micropulses with pulse-to-pulse stability of ± 2%.[405] The Er:YAG laser was first studied in this mode to determine whether it could be an effective resurfacing device.

When the coefficient of absorption for water is compared directly, that for the CO_2 laser (10.6 μm) is approximately 790 μm^{-1}, whereas the erbium laser peak at 2.94 μm is approximately 13,000 μm^{-1}, more than 16 times greater than that of the CO_2 laser (Fig. 7.35). This results in its energy being absorbed much more readily in a thinner layer of tissue than with the CO_2 laser. In fact, calculations of the absorption coefficient, assuming tissue to be 70% water, show this energy to be absorbed in about 1 μm of tissue.[11,24,400,402,405–409] This results in efficient tissue ablation with very little scattering of the beam and minimal residual thermal damage. However, actual clinical and experimental data reveal deeper tissue penetration than this calculated optical penetration.[409]

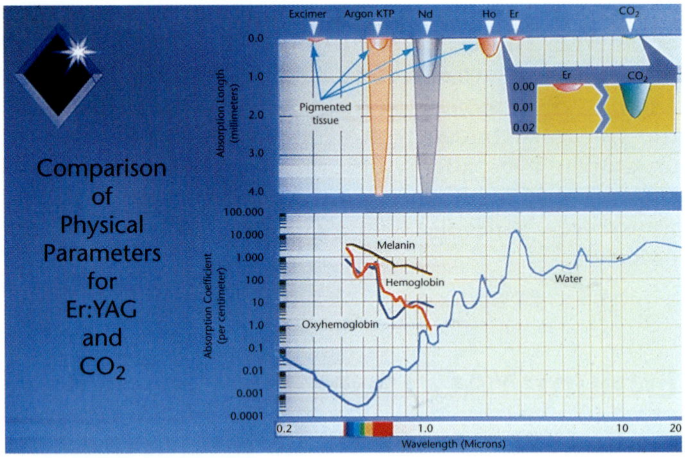

Figure 7.35 Erbium:YAG laser wavelength of 2.94 μm is absorbed 16 times more readily than that of CO_2 laser.

The ablation threshold for the Er:YAG laser is about 1.5 J/cm^2,[402,405,410] and the ablation efficiency about 2 to 3 μm/pulse/J/cm^2 up to about 10 J/cm^2.[24,402,405,407] However, ablation rates per pulse of 16 μm,[402] 30 μm,[408] and 400 μm (at 80 J/cm^2)[405] have been reported, which seem inconsistent with the reported optical penetration depth of the Er:YAG laser of about 1 μm.

This deeper ablation process occurs because ablation at 2.94 μm is an explosive process caused by rapid heating, vaporization, and consequent high-pressure expansion of irradiated tissue.[405,409] Explosive particle ejection occurs when a gradient exists between the atmospheric pressure of the environment and pressure within tissue. When tissue water is evaporated and prevented from escaping from tissue fast enough, tissue pressures may exceed atmospheric pressures when temperatures exceed 100°C. Because the tissue surface is cooled by expansion of the vapor, temperature and pressure may then be higher in a subsurface layer. The steam pressure of water increases rapidly with increasing temperature. Indeed, these high-temperature, high-pressure gases forming at the absorption site are thought to result in explosive tissue removal.[405,409] High-speed photography has shown ablated material to leave the surface at supersonic velocities (10^3 m/s).[411]

The ablation of tissue during the pulse of the Er:YAG laser is a dynamic process during which material heated at the beginning of the pulse is removed during the pulse, clearing a path for radiation to be deposited deeper in tissue during the same pulse.[405] High-speed photography has shown that tissue removal begins within 200 μs after the beginning of the pulse.[412] The explosive ejection of this ablated material removes it from the beam pathway. Furthermore, water vaporized by the pulse has a much lower coefficient of absorption than does liquid water and therefore does not interfere with the beam, because it is essentially transparent.[405,409] The explosive ejection of ablated material from the tissue surface causes the characteristic 'popping' sound heard during Er:YAG laser skin resurfacing.

Interestingly, lower fluences (less than 10 J/cm^2) of a thermal energy analyzer (TEA) CO_2 laser using 2-μs pulses result in the same ablation efficiency, supporting this instantaneous vaporization model.[405] This in-depth absorption explains the tearing of tissue seen in vascular tissue, the large ablation depths per pulse, and the zones of residual thermal damage that increase greatly at high fluences.[405,409]

Increasing pulse numbers applied to one spot results in decreasing the ablation efficiency and increasing the zone of thermal necrosis. Using 14 J/cm^2 and a 1-Hz repetition rate resulted in a decrease of the ablation rate from 30 to 22 μm when the pulse numbers increased from 20 to 120.[24] These effects are avoided clinically by moving the beam over the ablation area, and in fact, tissue necrosis of less than 50 μm is seen even with high fluences.[402,409]

The CO_2 laser is operated near its tissue ablation threshold (5 J/cm^2) in most resurfacing applications. This means that a large fraction of its energy is invested to heat, rather than ablate the target tissue. Therefore, the CO_2 laser produces relatively large residual thermal damage zones of up to 150 μm and causes significant dessication of the target tissue after only a few passes. With each subsequent pass of the CO_2 laser, the amount of vaporized tissue diminishes while the extent of thermal necrosis increases and a 'plateau' of ablation is typically reached after the fourth pass.

In contrast to the CO_2 laser, the Er:YAG laser has 16-times greater affinity for water and a significantly lower tissue ablation threshold (1.6 J/cm^2) which allows the Er:YAG to be operated at 8 to 10 times above its ablation threshold in most resurfacing applications.[6] Therefore, most of the energy delivered with the Er:YAG laser is utilized to ablate rather than heat the tissue and residual thermal damage zones not exceeding 30 to 50 μm have been confirmed both in vitro and in vivo with the Er:YAG laser.[23,24,402,408–410] Given the narrow zone of residual thermal damage produced by the Er:YAG laser, tissue dessication does not significantly increase with each subsequent and the ablation plateau characteristic of CO_2 laser resurfacing is not reached. In contrast to the coagulative, dessicating effect of the CO_2 laser on dermal blood vessels and dermal tissue, the Er:YAG laser causes vasodilation of dermal blood vessels and transudation of fluid that maintains a high water content in the target tissue and allows the Er:YAG laser to continue with efficient ablation.[10] The absence of tissue coagulation, however, results in bleeding as the vessels of the superficial dermal plexus are severed. This may limit the depth of ablation that is achievable.[23,24,410]

Clinical use of high-fluence, small-diameter beams is undesirable, because it may result in an irregular surface because of the deep instantaneous ablation.

This energy is delivered with a pulse duration that is far below the 1-ms thermal relaxation time calculated for that layer of human skin heated by the pulsed CO_2 laser, with the pulse generally 250 to 350 μs. However, because of the short penetration depth of the 2.94-μm wavelength, the laser-heated layer of tissue is only 1 μm thick and this layer has a thermal relaxation time of approximately 1 μs.[107,409,412] Single pulses of less than 1-μs duration are needed to minimize thermal diffusion during the laser

Table 7.8 *Er:YAG Laser Fluences (J/cm²)*

Spot size (mm)	Pulse energy (J)					
	0.5	1.0	1.2	1.7	2.0	3.0
0.2	1592.4	3184.7	3821.7	5414.0	6369.4	9554.1
0.5	254.8	509.6	611.5	866.2	1019.1	1528.7
1	63.7	127.4	152.9	216.6	254.8	382.2
2	15.9	31.8	38.2	54.1	63.7	95.5
3	7.1	14.2	17.0	24.1	28.3	42.5
4	4.0	8.0	9.6	13.5	15.9	23.9
5	2.5	5.1	6.1	8.7	10.2	15.3
6	1.8	3.5	4.2	6.0	7.1	10.6

pulse. In the normal-spiking mode, the Er:YAG laser emits approximately twenty 1-µsec micropulses in a macropulse burst of approximately 200µs. Because of efficient tissue vaporization and interpulse cooling time, minimal thermal damage occurs. Each micropulse can ablate tissue and act independently,[399,401] but in general the thermal damage from normal-spiking-mode irradiation is more extensive than that of Q-switched irradiation.

Most erbium lasers now available can deliver 1 to 3J per pulse, at repetition rates of 1 to 10Hz, so very high irradiances may be achieved, particularly with a focused beam. Although physicians and manufacturers typically report results as pulse energy and spot size, it would be much more meaningful and allow easier comparison if treatment parameters were discussed in fluence (J/cm²) (Table 7.8).

Thermally induced dermal collagen contraction is thought to underlie the superior clinical results achieved with the CO_2 laser. In contrast to the CO_2 laser (15 to 40% reported intraoperative collagen contraction), first-generation low-power short pulse Er:YAG lasers did not produce significant tissue contraction. The development of a second generation of more powerful Er:YAG lasers allowed investigators to demonstrate small but measurable degrees of tissue contraction after Er:YAG laser skin resurfacing. In 1998, Hughes et al demonstrated an immediate 4% linear tightening of the skin immediately after two or three passes with a short pulse (250µs) Er:YAG laser (5-mm spot diameter, fluences of up to 4.6J/cm²), which increased to a maximum of 14% 16 weeks postoperatively.[413]

Because of the high coefficient for absorption of water, very little tissue water is necessary for tissue reaction, allowing deep or very superficial vaporization, but both being done with minimal thermal injury. Its high affinity for tissue water and its ability to yield a narrow zone of residual thermal damage make the Er:YAG laser an exceptionally efficient and precise ablative laser with a side-effect profile that is considerably more favorable than that of the CO_2 laser.[11]

Erbium:YAG Laser: Indications

The indications for Er:YAG laser resurfacing include the following:

Rhytides

Mild to moderate photoinduced rhytides and mildly atrophic facial scars can be effectively treated with the short pulsed Er:YAG.[414] Severe rhytides (Fitzpatrick–Goldman Class III or greater) and severely photodamaged skin respond better to treatment with one of the modulated Er:YAG lasers with coagulative capabilities that facilitate deeper dermal ablation and induce a greater degree of collagen contraction and collagen remodeling. Static facial rhytides in the periorbital, perioral, cheek and forehead areas respond particularly well to Er:YAG laser resurfacing.[415] To preserve clinical correction of dynamic rhytides (e.g. periorbital, glabella, forehead), botulinum toxin A can be safely used (as previously described) in conjunction with Er:YAG laser resurfacing.[416]

Acne Scars

Modest improvement of mild to moderate acne scarring can be achieved with the short pulsed Er:YAG laser resurfacing. Deep acne scars have a better chance of improvement when resurfaced with a modulated Er:YAG laser. However, even with the modulated Er:YAG lasers, the reported improvement has been moderate at best.[28] Adjunctive treatment with other modalities (e.g. subcision, punch excision, fillers, grafts) is usually required to achieve significant correction of this difficult-to-treat condition.[417–419]

Posttraumatic and Surgical Scars

When performed during the phase of collagen remodeling (i.e. within 90 days of the original trauma) Er:YAG laser resurfacing can significantly improve the cosmetic appearance of posttraumatic and surgical scars. Linear facial scars tend to respond the best. Kwon et al reported 50% improvement of 9 of 12 hypertrophic scars, 17 of 20 depressed scars and 4 burn scars treated with a short pulsed Er:YAG laser (2-mm handpiece, 500–1200 mJ/pulse, 3.5–9 W).[29] Additionally, immediate postoperative resurfacing of Mohs surgery defects with the Er:YAG laser has been shown to significantly improve the outcome of second intention healing in anatomical areas that typically do not heal well by second intention (i.e. convex nasal surfaces).[420]

Benign Epidermal and Dermal Lesions

The Er:YAG laser has been used to safely and effectively treat a number of benign cutaneous lesions including: syringomas,[40] trichoepitheliomas, sebaceous hyperplasia, seborrheic keratoses,[421] actinic keratosis,[422] epidermal nevi,[423] Becker's nevus,[424] xanthelasma palpebrarum,[425,426] eruptive vellous hair cysts,[427] multiple military osteomas of the face,[428] colloid milium,[429] periungual warts,[430] rhynophyma,[431] Darier's disease and Hailey–Hailey disease,[432] Dowling–Degos disease[433] and Zoon's balanitis.[434]

Dyspigmentation

Superficial (epidermal) and deep (dermal) pigmentation problems can be addressed with Er:YAG laser resurfacing. Photoinduced dyspigmentation responds well to Er:YAG laser resurfacing. Melasma, on the other hand, tends to recur after Er:YAG resurfacing. Adjunctive therapy with topical bleaching agents (e.g. hydroquinone, azelaic acid, tretinoin, glycolic acid peel) and daily sunscreen is typically necessary when treating melasma. Additionally, the Er:YAG laser has been found useful for the preparation of recipient site prior to epidermal grafting in patients with vitiligo.[435]

Contraindications to Erbium:YAG Laser Resurfacing

The contraindications to Er:YAG laser resurfacing are the same as for CO_2 laser resurfacing and are listed in Box 7.2 (p. 207).

Clinical Situations Where the Erbium:YAG Laser Confers a Definite Technical Advantage

Given its relative lack of adnexal structures and delayed healing when compared to facial skin,[15,436] resurfacing of nonfacial skin in areas such as the neck, arms and hands must be approached with caution. Previous experience with CO_2 laser resurfacing of nonfacial skin has been plagued by a host of complications including permanent scarring and hypopigmentation. Fitzpatrick et al noted no improvement in wrinkling and four cases of permanent hypopigmentation (one with scarring) after single pass resurfacing of the neck with the UltraPulse CO_2 laser.[437] Another study by Rosenberg also reported scarring of the lower neck after resurfacing with the UltraPulse laser.[438]

Given the high rate of complications found in previous studies, resurfacing of the neck with the CO_2 laser is considered relatively contraindicated by most experts today. In contrast, resurfacing of the neck, arms and hands has been

A B

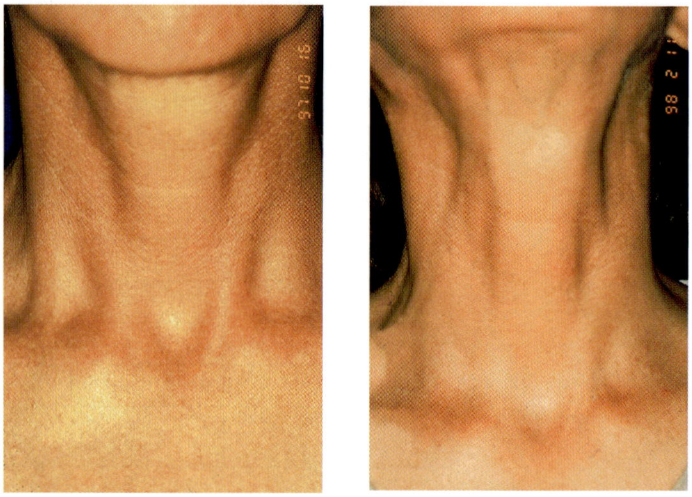

Figure 7.36 Treatment of neck using erbium laser allows removal of photodamaged epidermis without dermal injury. Improvement of skin texture and blending of color are reasonable goals. Improvement of 40% to 50% has been observed. (A) Before treatment; (B) 4 months postoperatively.

safely and effectively accomplished with Er:YAG laser systems (Fig. 7.36). Goldberg et al resurfaced the skin of the neck of ten patients with four passes of a short pulsed Er:YAG laser at a fluence of 3 to 4.5 J/cm^2. At 6-month follow-up, they noted at least a 25% improvement in wrinkling and 50% improvement in mottled dyspigmentation. No scarring or pigmentary complications occurred.[14] Goldman et al evaluated the results of neck resurfacing with an Er:YAG laser (Derma-20, ESC, Needham, MA) in 20 patients. Fluences of 8.7 to 13.5 J/cm^2 and spot sizes of 4- to 5-mm were used for the first pass and 2 to 9 J/cm^2 and 5- to 10-mm spot diameters for the second pass. In total, 51% of patients were satisfied with their results, and 39% improvement in texture and 37% improvement in skin color were noted. All patients healed within 7–10 days and no permanent adverse side effects occurred.[15] Jimenez and Spencer resurfaced the skin of the neck, hands and forearms of 12 patients with a 300-μs pulsed Er:YAG laser with a 5-mm spot size at a fluence of 5 J/cm^2. Two to three passes were performed on the arm and forearms and one or two passes were performed on the neck. Overall, they reported a mild improvement in photodamage and the majority of patients were pleased with their results. Healing took 2 to 3 weeks and two of seven patients who underwent resurfacing of the hands and forearms developed infections that were successfully treated. No scarring or permanent pigmentary alterations were observed.[439]

Pigmentary disturbances in patients with Fitzpatrick skin phototypes III and higher have been a frequent complication of CO_2 laser skin resurfacing.[16–18,77] The reported incidence of pigmentary alterations after Er:YAG laser skin resurfacing of patients with darker skin phototypes (Fitzpatrick skin phototype III or higher) is significantly lower than that reported after CO_2 laser skin resurfacing. The Er:YAG laser has shown a clear advantage over the CO_2 laser in the resurfacing of patients with darker (III–VI) Fitzpatrick skin phototypes.[2] Polnikorn et al utilized the

Er:YAG laser to treat 50 Asian patients (Fitzpatrick skin phototypes III–IV) with rhytides, photodamage, acne and varicella scars. Significant improvement was noted in all patients. Although 30% of patients experienced transient hyperpigmentation, only one patient developed transient hypopigmentation.[440]

The Er:YAG laser has also proven useful for removal of part of the zone of thermal damage left behind after CO_2 laser resurfacing, a technique that has been shown to decrease the duration of postoperative erythema and healing time. Several studies have documented the positive impact of Er:YAG laser resurfacing on postoperative recovery when performed immediately after CO_2 laser resurfacing. Goldman and colleagues randomized ten patients to receive three passes with the CO_2 laser alone (300 mJ, CPG settings of 596, 595, 584) to one side of the face and two CO_2 laser passes (300 mJ, CPG settings of 596 and 595) followed immediately by two passes with the Er:YAG laser (Derma-20 or Derma-K, ESC Medical systems, Needham, MA, 4-mm spot, 14 J/cm^2). They noted faster reepithelialization (1 to 2 days faster) and decreased duration of postoperative erythema (2 to 3 weeks versus more than 8 weeks) in those areas treated with the CO_2–Er:YAG laser combination (Fig. 7.37). This beneficial effect was accomplished without compromising clinical outcome.[31] McDaniel et al randomized 40 treatment sites on the upper lip of 20 patients to receive either two resurfacing passes with the UltraPulse CO_2 laser alone or a combination of two passes with the UltraPulse CO_2 laser (300 mJ, 95 Watts, CPG density of 6, 7.5 J/cm^2, spot diameter of 2.25 mm) followed by three passes with the Er:YAG laser (7-mm spot, 5.2 J/cm^2). Reduced duration of postoperative crusting (6.5 vs. 7.4 days), edema (6.0 vs. 6.3 days) and pruritus (4.8 vs. 5.5 days) was found in areas receiving the combined CO_2–Er:YAG laser treatment. Medium to deep rhytides were improved 70% with both treatments and there were no occurrences of permanent adverse side effects.[32]

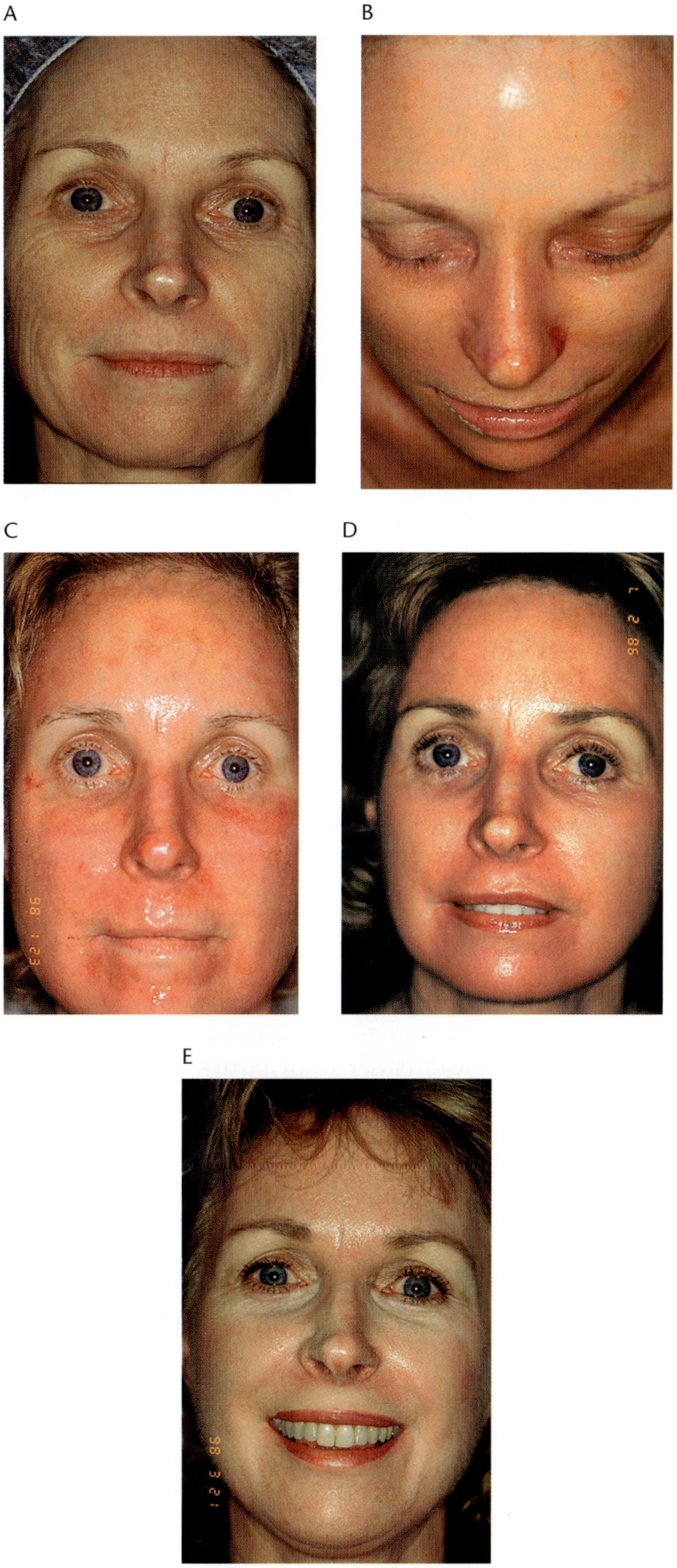

Figure 7.37 Combination Ultrapulse CO_2 (UPCO_2) and Er:YAG laser use (patients's right side) showing improvement equal to the left side treated with the UPCO_2 laser alone. (A) Before treatment. (B) Immediately after treatment (as described in the text). (C) 7 days after laser resurfacing. (D) 3 weeks after resurfacing. (E) 2 months after resurfacing. (From Fitzpatrick RE, Goldman M. Cosmetic laser surgery. Mosby, St Louis, 2000.)

Surgical Technique with the Erbium:YAG Laser

The depth of ablation is a function of the pulse energy and spot size or fluence. With the same pulse energy, a smaller spot size results in a higher fluence and therefore greater depth of vaporization. However, a smaller spot size also results in a tendency to create holes and an uneven texture. Also, the repetition rate and the pulse energy are inversely related, so a high pulse energy limits the repetition rate, at least within the limits of a 20-W laser. Virtually all systems that are currently available have an upper-limit repetition rate of 10 to 20 Hz, which limits the value of a pulse-scanning system, because these repetition rates can be manipulated by hand accurately by experienced laser surgeons.

Approximately 2 to 5 μm of tissue per J/cm^2 are ablated per pass with currently available Er:YAG laser systems. In contrast to CO_2 laser resurfacing, ablation depth does not diminish with each subsequent pass because the zone of residual thermal damage left behind by the Er:YAG laser is minimal (20 to 50 μm).[2]

Most often a spot size of 3 to 5 mm with a pulse energy of 1 to 2 J (fluences of 5.1 to 10.2 J/cm^2) is used. If a collimated beam is available, it is generally preferable at this stage. A repetition rate that can be easily handled is chosen (5 to 10 Hz), and spots are placed with 10% to 30% overlap. Therefore, with pulse energies of 1 to 2 Joules and a 5-mm spot size (fluence of 5.1 to 10.2 J/cm^2), two to three passes with a short pulsed Er:YAG laser are generally required to completely vaporize the epidermis (Fig. 7.38).

It is much more difficult to ascertain when the epidermis is completely removed with the erbium laser compared with the CO_2 laser, because the epidermis does not separate with a subepidermal vesicle as it does with the CO_2 laser. To determine the depth of vaporization into the skin, it is best to cover the skin in an orderly manner with relatively uniform passes rather than to treat with a random airbrush-type technique. This type of technique must be used cautiously because it leads to uneven results with much greater potential of inadvertent, deeper vaporization. Working in repetitive single passes allows better control and knowledge of depth.

It is best to remove the epidermis completely over the whole area to be treated and then to assess the dermal irregularities. Almost any patient being treated for photodamage will require some degree of dermal ablation, in addition to removal of the epidermis, because the textural irregularities and wrinkling originate in this layer. One to three passes are done in an even manner, just as was done with epidermal removal, with each pass ablating an additional 15 to 30 μm of tissue.

At this point, dermal irregularities may be removed in a tissue-sculpting mode. This is most easily accomplished with a focused handpiece having a focal spot size of 1 to 2 mm. The distance between the tissue and the handpiece will then determine the fluence delivered, and the handpiece may be moved closer to or farther from the tissue depending on the amount of tissue ablation desired. This is best done holding the handpiece at an acute angle to tissue in a manner such that tissue elevations above the desired plane are preferentially irradiated, thereby decreasing the risk of cutting holes or troughs in the tissue (Fig. 7.39).

Treatment using these techniques will result in maximal smoothing of tissue with minimal residual thermal damage. However, a second consequence of minimal thermal damage is that blood vessels are not cauterized, and therefore bleeding is encountered. Generally, the first dermal pass may result in scattered pinpoint bleeding at most as small dermal capillaries are encountered in the papillary dermis (Fig. 7.40). After an additional one to three passes, larger vessels are reached, which results in more significant bleeding requiring application of pressure. Bleeding that is brisk enough to interfere with treatment is usually encountered only with rhinophyma. In contrast to the smooth, glistening appearance of the papillary dermis, ablation into the reticular dermis typically produces an uneven surface as sebaceous gland lobules become visible.[441]

Although many physicians using the Er:YAG laser do not wipe away the fine tissue debris on the surface of

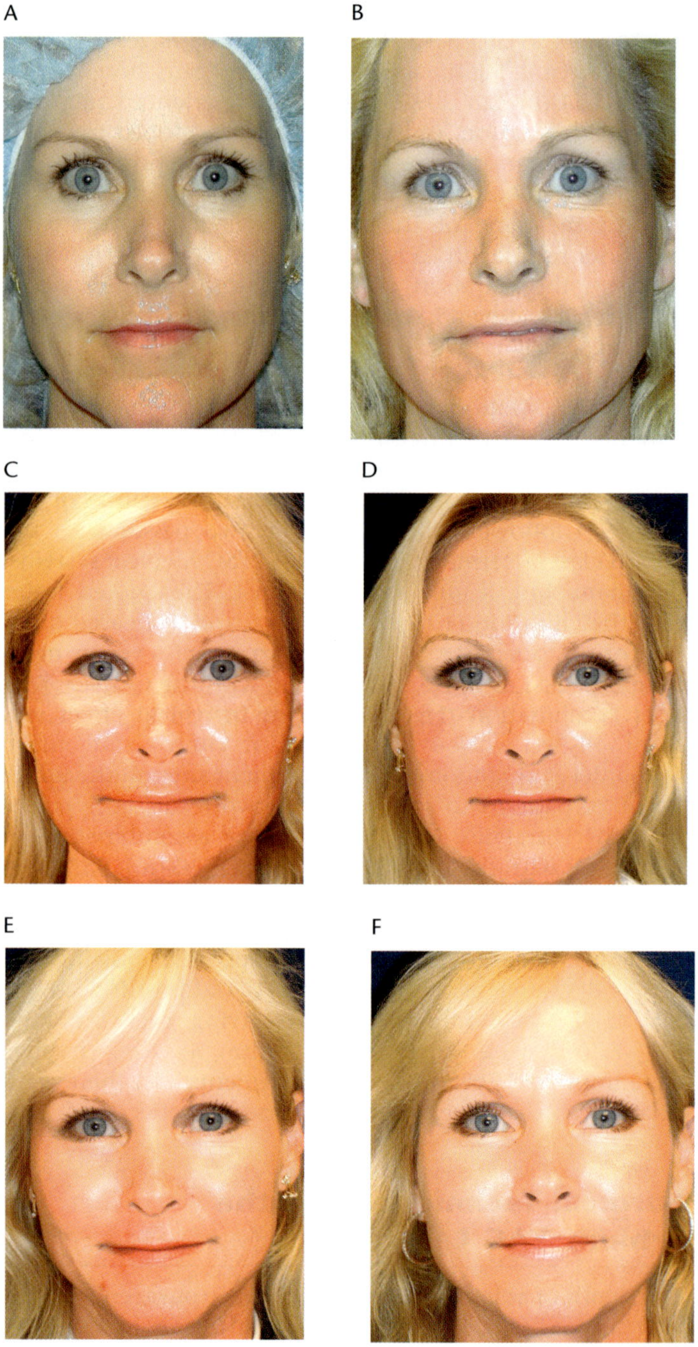

Figure 7.38 Microlaserpeel performed with 2 separate Er:YAG lasers. (A) 48 year-old women before treatment. (B) immediately after treatment. (C) 2 days after treatment with the Sciton Er:YAG laser on the left and CO_3 on the right side of the face, both at 2 J/cm^2 with a 0.5-ms pulse duration. Note squares of treated area on the left. (D) 2/3 days after treatment. (E) 8 days after treatment (F) 5 weeks after treatment. (Reproduced with permission from Avram DV, Goldman MP. The safety and effectiveness of single-pass Er:YAG laser in the treatment of mild to moderate photodamage. Dermatol Surg 2004; 30:1073–1076.)

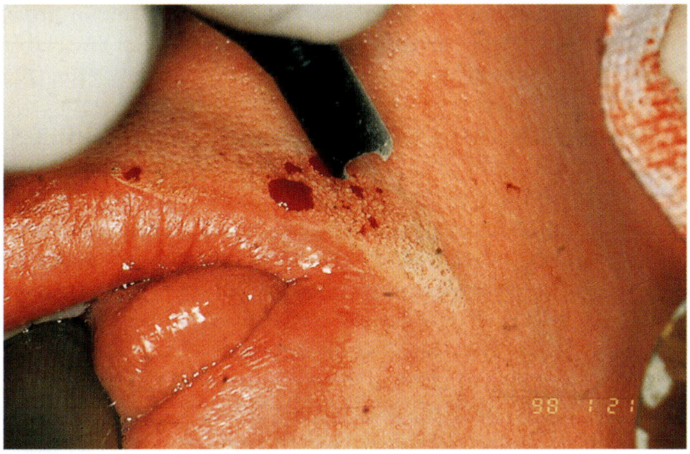

Figure 7.39 Tissue sculpting can be accomplished with the erbium laser, holding the beam at an acute angle to encounter higher tissue points selectively.

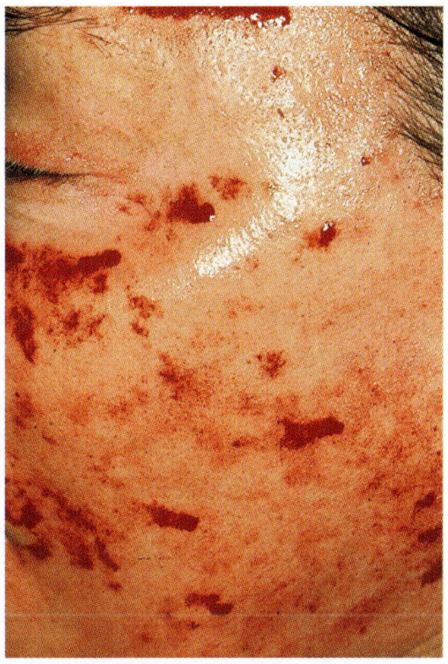

Figure 7.40 Because the erbium laser does not leave enough residual thermal necrosis to cauterize dermal vessels, bleeding will be encountered. Pinpoint bleeding is first seen in upper papillary dermis and becomes more significant as upper reticular dermis is reached.

treated skin between passes, using dry to damp gauze for this purpose is beneficial. By wiping this fine layer away, the laser has direct access to tissue to be treated, and the physician can more easily and more accurately visualize the anatomic location of the plane being treated. Wiping is particularly useful when performing epidermal passes, because it allows better identification of epidermis and dermis. Fragments of residual epidermis or lesional tissue that remain on the surface may be wiped cleanly away, avoiding the need to ablate these spots of tissue and providing a more even plane of tissue to be treated on the next pass.

Complications of Cutaneous Resurfacing with the Short Pulse Erbium:YAG Laser

Overall, the side effect profile of the short pulse Er:YAG laser has been found to be considerably more favorable than that of the CO_2 laser. As with CO_2 laser resurfacing, potential complications of resurfacing with the short pulse Er:YAG laser include erythema, dyspigmentation (hyperpigmentation and hypopigmentation), scarring and infection.

Prolonged Erythema

Prolonged erythema (greater than 4 months duration), reported in up to 20% of patients after CO_2 laser resurfacing, has a much lower incidence after resurfacing with the short pulse Er:YAG laser. The intensity of the erythema correlates well with depth of ablation and degree of residual thermal damage, hence its lower incidence when the short pulse Er:YAG laser is used. Katri et al performed a split-face study comparing multipass (three to five passes) resurfacing with a short pulse (300 μs) Er:YAG laser versus multipass (three passes) CO_2 laser resurfacing. At the 2-month follow up they reported a 24% incidence of erythema in the Er:YAG treated sites versus 62% for the CO_2 laser treated sites. At the 6 months follow up 10% of the CO_2 laser treated sites and none of the Er:YAG treated sites had remaining erythema.[20] Mean duration of erythema reported after multipass short pulse Er:YAG laser has ranged from 1 to 4 weeks in most studies as compared to 1–3 months for most patients after multipass treatment with CO_2 lasers.[2,5,12]

Hyperpigmentation

Transient hyperpigmentation has been reported in up to 37% of patients after CO_2 laser resurfacing, with a higher frequency in patients with Fitzpatrick skin types IV and above. Transient hyperpigmentation in patients with darker skin phototypes also occurs frequently 4 to 6 weeks after treatment with the short pulse Er:YAG laser.

In their large series of 625 patients treated with multiple passes of a short pulse Er:YAG laser, Weinstein et al observed a transient hyperpigmentation rate of 3.4%.[10] Ziering et al reported a 12% incidence of transient hyperpigmentation in his series of 50 patients resurfaced with multipass short pulse Er:YAG laser.[7] Three additional studies that treated with multiple passes of the short pulse Er:YAG reported transient hyperpigmentation rates of 24%[13,20] and 25% respectively.[5] Kye treated 30 patients with pitted facial scars and Fitzpatrick skin phototypes III–IV with multiple passes of a short pulse Er:YAG and noted only two cases of hyperpigmentation at the 3-month follow up. All of his patients, however, were treated preoperatively for 2 to 4 weeks with tretinoin 0.05% and postoperatively for 2 to 4 weeks with a combination of hydroquinone 4%, tretinoin 0.05% and hydrocortisone 1%.[419] In their series of 22 patients with Fitzpatrick skin phototype IV, Sriprachya-Anunt et al found no statistically significant difference in the rate of transient hyperpigmentation induced by treatment with either the CO_2 or the short pulse Er:YAG laser alone or a combination of both.[442] More recently, Kim et al resurfaced 190 patients with facial scars and Fitzpatrick skin phototypes III and above with either the short pulse Er:YAG laser or a modulated Er:YAG laser. They observed transient hyperpigmentation rates of 24.7%, 42.3% and 65.9% for the short pulse, variable-pulsed (CO_3, Cynosure, Chelmsford, MA) and the dual-mode (Contour, Sciton, Palo Alto, CA) lasers respectively.[443] Although hyperpigmentation in darker skin phototypes appears to occur just as frequently with both the CO_2 and Er:YAG lasers, it is often less severe and of shorter duration after Er:YAG laser resurfacing.[444]

Hypopigmentation

Delayed onset, permanent hypopigmentation is thought to be related to depth of ablation and the degree of residual thermal damage. Reported in up to 16% of patients after CO_2 laser resurfacing, hypopigmentation has a significantly lower incidence after short pulse Er:YAG laser resurfacing.

Alster resurfaced the face of 12 patients with Fitzpatrick skin phototypes I–IV with multiple passes of six different short pulse Er:YAG lasers and noted no instances of hypopigmentation.[5] Weinstein observed a 4% incidence of delayed onset permanent hypopigmentation in a series of 625 patients resurfaced with a short pulse Er:YAG laser.[10] In their series of 21 patients treated with multipass short pulse Er:YAG laser, Khatri et al noted a 5% incidence of hypopigmentation at the 6-month follow up.[20] Bass et al reported a 12% rate of hypopigmentation in their series of 25 patients treated with multipass short pulse Er:YAG laser.[13] In their series of 190 patients with Fitzpatrick skin phototypes III and above, Kim et al found hypopigmentation rates of 8.0%, 15.3% and 24.4% after resurfacing with the short pulsed Er:YAG, variable pulsed Er:YAG (CO_3, Cynosure) and dual-mode (Contour, Sciton) Er:YAG lasers respectively. The mean onset and duration of hypopigmentation in their patient populations were 2 months and 5.1 months. Only 15% of their patients had remaining hypopigmentation at the 12-month follow up.

Scarring

In contrast to CO_2 laser resurfacing, most series utilizing the short pulse Er:YAG for facial resurfacing have reported negligible rates of scarring.[5,7,11,13] In her large series of 625 patients, Weinstein observed a 0.8% incidence of scarring. In her study, scarring developed on the chest, lower eyelid and upper lip. All of these scars responded well to a 50/50 mixture of intralesional triamcinolone (10 mg/kg) and 5-fluorouracil.

Resurfacing of the neck and other nonfacial areas with the CO_2 laser has resulted in a high incidence of scarring and hypopigmentation in a number of studies. A study by Fitzpatrick and Goldman reported a 33% incidence of hypertrophic scarring after resurfacing of the lower neck with a single pass of the UltraPulse CO_2 laser. Another study by Rosenberg et al also reported scarring of the lower neck after single pass resurfacing with the UltraPulse CO_2 laser. The increased risk of scarring of nonfacial skin is thought to be due to the relative lack of pilosebaceous units in nonfacial skin as compared to facial skin.[438,444]

In contrast to CO_2, skin resurfacing of nonfacial areas including the neck, arms and hands with the Er:YAG laser has been demonstrated to be safe and moderately effective in several studies.

McDaniel et al used the short pulse Er:YAG with a 5-mm spot diameter and a fluence of 2.5 J/cm^2 to resurface the dorsal hands of three patients and the neck of one patient (two or three passes) and observed an improvement in appearance of 48% and 44% respectively and no cases of scarring or hypopigmentation.[406] Goldberg et al treated 11 necks and 4 dorsal hands with multiple passes of the short pulse Er:YAG laser at fluences of 4 to 5 J/cm^2 and reported significant clinical improvement of photodamage (25% to 100%) and no adverse sequelae.[14] Goldman et al treated the neck of 20 patients with two passes of the short pulse Er:YAG at higher fluences (up to 13.5 J/cm^2) and reported an overall patient satisfaction of 51%, an average improvement in skin texture of 39% and an average improvement in skin color of 37%. All their patients healed within 7 to 10 days, had resolution of their erythema within 2 weeks (except for 1 patient who developed an infection) and reported no permanent adverse effects.[15] Jimenez et al treated seven patients with photodamage of the forearms and hands and five patients with photodamage of the neck with one to three passes of the short pulse Er:YAG laser using a 5-mm spot size and a fluence of 5 J/cm^2. They reported no permanent adverse side effects with these laser parameters. However, they noted that the cosmetic improvement achieved was only mild, the healing time was significantly longer (2 to 3 weeks) than for Er:YAG facial resurfacing, topical anesthesia was inadequate and two of the seven patients who underwent hand and forearm resurfacing experienced infections that required oral antibiotics.[439]

Infection

As with any other cutaneous resurfacing method, infection is a potential risk of Er:YAG laser resurfacing. However, the reported infection rates have generally been low. Most infections occur during the first week, prior to re-epithelialization. *Staphylococcus aureus* and *Pseudomonas aeruginosa* are the most common bacterial pathogens and *Candida* is responsible for most fungal infections. Weinstein et al reported only one case of bacterial infection (on the neck) in their large series of 625 patients resurfaced with a short pulsed Er:YAG laser. Alster et al reported one instance of herpes simplex reactivation in a series of 12 patients who underwent facial cutaneous resurfacing with short pulse Er:YAG lasers. Teikemeier et al, Khatri et al, Ziering et al and Bass et al observed no infections in their respective series of 20, 21, 25 and 50 patients resurfaced with the short pulse Er:YAG laser.[5,7,10,11,13]

Note: a detailed discussion of the treatment of the complications described above is provided for the reader in the previous section of this chapter 'Complications of CO_2 Laser Resurfacing' (pp. 218–221).

Modulated (Coagulative and Ablative) Erbium:YAG Laser Systems

Despite the initial enthusiasm for the Er:YAG laser, clinicians quickly came to realize that clinical results achieved with the conventional short pulse Er:YAG lasers were considerably less impressive than those attained with CO_2 lasers. The hopes of those who had envisioned the Er:YAG laser as the resurfacing tool that would entirely replace the CO_2 laser were swiftly shattered.

There were a number of factors that limited the resurfacing potential of early generation Er:YAG lasers. First, early short pulse Er:YAG lasers were slow and underpowered. They had low repetition rates of only 1 to 2Hz, produced modest fluences no greater than 10J/cm² and had small beam diameters of 1 to 2mm. Multiple passes were required to achieve epidermal ablation with these systems.[413,445,446] Alster et al tested six different early generation short pulse Er:YAG lasers in skin resurfacing and found that with all of them, three passes were needed for complete epidermal ablation.[5]

The low ablation rates of early generation Er:YAG lasers, which typically hovered at around 20μm per second, represented a significant disadvantage when compared with the high peak-power, short pulsed CO_2 lasers.[445] Second, although early Er:YAG lasers proved efficacious for superficial ablation, their limited coagulative effect precluded good hemostasis and significantly limited depth of ablation.[23,24,447]

However, early Er:YAG lasers proved to be excellent tools for resurfacing of mild to moderate rhytides. Furthermore, postoperative erythema and reepithelialization time after Er:YAG resurfacing turned out to be significantly less than seen after CO_2 resurfacing.[11] Despite its advantageous side effect profile, clinicians quickly came to realize that skin resurfacing with the Er:YAG laser produced results that were considerably inferior to those attained with the CO_2 laser.[11,19–22,406,448]

A number or studies suggested that thermally induced effects on the dermal collagen contributed to the beneficial effects of CO_2 lasers in the treatment of facial rhytides and perhaps underlie the superior results achieved after CO_2 laser skin resurfacing. Tissue contraction, tightening of facial skin, synthesis of new collagen and collagen remodeling were demonstrated after CO_2 laser skin resurfacing in several studies.[2,6,449,450]

Therefore, a number of authors hypothesized that the relative lack of efficacy of traditional short pulse Er:YAG laser skin resurfacing was related to a relative lack of thermally mediated coagulative effects in the upper dermis.[52,6,19–22,448] Several studies demonstrated less coagulative effect and thermal residual damage after Er:YAG laser skin resurfacing as compared to CO_2 laser skin resurfacing.[32,449,450] Adrian et al compared the short pulse Er:YAG with a pulsed CO_2 laser in a bilateral comparison study and found that the Er:YAG was able to improve fine rhytides but showed less efficacy treating moderate to deep rhytides than the CO_2. In all instances, except for mild rhytids, the CO_2 laser produced superior and longer lasting results.[19]

With the notion that immediate tissue contraction and induction of thermally mediated changes in dermal collagen were important for long term laser skin resurfacing results, investigators began exploring ways to 'modulate' the Er:YAG laser to endow it with enhanced coagulative power while maintaining its powerful ablative capacity and extremely favorable side effect profile.[451]

Traditional Er:YAG lasers operated with pulse durations of 350μs and typically produced 10 to 20 microns of residual thermal damage. In 1998, Adrian et al studied the effect of increasing the pulse of the Er:YAG at a fluence of 5J/cm² during skin resurfacing procedures to 10ms (CO_3, Cynosure).[21] Histology revealed a 60μm residual thermal damage zone after multiple passes with this long-pulsed (10ms) Er:YAG laser. More significantly, this increased zone of residual thermal damage correlated well with increased tissue contraction when compared to the 350μs Er:YAG laser and the clinical results achieved were similar to those attained with the high peak power, short pulsed CO_2 laser. This and other subsequent studies[451] showed that as the pulse width increased, both the zone of residual thermal damage and the clinical effect approached the magnitudes seen after short pulsed CO_2 laser resurfacing.[21,116,452]

In an attempt to overcome the shortcomings of the conventional short pulse (350μs) Er:YAG laser, namely poor hemostasis which limited depth of ablation and its inability to resurface deep rhytides effectively, modulated Er:YAG lasers systems that conveniently combine long pulse (coagulative) and short pulse (ablative) capabilities in the same device were introduced in the late 1990s.

Currently there are two commercially available modulated Er:YAG laser systems with combined ablative and coagulative capabilities: a variable pulse Er:YAG laser (CO_3, Cynosure), which can deliver single pulses of variable widths and a dual-mode (ablation and subablative/coagulation modes) pulsed Er:YAG laser (Contour, Sciton). A third modulated Er:YAG laser system is a hybrid CO_2-Er:YAG laser (Derma-K, ESC Medical Systems, Needham, MA) that is no longer commercially available but, given that it is still in use by some clinicians, will be briefly reviewed below.

The variable pulsed CO_3 Er:YAG laser system can deliver pulse durations ranging from 500μs to 10ms. Short pulses are used for ablation, whereas longer pulses produce thermal effects mimicking the CO_2 laser–tissue response. With the longer pulse mode of 10ms and a fluence of 5J/cm², thermal damage zones of 30–40μm have been reported.

Rostan et al performed a split-face study comparing resurfacing with the variable pulsed (CO_3, Cynosure) Er:YAG laser versus the 950μs UltraPulse CO_2 laser. Sixteen patients were randomized to receive resurfacing with either UltraPulse CO_2 or CO_3 laser with a 10-ms pulse on one side of the face, followed immediately by a pass with the short pulse Er:YAG. Two passes with the CO_3 parameters set at 2J, 10 to 10.5J/cm², 10-ms pulse, 4 to 10Hz, 5-mm spot were performed. One additional pass with the CO_3 laser (same settings) over the areas of greatest scarring and photodamage was followed by a single pass with a 500μs

Er:YAG at 1.5 J, 7.7 J/cm^2, 5 to 7 mm spot and repetition rate of 10 Hz. UltraPulse CO_2 treatment was performed utilizing the CPG for two or three passes at settings of 596, 595 and 584 followed by a single pass with a short pulsed Er:YAG at 14 to 16 J/cm^2 with a 4-mm spot size and up to 50% overlap. Overall clinical improvement was found to be equal for both the UltraPulse CO_2 laser and variable pulse Er:YAG (CO_3) treated sides with an average improvement in photoaging scores of 57%. Moreover, decreased erythema and edema and faster healing were observed on the side treated with the variable pulse (CO_3) Er:YAG laser.[26]

Newman et al performed a side-by-side comparison study of the histologic and clinical effects of the variable pulse CO_3 Er:YAG versus the UltraPulse CO_2 laser after perioral resurfacing. Four ablative-mode passes with the CO_3 laser (5-mm spot size, fluence of 5.2 J/cm^2 and a 500 μsec pulse width) were followed by a single coagulative mode pass (5-mm spot, fluence of 2.6 J/cm^2 and a 10-ms pulse width). A final pass, designed to remove the thermally damaged tissue partially, used parameters identical to the initial ablative passes. Histology showed a 90-μm layer of ablation and a 10-μm layer of residual thermal damage. The authors postulated that the final ablative pass partly removed the zone of thermal necrosis generated by the 10 ms coagulative pulse. Two months after treatment there was a 54% improvement in rhytides treated with the variable pulse CO_3 Er:YAG laser, compared to 63% improvement with the CO_2 laser. Reduced duration of crusting (3.5 days vs. 7.8 days) was observed on the sides treated with the variable pulse CO_3 Er:YAG laser. They observed no cases of permanent hyperpigmentation, hypopigmentation or scarring.[27]

Christian et al conducted a six-patient, split-face study that evaluated the impact of single-pass resurfacing ('microresurfacing peel') at two different pulse durations (500 μs versus 4 ms) of the variable pulse (CO_3) modulated Er:YAG laser. Six of eight peels were performed at a fluence of 7.1 J/cm^2. Erythema was found to be significantly greater on the 4-ms side at postoperative days 3–4, but this difference was no longer significant at postoperative day 7. Average time to reepithelialization was found to be 3.6 days.[453]

The dual mode Contour Er:YAG laser (Sciton Corporation, Palo Alto, CA) uses a process called optical multiplexing that stacks together groups of individual Er:YAG laser pulses to create either short (200–300 μs) ablative pulses of high fluence or long duration pulses of low fluence (subablative and coagulative). These pulses can be delivered as purely ablative, purely coagulative, or a combination of both. Ablation depths of up to 200 μm can be achieved with a single pulse. At 50% overlap, high fluences of up to 100 J/cm^2 can be generated and the entire epidermis can be removed in a single pass. The coagulative component can produce thermal damage in the dermis and tissue contraction that approaches that seen with CO_2 laser skin resurfacing.[413,454] The Contour's touchscreen control panel allows the surgeon to 'dial in' the desired depths of ablation and coagulation and to choose the corresponding clinically appropriate laser parameters. The Contour has a built-in safety feature that automatically adjusts the displayed fluence to reflect the effect of changes in the degree of overlap. For example, an increase from 10% to 30% overlap will alert the surgeon to the fact that the delivered fluence has increased by approximately 65%. At 45 W, the Contour Er:YAG is a powerful laser that makes the use of a pulse scanner quite feasible and advantageous.[455] Several studies have investigated the histologic effects of dual-mode Er:YAG Contour laser resurfacing. A close correlation was found between the programmed and actual measured depths of ablation for single and multiple passes. It is clinically important to note that the chosen depth of coagulation correlates well with the histologic changes for the first pass but this correlation deteriorates with subsequent passes.[456–458]

Zachary et al achieved significant tissue contraction and good to excellent control of bleeding with the dual-mode Contour Er:YAG laser using 50% overlap, 84 μm of ablation (21 J/cm^2) and 50–100 microns of coagulation. 'CO_2-like' tissue contraction was observed during the second and subsequent passes with this laser.[454] Grekin and Zachary reported their experience resurfacing over 100 patients with the dual-mode Contour Er:YAG laser.[455,459] Average reepithelialization time for their patients was 3 to 5 days and they noted significant improvement in rhytides and acne scars. Full-face and regional resurfacing was accomplished in patients with all skin types. In comparison to the CO_2 laser, postoperative erythema cleared more rapidly and there were no cases of scarring. Transient hyperpigmentation was seen in most patients with darker skin phototypes, but it resolved in every case with the use of topical bleaching agents and sun protection. Of note, these authors reported two cases of delayed hypopigmentation that occurred in patients with lighter skin phototypes.

In another study, Tanzi and Alster utilized the dual-mode Contour Er:YAG laser to treat 25 patients with moderate to severe atrophic facial acne scars. Their laser parameters were 90 μm of ablation (22.5 J/cm^2) with 50% spot overlap and 50 μm of coagulation delivered with a rapid pulse scanner. Two to three passes were performed. The average clinical improvement score at the 12-month follow up was 2.16 (25 to 50% improvement). Side-effects were limited to transient erythema in all patients (mean duration of 3 weeks), one case of prolonged erythema, hyperpigmentation (44%) and acne flare-up that responded well to oral minocycline (32%). No cases of hypopigmentation or scarring occurred.[28]

Kwon et al evaluated the efficacy and safety of scar resurfacing with the dual-mode Contour Er:YAG laser. Nine of 12 hypertrophic scars, 17 of 20 depressed scars and 2 of 4 burn scars improved more than 50%. Side effects were minimal and included 1 case of postinflammatory hyperpigmentation and mild persistent erythema in all patients with burn scars.[29]

Until very recently a third laser, the Derma-K (ESC Medical Systems, Needham, MA) hybrid Er:YAG-CO_2 laser, was available commercially in the United States. Given that some clinicians continue to utilize the Derma-K system for skin resurfacing, and reports of its efficacy continue to appear in the literature,[460] we will briefly review this laser system as well.

The Derma-K laser is a hybrid laser system that delivers ablative Er:YAG laser pulses followed immediately by coagulative CO_2 laser pulses. The Er:YAG component produces a fluence of up to 28 J/cm^2 with a 350-µs pulse. The CO_2 component can deliver a subablative/coagulative pulse varying from 1 to 100 ms at 1 to 10 W power, providing excellent hemostasis. The CO_2 coagulative component can be programmed to be delivered during a fraction or all of the time between the ablative Er:YAG laser pulses. Energy can be delivered using either a CPG with a 3-mm spot or a noncollimated 0.2- to 8-mm spot. Zones of thermal necrosis of up to 50 µm in depth have been observed after resurfacing with this laser system.[30,461]

Goldman et al performed full-face resurfacing of 10 patients with the Derma-K hybrid laser. They performed four passes with a 4-mm spot, Er:YAG laser parameters of 350 µs, 1.7 J/cm^2 and the CO_2 component set at 5 W, 50 ms with a frequency of 10 Hz. Their patients experienced a 44% and 38% improvement in perioral and periorbital rhytides at their 3-month follow-up and an overall improvement of 39% in their facial photoaging score. Histology revealed a 20-µm zone of thermal damage immediately after treatment and an average depth of collagen of 54-µm (86% increase from baseline) 3 months postoperatively. Weinstein et al have also reported good to excellent results after facial resurfacing with the Derma-K Er:YAG/CO_2 hybrid laser. A mean reepithelialization time of 11.3 days and postoperative erythema that lasted an average of 8.3 weeks were noted in their study.[30]

Trelles et al recently performed single-pass resurfacing of 102 patients with skin phototypes I–V with the Derma-K hybrid laser. They used an ablative Er:YAG laser pulse (350 µs, 28 J/cm^2) followed immediately by a coagulative continuous wave CO_2 laser shot (4 to 6 W, 50 ms) through a 3-mm collimated handpiece (3-mm spot) with 50% overlapping and a repetition rate of 10 Hz. In total, 67 patients scored their results as very good, 25 as good and 10 as fair and the patient's rating correlated well with those of the treating physician and three independent observers. Mean duration of follow up in their study was 1.76 years. Mild, transient side effects were seen in only four of their 102 patients. Histology 2 months postoperatively demonstrated a band of well oriented newly synthesized collagen underneath a healthy epidermis.[462]

As previously described, one of the main benefits of cutaneous resurfacing with a CO_2 laser is tissue contraction, which is believed by a number of authors to underlie the superior resurfacing results achieved with the CO_2 laser. All of the new modulated Er:YAG laser systems have demonstrated the capability to produce 'CO_2-like' tissue contraction not only clinically, but histologically as well. Kist et al studied collagen contraction after CO_3 laser treatment in a bovine tendon collagen model. The depth of irreversible and reversible collagen fibril changes (measures of collagen contraction) were assessed by electron microscopy. With a constant fluence of 6.1 J/cm^2, the maximum irreversible collagen fibril change was achieved at the highest pulse duration (10 ms) and it measured 3.25 µm. The maximum depth of reversible collagen change at the same fluence was found to be 9.52 µm and it was attained at the 7-ms pulse duration. Their study showed that when pulse duration or fluence was increased while the other variable was held constant, there was a steady increase in the mean maximum tissue contraction and collagen fibril diameter. Remarkably, the degree of collagen contraction achieved in their study was consistent with that achieved with a pulsed CO_2 laser in a previous study using the same bovine tendon collagen model.[463]

Fitzpatrick et al compared the collagen tightening induced by a pulsed CO_2 laser and the modulated Derma-K laser. One eyelid, treated with three passes of a pulsed CO_2 (UltraPulse, Coherent Medical Group, Santa Clara, CA) was compared with the contralateral eyelid, treated with the Derma-K laser (ESC, Needham, MA) to an endpoint of early pinpoint bleeding. Intraoperative contraction of 43% after CO_2 resurfacing versus 12% after Derma-K laser resurfacing was measured. However, at 1 month and beyond, the degree of CO_2 and modulated Er:YAG-induced skin tightening were found to be identical.[25]

Modulated Erbium:YAG Lasers: Clinical Considerations

Their capability to produce precise ablation at highly efficient rates, provide excellent hemostasis with their coagulative pulses, generate 'CO_2-like' thermally induced changes in dermal collagen and their superior side-effect profile have made these powerful modulated Er:YAG lasers true alternatives to the CO_2 laser.

In contrast to CO_2 laser resurfacing, treatment with the modulated Er:YAG lasers can often be performed using local anesthesia. Topical anesthesia, nerve blocks and local infiltration typically are supplemented with a benzodiazepine (i.e. midazolam or diazepam) and/or an analgesic such as fentanyl or meperidine.

Currently available modulated Er:YAG lasers are powerful systems with efficient ablation rates that make the use of a scanner feasible. Alternatively, freehand ablation can be performed efficiently at a repetition rate of 5 Hz and with an overlap of 50% which produces the equivalent of two-pass ablation in a single pass. Single-passes are typically performed with a 20% to 30% overlap to prevent irregularities inherent to their Gaussian beam. Up to 40 um of tissue per pass can be ablated at a fluence of 10 J/cm^2 with both, the Contour and CO_3 lasers.[441,454,459]

Long pulse durations with the currently available modulated Er:YAG laser systems – CO_3 (Cynosure, Chelmsford, MA) and Contour (Sciton, Palo Alto, CA) – produce clinically evident, 'CO_2-like' intraoperative tissue contraction during and after the second pass. As a general rule, deeper rhytides and severe photodamage are optimally treated with the longest pulse durations available, while superficial rhytides and minimal photodamage are treated with short pulse durations. Wiping between passes, although not necessary, can afford a better view of rhytide effacement and depth of vaporization (Fig. 7.41).

The short pulsed mode of the modulated lasers can be used for purely ablative functions such as fine tissue sculpting and to remove the residual zone of thermal necrosis

A B

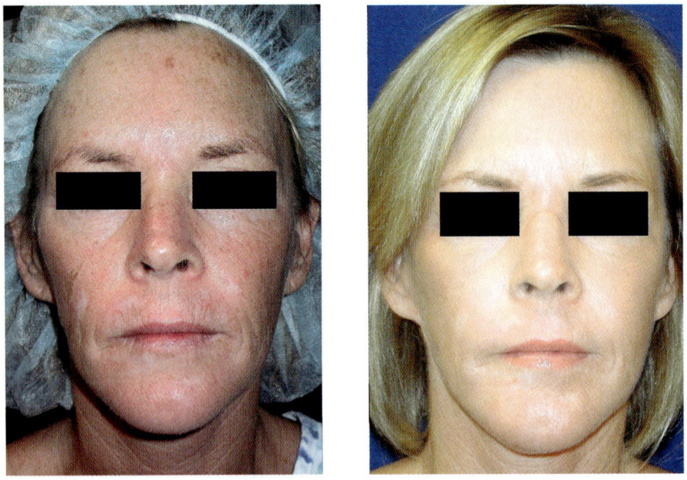

Figure 7.41 Treatment with the Cynosure CO_3 laser. (A) Before treatment; (B) 6 months after treatment with two passes at 10 J/cm^2 and 10 ms followed by two passes with 10 J/cm^2 and 0.5 ms.

left behind by the coagulative mode of these lasers. Removal of this zone of residual thermal damage after CO_2 laser resurfacing has been shown to improve postoperative healing.

The clinical endpoint during modulated Er:YAG laser skin resurfacing is not obvious. The long pulses (coagulative) of the modulated Er:YAG lasers produce excellent control of intraoperative hemostasis. Thus, punctate bleeding, which helps to signal the clinical endpoint during conventional short pulse Er:YAG resurfacing, does not occur when resurfacing with the modulated Er:YAG lasers. Furthermore, the typical depth-related color changes seen during CO_2 resurfacing also do not occur during modulated Er:YAG resurfacing. Therefore, when resurfacing with the modulated Er:YAG lasers, the surgeon must carefully choose clinically appropriate laser parameters based on anatomic considerations and the desired depth of tissue ablation. For example, the epidermal thickness of the eyelid is approximately 60 μm. Using the modulated Er:YAG lasers at a fluence of 15 J/cm^2 and 30% overlap, the entire epidermis of the eyelid can efficiently be removed in a single pass.

Modulated Erbium:YAG Lasers: Complications

Overall, the side effect profile of the modulated Er:YAG lasers has been reported to be slightly more than that of the short pulse Er:YAG laser but considerably more favorable than that of the CO_2 laser. As with the CO_2 laser, potential complications include prolonged postoperative erythema, pigmentary disturbances, scarring and infection.

Prolonged Erythema

Prolonged postoperative erythema, thought to be related to the degree of thermal damage and depth of ablation, can occur in up to 20% of patients treated with the CO_2 laser. Most studies have reported a decreased duration of postoperative erythema and a shortened recovery period after resurfacing with the modulated (coagulative-ablative) Er:YAG lasers as compared to CO_2 laser resurfacing. Alster et al resurfaced 50 patients with a dual mode Er:YAG laser (Contour, Sciton) and found that reepithelialization was complete in an average of 5 days, and only three patients (6%) experienced prolonged postoperative erythema.[464] In a split-face comparison of 16 patients following pulsed CO_2 and variable-pulse Er:YAG laser skin resurfacing, Rostan et al reported decreased erythema, less edema and faster reepithelialization on the side treated with the variable pulse (CO_3, Cynosure) Er:YAG laser.[26]

Postoperative Hyperpigmentation

Transient postinflammatory hyperpigmentation is not uncommon following modulated (coagulative-ablative) Er:YAG laser skin resurfacing. However, the reported duration of hyperpigmentation after modulated Er:YAG resurfacing has been shorter than that observed after CO_2 laser resurfacing.[16,465]

Jeong et al reported hyperpigmentation in 8 of 35 (29 %) patients (Fitzpatrick skin types III–V) treated with a variable-pulse Er:YAG laser for pitted acne scars. Similarly, Alster et al reported a 40% incidence of hyperpigmentation in their series of 50 patients resurfaced with a variable pulse Er:YAG laser. In both series the hyperpigmentation was transient and responded well to topical agents. In their series of 20 patients with pitted acne scars, Jeong et al reported an incidence of hyperpigmentation of 60% and an incidence of hypopigmentation of 5% following resurfacing with the dual mode Contour Er:YAG laser (Contour, Sciton). In all cases the hyperpigmentation was transient and resolved within 3 months postoperatively.[466]

Delayed Permanent Hypopigmentation

Delayed permanent hypopigmentation, a common side effect after CO_2 laser resurfacing (15–20% reported incidence) has not been reported in most series that utilized a modulated (coagulative-ablative) Er:YAG laser. One year postoperatively, Tanzi and Alster noted no cases of delayed hypopigmentation in their series of 50 patients resurfaced with the Contour (Sciton Corp.) Er:YAG laser.[464]

Sapijaszko and Zachary, however, reported two cases of hypopigmentation in their series of over 100 patients resurfaced with a modulated Er:YAG laser (Contour, Sciton).[455] Kim et al resurfaced 190 patients of Fitzpatrick skin type III–V with Er:YAG lasers and observed an incidence and mean duration of hyperpigmentation of 24.7% (6.5 weeks), 42.3% (7.3 weeks) and 65.9% (7.8 days) with the short pulsed, variable pulse (CO_3, Cynosure) and dual-mode (Contour Sciton), respectively. The incidence and mean duration of hypopigmentation observed was 8.0% (4.4 months), 15.3% (5.3 months) and 24.4% (5.7 months) for the short pulsed, variable pulse (CO_3, Cynosure) and dual mode (Contour, Sciton) Er:YAG lasers.[443] We are currently caring for a patient who presented to our practice with marked hypopigmentation of the lower face that manifested 5 months after aggressive resurfacing with the Derma-K CO_2-Er:YAG hybrid laser (ESC, Needham, MA).

In our practice we have resurfaced over 1000 patients with the variable pulse Er:YAG laser (CO_3, Cynosure) and have not yet seen a case of prolonged hypopigmentation resulting from treatment with this particular laser.

Topical photochemotherapy and the excimer laser have both been reported to be efficacious in the treatment of laser resurfacing-induced hypopigmentation. Grimes et al reported moderate to excellent repigmentation in five of seven patients (71%) treated biweekly with a mean number of 25 sessions of topical photochemotherapy with 0.001% methoxypsoralen.[53] Friedman and Geronemus reported 75% improvement of laser resurfacing-induced hypopigmentation in two patients treated with the 308 nm excimer laser for 8–10 treatment sessions. Initial treatment was performed at the minimal erythema dose minus 50 J/cm^2. If erythema was not seen 24 hours after the first treatment, the dose was increased by 50 mJ/cm^2 until erythema occurred. The average cumulative UVB dose was 1750 mJ/cm^2. They observed no complications and good retention of pigment at 1-month follow up.[54]

In summary, the modulated (coagulative and ablative modes) Er:YAG lasers have been able to produce 'CO_2-like' clinical results with a side-effect profile that has turned out to be considerably more favorable than that of the CO_2 lasers.

A B

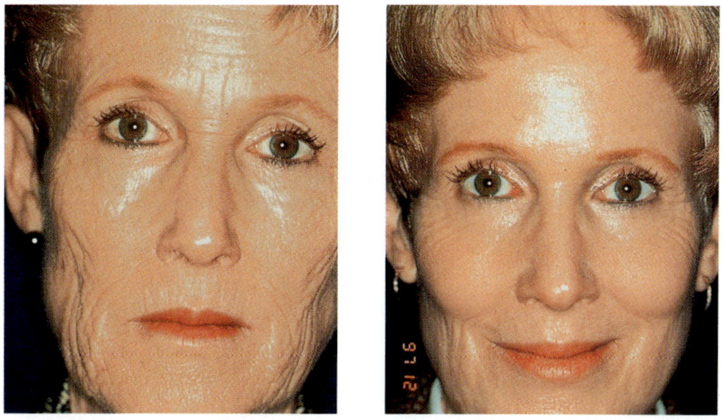

Figure 7.42 (A) With more advanced photodamage, full treatment with CO_2 laser is performed (two or three passes), then erbium laser is used to remove layer of thermal necrosis and selectively sculpt tissue. (B) This technique reduces residual erythema, quickens healing, and results in enhanced clinical results, as seen 2 months postoperatively. CO_2 laser provides tissue tightening periorbitally and on cheeks, while erbium laser sculpts deep lines of upper lip, glabella, and forehead.

Combination CO_2 and Erbium:YAG Laser Treatment

Necrotic tissue directly disregulates wound healing, induces proteases and inflammation. Many experts believe that the thermally induced zone of necrosis left behind by the CO_2 laser is one of the main factors contributing to its adverse sequelae including prolonged postoperative erythema, pain, delayed healing and scarring. Therefore, some authors have investigated the effect of removal of this residual zone of thermally damaged tissue after CO_2 laser resurfacing.

Goldman and colleagues studied the effect of Er:YAG laser resurfacing aimed to remove the residual zone of thermal damage left behind after CO_2 laser resurfacing.[31] They randomized 10 patients to receive resurfacing to one half of the face with a 950-μs pulsed CO_2 laser (three passes, 300 mJ, CPG settings of 596, 595, 584) and resurfaced the other side of the face with two passes of the same CO_2 laser at the same settings followed by two passes with a short pulse Er:YAG laser (4-mm spot, 1.7 J, 14 J/cm^2). They found that both reepithelialization time and the duration of erythema were significantly less for the side treated with the combination CO_2–Er:YAG as compared to the side treated with CO_2 laser alone (Figs 7.42 and 7.43). Moreover, this beneficial effect on postoperative healing was accomplished without compromising clinical efficacy. Biopsies taken at 2 to 3 days, 1 week, and 4 to 8 weeks showed that thermal necrosis was greatly reduced by adding the erbium laser treatment, speeding healing by 2 to 3 days without compromising new collagen production. In addition, inflammation was reduced at 1 week, and angiogenesis was decreased at 1 to 8 weeks, reflecting the decreased erythema that was seen clinically (Figs 7.44 and 7.45).

McDaniel et al compared resurfacing of the upper lip using a CO_2 laser alone (UltraPulse 5000-C, two passes, 300 mJ, 95 Watts, CPG density 6, spot diameter 2.25 mm, 7.5 J/cm^2) with the combination of the same CO_2 laser treatment followed by three passes with a short pulsed Er:YAG laser (7-mm spot, 2 J, 5.2 J/cm^2). Medium to deep (class III) rhytides were improved with both techniques. However, the duration of postoperative crusting, swelling and pruritus was significantly reduced at the sites treated with the CO_2–Er:YAG laser combination.[32]

Protocols for Combination CO_2-Erbium:YAG Laser Treatment

Both the CO_2 laser and the Er:YAG laser have unique qualities that can be exploited during resurfacing. The CO_2 laser is unique in the following ways:

- Hemostasis is achieved.
- A plateau of ablation is reached, limiting resurfacing depth if proper treatment protocols are followed.
- Collagen (skin) tightening occurs as a heat-related phenomenon, resulting in correction of loose tissue and atrophic scars.
- The first pass causes an epidermal/dermal split that allows easy and complete removal of the epidermis with a single pass.

The Er:YAG laser is unique in the following ways:

- Minimal residual thermal damage or tissue heating occurs.

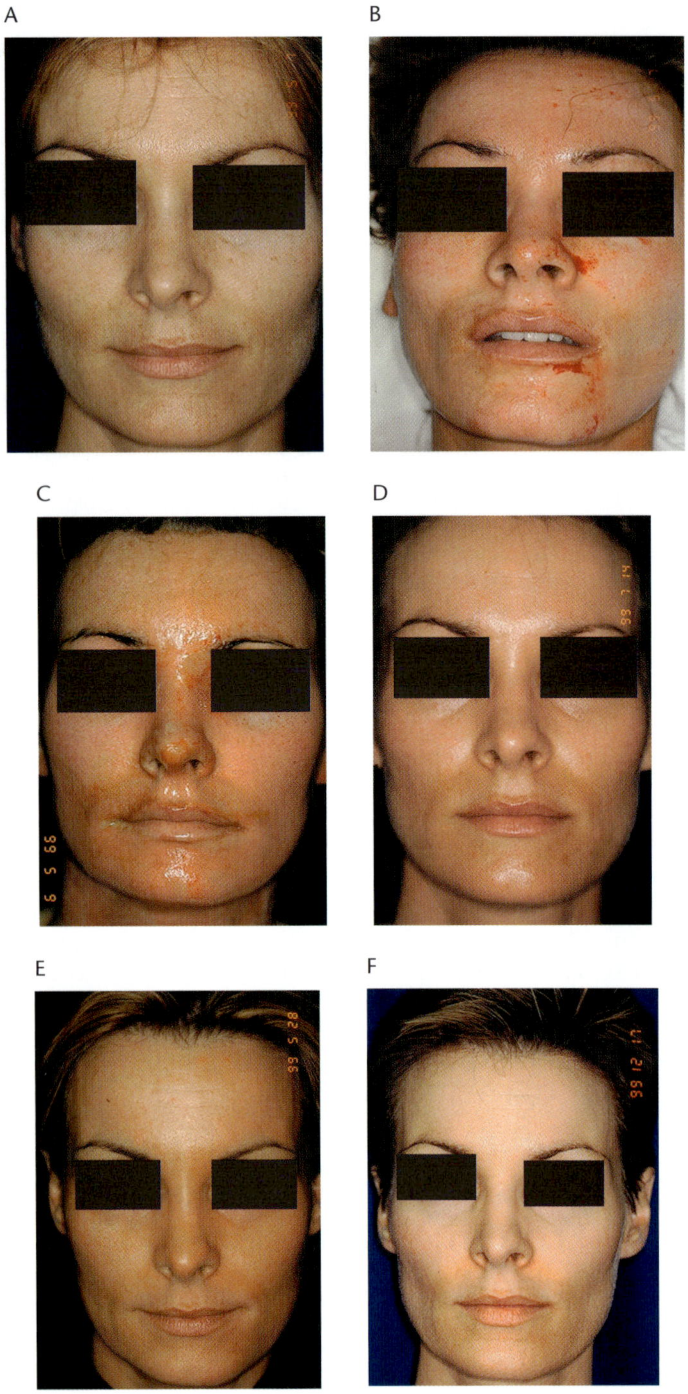

Figure 7.43 Laser resurfacing comparing the CO_2 laser to the Sciton Er:YAG laser. (A) 38-year-old women before treatment. (B) immediately after treatment with 2 passes of the UP CO_2 laser on the right side of the face at a setting of 300 mJ, CPG with a density of 5 followed by two passes with the Er:YAG at 5 J/cm^2. The left side was treated with the Sciton laser using a 50 μm of ablation and 100% coagulation for two passes followed by two passes with 0% coagulation and 5 J/cm^2. (C) 2 days after treatment the CO_2 laser treated side is more swollen and erythematous. (D) 1 week after treatment the CO_2 laser treated side is more swollen and erythematous. (E) 3 weeks after treatment the CO_2 laser side is more erythematous. (F) 30 weeks after treatment there is no appreciable difference between both sides of the face.

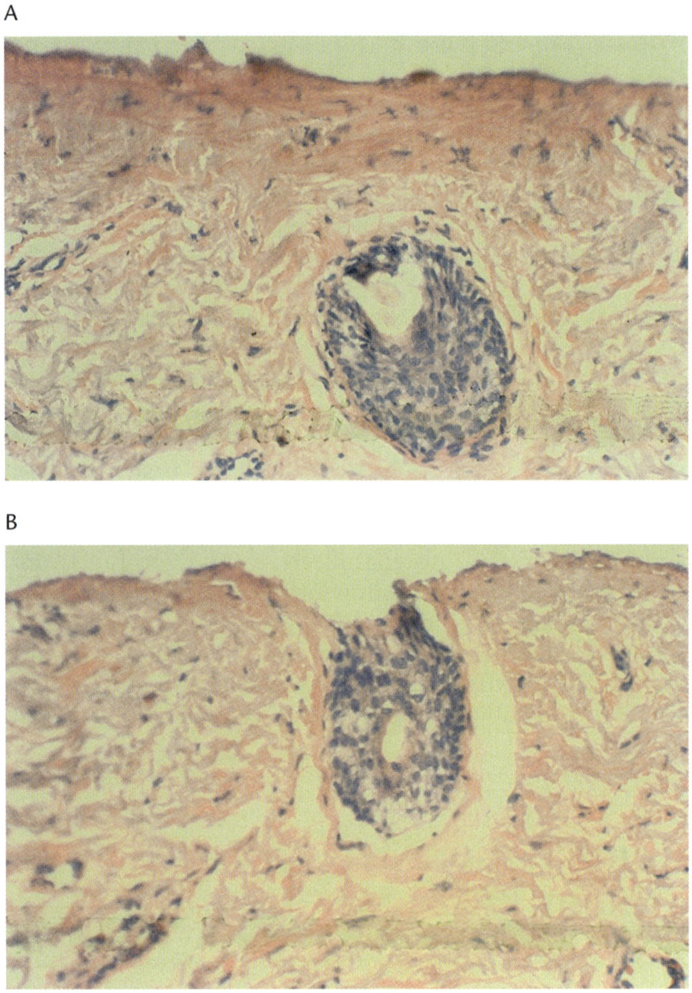

Figure 7.44 (A) Two passes of CO_2 laser at 7 J/cm^2 leaves approximately 70 μm of residual thermal necrosis. (B) Two passes of erbium laser at 10 J/cm^2 results in removal of approximately 50 μm of this necrotic tissue, resulting in faster wound healing.

- This pure-ablation laser continues to ablate with each pass and does not reach an ablation plateau with depth.
- Only minimal tissue water is required for laser–tissue interaction.

The most successful use of lasers for resurfacing would utilize each laser to take advantage of its unique benefit and to eliminate the disadvantages of each as much as possible. Accordingly, the following protocols are followed for early photodamage and for moderate to advanced photodamage.

Early Photodamage and Superficial Scars

When treating early photodamage or when patients desire a more superficial treatment allowing early return to work and as little healing time as possible (Fig. 7.46), the laser surgeon performs the following steps:

1. The epidermis is removed with a single pass of the CO_2 laser, usually with a density overlap of 20% to 30%. This can be accomplished very efficiently with the CO_2 laser, and biopsy studies have shown 0 to 10 μm of residual

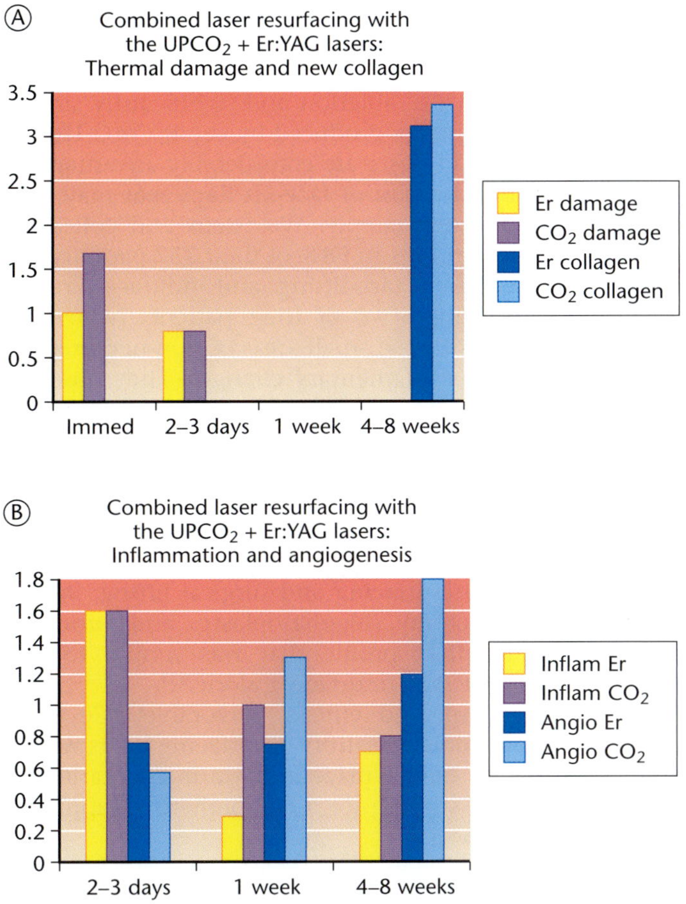

Figure 7.45 (A) Initial thermal necrosis was shown to be reduced significantly by adding erbium laser passes after use of ultrapulsed CO_2 laser (UPCO_2), without compromising new collagen formation at 4 to 8 weeks. (B) Inflammation was greatly reduced at 1 week postoperatively by removing thermal necrosis with erbium laser. Angiogenesis was also reduced at 1 to 8 weeks compared with use of UPCO_2 laser alone.

thermal necrosis with this single pass. If only epidermal removal is desirable, treatment is completed by using the Er:YAG laser to clean up any epidermal remnants and to feather the periphery. If dermal treatment of acne scars or photodamage is required, the areas of treatment are assessed with consideration of step 2.

2a. The CO_2 laser may be used with either the 3-mm spot or the CPG in small areas that will benefit from collagen tightening, such as the lower eyelids or medial cheeks and areas of atrophic acne scarring.

2b. The Er:YAG laser may be used uniformily in one or two passes to remove superficial photodamage and fine wrinkles and to feather the periphery.

Significant Photodamage and Scars

When treating patients who desire the maximal improvement in a single treatment and who have significant

A B

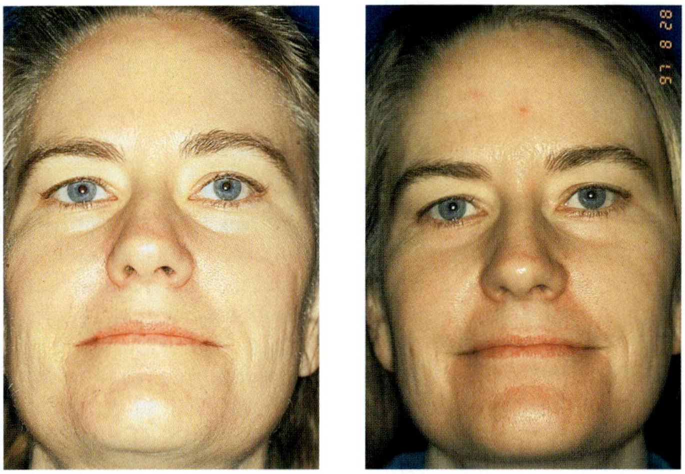

Figure 7.46 When treating early photodamage (A) especially if patient desires to return to work with as little healing time as possible, epidermis is removed with CO_2 laser and superficial dermal resurfacing performed with erbium laser (B). Although moderate improvement is seen, tissue tightening of cheeks and removal of deeper lines are not accomplished.

photodamage or acne scarring, the laser surgeon performs the following steps:

1. The epidermis is removed with a single pass of the CO_2 laser, usually with a density overlap of 30%.
2. A second pass of the CO_2 laser is done uniformly across the entire face, usually with a density overlap of 20% to 30%.
3. A third pass of the CO_2 laser is done in areas still having visible photodamage or scarring, generally the glabella and nose, middle lower forehead, middle to lateral cheeks and upper lip, and lateral chin areas, usually with a density overlap of 20% to 30%.
4. The 3 mm spot of the CO_2 laser is used to vaporize or induce thermal necrosis in areas of distinct photodamage or selectively to tighten loose photodamaged tissue, such as the eyelids, lateral cheeks, and atrophic scars. When used to induce thermal necrosis, the handpiece is moved slowly across the shoulder of a deep wrinkle line, the sharp edges of a scar crater, along the elevated portions of a linear scar, or over any dermal or epidermal growth, such as rhinophyma, syringoma, or seborrheic keratosis. The intent is to cause some superficial brownish char that will subsequently be ablated with the erbium laser.
5. The Er:YAG laser is used in a uniform manner, as in step 2b for early photodamage, removing the superficial portion of the 50 to 70 μm of residual thermal damage left by the CO_2 laser, thereby enhancing the reepithelialization process. This requires two passes at 1.7 J and a 4-mm pulse.
6. The Er:YAG laser is used with a small, focused spot size to sculpt tissue previously treated with the 3-mm CO_2 spot to smooth the tissue as uniformly as possible by ablating the necrotic tissue.

7. The periphery is feathered with the Er:YAG laser using a defocused energy of 1.0 to 1.7 J and a 5- to 8-mm diameter spot. This treatment protocol maximizes the benefit that can be achieved with each laser (see Fig. 7.40).

Future Trends

Over a decade of clinical literature has firmly established the ablative resurfacing lasers as reliable, effective, safe and versatile tools for cutaneous rejuvenation. Patient satisfaction from cutaneous laser resurfacing remains high. A recent prospective survey of patients who underwent full-face resurfacing 30 months before reported that 88% of these patients felt that their appearance had improved, 75% would recommend the procedure and 71% of them would undergo laser skin resurfacing again.[55]

Newer and more versatile technologies like the modulated (coagulative and ablative mode) Er:YAG lasers and improvements in treatment protocols and postoperative care regimens have improved clinical outcomes and increased the safety of laser skin resurfacing. This added margin of safety has made it appealing for cosmetic surgeons to begin exploring the potential benefits of simultaneously combining laser resurfacing with other surgical rejuvenation techniques.

Cosmetic surgeons now regularly, safely and effectively combine laser skin resurfacing with nonablative laser treatments in the same session. Pigmented lesions, tattoos and periorbital hyperpigmentation can be treated safely and more effectively when a Q-switched laser (i.e. ruby, alexandrite or Nd:YAG) is used following ablative laser resurfacing. A 100% improvement of facial telangiectasiae has been reported in patients treated with the pulsed dye laser (PDL) prior to ablative facial skin resurfacing.[33]

Moreover, in both of these clinical situations, combination treatment achieves cosmetic results that are superior to those attainable with either laser alone. By combining ablative laser skin resurfacing with other problem-specific nonablative laser technologies, cosmetic surgeons are now more effectively addressing multiple cosmetic concerns for their patient in a single treatment session.

Facial aging involves both, gravity-induced ptosis of soft tissue elements and photodamage of the overlying skin. Simultaneous rhytidectomy and full-face laser resurfacing addresses both of these components of facial aging and theoretically should produce superior cosmetic outcome than can be achieved with either treatment modality alone. Unfortunately, early reports of skin necrosis[34–36] after simultaneous undermining and chemical peeling, initially discouraged surgeons from exploring the benefits of this therapeutic combination.

However, as rhytidectomy and laser resurfacing techniques have improved, the combination of both of these techniques has become increasingly more popular. Cosmetic surgeons are now regularly combining laser resurfacing with transconjunctival blepharoplasty, endoscopic brow lifting and endoscopic face lifts.[39,467–470] A recent meta-analysis by Koch et al of ten series (493 patients) in which simultaneous treatment with rhytidectomy and full-face CO_2 laser resurfacing was performed found the complication rates to be no greater than those previously reported for rhytidectomy or CO_2 laser resurfacing alone.[37]

The precise depth of ablation and significantly smaller zone of thermal damage produced by the Er:YAG laser as compared to the CO_2 laser are considerably advantageous when resurfacing the skin of face-lift flaps that may have compromised vascular supply. Weinstein and colleagues reported excellent results in 98% of their 257 patients that underwent combined face-lifting and full-face Er:YAG laser skin resurfacing. Two of their patients, who were heavy smokers, developed small areas of skin necrosis that healed with residual pigmentary changes. They observed no additional cases of scarring, infection or pigmentary alterations in their large series.[38] In another large series of 242 patients treated with combined facelift and full-face resurfacing with a short pulsed Er:YAG laser, no flap complications were observed.[39] A more recent retrospective study of 34 patients who underwent combination CO_2 or Er:YAG laser skin resurfacing and surgical lifting, including S-lift rhytidectomy, blepharoplasty, and brow lift reported a side effect profile that was similar to that reported after laser skin resurfacing alone.[471]

Given their improved efficacy, favorable side effect profile and remarkable versatility, resurfacing lasers will no doubt continue to have a place in the armamentarium of cosmetic surgeons striving for a comprehensive approach to facial rejuvenation.

New Resurfacing Laser Technologies

The side effects of ablative skin resurfacing are unacceptable to many patients. To overcome some of the morbidity and complications associated with ablative skin resurfacing, a new concept of skin rejuvenation called fractional photothermolysis has been developed. In contrast to ablative skin resurfacing, which produces homogeneous thermal damage at a particular depth within the skin, fractional photothermolysis creates microscopic thermal wounds and specifically spares the tissue surrounding each wound. These microscopic treatment zones constitute the 'building blocks' for the macroscopic treatment effect. Manipulation of the laser parameters to produce different three-dimensional shapes, depths and densities of the microscopic treatment zones theoretically allows for fine adjustment of the macroscopic treatment effect and extent of the resurfacing.

A pilot study with a prototype laser implementing the concepts of fractional photothermolysis was recently carried out by Anderson et al,[56] who treated the lateral periorbital area of 30 subjects with a 1.5-μm laser that created a final microscopic treatment zone (MTZ) density of $2500\,cm^2$ and delivered a mean fluence per pass of 1.5 to $3\,J/cm^2$ depending on the energy per MTZ which varied from 6 to 12 mJ. Pulse duration ranged from 1.5 to 5 milliseconds and produced a single MTZ. The rate of MTZ deposition was approximately 120 per second. Ten passes were performed at each of four total treatment sessions spaced 4 to 7 days apart. Average treatment pain intensity was reported as a 3.2 ± 0.97 (scale of 0–10) and typically subsided within 10 to 60 minutes. Side effects of treatment included erythema which 33% of the patients experienced at day 1 and persisted in 10% after the first week. Post-treatment edema scores ranged from 0 to 3 (scale of 0 to 6) and typically subsided within 6 to 24 hours but persisted for one week in 10% of patients. During the first 2 weeks after treatment, the patients developed a slight 'bronzing' of the skin. Epiluminescence microscopy revealed this discoloration was due to thousands of individual brown spots on the skin surface, which disappeared with desquamation within 2 weeks. There were no instances of permanent pigmentary alterations. At their 3 month follow up, 34% of subjects showed moderate or better improvement in appearance of wrinkles and 47% of subjects showed moderate or better improvement in quality of skin texture. The Fitzpatrick–Goldman wrinkle score improved by an average of 0.9 ± 0.7 points from baseline to the 3-month follow up visit.

The concepts of fractional photothermolysis were recently implemented in the 1550 nm FRAXEL laser developed and made available commercially by Reliant Technologies (Palo Alto, CA). Optimal treatment parameters have not yet been defined for this laser. Clinical data presented at the most recent annual meeting of the American Academy of Cosmetic Surgery (San Diego, California, January 2005), suggests that the FRAXEL laser may be advantageous in the treatment of dyschromias (i.e. melasma) and the resurfacing of patients with darker skin phototypes. Additionally, the FRAXEL promises to be a therapeutic option for those patients who find any 'downtime' unacceptable and are otherwise unwilling to undergo a laser resurfacing procedure. Of note, studies comparing the clinical efficacy of this new resurfacing laser versus that of the Er:YAG or CO_2 lasers have not yet been performed.

References

1. Welch AJ. The thermal response of laser irradiated tissue. IEEEJ Quantum Electron 1984; 20:1471.
2. Alster TS. Cutaneous resurfacing with CO_2 and erbium:YAG lasers: preoperative, intraoperative and postoperative considerations. Plast Reconstr Surg 1999; 103:619.
3. Weinstein C. Ultrapulse CO_2 laser removal of periocular wrinkles in association with laser blepharoplasty. J Clin Laser Med Surg 1994; 12:205.
4. Lowe NJ, Lask G, Griffin ME et al. Skin resurfacing with the UltraPulse CO_2 laser: observations on 100 patients. Dermatol Surg 1995; 21:1025.
5. Alster TS. Clinical and histologic evaluation of six Er:YAG lasers for cutaneous resurfacing. Lasers Surg Med 1999; 24: 87.
6. Ross VE, McKinlay JR, Anderson RR. Why does CO_2 resurfacing work: a review. Arch Dermatol 1999; 135(4):444.
7. Ziering CL. Cutaneous laser resurfacing with the Er:YAG laser and the char-free CO_2 laser: a clinical comparison of 100 patients. Int J Aesthetic Rest Surg 1997; 5:29.
8. Alster TS, Lupton JR. Erbium:YAG cutaneous laser resurfacing. Dermatol Clin 2001; 19:453.
9. Kauvar ANB, Waldorf HA, Geronemus RG. A histolopathological comparison of 'char-free' CO_2 lasers. Dermatol Surg 1996; 22:343.
10. Weinstein C. Erbium laser resurfacing: current concepts. Plast Reconstr Surg 1999; 103(2):602.
11. Teikemeier G, Goldberg DJ. Skin resurfacing with the Er:YAG laser. Dermatol Surg 1997; 23:685.
12. Papadavid E, Katsambas A. Lasers for facial rejuvenation: a review. Int J Dermatol 2003; 42:480.
13. Bass LS. Erbium:YAG laser skin resurfacing: preliminary clinical evaluation. Ann Plast Surg 1998; 40:328.
14. Goldberg DJ, Meine JG: Treatment of photoaged neck skin with the pulsed erbium:YAG laser. Dermatol Surg 1998; 24:619.
15. Goldman MP, Fitzpatrick RE, Manuskiatti W. Laser resurfacing of the neck with the Er:YAG laser. Dermatol Surg 1999; 25:164.
16. Nanni CA, Alster TS. Complications of CO_2 laser resurfacing. An evaluation of 500 patients. Dermatol Surg 1998; 24:315.
17. Nanni CA, Alster TS. Complications of cutaneous laser surgery: a review. Dermatol Surg 1998; 24:209.
18. Alster TS, West TB. Resurfacing of atrophic facial acne scars with a high-energy, pulsed CO_2 laser. Dermatol Surg 1996; 22:151.
19. Adrian RM. Pulsed CO_2 and erbium-YAG laser resurfacing: a comparative clinical and histologic study. J Cutan Laser Ther 1999; 1:29.
20. Khatri KA, Ross V, Grevelink J, Magro C, Anderson RR. Comparison of Er:YAG and CO_2 lasers in resurfacing of facial rhytides. Arch Dermatol 1999; 135:391.
21. Adrian RM. Pulsed CO_2 and long-pulsed 10-ms erbium-YAG laser resurfacing: a comparative clinical and histologic study. J Cutan Laser Ther 1999; 1(4):197.
22. Khatri KA, Ross V, Grevelink JM, Magro CM, Anderson RR. Comparison of erbium:YAG and CO_2 lasers in resurfacing of facial rhytides. Arch Dermatol 1999; 135(4):391.
23. Kaufmann R, Hibst R. Pulsed 2.94 µm Er:YAG laser skin ablation: experimental results and first clinical application. Clin Exp Dermatol 1990; 15:389.
24. Kaufmann R, Hibst R. Pulsed Er:YAG and 308 nm UV-excimer laser: an in vitro and in vivo study of skin ablative effects. Lasers Surg Med 1989; 9:132.
25. Fitzpatrick RE, Rostan EF, Marchell, N. Collagen tightening induced by CO_2 laser versus Er:YAG laser. Lasers Surg Med 2000; 27:395.
26. Rostan EF, Fitzpatrick RE, Goldman MP. Laser resurfacing with a long pulse Er:YAG laser compared to the 950 µs pulsed CO_2 laser. Lasers Surg Med 2001; 29:136.
27. Newman JB, Lord JL, Ash K, McDaniel DH. Variable pulse Er:YAG laser skin resurfacing of perioral rhytides and side-by-side comparison with CO_2 laser. Lasers Surg Med 2000; 26:208.
28. Tanzi EL, Alster TS. Treatment of atrophic facial acne scars with a dual-mode Er:YAG laser. Dermatol Surg 2002; 28:551.
29. Kwon SD, Kye YC. Treatment of scars with a pulsed Er:YAG laser. J Cutan Laser Ther 2000; 2(1):27.
30. Weinstein C, Scheflan M. Simultaneously combined Er:YAG and CO_2 laser (Derma K) for skin resurfacing. Clin Plast Surg 2000; 27(2):273.
31. Goldman MP, Manuskiatti W. Combined laser resurfacing with the 950 µsec pulsed CO_2 + Er:YAG lasers. Dermatol Surg 1999; 25:160.
32. McDaniel DH, Lord J, Ash K, Newman J. Combined CO_2/Erbium:YAG laser resurfacing of peri-oral rhytides and side-by-side comparison with CO_2 laser alone. Dermatol Surg 1999; 25:285–293
33. Manuskiatti W, Fitzpatrick RE, Goldman MP. Treatment of facial skin using combinations of CO_2, Q-switched alexan-

drite, flashlamp-pumped pulsed dye and Er:YAG lasers in the same treatment session. Dermatol Surg 2000; 26:114–120.
34. Spira M, Gerow FJ, Hardy SB. Complications of chemical face peeling. Plast Reconstr Surg 1974; 54:397.
35. Litton C. Chemical face lifting. Plast Reconstr Surg 1962; 29:371.
36. Baker TL, Gordon HL. Chemical face peeling: an adjunct to surgical facelifting. South Med J 1963; 56:412.
37. Koch BB, Perkins SW. Simultaneous rhytidectomy and full-face CO_2 laser resurfacing: a case series and meta-analysis. Arch Facial Plast Surg 2002; 4(4):227.
38. Weinstein C, Poszner J, Scheflan M. Combined Er:YAG laser resurfacing and face lifting. Plast Reconstr Surg 2001; 107:586.
39. Roberts TL III, Pozner JN. Lasers, facelifting and the future. Clin Plast Surg 2000; 2:293.
40. Weinstein C, Ramirez OM, Pozner JN. Postoperative care following CO_2 laser resurfacing: avoiding pitfalls. Plast Reconstr Surg 1997; 100:1855.
41. Sriprachya-Anunt S, Fitzpatrick RE, Goldman MP et al. Infections complicating CO_2 laser resurfacing. Dermatol Surg 1997; 23:527.
42. Monheit GD. Facial resurfacing may trigger the herpes simplex virus. Cosmetic Dermatol 1995; 8:9.
43. Manuskiatti, W, Fitzpatrick RE, Goldman MP, Krejci-Papa N. Propylactic antibiotics in patients undergoing laser resurfacing of the skin. J Am Acad Dermatol 1999; 40:77.
44. Ross VE, Amesbury EC, Barile A et al. Incidence of postoperative infection or positive culture after facial laser resurfacing: a pilot study, a case report, and a proposal for a rational approach to antibiotic prophylaxis. J Am Acad Dermatol 1998; 39:975.
45. Alster TS, Nanni CA. Famciclovir prophylaxis of herpes simplex virus reactivation after laser skin resurfacing. Dermatol Surg 1999; 25:242.
46. Batra RS, Ort RJ, Jacob C et al. Evaluation of a silicone occlusive dressing after laser skin resurfacing. Arch Dermatol 2001; 137(10):1317.
47. Goldman MP, Roberts TL 3rd, Skover G et al. Optimizing wound healing in the face after laser ablation. J Am Acad Dermatol 2002; 46(3):399.
48. Newman JP, Fitzgerald, P, Koch, RJ. Review of closed dressings after laser resurfacing. Dermatol Surg 2000; 26:562.
49. Newman JP, Koch RJ, Goode RL. Closed dressings after laser skin resurfacing. Arch Otolaryngol Head Neck Surg 1998; 124(7):751.
50. Eaglstein, WH. Occlusive dressings. J Dermatol Surg Oncol 1993; 19:716.
51. Horton S, Alster TS. Preoperative and postoperative considerations for CO_2 laser resurfacing. Cutis 1999; 64:399.
52. West TB, Alster TS. Effect of pretreatment on the incidence of hyperpigmentation following cutaneous CO_2 laser resurfacing. Dermatol Surg 1999; 25:15.
53. Grimes PE, Bhawan J, Kim J et al. Laser resurfacing-induced hypopigmentation: histologic alterations and repigmentation with topical photochemotherapy. Dermatol Surg 2001; 27:515.
54. Friedman PM, Geronemus RG. Use of the 308-nm laser for postresurfacing leukoderma. Arch Dermatol 2001; 137:824.
55. Batra RS, Jacob C, Hobbs L et al. A prospective survey of patient experiences after laser skin resurfacing. Results from 2.5 years of follow up. Arch Dermatol 2003; 139:1295.
56. Manstein D, Herron GS, Kink RK et al. Fractional photothermolysis: a new concept for cutaneous remodeling using microscopic patterns of thermal injury. Lasers Surg Med 2004; 34:426.
57. Dover JS, Smoller BR, Stern RS et al. Low-fluence CO_2 laser irradiation of lentigines. Arch Dermatol 1988; 124:1219.
58. Kamat BR, Tang SV, Arndt KA et al. Low-fluence CO_2 laser irradiation: selected epidermal damage to human skin. J Invest Dermatol 1985; 85:274.
59. Wheeland RG. Revision of full-thickness skin grafts using the CO_2 laser. J Dermatol Surg Oncol 1988; 14:130.
60. Garrett AB, Dufresne RG, Ratz JL, Berlin AJ. CO_2 laser treatment of pitted acne scarring. J Dermatol Surg Oncol 1990; 16:737.
61. Goldman L, Shumrick DA, Rockwell J. The laser in maxillofacial surgery: preliminary investigative surgery. Arch Surg 1968; 96:397.
62. David LM. Laser vermilion ablation for actinic cheilitis. J Dermatol Surg Oncol 1985; 11:605.
63. Brauner G, Schliftman A. Laser surgery for children. J Dermatol Surg Oncol 1987; 13:178.
64. David LM, Lask GP, Glassberg E et al. Laser ablation for cosmetic and medical treatment of facial actinic damage. Cutis 1989; 43:583.
65. Anderson RR, Parrish JA. Selective photothermolysis: precise microsurgery by selective absorption of pulsed radiation. Science 1983; 220:524.
66. Fitzpatrick RE et al. Lasers Surg Med, 1989 (abstract).
67. Fitzpatrick RE, Ruiz-Esparza J, Goldman MP. The clinical advantage of the superpulse CO_2 laser. Lasers Surg Med 1990; Suppl 2:52.
68. Fitzpatrick RE, Ruiz-Esparza J, Goldman MP. The depth of thermal necrosis using the CO_2 laser: a comparison of the superpulsed mode and conventional mode. J Dermatol Surg Oncol 1991; 17:340.
69. Fitzpatrick RE: The UltraPulse CO_2 laser: selective photothermolysis of epidermal tumors. Lasers Surg Med 1993; Suppl 5:56.
70. Fitzpatrick RE, Goldman MP, Ruiz-Esparza JR. Clinical advantage of the CO_2 laser superpulsed mode: treatment of verruca vulgaris, seborrheic keratoses, lentigines and actinic cheilitis. J Dermatol Surg Oncol 1994; 20:449.
71. Fitzpatrick RE, Ruiz-Esparza J. The superpulsed CO_2 laser. In: Roenigk RK, Roenigk H, eds New trends in dermatologic surgery. Dunitz, London, 1993.
72. Green HA, Burd E, Nishioka NS et al. Skin graft take and healing ablation of graft beds. J Invest Dermatol 1989; 92:436 (abstract).
73. Green HA, Burd E, Nishioka NS. Pulsed CO_2 laser ablation of burned skin: in vitro and in vivo analysis. Lasers Surg Med 1990; 10:476.
74. Green HA, Burd E, Nishioka NS et al. Mid-dermal wound healing: a comparison between dermatomal excision and pulsed CO_2 ablation. Arch Dermatol 1992; 128:639.
75. Smalley P: Personal communication, 1991.
76. Fitzpatrick RE, Tope WD, Goldman MP, Satur NM. Pulsed CO_2 laser, tricholoroacetic acid, Baker-Gordon phenol, and dermabrasion: a comparative clinical and histological study of cutaneous resurfacing in a porcine model. Arch Dermatol 1996; 132:469.
77. Fitzpatrick RE, Goldman MP, Satur NM, Tope WD. Pulsed CO_2 laser resurfacing of photoaged skin. Arch Dermatol 1996; 132:395.
78. Arnold D, Slatkine M, Eliezer Z. Swiftlaser: a new technology for char-free ablation in rectal surgery. J Clin Laser Med Surg 1993; 11:309.

79. Krespi YP, Keidar A, Khosh MM et al. The efficacy of laser-assisted uvuloplasty in the management of obstructive sleep apnea and upper airway resistance syndrome. Oper Tech Otolaryngol Head Neck Surg 1994; 5:235.
80. Grevelink JM, Brennick JB. Hair transplantation facilitated by flashscanner-enhanced CO_2 laser. Oper Tech in Otolaryngol Head Neck Surg 1994; 5:278.
81. Chernoff WG, Shoenrock L. Cutaneous laser resurfacing. Oper Tech Otolaryngol Head Neck Surg 1994; 5:281.
82. Waldorf HA, Kauvar ANB, Geronemus RG. Skin resurfacing of fine to deep rhytides using char-free CO_2 laser in 47 patients. Dermatol Surg 1995; 21:940.
83. Lask G, Keller G, Lowe N, Gormley D. Laser skin resurfacing with the SilkTouch flashscanner for facial rhytides. Dermatol Surg 1995; 21:1021.
84. Alster TS. Comparison of two high-energy pulsed CO_2 lasers in the treatment of periorbital rhytides. Dermatol Surg 1996; 22:541.
85. Alster TS, Garg S. Treatment of facial rhytides with the UltraPulse high energy CO_2 laser. Plast Reconstr Surg 1996; 98:791.
86. Ho C, Nguyen Q, Lowe NJ et al. Laser resurfacing in pigmented skin. Dermatol Surg 1995; 21:1035.
87. Goldman MP, Fitzpatrick RE, Smith SS. Resurfacing complications and their management. In: Coleman WP, Lawrence N, eds Laser resurfacing. Williams and Wilkins, Baltimore, MD, 1997.
88. Chernoff G, Shoenrock L, Cramer H et al. Cutaneous laser resurfacing. Int J Aesthetic Rest Surg 1995; 3:57.
89. Chernoff WG, Cramer H. Rejuvenation of the skin surface: laser exfoliation. Facial Plast Surg 1996; 12:135.
90. Dover JS. CO_2 laser resurfacing: why all the fuss? Plast Reconstr Surg 1996; 98:506 (editorial).
91. Goodman GJ. Facial resurfacing using a high-energy, short pulsed CO_2 laser. Aust J Dermatol 1996; 37:125.
92. Trelles MA, Kaplan I, Rigau J, Buezo O. Periocular skin reshaping by CO_2 laser coagulation. Aesthetic Plast Surg 1996; 20:327.
93. Fulton JE Jr. Dermabrasion, chemabrasion, and laserabrasion: Historical perspectives, modern dermabrasion techniques, and future trends. Dermatol Surg 1996; 22:619.
94. Chernoff G, Slatkine M, Zair E, Mead D. SilkTouch: a new technology for skin resurfacing in aesthetic surgery. J Clin Laser Med Surg 1995; 13:97.
95. Walsh JJ, Deutsch TF. Pulsed CO_2 laser tissue ablation: measurement of the ablation rate. Lasers Surg Med 1988; 8:264.
96. Olbricht SM. Use of the CO_2 laser in dermatologic surgery: a clinical relevant update for 1993. J Dermatol Surg Oncol 1993; 93:364.
97. Fitzpatrick RE, Goldman MP. CO_2 laser surgery. In: Cutaneous laser surgery: the art and science of selective photothermolysis. CV Mosby, St Louis, 1994.
98. Kauver ANB, Waldorf HA, Geronemus RG. A histopathological comparison of 'char-free' CO_2 lasers. Dermatol Surg 1996; 22:343.
99. Cotton J, Hood AF, Gonin R et al. Histologic evaluation of preauricular and postauricular human skin after high-energy, short pulse CO_2 laser. Arch Dermatol 1996; 132:425.
100. Stuzin JM, Baker TJ, Baker TM, Kligman AM. Histologic effects of the high energy pulsed CO_2 laser on photoaged facial skin. Plast Reconstr Surg 1997; 97:2036.
101. Alster TS. Histology of CO_2 resurfacing. Semin Cutan Med Surg 1996; 15:189.
102. Ross EV, Domankevitz Y, Skrobal M, Anderson RR. Effects of CO_2 laser pulse duration in ablation and residual thermal damage: implications for skin resurfacing. Lasers Surg Med 1996; 19:123.
103. Venugopalan V, Nishioka N, Mikic B. The effect of laser parameters on the zone of thermal injury produced by laser ablation of biological tissue. ASME Biomech Eng 1994; 116:62.
104. Gardner ES, Reinisch L, Stricklin GP et al. In vitro changes in non-facial human skin following laser resurfacing: a comparison study. Lasers Surg Med 1996; 19:379.
105. Schomacker K, Walsh J, Flott T, Deutsch T. Thermal damage produced by high-irradiance continuous wave CO_2 laser cutting of tissue. Lasers Surg Med 1990; 10:74.
106. McKenzie A. How far does thermal damage extend beneath the surface of CO_2 laser incisions? Phys Med Biol 1983; 28:905.
107. Walsh J, Flotte T, Anderson R, Deutsch T. Pulsed CO_2 laser tissue ablation: effects of tissue type and pulse duration on thermal damage. Lasers Surg Med 1988; 8:108.
108. Hobbs E, Bailin P, Wheeland R, Ratz J. Superpulsed lasers: minimizing thermal damage with short duration, high irradiance pulses. J Dermatol Surg Oncol 1987; 13: 955.
109. Apfelberg DB. The UltraPulse CO_2 laser with computer pattern generator automatic scanner for facial cosmetic surgery and resurfacing. Ann Plast Surg 1996; 36:522.
110. Rubach BW, Schoenrock LD. Histological and clinical evaluation of facial resurfacing using a CO_2 laser with the computer pattern generator. Arch Otolaryncol Head Neck Surg 1997; 123:929.
111. Apfelberg DB. UltraPulse CO_2 laser with CPG scanner for full-face resurfacing for rhytids, photoaging, and acne scars. Plast Reconstr Surg 1997; 99:1817.
112. Apfelberg DB, Smoller B. UltraPulse CO_2 laser with CPG scanner for deepithelialization: clinical and histologic study. Plast Reconstr Surg 1997; 99:2089.
113. Hruza GJ, Fitzpatrick RE, Dover JS. Laser skin resurfacing. In: Arndt KA, Olbricht SM, Dover JS, eds Cutaneous laser surgery. Lippincott-Raven, Philadelphia, 1997.
114. Stuzin JM, Baker TJ, Baker TM, Kligman AM. Histologic effects of the high-energy pulsed CO_2 laser on photoaged facial skin. Plast Reconstr Surg 1997; 99:2036.
115. Rein R. Physical and surgical principles governing CO_2 laser surgery on the skin. Dermatol Clin 1991; 9:297.
116. Fitzpatrick RE, Smith SR, Sriprachya-Anunt S. Depth of vaporization and the effect of pulse stacking with a high energy, pulsed CO_2 laser. J Am Acad Dermatol 1999; 40(4):615.
117. Nelson BR, Majmudar G, Griffiths CEM et al. Clinical improvement following dermabrasion of photoaged skin correlates with synthesis of collagen I. Arch Dermatol 1994; 130:1136.
118. Goldman MP, Fitzpatrick RE. New collagen. J Clin Laser Med Sur.
119. Flor PJ, Garrett RR. Phase transition in collagen and gelatin systems. J Am Chem Soc 1958; 80:4836.
120. Flor PJ, Spurr OK. Melting equilibrium for collagen fibers under stress: elasticity in the amorphous state. J Am Chem Soc 1960; 83:1308.
121. Flor PJ, Weaver ES. Helix coil transition in dilute aqueous collagen solutions. J Am Chem Soc 1959; 82:4518.
122. Stryer L. The stability of the collagen helix depends on cooperative interactions. In: Stryer L ed Biochemistry, 2nd edn. Freeman, New York, 1981.
123. Gross J. Thermal denaturation of collagen in the dispersed and solid state. Science 1964; 143:960 (abstract).

124. Bourne G ed. The biochemistry and physiology of bone. Academic Press, New York, 1956.
125. Horn DJ, King NL, Kurth LB et al. Collagen crosslinks and their relationship to the thermal properties of calf tendons. Arch Biochem Biophys 1980; 28:21.
126. Gelman RA, Blackwell J, Kefalides NA et al. Thermal stability of basement membrane collagen. Biochim Biophys Acta 1976; 427:492.
127. Tanzer ML. Cross-linkage of collagen. Science 1973; 180:561.
128. Boedtker H, Doty P. The native and denatured states of soluble collagen. J Am Chem Soc 1956; 79:4267.
129. Boedtker H, Doty P. On the nature of the structural element of collagen. J Am Chem Soc 1955; 77:248 (editorial).
130. Sarkar SK, Hiyama Y, Niu CH et al. Molecular dynamics of collagen side chains in hard and soft tissues: a multicenter magnetic resonance study. Biochemistry 1987; 26:6793.
131. Mosler E, Foldhard W, Knorzer W et al. Stress-induced molecular arrangement in tendon collagen. J Mol Biol 1985; 182:589.
132. Gustavson KH. The chemistry and reactivity of collagen. Academic Press, New York, 1956.
133. Pearce JA, Thomsen S. Kinetic models of laser-tissue fusion processes. Biomed Sci Instrum 1993; 29:355.
134. Guthrie CR, Murray LW, Kopchok GE. Biochemical mechanisms of laser vascular tissue fusion. J Invest Surg 1991; 4:3.
135. Schmid TM, Linsenmayer TF. Denaturation-renaturation properties of two molecular forms of short-chain cartilage collagen. Biochemistry 1984; 23:553.
136. Tanaka S, Avigad G, Eikenberry EF et al. Isolation and partial characterization of collagen chains dimerized by sugar-derived cross-links. J Biol Chem 1988; 263:17650.
137. Lennox FG. Shrinkage of collagen. Biochim Biophys Acta 1949; 3:170.
138. Lloyd DJ, Garrod M. A contribution to the theory of the structure of protein fibres with special reference to the so-called thermal shrinkage of the collagen fibre, 1947.
139. Theis ER. Relation of swelling to shrinkage temperature of collagen, 1946.
140. Allain JC, Le Lous M, Cohen-Solal L et al. Isometric tensions developed during the hydrothermal swelling of rat skin. Connect Tissue Res 1980; 7:127.
141. Verzar F, Nagy IZ. Electronmicroscopic analysis of thermal collagen denaturation in rat tail tendons. Gerontologia 1970; 16:77.
142. Thomsen S. Pathologic analysis of photothermal and photomechanical effects of laser–tissue interactions. Photochem Photobiol 1991; 53:825.
143. Pearce JA. Thermodynamic principles of laser–tissue interaction. Proc IEEE BME, November 1990.
144. Sand BJ. Method for collagen treatment. US Patent No. 4 976 709, 1990.
145. Smelser GK, Polack FM, Ozanics V. Persistence of donor collagen in corneal transplants. Exp Eye Res 1965; 4:349.
146. Stringer HCW, Highton TC. The shrinkage temperature of skin collagen. Aust J Dermatol 1960; 5:230.
147. Vangsness CT Jr, Mitchell W III, Nimni M et al. Collagen shortening: an experimental approach with heat. Clin Orthop Rel Res 1997; 337:267.
148. Hayashi K, Thabit III, Massa KL et al. The effect of thermal heating on the length and histologic properties of the glenohumeral joint capsule. Am J Sports Med 1997; 25: 107.
149. Ross EV, Naseef M, Skrobal JM et al. In vivo dermal collagen shrinkage and remodeling following CO_2 laser resurfacing. Lasers Surg Med 1996; 19(suppl 8):38.
150. Kirsch KM, Zelickson BD, Zachary CB et al. Ultrastructure of collagen thermally denatured by microsecond domain pulsed CO_2 laser. Paper presented at 17th Annual Meeting of American Society of Lasers in Medicine and Surgery, Phoenix, April 1997.
151. Brugmans MJP, Kemper J, Gijsbers GHM et al. Temperature response of biological materials to pulsed non-ablative CO_2 laser irradiation. Lasers Surg Med 1991; 11:587.
152. Polatnick J, La Tessa AJ, Katzin HM. Comparison of collagen preparations from beef cornea and sclera. Biochim Biophys Acta 1957; 26:365.
153. Lans LJ. Experimentelle Untersuchungen über Entstehung von Astigmatismus durch nicht-perforirende Corneawunden. Graefes Arch Ophthalmol 1898; 45:117.
154. Wray C. Case of 6 D of hypermetropic astigmatism cured by the cautery. Trans Ophthalmol Soc UK 1914; 34:109.
155. O'Connor R. Corneal cautery for high myopic astigmatism. Am J Ophthalmol 1933; 16:337.
156. Shaw EL, Gasset AR. Thermokeratoplasty (TKP) temperature profile. Invest Ophthalmol 1974; 13:181.
157. Gasset AR, Shaw EL, Kaufman HE et al. Thermokeratoplasty. Trans Acad Ophthalmol Otol 1973; 77:OP441.
158. Stringer H, Parr J. Shrinkage temperature of eye collagen. Nature 1964; December:1307.
159. Horn G, Spears KG, Lopez O et al. New refractive method for laser thermal keratoplasty with the Co:MgF2 laser. J Cataract Refract Surg 1990; 16:611.
160. Parel JM, Ren Q, Simon G. Noncontact laser photothermal keratoplasty. I. Biophysical principles and laser beam delivery system. J Refract Corneal Surg 1994; 10:511.
161. Aquavella JV. Thermokeratoplasty. Ophthal Surg 1974; 5: 39.
162. Aquavella JV, Buxton JN, Shaw EL. Thermokeratoplasty in the treatment of persistent corneal hydrops. Arch Ophthalmol 1977; 95:81.
163. Keates RH, Dingle J. Thermokeratoplasty for keratoconus. Ophthal Surg 1975; 6:89.
164. Fogle JA, Kenyon KR, Stark WJ. Damage to epithelial basement membrane by thermokeratoplasty. Am J Ophthalmol 1977; 83:392.
165. Aquavella JV, Smith RS, Shaw EL. Alterations in corneal morphology following thermokeratoplasty. Arch Ophthalmol 1976; 94:2082.
166. Arenstein JJ, Rodrigues MM, Laibson PR. Histopathologic changes after thermokeratoplasty for keratoconus. Invest Ophthalmol Vis Sci 1977; 16:32.
167. Itoi M. Computer photokeratometry changes following thermokeratoplasty. In: Schachar RA, Levy NS, Schachar L eds Refractive modulation of the cornea. LAL, Denison, TX, 1981.
168. Rowsey JJ, Gaylor JR, Dahlstrom R et al. Los Alamos keratoplasty techniques. Contact Intraocular Lens Med J 1960; 6:1.
169. Rowsey JJ, Doss JD. Preliminary report of Los Alamos keratoplasty techniques. Ophthalmology 1981; 88:755.
170. Neumann AC, Fyodorov S, Sanders DR. Radial thermokeratoplasty for the correction of hyperopia. J Refract Corneal Surg 1990; 6:404.
171. Neumann AC, Sanders D, Raanan M et al. Hyperopic thermokeratoplasty: clinical evaluation. J Cataract Refract Surg 1991; 17:830.
172. Neumann AC. Thermokeratoplasty for hyperopia. Ophthalmol Clin North Am 1992; 5:753.
173. Rowsey JJ. Electrosurgical keratoplasty: update and retraction. Invest Ophthalmol Vis Sci 1987; 28(suppl):224.

174. Feldman ST, Ellis W, Frucht-Pery J et al. Regression of effect following radial thermo-keratoplasty in humans. J Refract Corneal Surg 1989; 5:288.
175. Thompson VM, Seiler T, Durrie DS et al. Holmium:YAG laser thermokeratoplasty for hyperopia and astigmatism: an overview. J Refract Corneal Surg 1993; 9:134.
176. Mainstern MA: Ophthalmic applications of infrared lasers: thermal considerations. Invest Ophthalmol Vis Sci 1979; 18:414.
177. Beckman H, Fuller TA, Boyman R et al. CO_2 laser surgery of the eye and adnexa. Ophthalmology 1980; 87:990.
178. Peyman GA, Larson B, Raichand M et al. Modification of rabbit corneal curvature with use of CO_2 laser burns. Ophthal Surg 1980; 11:325.
179. Householder J, Horwitz LS, Lowe K, Murillo A. Laser induced thermal keratoplasty. SPIE Proc 1989; 1066:18.
180. McCally RL, Bargeron CB, Green WR et al. Stromal damage in rabbit corneas exposed to CO_2 laser radiation. Exp Eye Res 1983; 37:543.
181. Kanoda AN, Sorokin AS. Laser correction of hypermetropic refraction. In: Fyodorov SN ed Microsurgery of the eye: main aspects. MIR, Moscow, 1987.
182. Spears KG, Horn G, Serafin J. Corneal refractive correction by laser thermal keratoplasty. Proc SPIE 1990; 1202:334.
183. Zhou Z, Ren QS, Simon G et al. Thermal modeling of laser photothermokeratoplasty (LPTK). SPIE Proc 1992; 1644:61.
184. Durrie DS, Seiler T, King MC et al. Application of the holmium:YAG laser for refractive surgery. SPIE Proc 1992; 1644:56.
185. Seiler T. Ho:YAG laser thermokeratoplasty for hyperopia. Ophthalmol Clin North Am 1992; 5:773.
186. Koch DD, Berry MJ, Vassiliadis A et al. Non-contact holmium:YAG laser thermal keratoplasty. In: Salz JJ ed Corneal laser surgery. CV Mosby, Philadelphia, 1994.
187. Ariyasu RG, Sand B, Menefee R et al. Holmium laser thermal keratoplasty of 10 poorly sighted eyes. J Refract Surg 1995; 11:358.
188. Koch DD, Abarca A, Villarreal R et al. Hyperopic correction by non-contact holmium:YAG laser thermal keratoplasty: clinical study with two year follow-up. Ophthalmology 1996; 22:362.
189. Koch DD, Kohnen T, McDonnell PJ et al. Hyperopia correction by non-contact holmium:YAG laser thermal keratoplasty: US Phase IIA clinical study with 1-year follow-up, Ophthalmology 1998 (in press).
190. Moreira H, Campos M, Sawusch MR et al. Holmium laser thermokeratoplasty. Ophthalmology 1993; 100:752.
191. Seiler T, Matallana M, Bende T. Laser thermokeratoplasty by means of a pulsed holmium:YAG laser for hyperoptic correction. Refract Corneal Surg 1990; 6:335.
192. Koch DD. Histological changes and wound healing response following non-contact holmium:YAG laser thermal keratoplasty. Trans Am Ophthalmol Soc 1996; 94:745.
193. Koch DD, Kohnen T, Anderson JA et al. Histologic changes and wound healing response following 10-pulse non-contact holmium:YAG laser thermal keratoplasty. J Refract Surg 1996; 12:623.
194. Ren Q, Simon G, Parel JM. Non-contact laser photothermal keratoplasty. III. Histological study in animal eyes. J Refract Corneal Surg 1994; 10:529.
195. Farrell RA, Bargeron CB, McCally RL et al. Corneal effects produced by IR laser radiation: laser safety, eyesafe laser systems, and laser eye protection. SPIE Proc 1990; 1207:59.
196. Fing PT, Richards R, Iwamoto T et al. Heat shrinkage of extraocular muscle tendon. Arch Ophthalmol 1987; 105:716.
197. Hayashi K, Markel MD, Thabit G III et al. The effect of non-ablative laser energy on joint capsular properties: an in-vitro mechanical study using a rabbit model. Am J Sports Med 1995; 23:482.
198. Dillingham MF, Price JM, Fanton GS. Holmium laser surgery. Orthopedics 1993; 16:563.
199. Sherk HH. Current concepts review: the use of lasers in orthopaedic procedures. J Bone Joint Surg 1993; 75A:768.
200. Thabit G. Treatment of unidirectional and multidirectional glenohumeral instability by an arthroscopic holmium:YAG laser-assisted capsular shift procedure: a pilot study. In: Laser application in arthroscopy. International Musculo-skeletal Laser Society, Neuchatel, Switzerland, 1994.
201. Hayashi K, Thabit G III, Massa KL et al. The effect of thermal heating on the length and histologic properties of the glenohumeral joint capsule. Am J Sports Med 1997; 25:107.
202. Tang J, Godlewski G, Rouy S et al. Morphologic changes in collagen fibers after 830 nm diode laser welding. Lasers Surg Med 1997; 21:438.
203. Tang J, O'Calaghan D, Rouy S et al. Quantity change in collagen following 830 nm diode laser welding. Proc SPIE 1996; 2922:432.
204. Bass LS, Moazami N, Procsidio J et al. Changes in type I collagen following laser welding. Lasers Surg Med 1992; 12:500.
205. Bass LS, Treat MR, Dzakonski C, Trokel SL. Sutureless microvascular anastomosis using the THC:YAG laser: a preliminary report. Microsurgery 1989; 10:189.
206. Murray LW, Su L, Kopchok GE et al. Cross-linking of extracellular matrix proteins: a preliminary report on possible mechanism of argon laser welding. Lasers Surg Med 1989; 9:490.
207. Schober R, Ulrich F, Sander T et al. Laser-induced alteration of collagen substructure allows microsurgical tissue welding. Science 1986; 232:1421.
208. Oz MC, Bass LS, Popp HW et al. In vitro comparison of thulium-holmium-chromium:YAG and argon lasers for welding of biliary tissue. Lasers Surg Med 1989; 9:248.
209. Oz MC, Chuck RS, Johnson JP et al. Indocyanine green dye-enhanced welding with a diode laser. Surg Forum 1989; 40:316.
210. Anderson RR, Lemole GM Jr, Kaplan R et al. Molecular mechanisms of thermal tissue welding. Part 2. Lasers Surg Med 1994; Suppl 6:56 (abstract).
211. Lemole GM, Anderson RR, DeCoste S. Preliminary evaluation of collagen as a component in the thermally induced 'weld'. Proc SPIE 1991; 1422:116.
212. Solhpour S, Weldon E, Foster TE et al. Mechanism of thermal tissue 'welding'. Part I. Lasers Surg Med 1994; Suppl 6:56 (abstract).
213. White RA, Kopchok GE, White GH et al. Laser vascular anastomotic welding. In: White RA, Grundfest WS eds Lasers in cardiovascular disease. Year Book, Chicago, 1987.
214. White RA, Kopchok G, Donayre C et al. Argon laser-welded arteriovenous anastomosis. J Vasc Surg 1987; 6:447.
215. White RA, Kopchok G, Donarye C et al. Comparison of laser-welded and sutured arteriotomies. Arch Surg 1996; 121: 1133.
216. White RA, Abergel RP, Klein SR et al. Laser welding of venotomies. Arch Surg 1986; 121:905.
217. White RA, Kopchok G, Donayre CE et al. Mechanism of tissue fusion in argon laser welded vein–artery anastomosis. Lasers Surg Med 1988; 8:83.
218. Popp HW, Oz MC, Bass LS et al. Welding of gallbladder tissue using a pulsed 2.15 micron thulium-holmium-chromium: YAG laser. Lasers Surg Med 1989; 9:155.

219. Quigley MR, Bailes JE, Kwaan HC, Heiferman K. Microvascular laser-assisted anastomosis: results at one year. Lasers Surg Med 1986; 6:179 (abstract).
220. Quigley MR, Bailes JE, Kwaan HC et al. Microvascular anastomosis using the milliwatt CO_2 laser. Lasers Surg Med 1985; 5:357.
221. Abergel RP, Lyons RF, White RA et al. Skin closure by Nd: YAG laser welding. J Am Acad Dermatol 1986; 14:810.
222. Abergel RP, Lyons RF, Dwyer R et al. Use of lasers for closure of cutaneous wounds: experience with Nd:YAG, argon, and CO_2 lasers. J Dermatol Surg Oncol 1986; 12:1181.
223. Jain KK. Sutureless microvascular extra-intracranial anastomosis with Nd:YAG laser. Lasers Surg Med 1984; 3:311 (abstract).
224. Ashworth EM, Dalsing MC, Olson JF et al. Large-artery welding with a milliwatt CO_2 laser. Arch Surg 1987; 122:673.
225. Chuck RS, Oz MC, Delohery TM et al. Dye-enhanced laser tissue welding. Lasers Surg Med 1989; 9:471.
226. Pribil S, Powers SK. Carotid artery end-to-end anastomosis in the rat using the argon laser. J Neurosurg 1985; 63:771.
227. McCarthy WJ, Hartz RS, Yao JST et al. Vascular anastomoses with laser energy. J Vasc Surg 1986; 3:32.
228. Frazier OH, Painvin GA, Morris JR et al. Laser-assisted microvascular anastomoses: angiographic and anatomopathological studies on growing microvascular anastomoses: preliminary report. Surgery 1985; 97:585.
229. Sigel B, Dunn MR. The mechanism of blood vessel closure by high frequency electrocoagulation. Surg Gynecol Obstet 1965; 121:823.
230. Guthrie CR, Murray LW, Kopchok GE et al. Biochemical mechanisms of laser vascular tissue fusion. J Invest Surg 1991; 4:3.
231. Serure A, Wither EH, Thomsen S, Morris J. Comparison of CO_2 laser-assisted microvascular anastomosis and conventional microvascular sutured anastomosis. Surg Forum 1983; 34:634.
232. White RA, Kopchok G, Peng SK et al. Laser vascular welding: how does it work? Ann Vasc Surg 1986; 1:461.
233. Kopchok G, White RA, Grundfest WS et al. Thermal studies in in-vivo vascular tissue fusion by argon laser. J Invest Surg 1988; 1:5.
234. Kopchok WS, Grundfest WS, White RA et al. Argon laser vascular welding: the thermal component. SPIE Lasers Med 1986; 712:260.
235. Epstein M, Cooley CB. Electron microscopic study of laser dosimetry for microvascular tissue welding. Lasers Surg Med 1986; 6:202.
236. Weinstein C. CO_2 laser resurfacing: long-term follow-up in 2123 patients. Clin Plast Surg 1998; 25:109.
237. Fitzpatrick RE, Manuskiatti W, Goldman MP. Long-term effectiveness and side effects of CO_2 laser resurfacing for photoaged facial skin. J Am Acad Dermatol, 1998 (submitted for publication).
238. Ross EV, Grossman MC, Duke D, Grevelink JM. Long-term results after CO_2 laser skin resurfacing: a comparison of scanned and pulsed systems. J Am Acad Dermatol 1997; 37:709.
239. Reed JT, Joseph AK, Bridenstine JB. Treatment of periorbital wrinkles: a comparison of the SilkTouch CO_2 laser with a medium-depth chemical peel. Dermatol Surg 1997; 23: 643.
240. Abergel RP, Dahlman CM. The CO_2 laser approach to the treatment of acne scarring. Cosmet Dermatol 1995; 8:33.
241. Hruza JG. Skin resurfacing with lasers. Fitzpatrick's J Clin Dermatol 1995; 3:38.
242. Alamillos-Granados FJ, Naval-Gias L, Dean-Ferrer A et al. CO_2 laser vermilionectomy for actinic cheilitis. J Oral Maxillofac Surg 1993; 51:118.
243. Stanley RJ, Roenigk RK. Actinic cheilitis: treatment with the CO_2 laser. Mayo Clin Proc 1988; 63:230.
244. Robinson JK. Actinic cheilitis: a prospective study comparing four treatment methods. Arch Otolaryngol Head Neck Surg 1989; 115:848.
245. Zelickson BD, Roenigk RK. Actinic cheilitis: treatment with the CO_2 laser. Cancer 1990; 65:1307.
246. Dufresne RJ, Garrett AB, Bailin PL et al. CO_2 laser treatment of chronic actinic cheilitis. J Am Acad Dermatol 1988; 19:876.
247. Johnson TM, Sebastien TS, Lowe L et al. CO_2 laser treatment of actinic cheilitis: clinicohistopathologic correlation to determine the optimal depth of destruction. J Am Acad Dermatol 1992; 27:737.
248. Ries WR, Duncavage JA, Ossoff RH. CO_2 laser treatment of actinic cheilitis. Mayo Clin Proc 1988; 63:294.
249. Scheinberg RS. CO_2 laser treatment of actinic cheilitis. West J Med 1992; 156:192.
250. Whitaker DC. Microscopically proven cure of actinic cheilitis by CO_2 laser. Lasers Surg Med 1987; 7:520.
251. Frankel DH. CO_2 laser vermilionectomy for chronic actinic cheilitis. Facial Plast Surg 1989; 6:158.
252. Goldman MP, Fitzpatrick RE, Smith SS. Resurfacing complications and their management. In: Coleman WP, Lawrence N eds Laser resurfacing. Williams & Wilkins, Baltimore, MD, 1997.
253. Lowe NJ, Lask G, Griffin ME. Laser skin resurfacing: pre- and post-treatment guidelines. Dermatol Surg 1995; 21: 1017.
254. Fitzpatrick RE, Goldman MP. Laser treatment of benign pigmented lesions using a 300 nanosecond pulse and 510nm wavelength. J Dermatol Surg Oncol 1993; 19:341.
255. Goldberg D. Benign pigmented lesions of the skin: treatment with the Q-switched ruby laser. J Dermatol Surg Oncol 1993; 19:376.
256. Brauner GJ, Schliftman AB. Treatment of pigmented lesions of the skin with the alexandrite laser. Lasers Surg Med 1992; 4:72.
257. Monheit GD. The Jessner's TCA peel: a medium-depth chemical peel. J Dermatol Surg Oncol 1989; 15:945.
258. Brody HJ, Hailey CW. Medium-depth chemical peeling of the skin: a variation of superficial chemosurgery. J Dermatol Surg Oncol 1986; 12:1268.
259. Taylor CR, Anderson RR. Ineffective treatment of refractory melasma and post-inflammatory hyperpigmentation by Q-switched ruby laser. J Dermatol Surg Oncol 1994; 20: 592.
260. Greenbaum SS, Krull EA, Watnich K. Comparison of CO_2 laser and electrosurgery in the treatment of rhinophyma. J Am Acad Dermatol 1988; 18:363.
261. Wheeland RG, Bailin PL, Ratz JL. Combined CO_2 laser excision and vaporization in the treatment of rhinophyma. J Dermatol Surg Oncol 1987; 13:172.
262. Apfelberg DB, Maser MR, Lash H et al. Superpulse CO_2 laser treatment of facial syringomata. Lasers Surg Med 1987; 7:533.
263. Wheeland RG, Bailin PL, Kronberg E. CO_2 (CO_2) laser vaporization for the treatment of multiple trichoepithelioma. J Dermatol Surg Oncol 1984; 10:470.
264. Apfelberg DB, Maser MR, Lash H et al.Treatment of xanthelasma palpebrum with the CO_2 laser. J Dermatol Surg Oncol 1987; 13:149.

265. Wheeland RG, Bailin PL, Kantor GR et al. Treatment of adenoma sebaceum with CO_2 laser vaporization. J Dermatol Surg Oncol 1985; 11:861.
266. Ratz JL, Bailin PL, Wheeland RG. CO_2 laser treatment of epidermal nevi. J Dermatol Surg Oncol 1986; 12:567.
267. Hohenleutner U, Landthaler M. Laser therapy of verrucous epidermal nevi. Clin Exp Dermatol 1993; 18:124.
268. Blitzer A, Brin MF, Keen MS et al. Botulinum toxin for the treatment of hyperfunctional lines of the face. Arch Otolaryngol Head Neck Surg 1993; 119:1018.
269. Carruthers JDA, Carruthers JA. Treatment of glabellar frown lines with C. botulinum-A exotoxin. J Dermatol Surg Oncol 1992; 18:17.
270. Garcia A, Fulton JE. Cosmetic denervation of the muscles of facial expression with botulinum toxin: a dose-response study. Dermatol Surg 1996; 22:39.
271. Keen M, Blitzer A, Aviv J et al. Botulinum toxin-A for hyperkinetic facial lines: results of a double-blind, placebo-controlled study. Plast Reconstr Surg 1994; 94:94.
272. Bhawan J, Gonzales-Serva A, Nehal K et al. Effects of tretinoin on photodamaged skin: a histologic study. Arch Dermatol 1991; 127:666.
273. Kang S, Fisher GJ, Voorhees JJ. Photoaging and topical tretinoin: therapy, pathogenesis and prevention. Arch Dermatol 1997; 133:1280.
274. Orringer JS, Kang S, Johnson TM et al. Tretinoin treatment before carbon-dioxide laser resurfacing: a clinical and biochemical analysis. J Am Acad Dermatol 2004; 51:940.
275. Ruiz-Esparza J, Barba Gomez JM, Labastida Gomez de la Torre O. Erythema after laser skin resurfacing. Dermatol Surg 1998; 24:79.
276. Ruiz-Esparza J, Lupton JR. Laser resurfacing of darkly pigmented patients. Dermatol Clin 2002; 20(1):113.
277. Alster TS. Combined laser resurfacing and tretinoin treatment of facial rhytides. Cosmet Dermatol 1997;10:39–42.
278. Friedman PM, Geronemus RG. Antibiotic prophylaxis in laser resurfacing patients. Dermatol Surg 2000; 26:695.
279. Bernstein LJ, Kauvar ANB, Grossman MC, Geronemus RG. The short- and long-term side effects of carbon dioxide laser resurfacing. Dermatol Surg 1997; 23:519–525.
280. Nanni CA, Alster TS. Complications of carbon dioxide laser resurfacing. Dermatol Surg 1998; 24:315–320.
281. Waldorf HA, Kauvar ANB, Geronemus RG. Skin resurfacing of fine to deep rhytides using a char-free carbon dioxide laser in 47 patients. Dermatol Surg 1995; 21:940–946.
282. Gaspar ZE, Vincuillo C, Elliott T. Antibiotic prophylaxis for full-face laser resurfacing: is it necessary? Arch Dermatol 2001; 137(3):313–315.
283. Walia S, Alster TS. Cutaneous CO_2 laser resurfacing infection rate with and without prophylactic antibiotics. Dermatol Surg 1999; 25(11):857.
284. Grekin RC. Cutaneous CO_2 laser resurfacing infection rate with and without prophylactic antibiotics. Dermatol Surg 1999; 25:51.
285. Raz R, Miron D, Colodner R et al. A 1-year trial of nasal mupirocin in the prevention of recurrent staphylococcal nasal colonization and skin infection. Arch Intern Med 1996; 156:1109.
286. Russell SW, Dinehart SM, Davis I, Flock ST. Efficacy of corneal shields in protecting patients' eyes from laser irradiation. Dermatol Surg 1996; 22:613.
287. Fitzpatrick RE, Williams B, Goldman MP. Preoperative anesthesia and postoperative considerations in laser resurfacing. Semin Cutan Med Surg 1996; 15:170.
288. Dvork HF. Tumors: wounds that do not heal: similarities between tumor stroma generation and wound healing. N Engl J Med 1986; 315:1650.
289. Peacock EE Jr. Inflammation and the cellular response to injury. In: Peacock EE Jr ed Wound repair. WB Saunders, Philadelphia, 1984.
290. Peacock EE Jr. Biological and pharmacological control of scar tissue. In: Peacock EE Jr ed Wound repair. WB Saunders, Philadelphia, 1984.
291. Kanzler MH, Gorsulowsky DC, Swanson NA. Basic mechanisms in the healing cutaneous wound. J Dermatol Surg Oncol 1986; 12:1156.
292. Goslen JB. Wound healing for the dermatologic surgeon. J Dermatol Surg Oncol 1988; 14:959.
293. Stenn KS, Malhotra R. Epithelialization. In: Cohen IK, Diegelmann RF, Lindblad WJ eds Wound healing: biochemical and clinical aspects. WB Saunders, Philadelphia, 1992.
294. Waldorf H, Fewkes J. Wound healing. Adv Dermatol 1995; 10:77.
295. Bach R, Nemerson Y, Konigsberg W. Purification and characterization of bovine tissue factor. J Biol Chem 1981; 256:8324.
296. Leibovich SJ, Ross R. A macrophage-dependent factor that stimulates the proliferation of fibroblasts in vitro. Am J Pathol 1976; 84:501.
297. Leibovich SJ, Ross R. The role of the macrophage in wound repair: a study with hydrocortisone and antimacrophage serum. Am J Pathol 1975; 78:71.
298. Shavit ZB, Ray A, Goldman R. Complement and Fc receptor-mediated phagocytosis of normal and stimulated mouse peritoneal macrophages. Eur J Immunol 1979; 9:385.
299. Littman BH, Ruddy S. Production of the second component of complement by human monocytes: stimulation by antigen-activated lymphocytes or lymphokines. J Exp Med 1979; 145:1344.
300. Clark RAF. Cutaneous tissue repair: basic biologic considerations. J Am Acad Dermatol 1985; 13:701.
301. Clark RAF. Basics of cutaneous wound repair. J Dermatol Surg Oncol 1993; 19:693.
302. Krummel TM, Nelson JM, Diegelmann RF et al. Fetal response to injury in the rabbit. J Pediatr Surg 1987; 22:640.
303. DePalma RL, Krummel TM, Nelson JM et al. Fetal wound matrix is composed of proteoglycan rather than collagen. Surg Forum 1987; 38:626.
304. Longaker MT, Adzick NS, Hall JL et al. Studies in fetal wound healing. VII. Fetal wound healing may be modulated by hyaluronic acid stimulating activity in amniotic fluid. J Pediatr Surg 1990; 25:430.
305. Mast BA, Diegelmann RF, Krummel TM, Cohen IK. Hyaluronic acid modulates proliferation, collagen and protein synthesis of cultured fetal fibroblasts. Matrix 1993; 13:441.
306. Mast BA, Haynes JH, Krummel TM et al. In vivo degradation of fetal wound hyaluronic acid results in increased fibroplasia, collagen deposition, and neovascularization. Plast Reconstr Surg 1992; 89:503.
307. Hellstrom S, Laurent C. Hyaluronan and healing of tympanic membrane perforations: an experimental study. Acta Otolaryngol 1987l; Suppl (Stockh) 442:54.
308. Bertheim U, Hellstrom S. The distribution of hyaluronan in human skin and mature, hypertrophic and keloid scars. Br J Plast Surg 1994; 47:483.
309. Passarini B, Tosti A, Fanti PA, Varotti C. [Effect of hyaluronic acid on the reparative process of non-healing ulcers: comparative study]. G Ital Dermatol Venereol 1982; 117:XXVII.

310. Torregrossa F, Caroti A. [Clinical verification of the use of topical hyaluronic acid under non-adhesive gauze in the therapy of torpid ulcers]. G Ital Dermatol Venereol 1983; 118:XLI.
311. Venturini D. [Clinical observations on the use of hyaluronic acid in dermatologic therapy]. G Ital Dermatol Venereol 1985; 120:V.
312. Celleno L, Piperno S, Bracaglia R. [Clinico-experimental studies on the use of hyaluronic acid in skin healing processes: preliminary data]. G Ital Dermatol Venereol 1985; 120:XLVII.
313. Retanda G. [Hyaluronic acid in the process of reparation of cutaneous ulcers: clinical experience]. G Ital Dermatol Venereol 1985; 120:LXXI.
314. Abatangela G, Martelli M, Vecchia P. Healing of hyaluronic acid-enriched wounds: histological observations. J Surg Res 1983; 35:410.
315. Trabucchi E, Preis-Baruffaldi F, Baratti C, Montorsi W. Topical treatment of experimental skin lesions in rats: macroscopic, microscopic and scanning electron-microscopic evaluation of the healing process. Int J Tissue React 1986; 8:533.
316. King SR, Hickerson WL, Proctor KG. Beneficial actions of exogenous hyaluronic acid in wound healing. Surgery 1991; 109:76.
317. Laurent C, Hellstrom S, Fellenius E. Hyaluronan improves the healing of experimental tympanic membrane perforations: a comparison of preparations with different rheologic properties. Arch Otolaryngol Head Neck Surg 1988; 114: 1435.
318. Doillon CJ, Dunn MG, Berg RA, Silver FH. Collagen deposition during wound repair. Scanning Electron Microsc 1985; pt 2:897.
319. Doillon CJ, Silver FH. Collagen-based wound dressing: effects of hyaluronic acid and fibronectin on wound healing. Biomaterials 1986; 7:3.
320. Burd DA, Greco RM, Regauer S et al. Hyaluronan and wound healing: a new perspective. Br J Plast Surg 1991; 44:579.
321. Borgognoni L, Reali UM, Santucci M. Low molecular weight hyaluronic acid induces angiogenesis and modulation of the cellular infiltrate in primary and secondary healing wounds. Eur J Dermatol 1996; 6:127.
322. Bailey AJ, Bazin S, Sims TJ et al. Characterization of the collagen of human hypertrophic and normal scars. Biochim Biophys Acta 1974; 21:404.
323. Oliver N, Baba M, Diegelmann R. Fibronectin gene transcription is enhanced in abnormal wound healing. J Invest Dermatol 1992; 99:579.
324. Skuta GL, Parrish RK II. Wound healing in glaucoma filtering surgery. Surv Ophthalmol 1987; 32:149.
325. Ross R, Raines EW, Bowen-Pope DR. The biology of platelet-derived growth factor. Cell 1986; 46:155.
326. Ross R. Fibroblast proliferation induced by blood cells. Agents Actions Suppl 1980; 7:81.
327. Bijrkedal-Hansen H. Catabolism and turnover of collagens: collagenases. Methods Enzymol 1987; 144:140.
328. Liu X, Wu H, Byrne M et al. A targeted mutation at the known collagenase cleavage site in mouse type I collagen impairs tissue remodeling. J Cell Biol 1995; 130: 227.
329. Matrisian LM, Hogan BL. Growth factor-regulated proteases and extracellular matrix remodeling during mammalian development. Curr Top Dev Biol 1990; 24:219.
330. Prockop D, Kivirikko K. Heritable diseases of collagen. N Engl J Med 1984; 311:376.
331. Mast BA. The skin. In: Cohen IK, Diegelmann RF, Lindblad WJ eds Wound healing: biochemical and clinical aspects. WB Saunders, Philadelphia, 1992.
332. Lamberg SI, Stoolmiller AC. Glycosaminoglycans: a biochemical and clinical review. J Invest Dermatol 1974; 63:433.
333. VanLis JM, Kalsbeek GL. Glycosaminoglycans in human skin. Br J Dermatol 1973; 88:355.
334. Levensen SM, Geever EG, Crowley LV et al. The healing of rat skin wounds. Ann Surg 1965; 161:293.
335. Rudolph R. Contraction and the control of contraction. World J Surg 1980; 4:279.
336. Gabbiani G, Ryan GB, Majne G. Presence of modified fibroblasts in granulation tissue and their possible role in wound contraction. Experientia 1971; 27:549.
337. Majno G. Contraction of granulation tissue in vitro: similarity to smooth muscle. Science 1971; 173:543.
338. Rudolph R, Berg JV, Ehrlich HP. Wound contraction and scar contracture. In: Cohen IK, Diegelmann RF, Linblad WJ eds Wound healing: biochemical and clinical aspects. WB Saunders, Philadelphia, 1992.
339. Schaffer CJ, Reinisch L, Polis SL et al. Comparisons of wound healing among excisional, laser-created, and standard thermal burns in porcine wounds of equal depth. Wound Rep Reg 1997; 5:52.
340. Fisher AA. Lasers and allergic contact dermatitis to topical antibiotics, with particular reference to bacitracin. Cutis 1996; 58:252.
341. Dooms-Goossens A, Degreef H. Contact allergy to petrolatums. II. Attempts to identify the nature of allergens. Contact Dermatitis 1983; 9:247.
342. Hinman CC, Maibach H, Winter GD. Effect of air exposure and occlusion on experimental human skin wounds. Nature 1963; 200:377.
343. Schilling RSF, Roberts M, Goodman N. Clinical trial of occlusive plastic dressings. Lancet 1950; 1:293.
344. Smack DP, Harrington AC, Dunn C et al. Infection and allergy incidence in ambulatory surgery patients using white petrolatum vs. bacitracin ointment. JAMA 1996; 276: 972.
345. Hunter GR, Change FC. Outpatient burns: a prospective study. J Trauma 1976; 16:191.
346. Eaglstein WH, Mertz PM. 'Inert' vehicles do affect wound healing. J Invest Dermatol 1980; 74:90.
347. Martin A. The use of antioxidants in healing. Dermatol Surg 1996; 22:156.
348. O'Donnell-Torney J, Nathan CF, Lanks K. Secretion of pyruvate: an antioxidant defense of mammalian cells. J Exp Med 1987; 165:500.
349. Shacter E. Serum-free medium for growth factor-dependent and independent plastocytomas and hybridomas. J Immunol Meth 1987; 99:259.
350. Winter GD. Formation of scab and rate of epithelialization of superficial wounds in the skin of the domestic pig. Nature 1962; 193:293.
351. Rovee DY, Kurowsky CA, Lobun J et al. Effect of local wound environment on epidermal healing. In: Maibach HL, Rovee DT eds Epidermal wound healing. Year Book, Chicago, 1972.
352. Geronemus RG, Robins P. The effect of two new dressings on epidermal wound healing. J Dermatol Surg Oncol 1982; 8:850.
353. Mandy S. A new primary wound dressing made of polyethylene oxide gel. J Dermatol Surg Oncol 1983; 9:153.
354. May SR. Physiology, immunology and clinical efficacy of an adherent polyurethane wound dressing: Op-Site. In:

Wise DL ed Burn wound coverings, vol 2. CRC, Boca Raton, FL, 1984.
355. Eaglstein WH, Mertz PM. New methods for assessing epidermal wound healing: the effects of triamcinolone acetonide and polyethylene film occlusion. J Invest Dermatol 1978; 71:382.
356. Barnett A, Berkowitz RL, Mius R et al. Comparison of synthetic adhesive moisture vapor permeable and fine mesh gauze dressings for split-thickness skin graft donor sites. Am J Surg 1983; 145:379.
357. Van Rijswijk L, Brown D, Friedman S et al. Multicenter clinical evaluation of hydrocolloid dressing for leg ulcers. Cutis 1985; 35:173.
358. Eaton AC. A controlled trial to evaluate and compare a sutureless skin closure technique (Op-Site skin closure) with conventional skin suturing and clipping in abdominal surgery. Br J Surg 1980; 67:857.
359. Kannon GA, Garrett AB. Moist wound healing with occlusive dressings: a clinical review. Dermatol Surg 1995; 21: 583.
360. Eaglstein WH. Experiences with biosynthetic dressings. J Am Acad Dermatol 1985; 12:434.
361. Bolton LL, Johnson CL, Rijswijk LV. Occlusive dressings: therapeutic agents and effects on drug delivery. Clin Dermatol 1992; 9:573.
362. Winter GD. Epidermal regeneration studied in the domestic pig. In: Maibach HL, Rovee DT eds Epidermal wound healing. Year Book, Chicago, 1972.
363. Alvarez OM, Mertz PM, Eaglstein WH. The effect of occlusive dressings on collagen synthesis and re-epithelialization in superficial wounds. J Surg Res 1983; 35:142.
364. Brown GL, Curtsinger L III, Brightwell JR et al. Enhancement of epidermal regeneration by biosynthetic epidermal growth factor. J Exp Med 1986; 163:1319.
365. Eaglstein WH, Davis SC, Mehle AL, Mertz PM. Optimal use of an occlusive dressing to enhance healing: effect of delayed application and early removal on wound healing. Arch Dermatol 1988; 124:392.
366. Michelow BJ, Varghai A, Kiumars M, Guyuron B. A new dressing for laser treated areas. Plast Reconstr Surg 2002; 110(4): 1150.
367. Concannon MJ, Malaney KB, Wiemer MS, Puckett CL. Omiderm: an inexpensive dressing after CO_2 laser resurfacing. Plast Reconstr Surg 1998; 101(7):1981.
368. Raab B. A new hydrophilic copolymer membrane for dermabrasion. J Dermatol Surg Oncol 1991; 17:323.
369. Wheeland RG. Wound healing and the newer surgical dressings. In: Moschella SL et al eds Dermatology. WB Saunders, Philadelphia, 1992.
370. Afilalo M, Guttman A, Lloyd J. DuoDerm hydroactive dressing versus silver sulphadiazine/Bactigras in the emergency treatment of partial skin thickness burns. Burns 1992;18:313.
371. Liu HT. Wound care following CO_2 laser resurfacing using Kaltostat, Duoderm and Telfa for dressings. Dermatol Surg 2000; 26(4):341.
372. Thomas S. Wound management: use of a calcium alginate dressing. J Wound Care 2000; 9:56.
373. Passe ER, Blaine G. Lancet 1948; 2:651.
374. Oliver LC, Blaine G. Br J Surg 1950; 147:307.
375. Frantz VK. Ann Surg 1948; 127:1165.
376. Levy PM, Salomon D. Use of Biobrane after laser resurfacing. Dermatol Surg 1998; 14(7):729.
377. Oliveria-Gandia M, Davis SC, Mertz PM. Can occlusive dressing composition influence proliferation of bacterial wound pathogens? Wounds 1998; 10:4.
378. Reynolds JEF. The extra pharmacopocia, 29th edn. Pharmaceutical Press, London, 1989.
379. Ahmed K, Roberts ML, Mammion PT. Antimicrobial activity of glycerine-ichthammaol in otitis externa. Clin Otolaryngol 1995; 20:201.
380. Mertz PM, Eaglstein WH. The effect of semi-occlusive dressing on the microbial population in superficial wounds. Arch Surg 1984; 119:287.
381. Geronemus RG, Mertz PM, Eaglstein WH. The effects of topical antimicrobial agents. Arch Dermatol 1979; 115:1311.
382. Linsky CB, Rovee DT, Dow T. Effect of dressing on wound inflammation and scar tissue. In: Dineen P, Hildick-Smith G eds The surgical wound. Lea & Febiger, Philadelphia, 1981.
383. Marples RR. The effect of hydration on the bacterial flora of the skin. In: Maibach HI, Hildick-Smith G eds Skin bacteria and their role in infection. McGraw-Hill, New York, 1963.
384. Buchan IA, Andrews JK, Lang SM. Laboratory investigation of the composition and properties of pig skin wound exudate under Op-Site. Burns 1981; 8:39.
385. Buchan IA, Andrews JK, Lang SM. Clinical and laboratory investigation of the composition and properties of human skin wound exudate under semi-permeable dressing. Burns 1981; 7:326.
386. Hutchison JJ, McGuckin M. Occlusive dressings: a microbiologic and clinical review. Am J Infect Control 1990; 18:257.
387. Handfield-Jones SE, Grattan CEH, Simpson RA et al. Comparison of a hydrocolloid dressing and paraffin gauze in the treatment of venous ulcers. Br J Dermatol 1988; 118:425.
388. Gilchrist B, Reed C. The bacteriology of chronic venous ulcers treated with occlusive hydrocolloid dressings. Br J Dermatol 1989; 121:337.
389. Leydon JL, Steward R, Kligman AM. Updated in vivo methods for evaluating topical antimicrobial agent on human skin. J Invest Dermatol 1979; 72:165.
390. Mertz PM, Ovington LG. Wound healing microbiology. Dermatol Clin 1993; 11(4):739.
391. Christian MM, Behroozan DS, Moy RI. Delayed infections following full-face CO_2 laser resurfacing and occlusive dressing use. Dermatol Surg 2000; 26:32.
392. Fitzpatrick RE, Geronemus RG, Grevelink JM et al. The incidence of adverse healing reactions occurring with UltraPulse CO_2 resurfacing during a multicenter study. Lasers Surg Med 1996; Suppl 8:34.
393. Goldman MP, Fitzpatrick RE.
394. Yurt RW. Burns. In: Mandell GL, Bennett JE, Dolin R eds Mandell, Douglas and Bennett's Principles and practice of infectious diseases. Churchill Livingstone, New York, 1995.
395. Phillips LG, Heggers JP, Robson MC et al. The effect of endogenous skin bacteria on burn wound infection. Ann Plast Surg 1989; 23:35.
396. Husain MT, Karim QN, Tajuri S. Analysis of infection in a burn ward. Burns 1989; 15:299.
397. Shalita A: Personal communication, 1997.
398. Roberts TL, Lettieri JT, Ellis LB. CO_2 laser resurfacing: recognizing and minimizing complications. Aesth Surg Q 1996; 16:141.
399. Coates J. Basic physics of erbium laser resurfacing. J Cutan Laser Ther 1999; 1:71.
400. Hibst R, Kaufmann R. Fundamentals of pulsed UV and mid-infrared laser skin ablation. In: Steiner R, Kaufmann R, Landthaler M, Braun-Falco O eds Lasers in dermatology. Springer-Verlag, Berlin, 1991.
401. Kaufmann R, Hibst R. Pulsed UV and mid-infrared laser skin ablation: experimental and first clinical results. In: Steiner R,

Kaufmann R, Landthaler M, Braun-Falco O eds Lasers in dermatology. Springer-Verlag, Berlin, 1991.

402. Hohenleutner U, Hohenleutner S, Bäumler Landthaler M. Fast and effective skin ablation with an Er:YAG laser: determination of ablation rates and thermal damage zones. Lasers Surg Med 1997; 20:242.
403. Drnovsvek-Olup B, Vedlin B. Use of Er:YAG laser for benign skin disorders. Lasers Surg Med 1997; 21:13.
404. Kaufmann R, Hibst R. Pulsed Er:YAG laser ablation in cutaneous surgery. Lasers Surg Med 1996; 19:324.
405. Walsh JT, Deutsch TF. Er:YAG laser ablation of tissue: measurement of ablation rates. Lasers Surg Med 1989; 9:327.
406. McDaniel DH, Ash K, Lord J et al. The Er:YAG laser: a review and preliminary report on resurfacing of the face, neck and hands. Aesthetic Surg J 1997; 17:157.
407. Hibst R, Kaufmann R. Effects of laser parameters on pulsed Er:YAG laser skin ablation. Lasers Med Sci 1991; 6:391.
408. Kaufmann R, Hartmann A, Hibst R. Cutting and skin ablative properties of pulsed mid-infrared laser surgery. J Dermatol Surg Oncol 1994; 20:112.
409. Walsh JT, Flotte TJ, Deutsch TF. Er:YAG laser ablation tissue: effect of pulse duration and tissue type on thermal damage. Lasers Surg Med 1989; 9:314.
410. Kaufmann R, Hibst R. Vergleich verschildener Mittelin-frafot: Laser für die ablation der Hauset. Lasermedizin 1995; 11:19.
411. Walsh JT. Pulsed laser ablation of tissue: analysis of the removal process and tissue healing. PhD thesis, MIT archives, Cambridge, MA, 1988.
412. Wolbarsht ML. Laser surgery: CO_2 or HF.IEEE. J Quantum Electronics 1984; 20:1427.
413. Hughes PS. Skin contraction following Er:YAG laser resurfacing. Dermatol Surg 1998; 24(1):109.
414. Goldberg DJ, Cutler KB. The use of the Er:YAG laser for the treatment of class III rhytids. Dermatol Surg 1999; 25:713.
415. Weinstein C. Computerized scanning Er:YAG laser for skin resurfacing. Dermatol Surg 1998; 24:83.
416. Ymauchi PS, Lask G, Lowe NJ. Botulinum toxin type A gives adjunctive benefit to periorbital laser resurfacing. J Cosmet Laser Ther 2004; 6(3):145.
417. Rostan EF, Goldman MP, Fitzpatrick RE. Laser resurfacing with a dual mode, long-pulse Erbium:YAG laser compared to the 950μs pulsed CO_2 laser. Am J Cos Surg 2000; 17(4): 227.
418. Jeong JT, Kye YC. Resurfacing of pitted facial acne scars with a long-pulsed Er:YAG laser. Dermatol Surg 2001; 27:107.
419. Kye YC. Resurfacing of pitted facial scars with a pulsed Er:YAG laser. Dermatol Surg 1997; 23:880.
420. Ammirati CT, Cottingham TJ, Hruza GJ. Immediate postoperative laser resurfacing improves second intention healing on the nose: 5-year experience. Dermatol Surg 2001; 27:147.
421. Khatri KA. Ablation of cutaneous lesions using an Er:YAG laser. J Cosmet Laser Ther 2003; 5(3–4):150.
422. Jiang SB, Levine VJ, Nehal KS et al. Er:YAG laser for the treatment of actinic keratoses. Dermatol Surg 2000; 26:437.
423. Park JH, Hwang ES, Kim SN, Kye YC. Er:YAG laser treatment of verrucous epidermal nevi. Dermatol Surg 2004; 30:378.
424. Trelles MA, Moreno-Arias GA. Becker's nevus: erbium:YAG versus Q-switched neodinium:YAG? Lasers Surg Med 2004; 34:295.
425. Borelli C, Kaudewitz P. Xanthelasma palpebrarum: treatment with the Er:YAG laser. Lasers Surg Med 2001; 29:260.
426. Drnovsek-Olup B, Vedlin B. Use of Er:YAG laser for benign skin disorders. Lasers Surg Med 1997; 21:13.
427. Kageyama N, Tope W. Treatment of multiple eruptive hair cysts with erbium:YAG laser. Dermatol Surg 1999; 25:819.
428. Hughes PSH. Multiple military osteomas of the face ablated with the Er:YAG laser. Arch Dermatol 1999; 135:378.
429. Ammirati CT, Giancola JM, Hruza GJ. Adult-onset facial colloid milium successfully treated with the long-pulsed Er: YAG laser. Dermatol Surg 2002; 28:215.
430. Langdon R. Erbium:YAG laser enables complete ablation of periungual verrucae without the need for injected anesthetics. Dermatol Surg 1998; 24:157.
431. Orenstein A, Haik J, Tamir J et al. Treatment of rhynophyma with Er:YAG laser. Lasers Surg Med 2001; 29:230.
432. Beier C, Kaufmann R. Efficacy of Er:YAG laser ablation in Darier's disease and Hailey–Hailey disease. Arch Dermatol 1999; 135:423.
433. Wenzel J, Petrow W, Tappe K, Gerdsen R. Treatment of Dowling–Degos disease with Er:YAG laser: results after 2.5 years. Dermatol Surg 2003; 29:1161.
434. Albertini JG, Holck DEE, Farley MF. Zoon's balanitis treated with Er:YAG laser ablation. Lasers Surg Med 2002; 30:123.
435. Yang JS, Kye YC. Treatment of vitiligo with autologous epidermal grafting by means of pulsed Er:YAG laser. J Am Acad Dermatol 1999; 38(2):280.
436. Brody HJ. Complications of chemical peels. In: Brody HM ed Chemical peeling. Mosby Yearbook, St Louis, 1992.
437. Fitzpatrick RE, Goldman MP, Sriprachya-Anunt S. Resurfacing of photodamaged skin on the neck with an UltraPulse® CO_2 laser. Lasers Surg Med 2001; 28:145.
438. Rosenberg JR. Full-face and neck laser skin resurfacing. Plast Reconstr Surg 1997; 100:1846.
439. Jimenez G, Spencer J. Erbium:YAG laser resurfacing of the hands, arms and neck. Dermatol Surg 1999; 25:831.
440. Polnikorn N, Goldberg DJ, Suwanchinda A, Ng SW. Erbium: YAG laser resurfacing in Asians. Dermatol Surg 1998; 24:1303.
441. Airan LE, Hruza G. Current lasers in resurfacing. Facial Plast Surg Clin North Am 2005; 13:127.
442. Sriprachya-Anunt S, Marchell NL, Fitzpatrick RE et al. Facial resurfacing in patients with Fitzpatrick skin type IV. Lasers Surg Med 2002; 30:86.
443. Kim YJ, Lee HS, Son SW et al. Analysis of hyperpigmentation and hypopigmentation after Er:YAG laser skin resurfacing. Lasers Surg Med 2005; 36:47.
444. Fitzpatrick RE, Goldman MP. Resurfacing of photodamage on the neck with an Ultrapulse CO_2 laser. Lasers Surg Med 1997; Suppl 9:33.
445. Walsh JT Jr, Deutsch TF. Erbium:YAG laser ablation of tissue: measurement of ablation rates. Lasers Surg Med 1989; 9: 327.
446. Perez MI, Bank DE, Silvers D. Skin resurfacing of the face with the erbium:YAG laser. Dermatol Surg 1998; 24: 653.
447. Kaufmann R, Hibst R. [Vergleich verschildener Mittelin-frafot: Laser für die ablation der Hauset]. Lasermedizin 1995; 11:19 (abstract).
448. Venugopalan V, Nishioka NS, Mikic BB. Thermodynamic response of soft biological tissues to pulsed infrared-laser irradiation. Biophys J 1996; 70:2981.
449. Ross EV, Naseef GS, McKinlay JR et al. Comparison of CO_2 laser, Er:YAG laser, dermabrasion and dermatome: a study of thermal damage, wound contraction and wound healing in a live pig model: implications for skin resurfacing. J Am Acad Dermatol 2000; 42:92.
450. Smith KJ, Skelton HG, Graham JS et al. Depth of morphologic skin damage and viability after one, two and three passes of a high-energy, short pulse CO_2 laser (TruPulse) in pig skin. J Am Acad Dermatol 1997; 37(2 Pt 1):204.

451. Zelickson R, Kist D. Effect of varied pulse duration and fluence of the CO_3 laser on coagulation and depth of collagen contraction. Lasers Surg Med 2000; 12:14.
452. Woo SH, Park JH, Kye YC. Resurfacing of different types of facial acne scar with short pulsed, variable-pulsed and dual-mode Er:YAG laser. Dermatol Surg 2004; 30(4 Pt 1):488.
453. Christian MM. Microresurfacing using the variable pulse erbium:YAG laser: a comparison of the 0.5 and 4-ms pulse durations. Dermatol Surg 2003; 29(6):605.
454. Zachary CB. Modulating the Er:YAG laser. Lasers Surg Med 2000; 26:223.
455. Sapijaszko MJ, Zachary CB. Er:YAG laser skin resurfacing. Dermatol Clin 2002; 20:87.
456. Pozner JM, Goldberg DJ. Histologic effect of a variable pulsed Er:YAG laser. Dermatol Surg 2000; 26:733.
457. Pozner JN, Roberts TL 3rd. Variable-pulsed width ER:YAG laser resurfacing. Clin Plast Surg 2000; 27:263.
458. Ross EV, McKinlay JR, Sajben FP et al. Use of a novel erbium laser in a Yucatan minipig: a study of residual thermal damage (RTD), ablation, and wound healing as a function of pulse duration. Lasers Surg Med 2002; 30:93.
459. Zachary CB, Grekin RC. Dual mode Er:YAG laser systems for skin resurfacing. Online. Available: http://www.LaserNews.net
460. Mueller DF, Zimmermann A, Borelli C. The efficiency of laser for the treatment of Ehlers–Danlos syndrome. Lasers Surg Med 2005; 36:76.
461. Goldman MP, Marchell N, Fitzpatrick RE. Laser skin resurfacing of the face with a combined CO2/Er:YAG laser. Dermatol Surg 2000; 26:102.
462. Trelles MA, Allones I, Luna R. One-pass resurfacing with a combined-mode Er:YAG/CO_2 laser system: a study of 102 patients. Br J Dermatol 2002; 146:473.
463. Kist DA, Sierra R, Sherr E, Zelickson BD. Collagen fibril contraction in bovine tendon and poultry skin after CO_3 laser exposure. Online. Available: http://www.LaserNews.net [accessed March 2000].
464. Tanzi EL, Alster TS: Side effects and complications of variable pulsed erbium: yttrium-aluminum-garnet laser skin resurfacing: extended experience with 50 patients. Plast Reconstr Surg 2003; 111(4):1524.
465. Tanzi EL, Alster TS. Treatment of atrophic facial acne scars with dual mode Er:YAG laser. Dermatol Surg 2002; 28:551.
466. Jeong JT, Park JH, Kye YC. Resurfacing of pitted facial acne scars using Er:YAG laser with ablation and coagulation mode. Aesthetic Plast Surg 2003; 27:130.
467. Roberts TL III. Laser blepharoplasty and laser resurfacing of the periorbital area. Clin Plast Surg 1998; 25:95.
468. Roberts TL III. In pursuit of optimal rejuvenation of the forehead: endoscopic browlift with CO_2 laser resurfacing. Plast Reconstr Surg 1998; 101:1075.
469. Ramirez OM, Pozner JN. Laser resurfacing as an adjunct to endoforehead lift, endofacelift and biplanar facelift. Ann Plast Surg 1997; 38:315.
470. Ramirez OM, Pozner JN. Subperiosteal minimally invasive laser endoscopic rhytidectomy: the SMILE facelift. Aesthetic Plast Surg 1996; 20:463.
471. Alster TS, Doshi SN, Hopping SB. Combination surgical lifting with ablative laser skin resurfacing of facial skin: a retrospective analysis. Dermatol Surg 2004; 30:1191.

Portions of this chapter were updated from the following previously published chapters:

Fitzpatrick RE, Goldman MP. CO_2 Laser surgery. In: Goldman MP, Fitzpatrick RE, eds. Cutaneous laser surgery, 2nd edn. Mosby-Yearbook, Inc., St Louis, 1999, p 279–338.
Fitzpatrick RE, Goldman MP. CO_2 and erbium laser resurfacing. In: Goldman MP, Fitzpatrick RE, eds. Cutaneous laser surgery, 2nd edn. Mosby-Yearbook, Inc., St Louis, 1999, p 339–436.
Fitzpatrick RE, Goldman MP. CO_2 resurfacing of the face. In: Fitzpatrick RE, Goldman MP eds Cosmetic laser surgery. Mosby, St Louis, 2000, p 45–70.
Goldman MP, Manuskiatti W, Fitzpatrick RE. Combined laser resurfacing with the UltraPulse CO_2 and Er:YAG lasers. In: Fitzpatrick RE, Goldman MP eds Cosmetic laser surgery. Mosby, St Louis, 2000, p 88–103.
Goldman MP, Fitzpatrick RE. Laser resurfacing of the neck. In: Fitzpatrick RE, Goldman MP eds Cosmetic laser surgery. Mosby, St Louis, 2000, p 104–112.
Goldman MP, Fitzpatrick RE. Resurfacing complications and their management. In: Fitzpatrick RE, Goldman MP eds Cosmetic laser surgery. Mosby, St Louis, 2000, p 113–145.

Chapter 8

Devices for Nonablative Photorejuvenation

Robert A. Weiss and Margaret A Weiss

Introduction

This chapter outlines technologies utilized for nonablative skin rejuvenation also termed photorejuvenation. Although many technologies have been available for a number of years, an explosion of newer technologies has recently appeared. These are discussed in terms of how they may play a role in treatment of photoaged skin. A discussion on radiofrequency (RF) devices can also be found in Chapter 14. The principles behind these technologies are also discussed.

Photorejuvenation is the process whereby light energy sources are utilized to reverse the process of photo or sun induced aging or environmental damage to the skin. Nonablative photorejuvenation accomplishes this without disturbance of the overlying epidermis. Nonablative typically refers to controlled wounding by thermal means inducing photothermolysis of targeted structures. This compares to a new modality of nonwounding/nonthermal, also termed photomodulation. A reorganization in dermal structural elements and an increase in dermal volume is the goal of photorejuvenation.

The key feature of nonablative therapy is the prevention of the epidermal injury. The thermal aspect of inducing changes to the dermis structurally with increased collagen in the dermis, reduced telangiectasias in the dermis and reduced melanin in the dermis and epidermis is the goal without epidermal thermal injury. The concept of causing these changes in a noninvasive way can be traced back to chemical peels. Although the exact mechanism is unknown, it was believed that application of glycolic acid for skin peeling induced a small amount of collagen production by stimulating a more rapid epidermal turnover rate. Its use has been shown to improve the dermal scarring of striae. Deeper chemical peels, such as phenol and 50% or greater trichloroacetic acid, promote photorejuvenation effects by a combination of several elements: destruction of the epidermis and dermal injury which leads to a reorganization in dermal structural components mediated by wound healing mechanisms and an increase in dermal volume.[1] This has also been the basis for improvements seen following ablative dermabrasion.

The thought processes in increased epidermal turnover leading to increase in dermal volume with chemical peels and dermabrasion led directly to the use of ablative lasers such as CO_2 and erbium:YAG (Er:YAG; see Chapters 6 and 7). By removing the epidermis and heat wounding the dermis, these helped to promote understanding of an enhanced mechanism by which the ability to remove photodamaged epidermis and dermis of the skin in a precise and reproducible manner while leaving behind a narrow zone of thermal damage led to reversal of photoaging.[2] Each pass of the CO_2 after ablation leaves 50–125 microns of residual dermal thermal damage whereas the other major ablative laser – the Er:YAG – produces 5–20 microns of thermal damage per pass.[3] Both these levels of injury leave some thermal necrotic tissue, which must slough, and also another component of non-necrotic thermal injury. It is probably this latter zone of potentially reversible thermal injury that triggers new collagen synthesis by repair of thermal damage and replacement with a new collagen and extracellular matrix (ECM).

The Er:YAG laser results in major epidermal damage, but far less dermal injury has been shown to significantly improve skin appearance with new collagen formation.[4] This has defined a primary goal of rejuvenation; a reorganization in dermal structural elements and an increase in dermal volume replacing the elastotic dermal UV-induced photodamage. This results in the improvement in the appearance of the skin and also alters the structure and sometimes the function of the skin subsurface – hence the term 'subsurface remodeling' really refers to wound remodeling that occurs without the removal of the epidermis and without the necessity of wound care or recovery time.[5] Experience with attempts to reduce thermal damage by using devices other than the CO_2 laser has led to the belief that induction of collagen and ECM is possible with less injury. This has led to the development of the 1319/1320 nm, 1450 nm and 1540 nm infrared lasers with cryogen cooled epidermal protection and low fluence pulsed dye lasers, but these nonablative techniques remain thermal in nature. A new theory of photomodulation proposes that such improvements in skin appearance, structure and function may be achieved via a different nonthermal pathway, thus accomplishing nonablative skin rejuvenation without the use of a thermal injury and thus without the traditional activation of the wound healing mechanism.

The primary goal of nonablative rejuvenation is therefore the induction of new collagen and ECM synthesis to reverse or reduce the appearance of rhytids of photoaging without disturbance or damage to the overlying epidermis. A secondary goal is the remodeling of scars such as acne scars (see Chapter 10). Total nonablative rejuvenation, however, must also include reversal of some of the visible changes that occur from photoaging, not entirely relating to structural changes. These include reduction of superficial dyspigmentation (both dermal and epidermal), reduction of dermal telangiectasias and the appearance of an overall smoother texture and tone. Thus, two types of photorejuvenation have been described: Type I deals with the elements of vascular and pigmentary changes associated with photoaging, lentigines, telangiectasias, dull skin tone, diffuse redness and rosacea; type II involves the structural changes in collagen and connective tissue and can be associated with improvement in pore size, elastosis, and rhytides. Type I and II skin rejuvenation represent photothermal nonablative therapies as traditionally described.

Mechanisms of Action of Photorejuvenation

Photorejuvenation can span a broad range of wavelengths, light sources and target chromophores but may be generally divided into mechanisms based on absorption characteristics of the laser or light source. Nonablative skin rejuvenation techniques produce dermal remodeling without the obvious epidermal injury and the wound created with earlier ablative approaches.[6–8] The popularity of these new techniques lies significantly in the lack of wound care and down time as well as reduced costs. However, the current embodiments produce rather variable clinical results even when utilizing a series of treatments. Although not requiring general anesthesia like former methods, some – but not all – of the newer nonablative thermal techniques produce considerable discomfort, even with optimal topical anesthesia. Treatment times vary, but typically require 15–20 minutes or more to perform treatment to an entire face.

New collagen formation following dermal wounding is a primary mechanism for restoration of collagen observed following laser resurfacing. It follows that techniques that induce a dermal wound without concomitant epidermal ablation should allow for improvement of dermal photodamage as long as new collagen growth is stimulated.

Thermal injury with subsequent wound healing is still believed to be the primary mechanism for photorejuvenation. Ideally, this thermal injury could be confined to specific levels of the dermis so that deeper scars or rhytids could be treated by a deeper level of heating while with further penetration into ligaments, fascia or subcutaneous fat entire regions of skin could be 'tightened'. Creation of this heat energy (whether by lasers, light sources, RF, ultrasound or microwave energy), would cause collagen injury and contraction.

For all these energy sources being investigated for photorejuvenation, the currently popular methods all have as a common denominator their primary stimulus for new collagen production thermal injury and subsequent repair of collagen injury with both activation and recruitment of fibroblasts. However, many have speculated that there are almost certainly other mechanisms. Inflammatory cytokines of various origins influence expression of extracellular matrix proteins, such as type I collagen, fibronectin, and decorin, in human skin fibroblasts.[9] Some suggest these cytokines are released from immune system cells, which infiltrate following superficial capillary damage.[10] These cell-signaling pathways arise from cell injury or death and signal wound healing mechanisms in the skin. Additionally, skin enzymes such as matrix metalloproteinases (MMP) are also produced and may paradoxically degrade some of the newly formed collagen and ECM (e.g. MMP-1, also known as collagenase, may negate the net increase in dermal collagen by degrading some of the newly formed collagen I). This potentially contributes to the variability of these techniques seen in clinical practice.

In contrast to these thermal mechanisms, there is another possible means to alter cellular activity by light which includes the emerging field of nonablative, nonthermal photomodulation. This is the process in which low-level light energy is used to modulate – that is activate or inhibit – the normal activities of a cell. It has been proposed that this occurs by modulating the energy production of the mitochondria and/or by signaling the up-/downregulation of receptors. The goal for photorejuvenation by photomodulation is to activate fibroblast activity and perhaps also to modulate melanocyte activity, inflammatory responses, blood flow or even stem cell activity in the skin by using low level energy of certain wavelengths to 'energize' and amplify the cell signal transduction and thus increase collagen and ECM synthesis machinery. Some early data will be presented below.

Classification and Use of Lasers/Light Sources for Photorejuvenation

The main classifications of lasers and light sources utilized for photorejuvenation are outlined in Box 8.1. All such classifications are arbitrary as many devices are capable of delivering multiple wavelengths.

The first category is visible light lasers or light sources that have more absorption by hemoglobin and melanin. These visible light sources and lasers have more influence on the telangiectatic and melanocytic components of photoaging. These sources can be subdivided into coherent, single wavelength, broadband (flashlamps) or narrowband such as light-emitting diodes (LED). Intense pulsed light is a broadband light source with filters used to limit the lower end of the emitted spectrum.

The next category is infrared with absorption predominantly by water. Infrared wavelengths with primarily water absorption are used to create thermal dermal and collagen injury. The most commonly employed devices are 1320 nm, 1450 nm and 1540 nm lasers, although narrowband infrared LED devices, other filtered light sources and possibly ultrasound may be available in the future.

Another category is the near infrared lasers or light sources which are absorbed by a combination of melanin, hemoglobin and water. The tradeoff is that these wavelengths are absorbed at a lesser intensity but cover more targets. The flashlamp pumped 1064 nm Nd:YAG laser is the most commonly used example. The broadband flashlamp pumped light sources also have a number of effects for structural photorejuvenation in that they emit not only wavelengths absorbed by melanin and hemoglobin, but wavelengths absorbed by water as well. IPL broadband sources emit 515 nm to 1200 nm with high energy available for thermal absorption although the output is nonlinear and is stronger in the visible light spectrum than the infrared.

Other devices on the market use RF to heat tissue. Depending on the delivery system and frequency, deep or superficial heating can be produced. Monopolar RF has a very different and deeper penetration (as the result of the patient being grounded) than bipolar RF devices, in which the RF travels from one electrode to another over relatively short distances. Microwave devices have been used to heat specific targets such as blood vessels or hair but none have been commercialized. Use of nondiagnostic ultrasound frequencies may also have future applications in skin tightening but ultrasound is omnidirectional unless special methods to focus the energy are employed.

A new method for photorejuvenation is called fractional resurfacing. This method is basically microablative, namely, small areas of skin are ablative in a pixel like fashion. The present device uses a 1550 nm wavelength to make small 'punctures' into the skin about 50 microns in diameter. It is speculated that this pixel puncture microablation will result in skin contraction, dermal collagen thickening and improvement in the rhytid portion of photoaging. This technology is at the very early stages.

When selecting a thermal photorejuvenation system it is therefore critical to understand the physics behind the wavelength and the method of delivery rather than exaggerated manufacturer's claims. Having knowledge of the output of a device, understanding whether the target is hemoglobin, melanin or water (or all three) and understanding spot size and method of delivery, the physician may be better able to choose the correct system for the correct application. For example, photorejuvenation of pigmented lesions would not be possible with a unit emitting 1450 nm, for which the target is water and not melanin. This knowledge is also vital if the clinician is to minimize possible adverse clinical events in darker ethnic skin types. Visible light, more strongly absorbed by melanin, must therefore be used with greater caution in darker skin. An algorithm for approaches to specific patient problems with specific treatments is outlined in Box 8.2.

Box 8.1 ***Lasers and Light Sources Used for Photorejuvenation***

- Visible laser light sources:
  - frequency doubled Nd:YAG, KTP (green 532 nm)
  - pulsed dye (yellow 585–595 nm): long pulse versus short PDL
- Visible non-laser light sources:
  - intense pulsed light (IPL) – broadband filtered light of various orgins: visible infrared
  - LED (light-emitting diodes) – narrowband: UV, visible, infrared
- Infrared lasers (target pigment, hemoglobin and water):
  - Q-switched and millisecond domain Nd:YAG 1064 nm: infrared lasers (target is water only)
  - 1320 nm Nd:YAG laser
  - 1450 nm diode laser
  - 1540 nm erbium glass laser
- Radiofrequency (RF), microwave and ultrasound.

Visible Light Lasers

Frequency Doubled Nd:YAG, KTP (Green 532 nm)

This has been reported to be used for the pigment and telangiectatic component of photoaging. Most recently for more comprehensive photorejuvenation the simultaneous use of 1064 nm has been employed.[11] The original use of this device was very technique dependent as the 532 nm was delivered via a relatively small spot size of 4–5 mm and required a specific pattern of delivery. The newest version of this device allows implementation of a 10-mm spot size of 532 nm green so that a specific technique to treat a cheek in one to three passes can be employed with reproducible results. This now compares favorably to some of the broadband devices which deliver energy in large spot sizes so that the entire face can be treated quickly. In a

Box 8.2 ***Algorithm by Photoaging Problem for Nonablative Skin Photorejuvenation***

- Telangiectasias:
  - IPL
  - PDL LP (long-pulse)
  - Nd:YAG LP 532nm
- Diffuse redness (nonvisible telangectasia):
  - IPL
  - LED photomodulation
- Mottled pigmentation:
  - IPL
  - Nd:YAG LP 532nm
  - LED photomodulation
- Mild rhytides:
  - LED photomodulation
  - IPL
  - PDL
  - Non-ablative infrared lasers
- Moderate rhytides:
  - Infrared
- Deeper rhytids:
  - Infrared wavelengths beyond main hemoglobin and melanin absorption: 1320nm, 1450nm, 1540nm
  - Radiofrequency (more effective for skin tightening)
- Acne scars (worsened by actinic damage; acne scars are generally included in a discussion of this topic. Although they are not induced by actinic damage, they are worsened by photoaging):
  - Erythematous:
    - IPL
    - PDL
    - LED photomodulation
  - Nonerythematous:
    - 1320nm, 1450nm, 1540nm infrared lasers and IPL
    - LED photomodulation

A

B

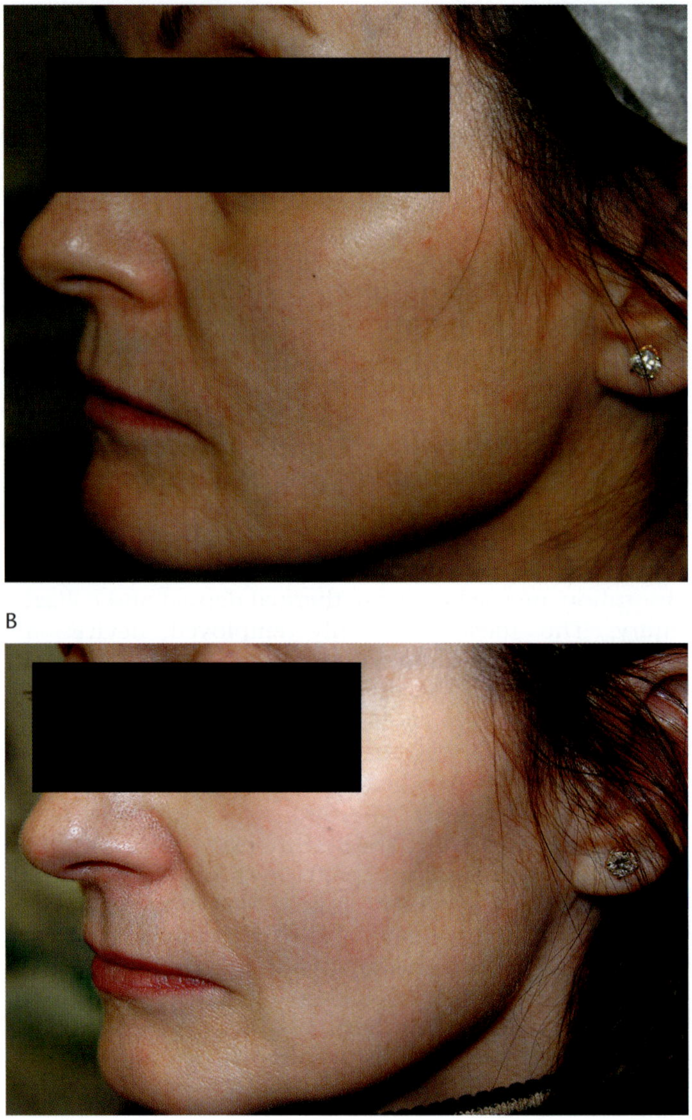

Figure 8.1

bilateral comparison of IPL versus large spot 532nm, the large spot 532nm was actually a little bit faster than the IPL and delivered slightly better results on pigmentation.[12] This is predicted by the higher absorption of 532nm by melanin over wavelengths cut off at 560nm with the IPL device. This is an example of a new photorejuvation device appearing on the market using a relatively abandoned wavelength but brought back for practical use by increasing the spot size and improving the speed of treatment. Parameters used on the large spot size 532nm/1064nm device (Gemini, Laserscope, San José, CA) are 6–9J/cm^2, 20–30ms pulse duration and two to three passes until uniform erythema of the treated surface is noted. Some argue that the addition of an additional pass of 1064nm Nd:YAG from the same device will yield better results for rhytids,[13] yet for resistant pigmentation this method of photorejuvenation shows some promise.

In combinations of both 532nm and 1064nm, the use of 532nm alone leads to 80% improvement of redness and pigmentation, 20–40% improvement in skin textural improvement and 20–30% improvement in rhytids.[14] By the addition of 1064nm as a second pass, the improvement in skin texture and rhytids is increased by 20–30%. Use of 1064nm alone has minimal effect on pigmentation and telangiectasias as predicted by the absorption characteristics.

> ***Case 1***
>
> *Photorejuvenation with the Gemini 10-mm spot 532nm laser*
>
> This 42-year-old patient (Fig. 8.1A) was treated with two passes of 10-mm spot size, 532nm green. The 'after' shot (Fig. 8.1B) was at 1 month, with textural improvement as well as reduction in telangiectasias and pigmentation.

Pulsed Dye (yellow 585nm–595nm)

Cleared by the FDA for periocular wrinkling for both the 585nm and 595nm wavelengths, these have become popular devices for several components of photoaging with the newer longer pulse durations. By avoiding the purpura of the original 0.45 millisecond (ms), pulse durations, pulse durations from 6 ms to 40 ms or low fluences of 2–3 J/cm^2 are being utilized for the thermal remodeling effects on the dermis at lower energies, but are also utilized at higher energies for the reduction of telangiectasias. These longer pulse durations are achieved not by producing a single continuous pulse, but rather by assembling a 'train' of smaller pulselets, and thus different brands of device may produce different clinical effects even though using similar pulse durations on the control panels. Studies with the original short pulse pulsed dye laser (PDL) at 6–7 J/cm^2 revealed that although all patients had purpura and swelling, biopsies showed thickening of collagen and increased dermal mucin.[15] Zelickson also has reported the presence of increased extracellular matrix proteins in patients after periorbital treatments with both PDL and IPL. Stains for types I and III collagen, procollagen, elastin receptors and collagenase were increased in all posttreatment specimens at 6 weeks.

Bjerring et al utilized the 585 nm pulsed dye at 0.35 ms at subpurpuric doses of 2.4 J/cm^2 and reported improvements in wrinkle scores in periocular wrinkles with just one treatment.[16] This therapy had apparently little or no effect on the telangiectatic and pigmented component of photoaging as the authors described no pigmentary changes. Recent electron microscopy of skin lesions treated with 3.0 J/cm^2 at 350 microseconds demonstrated vascular injury and fibrosis compatible with a thermal mechanism of action.[17]

Long Pulse Versus Short Pulse PDL

In addition to minimizing the purpuric side effects of short pulse, longer pulses theoretically allow more heating of larger capillaries, multiple passes to obtain more overall heating of the dermis with less risk and greater patient comfort. The longer pulses also allow treatment of the surface telangiectasias with less risk of purpura. The authors' experience indicates that the use of 2-, 6-, or 10-ms pulse durations is ideal for treatment of the telangiectatic component of photoaging, while stimulation of new collagen is quite variable, the optimal pulse durations and energy fluences are presently unknown for these longer pulse durations. The ideal fluence has not yet been determined. We typically utilize 10 ms, 6–8 J/cm^2, forced air cooling and a 10-mm spot size with the Cynosure V-Star (Cynosure, Chelmsford, MA) or 6 ms, 7.5 J, 30 ms of cryogen and a 10-mm spot with the Candela V-beam. (Candela, Waymouth, MA).

> ***Case 2***
> *Use of Extended Pulsed Dye Laser for Photorejuvenation*
> This 39-year-old male was treated with the extended pulsed dye laser (V-Star, Cynosure, Chelmsford, MA). He complained of flushing episodes and facial telangiectasia (Fig. 8.2A). He was treated with stacked pulsing, three pulses per stack, of 595 nm, 10 mm spot, 7 J/cm^2 and use of forced air cooling. At 1 month after one treatment there was a 75% reduction of telangiectasia; his facial flushing intensity and frequency was reduced (Fig. 8.2B).

A
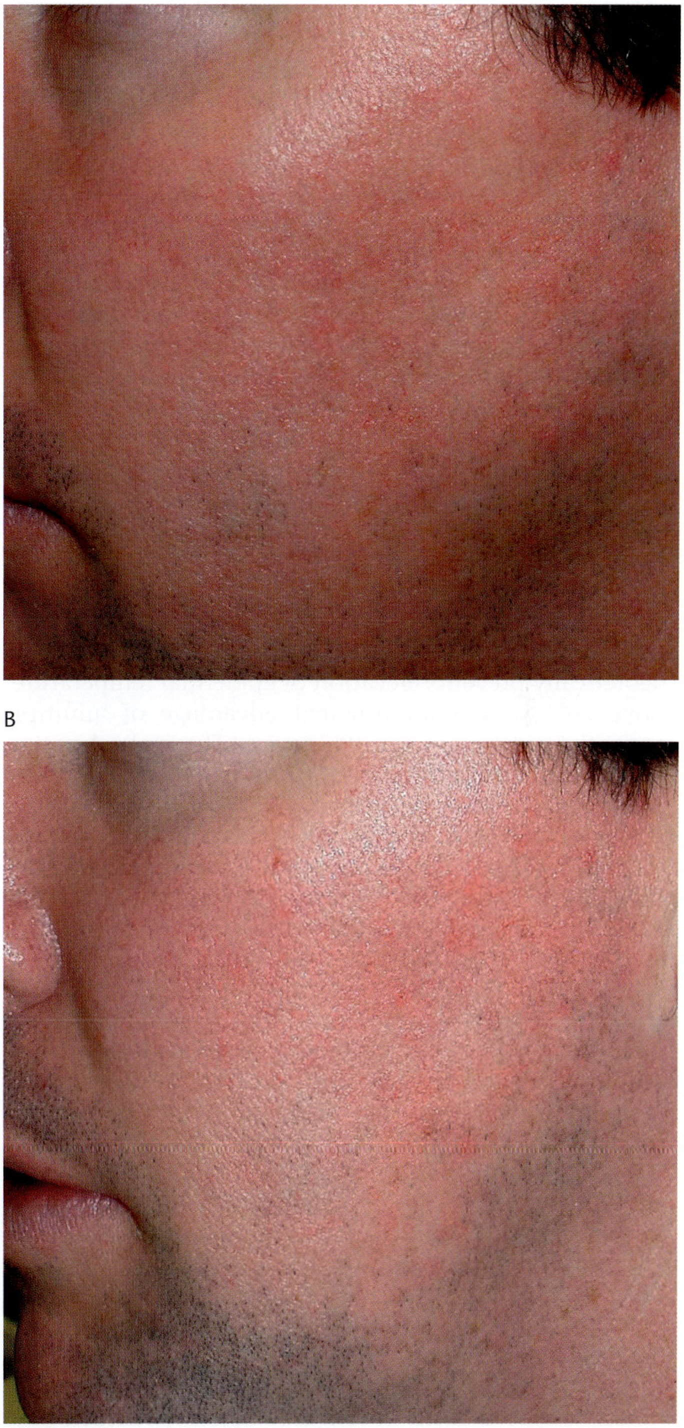
B

Figure 8.2

Light Sources

Intense Pulsed Light

One of the most controversial light-based technologies, first introduced for clinical studies in 1994 and cleared by the US FDA in late 1995 as the Photoderm™ (Lumenis, Santa Clara, CA), is the noncoherent filtered flashlamp intense pulsed light (IPL) source. It was initially launched and promoted as a radical improvement over existing methods for elimination of leg telangiectasias and as a specific modality to minimize the possibility of purpura common to PDL. In reality, the device turned out to be of greater utility for other indications than leg telangiectasias, and the road to usability, reproducibility and good results was a long one. Present-day indications have expanded far beyond the initial ones to include hair removal, facial telangiectasias, pigmentation, poikiloderma of Civatte, scars and most all encompassing domain of nonablative facial rejuvenation or photorejuvenation.

Intense pulsed light is produced by a noncoherent flashlamp pumped light source that is capable of emitting light from 500–1200 nm. The use of cutoff filters allows the elimination of some of the shorter wavelengths of the visible light spectrum. The device is best thought of as capable of emitting yellow, red and infrared simultaneously so that multiple components of photoaging can be treated concurrently. These include the pigmented, telangiectatic and fine wrinkling components of photoaging. The advantage of a large spot size is inherent in the design of a system in which the flashlamp resides in the treatment head.

Allowing proper thermal relaxation time between pulses theoretically prevents elevation of epidermal temperatures above 70°C and is an inherent advantage of 'multiple sequential pulsing' of the IPL device. Thermal relaxation time is the amount of time it takes for the temperature of a tissue to decrease by a factor of $\varepsilon = 2.72$ as a result of heat conductivity. For a typical epidermis thickness of 100 microns, thermal relaxation time is approximately 10 ms. For a typical vessel 100 microns (0.1 mm), thermal relaxation time is approximately 4 ms, for a vessel of 300 microns (0.3 mm), thermal relaxation time is approximately 10 ms. Therefore vessels greater than 0.3 mm cool more slowly than the epidermis with a single pulse. For larger vessels, however, multiple pulses may be advantageous with delay times of 10 ms or more between pulses for epidermal cooling. This delay time must be increased with larger vessels as thermal diffusion across a larger vessel elongates the thermal relaxation time. Multiple sequential pulsing with delay times permits successive heating of targeted vessel(s) with adequate cooling time for epidermis and surrounding structures.

These theoretical considerations imply: (1) vessels smaller than 0.3 mm should theoretically only require a single pulse, although a double pulse should have no adverse effect on treatment; (2) double or triple pulses should be spaced 10 ms or longer to accommodate normal epidermal thermal relaxation times (an even safer setting might be a 15-ms thermal relaxation time); (3) bright red lesions (oxyhemoglobulin) are better treated with 515–590 nm filters; (4) violaceous lesions (deoxyhemoglobulin) should be treated with 590 nm or higher filters; (5) darker skin (melanin) should always be treated with the highest filter available accompanied by increasing delay times between pulses to allow for increased skin thermal relaxation times. The treatment of darker-skinned individuals is of greater concern when performing photoepilation. In these cases the 755 nm filter is used primarily with delay times between pulses from 50 to 100 ms to allow plenty of time for the skin to cool down avoiding thermal damage.

Most commonly employed pulse durations and pulse combinations in our practice are an initial pulse of 2.4 ms followed by a second pulse delivered after a delay or rest interval of 10–20 ms. The second coupled or synchronized pulse is set for 2.4 to 8 ms, depending on the diameter of the vascular target with smaller diameter (0.1–0.2 mm) bright red vessels treated with the shorter second pulse duration of 2.4 to 4.0 ms and larger vessels (0.3–0.5 mm) treated with the second pulse duration of 5 to 8 ms. These are adjusted based upon the immediately observed clinical response. For small vessels, we wish to see immediate clearing with slight background erythema as our clinical endpoint. The concept for double pulsing of larger telangiectasias is to allow preheating of vessels with absorption by smaller vessels with the first pulse, then allow surrounding structures to cool. The second coupled longer pulse then heats up the larger vessels in the area under the crystal.

IPL is frequently used to treat photoaging. As a model for photoaging, poikiloderma involving the neck includes fine telangiectasias, irregular pigmentation and epidermal and dermal atrophy. In studies of the use of IPL for poikiloderma, Weiss et al reported on treatment of 135 patients randomly selected with typical changes of poikiloderma of Civatte on the neck and/or upper chest treated with one to five treatments using IPL. Results indicated clearance of more than 75% of telangiectasias and hyperpigmentation.[18] The incidence of side effects was 5%, including pigment changes. In many cases, improved skin texture was noted both by physician and patient. The authors concluded that IPL was an effective mode of therapy for poikiloderma of Civatte. Cutoff filters utilized in these treatments included primarily 550 nm–570 nm. Median number of treatments to achieve results was 3.

Bitter reported facial rejuvenation in 49 patients using similar parameters and cutoff filters, with 550–570 nm cutoff filters and double pulsing of 2.4 to 4.7 pulses with varying interpulse intervals.[19] Subjects were treated with a series of four or more full-face treatments at 3-week intervals with fluences varying from 30 to 50 J/cm^2. Subject evaluation and skin biopsies were used to assess treatment results. The results reported were that all aspects of photodamage including telangectasia, irregular pigmentation, wrinkling, skin coarseness, and pore size showed visible improvement in more than 90% of subjects with minimal downtime and no scarring. In total, 88% of subjects were satisfied with the overall results of their treatments. Side effects of edema, mild blistering and transient pigmentation changes were observed in a small percentage of patients. Collagen synthesis was noted in the biopsy sample.

The importance of the lower wavelengths is illustrated by the study of Goldberg, who utilized a 645 nm cutoff filter, relatively high fluence of 40–50 J/cm^2 and a series of one to four treatments.[5] In this study, only about 30% of patients showed improvement in wrinkle appearance. Pigmentation and telangiectatic components of photoaging responded poorly to the technique. Visible wavelengths of

IPL from 550 nm to 645 nm are thought to lead to improvement in the telangiectatic and pigmentation components, whereas the longer wavelengths absorbed by water allow heating of the dermis with resultant thermal effects. Ross has speculated that the shorter filters favor hemoglobin and melanin heating, while the effect on dermal collagen is caused by heat diffusion from the vasculature and by discharge of inflammatory mediators induced by direct vessel heating.[20] Thermal effects of tissue water heating probably also play a role.

The longevity of improvement with light based devices has always been questioned. A recent study demonstrated that a 5-year follow-up of 80 randomly selected patients with skin types I–IV who were treated by IPL during 1996 and 1997 showed that at 5 years after initial treatment, skin textural improvement was noted in 83% of the subjects.[21] Photos and patient self-assessment were also graded for telangiectasia severity and dyspigmentation. For those patients practicing rigorous UV blocking methods, telangiectasias were improved in 82% of subjects; pigmentation remained improved in 79% over the 5-year period.

Case 3

Photorejuvenation of the Chest with IPL

IPL is well suited for rejuvenation of large surface areas due to the large crystal size, which often ranges to several cm^2. This 52-year-old female presented with extensive photodamage of the face, chest and neck. The images are before (Fig. 8.3A) and after one treatment at 1 month (Fig. 8.6B). The settings on the Quantum IPL (Lumenis, Santa Clara, CA) device were Program 1 with a slight modification. The 560 nm filter with a setting of 2.4 ms, 10 ms delay and 4 ms second pulse shows a dramatic reduction in pigmentation, telangiectatic and hemangioma lesions. After one treatment some rectangular footprints can still be seen. These are eliminated during the next treatment in which the treatment head is rotated 90 degrees across the chest. This treatment is also excellent for the arms and legs.

A

B

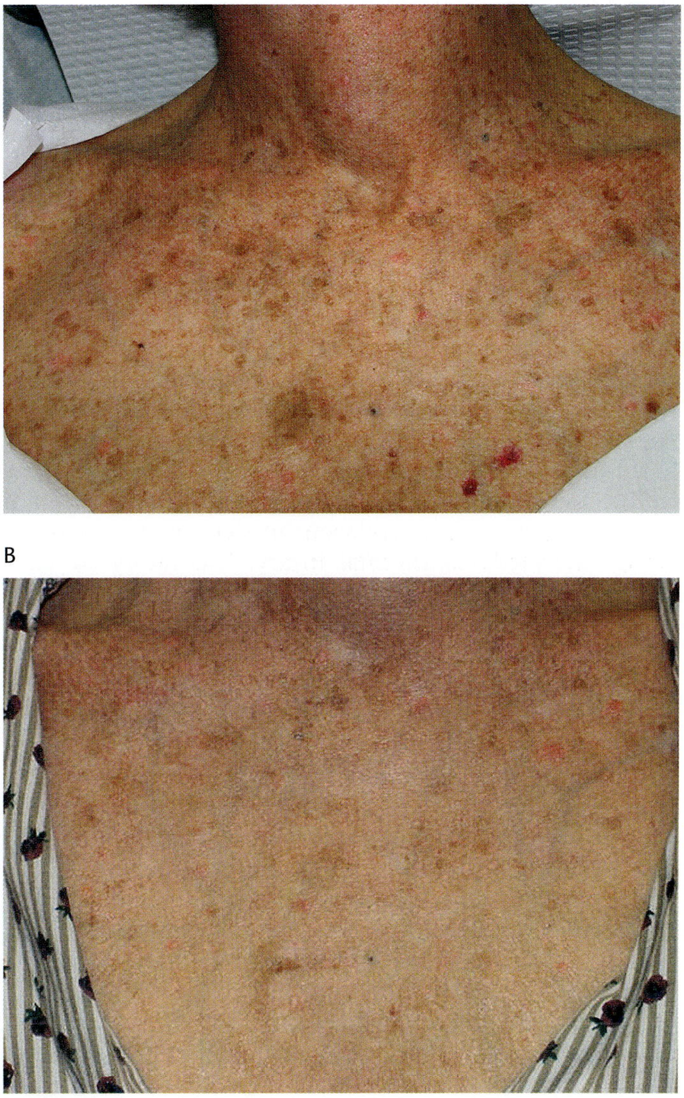

Figure 8.3

Intense Pulsed Light plus Bipolar Radiofrequency

The use of IPL plus RF has been designated as a trademark of ELOS™ (electrooptical synergy) technology. It has recently been reported that the addition of bipolar RF through electrodes separately by 8 mm possibly enhances the results of IPL photorejuvenation.[22] A study at five sites with a total of 108 patients showed changes similar to the use of IPL alone, with improvement in telangiectasias, pigmentation and skin texture. No comparison of IPL alone with IPL plus RF (ELOS™) was performed, therefore no conclusion about the enhanced efficacy of RF in addition to IPL could be made. The device performed similarly to other devices based on IPL alone.

Photomodulation and Low-energy Light-emitting Diodes

Light-emitting diodes (LEDs) are narrow band emitters of a broad range of electromagnetic radiation ranging from UV to visible to infrared (IR). LEDs themselves are typically assembled on small chips or equipped with tiny lenses and assembled into small lamps (typically up to 3–5 mm in diameter but 10 mm and larger lamps are available). These LEDs typically emit a low intensity of light in the milliwatt domain. LEDs may be assembled, however, into larger arrays or panels. Higher energy intensities may also be generated, although the life of the LED is typically shortened. LEDs are extremely versatile and durable exhibiting good resistance to temperature, dirt, vibration, and other environmental insults, with a typical lamp life of up to 100,000 hours. They also do not require expensive or dangerous high voltage power supplies or complex optics and thus alignment issues and maintenance tend to be very minimal. This therapy is painless and large LED panel arrays can be assembled so that the entire face may be treated in a few minutes or less.

While the exact mechanisms of action are still under study, LED photomodulation is thought to occur by the illumination of certain 'receptors' within cells or subcellular components. The net result is to activate or to inhibit (or have no discernible effect on) the function of a given cell type depending on the treatment parameters and wavelengths selected; hence the use of the term 'modulation'. It is important to recognize the specificity of the photomodulation 'code' or parameter protocol for a particular cell target because it is possible, using an identical LED light source and an identical energy fluence, to obtain either an increase in synthesis of collagen or no increase in collagen synthesis. Thus the modulation parameters represent one of the unique features of this process.

Typically LEDs emit light in a ±10–20 nm band around the dominant emitted wavelength. One proposal is that these photons are absorbed by the 'antenna molecules' in mitochondria, thus activating the electron transport system that amplifies the cell signals, eventually resulting in an increased production of the cell's normal products. In the case of fibroblasts, this translates into production of ECM proteins such as collagen and elastin but without being mediated via thermal injury. Laboratory in vitro testing suggests that a greater net increase in total collagen may be created using nonthermal LED photomodulation than with thermal injury techniques. Initial studies of 47 patients treated with the LED device showed an average of 44% improvement in the appearance of wrinkles and skin tone and texture.

A multicenter clinical trial was conducted on 90 photoaged females.[23] One week after the last treatment, the global improvement in appearance of skin in the periorbital region was 62%. Upper lip improvement was 36%. Other observations in the periorbital area included reduction of 27% in skin roughness, 30% in elastosis, 14% in pore size, 25% in redness. Histopathology and immunohistopathology showed increase in several key extracellular matrix proteins associated with clinical improvement in wrinkles. Data up to 1 year posttreatment in these same subjects indicates that improvement peaked at 4–6 months but that, without further treatments of photomodulation, the results decline from 6–12 months. Based on this study, the FDA cleared the Gentlewaves™ (LightBioScience, Virginia Beach, VA) LED photomodulation device for improvement of periocular rhytids. We have our patients perform a series of eight treatments over a 4-week interval and then perform maintenance treatments once a month. We have also found that the use of LED photomodulation after other photorejuvenation procedures such as IPL improves results of textural smoothing and more rapidly reduces the thermal effects of erythema and edema.

Case 4

Gentlewaves™ LED Photomodulation for Mild Photoaging

A 38-year-old female presents with mild photoaging changes including mild periocular rhytids and slight dyspigmentation (Fig. 8.4A). The 'after' image was taken at 4 months following eight treatments given over 4 weeks (Fig. 8.4B). Each treatment was delivered as 100 pulses of 250 ms each, at an extremely low fluence of 0.1 J/cm^2. Treatments are easily tolerated because no heat is involved. This device is cleared by the FDA for improvement of periocular rhytids. This treatment regimen used alone is best for mild or early onset photoaging. Strict sun protection measures must be enforced for patients to benefit from photomodulation

A B

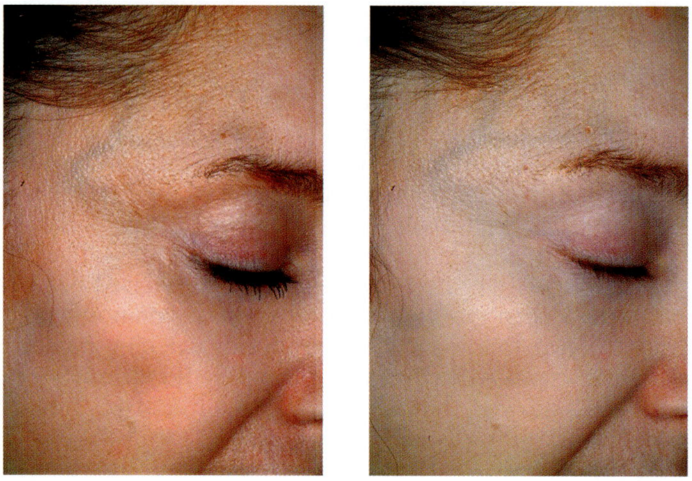

Figure 8.4

Infrared Lasers (Melanin, Hemoglobin and Water Absorbing)

Long Pulse Nd:YAG (1064 nm)

The wavelength primarily available in this category of lasers is 1064 nm. The chromophores absorbed at 1064 microns of infrared light include melanin, hemoglobin and water. The laser results in thermal effects by targeting all three chromophores. Due to the relatively poor absorption by all three chromophores, 1064 nm has a characteristic of deep penetration. Effects on blood vessels were observed at 3 mm below the skin surface, confirming the deep penetration.[24] As a result, there is a diffuse heating of dermal tissue by 1064 nm, which has an optical penetration depth of 5–10 mm. Heat diffusion from these depths is slower so that the heat effect remains for seconds rather than milliseconds. The depth and duration of heating can be varied by the pulse duration although the parameters and effects are still being investigated. Results may yet show that 1064 nm used with the correct pulse durations and fluence is capable of inducing collagen remodeling by thermal effects on dermal water heating. There has been no definitive study published with fully objective data, although results of reduction of skin laxity and rhytids using pulses in the millisecond range have been reported.[25] As mentioned above, in the section on 532 nm, the combination of 532 nm and 1064 nm appears to work better on collagen remodeling than 532 nm alone, although this has not been confirmed by more than one investigator.[13]

Short Pulse Q-switched Nd:YAG (1064nm)

Although 1064nm is typically used in the millisecond domain, it has been on the market for over a decade as Q-switched laser for tattoos and pigmented lesions. Due to the deep penetration of 1064nm and the safety with very small amounts of heat generated in the nanosecond pulse domain, the Q-switched nanosecond domain 1064nm laser was actually one of the first lasers used for nonablative skin rejuvenation. Used at a fluence of 5.5J/cm^2 at around 40 nanosecond pulse duration, Q-switched 1064nm was employed in an attempt to smooth the skin of 11 patients.[26] This initial group demonstrated pinpoint bleeding at this fluence, thus making this more of an epidermal ablative treatment rather than a nonablative one. Newer parameters were tried to avoid the pinpoint bleeding by keeping fluence below this threshold, athough this was never published (D. McDaniel, personal communication). Rhytid improvement was scored at about 25% by relatively nonobjective means. Fluences utilized were low at 2.5J/cm^2 and so the goals of a nonablative were achieved.

900nm to 980nm Diode Lasers

Like 1064nm, the diode lasers in the 900 to 980nm range are absorbed by all three chromophores: melanin, hemoglobin and water. In a study designed to measure tissue shrinkage, the 980nm diode was used at a pulse duration of 400ms, with best results at 8W showing 16% tissue shrinkage. Biopsies performed in two patients at 6 and 21 days posttreatment showed denatured collagen with subsequent digestion and new collagen deposition.[27] From the biopsies, the thermal destruction of collagen with subsequent repair appeared to be the primary mechanism. Most studies on these diode lasers are for hair removal with very few reported for nonablative rejuvenation.[28] A recent study used a 915nm diode combined with bipolar RF for treatment of leg veins, not for rejuvenation.[29] For photorejuvenation, these wavelengths have neither been widely studied nor used in clinical applications, with or without accompanying other energy sources.

Infrared Lasers (Water Absorbing Only)

1320nm Nd:YAG

The 1320nm wavelength is thought to accomplish collagen production by scattering thermal energy throughout the laser irradiated dermis after nonspecific absorption by dermal water. Typical pulse durations are 30–50 milliseconds with fluence ranging from 15 to 30J/cm^2. Once slight thermal damage of collagen has been induced, the same mechanisms are triggered for collagen regeneration as for other collagen damaging lasers. The 1320nm wavelength has an advantage in that inherent scatter allows penetration to at least 500 microns with some estimates of up to 2mm into the dermis.[30] Theoretically, this wavelength has the deepest penetration into the dermis because its water absorption is the least of the available water-only-targeted infrared lasers. This penetration is unimpeded by absorption by hemoglobin or melanin, which occurs at lower wavelengths. Deeper heating than 200–300 microns, however, may be detrimental to collagen synthesis as reported with the erbium glass laser.[31]

In the latest form of the 1320nm delivery system (CoolTouch3, CoolTouch Corp, Roseville, CA), the epidermis is thermally protected from injury with a 20–30-ms cryogen spray delivered 10ms pre-pulse, mid-pulse and postlaser pulse. Typical parameters are 13–15J/cm^2, fixed 50ms pulse duration, 10ms precooling, 5–10ms mid-cooling and 10ms postcooling. The goal of this system, like that of other nonablative systems, is improvement of rhytids without the creation of a visible epidermal wound. In a study with 1320nm without coordinated epidermal cooling, ten patients received laser treatments of their periocular rhytids and postauricular skin.[32] Postauricular skin biopsies from before treatment and 3 months posttreatment showed a small posttreatment increase in the amount of dermal collagen in three patients. Without epidermal cooling, complications included hyperpigmentation in three patients and pitted scarring in three patients. More recently, Nelson using the dynamic cryogen cooling technique before the laser pulse showed that one or more passes of a 1320nm Nd:YAG laser on photoaged skin led to improved facial rhytids at 2 months after treatment.[33] Immediately after treatment, mild edema and erythema appeared in the treated skin which disappeared within hours.

A recent histologic study was reported on the preauricular cheek of 10 patients who were biopsied following one to three laser passes of dynamically cooled millisecond domain Nd:YAG 1320nm laser.[8] Biopsies were performed at 1 hour and at 3 days after a single treatment. The number of passes was varied from one to three and Tmax (peak temperature measured by integrated radiometer) during treatment was targeted for 45–48°C. At 1 hour posttreatment, epidermal spongiosis and edema of the basal cell layer were present in all the specimens treated with three passes. At 3 days, the three pass samples also showed microthrombosis, widened vessels, sclerosis of the vessel walls, and infiltration of neurophilic granulocytes. The occurrence of these histologic findings correlated well with the presence of clinical improvement at 8 weeks posttreatment. Acute histologic changes and clinical improvement were not observed below treatment temperatures of Tmax 45°C or after one pass alone. Repeated temperatures above Tmax of 48°C incurred risk of epidermal injury.

The authors concluded that whereas longer-term histologic findings have confirmed the collagen synthesis component of 1320nm Nd:YAG laser, the short-term histologic data indicate that there may be some additional factors other than dermal collagen heating with subsequent collagen repair. The clinical findings in our experience with the 1320nm wavelength are improvement in rhytids, more effectively on nondynamic lines as well as significant improvement in acne scarring. The concept of true ‘nonablative resurfacing’ may involve some form of subclinical epidermal injury that improves the clinical outcome.

Case 5

CoolTouch Collagen Remodeling

A 44-year-old female presents with periocular rhytids and lower lid laxity (Fig. 8.5A). The postimage shows the eye after three treatments with 1320nm to the point of erythema (Fig. 8.5B). Three passes were performed for each treatment at a fluence of 17J/cm^2. The spot size and pulse duration are fixed at 10mm and 50ms, respectively. The parameters of cooling utilized were 20ms precooling to a final skin temperature of 45°C after three passes. Prior treatment for 30 minutes with a topical anesthetic such as LMX (Ferndale Labs, Ferndale, MI) makes the treatment tolerable. Enhancement of results can be obtained with administration of botulinum toxin immediately after the first treatment.

1450nm Diode

This mid-infrared wavelength is thought to penetrate the skin to a maximum of 500 microns. It is sold as a low-power diode system with pulsed cryogen cooling delivered in small pulses throughout the typical delivery cycle of 250ms (Smoothbeam, Candela, Wayland, MA) Relatively long 'on' times are required to achieve dermal heating; these range up to 250ms. Fluence typically ranges from 10 to 20J/cm^2. Preliminary results have shown improvement in mean wrinkle score.[34] Rhytid scores improved from a baseline score of 2.3 to 1.8 at 6 months after treatment ($p > 0.05$). Patient acceptance of the treatment was high but most felt that there was little improvement of the treated rhytids. The device has also recently received FDA clearance for the treatment of active acne, as sebaceous activity seems to be diminished by this device. We find this device most useful for sebaceous hyperplasia and acne scarring on the chin. It is also effective and FDA cleared for active acne. It shares this in common with the 1320nm wavelength.

A

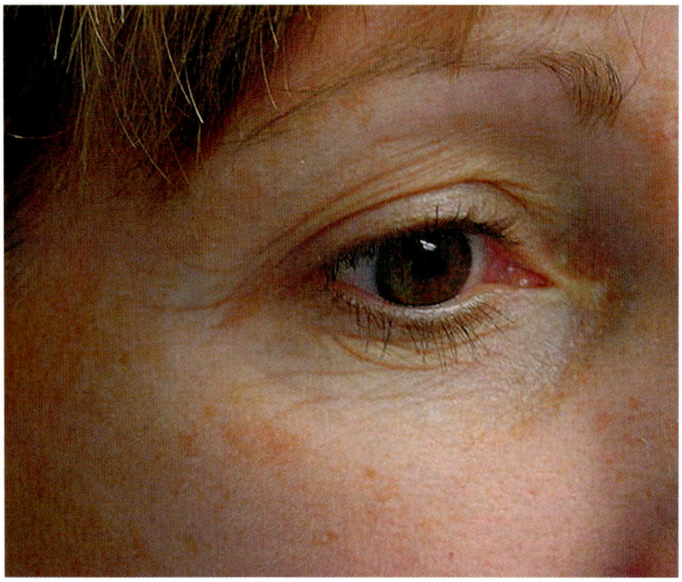

B

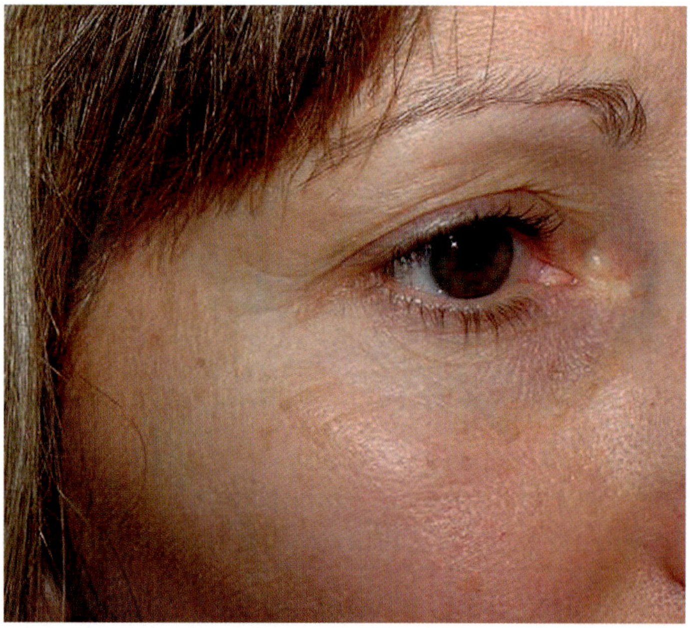

Figure 8.5

Case 6

Smoothbeam Sebaceous Hyperplasia and Collagen Remodeling Treatment

Sebaceous hyperplasia can be a significant component of photoaging. This 54-year-old male presents with multiple sebaceous hyperplasia on the forehead (Fig. 8.6A). This is shown after two treatments with the 1450 nm Smoothbeam (Fig. 8.6B). The settings that were used include the 4-mm spot size, 13 J/cm^2 and 40 ms of cooling. The pulse duration is fixed. It is believed that the mechanism is nonselective heating of sebaceous glands at 100–200 microns. There is also accompanying smoothing of the forehead surface texture.

A

B

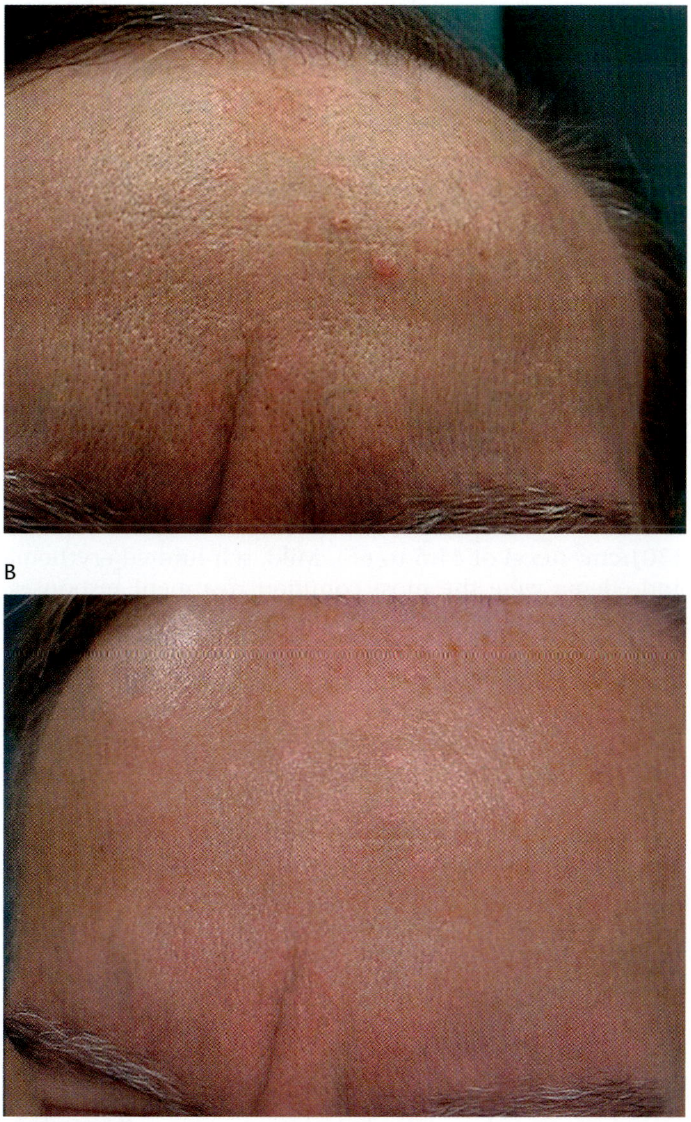

Figure 8.6

1540 nm Erbium Glass

Like the other target water-only midinfrared lasers, the 1540 nm erbium glass laser is delivered in 10–100 ms pulses with fluences ranging from 20 to 30 J/cm^2, although relatively long pulses comprising pulselets are necessary to effect dermal heating. The biggest problems for clinical treatment are the small spot size (4 mm), very long pulse length (1–2 s for the entire pulse train envelope) and uncontrolled contact cooling. In one study, immediate posttreatment biopsies demonstrated thermal damage in a band 333 microns thick (mean range from 311 microns to 644 microns deep in the dermis). Finally, dermal fibrosis was observed 2 months after treatment in a band 272 microns thick (mean range from 148 to 420 microns deep in the dermis).[35] In earlier experiments with less sophisticated cooling, heat effects were seen at up to 1.3 mm deep with some scarring-like effect, but this effect was considered a bit too deep for optimal results with rhytids.[35] The authors felt that the optimal depth for thermal effects on rhytids was a 0.1- to 0.4-mm band of the dermis just below the epidermis. A clinical study of ten patients demonstrated some improvement in periocular rhytids but some changes in pigmentation led the authors to conclude that this wavelength had the potential to be used for collagen remodeling under the right conditions.[36]

Microablative (Fractional) Resurfacing (1550 nm)

Fractional photothermolysis creates multiple arrays of 50-micron surface and subsurface thermal punctures in a pixilated pattern. Microablation of epidermis and dermis is theoretically able to improve skin texture and reduce fine to moderate rhytids over a few treatment sessions. By penetrating to depths of several hundred microns, these microthermal zones (MTZs) are anticipated to stimulate renewal of deeper collagen and elastin tissues. The effect visible to the eye is erythema and urtication, which can last for several hours to several days. We have been using this technology for 6 months at the time of writing. We have seen some patients with bruising, bleeding or crusting but typically we see 1–3 days of erythema and scaling. Most treatments have been performed 1 month apart for a total series of five treatments. Our preliminary observations are improvement in skin texture, some improvement in superficial acne scarring and reduction of periocular rhytids. The biggest downside is the application of blue dye and the subsequent removal, which can take 30 minutes or at worst will be visible to some extent for 3 days. The treatment requires multiple passes, typically eight, to insure uniformity of MTZ application as the head of the device delivers a single row of 50 microns microablative points. Clinical studies are underway and a consensus view of this technology is forthcoming. It is important that this technology is also based on microareas of contraction based on a water-only absorbing wavelength.

A

B

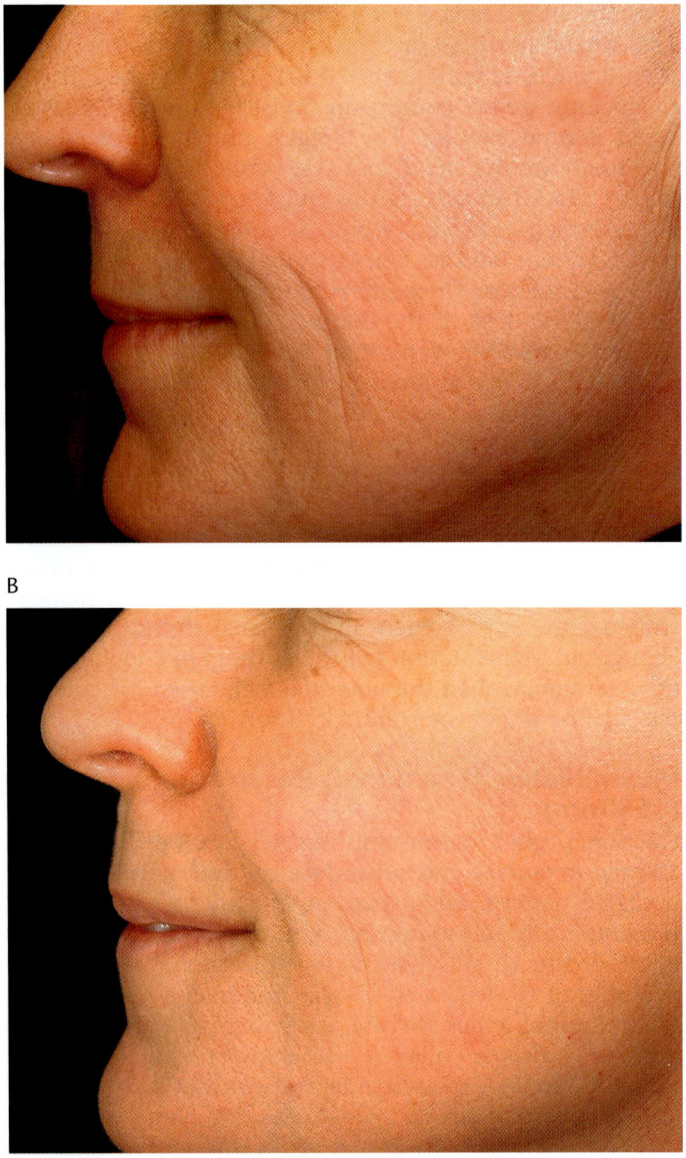

Figure 8.7

> ### *Case 7*
> *Fraxel Resurfacing for Superficial Wrinkling*
> A relatively new device still in the process of evaluation and developing parameters shows promise for less invasive skin resurfacing or retexturing. The patient (shown in lateral view; Fig. 8.7A) has moderate improvement in surface texture and some slight skin tightening after three treatments 3 weeks apart with the Fraxel microablative laser (Reliant Technology, San Diego, CA; Fig. 8.7B). The treatment settings used were four passes with 8 mJ at 250 microthermal zones (MTZ) followed by four passes with 14 mJ at 125 MTZs for a total energy delivery of 4 kJ. The patient had erythema lasting for 48 hours after each treatment. Treatment must be performed using the forced air cooling system (Cynosure SmartCool, Cynosure, Chelmsford, MA); it is too painful to tolerate with topical anesthesia alone.

Radiofrequency (RF)

Radiofrequency (RF; also discussed in Chapter 14) and microwave (MW) radiation are electromagnetic radiation in the frequency range 3 kilohertz (kHz) to 300 gigahertz (GHz). Microwave radiation is considered a subset of RF radiation. An alternative convention treats RF and MW radiation as two spectral regions. Microwaves occupy the spectral region between 300 GHz and 300 MHz, while RF or radiowaves include 300 MHz to 3 kHz. RF/MW radiation are nonionizing in that there is insufficient energy (less than 10 eV) to ionize biologically important atoms. Primary effects of RF/MW energy on living tissue are considered to be thermal. Therefore the goal of the new devices based on these frequency ranges is to heat up specific layers of the skin. Clinical tissue tightening following RF treatment is thought to result from heat-induced immediate collagen contraction, subsequent collagen remodeling, neocollagenesis, and the normal wound healing response. The most frequently utilized device is a monopolar RF device in which the patient has a grounding pad placed on the back or flank and RF energy is delivered through an inductive capacitance membrane which distributes RF evenly over a 1.5 cm^2 area. Patients experience heat in the region of each pulse. It is thought that the RF energy not only causes dermal heating but also heating in the fibrous septae attaching the dermis to the facial fascia below, thus causing contraction and lifting of the skin. In a recent study, 362 patients with facial and/or neck skin laxity were treated with a monopolar RF device (Thermacool, Thermage Corp., Haywood, CA) beginning in May 2002.[37] Treatment was delivered with one of three different tips as each became available. Tips included the 1 cm^2 standard tip at fluences of 81 to 124 J/cm^2 (level of 12.5 to 15), the 1 cm^2 fast tip at fluences of 62 to 109 J/cm^2 (level of 72.0 to 76.0), and the 1.5 cm^2 big fast tip at fluences of 75 to 130 J/cm^2 (level of 61.5 to 65). Mild, self-limited erythema and edema were the most common treatment responses. Complications included one patient with a slight 1 cm^2 depression, which resolved without intervention at 6 weeks. Although depressions have been reported with the 1 cm^2 standard tip, we believe they are due to higher fluence, use of injectable anesthetics and/or IV sedation and the slower cycle tip.

When surveyed, 80% of patients were satisfied with the procedure, thus allowing the authors to conclude that monopolar RF treatment of the face and neck is an extremely safe procedure with minimal adverse sequelae. The authors' experience has been that treatment to a specific endpoint of tightening using a specific algorithm of multiple passes at low energy has led to consistent tightening of the jowls and chin on appropriately selected candidates in a predictable way.

Other methods of delivering RF include using bipolar, with the RF not penetrating deeply but traveling from one electrode to the other. The ELOS™ system by Syneron uses electrodes 8 mm apart to cause slight superficial heating. Lumenis has developed a system in which suction is used to pull skin between two RF electrodes. Skin tightening and reduction of rhytids is claimed for both bipolar systems and definitive studies are pending.

A B

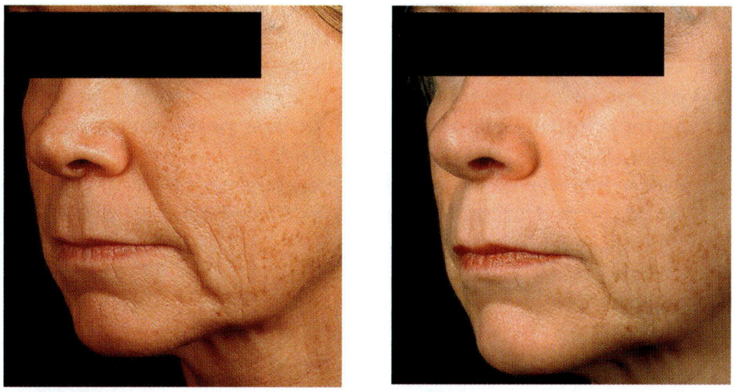

Figure 8.8

Case 8

Monopolar Radiofrequency Skin Tightening

Monopolar RF (Thermacool, Thermage, Haywood, CA) skin tightening. This 62-year-old patient presented with sagging of the lower face that could have been treated surgically, but she preferred a noninvasive procedure (Fig. 8.8A). She has a grounded pad placed on the lower back to complete the RF circuit. The treatment regimen utilized in this patient was three passes at a setting of 62.5 over the lower part of the face using the 1.5 cm^2 tip and following a grid applied to the face. An additional two passes were performed at a setting of 61.5 both lateral to the nasolabial folds and just above but all along the mandible. The results are shown 2 months after treatment with visible improvement in nasolabial and melolabial folds. There is slight improvement of the periocular rhytids as well with slight elevation of the malar eminence. The improvement is expected to continue for a period of 6 months posttreatment (Fig. 8.8B). Most patients will experience a 20% improvement in lower face sagging after one treatment. Multiple treatments at least 6 months apart may be necessary for the maximal result. Pain during treatment is controlled by minimizing energy levels and performing multiple passes. This regimen is also much safer and minimizes heat build-up in subcutaneous tissue. Patients typically require oral valium and oral oxycodone, as treatment requires 300–400 pulses over 45 minutes.

Adverse Effects

Visible light, which is more strongly absorbed by melanin, must therefore be used with greater caution in darker skin. Therefore, wavelengths from lower wavelength filters with IPL devices, green light 532 nm and yellow light at 585–595 nm must be used with far lower fluence in skin types IV–VI to minimize epidermal blistering or changes in pigmentation. Using IPL, for example, the treatment of darker skin individuals becomes of increasing concern when performing pigment abnormalities. In these cases a filter above 620 nm is typically utilized with delay times between pulses from 50 to 100 ms to allow plenty of time for the skin to cool down, avoiding thermal damage. The use of LED photomodulation, even though it is yellow light (590 nm) has no adverse events due to the extremely low light energies utilized; it is a nonthermal process stimulating mitochrondrial DNA.

RF skin tightening using the monopolar device rarely leads to adverse effects when correct conditions are met (as with the other devices). Complications seen in our practice are one patient with a slight 1 cm^2 depression, which resolved without intervention at 6 weeks. Use of injectable anesthetics and/or IV sedation – thus minimizing patient feedback about pain as well as use of the slower cycle tip were responsible for the depressions seen with this device. Another new device, microablative (fractional or pixillated) resurfacing can lead to epidermal vesicles, crusting or prolonged erythema lasting for 7 days when the dots of thermal energy are spaced too closely and delivered with too much fluence. Parameters are presently being worked out.

Conclusions

Nonablative skin rejuvenation techniques produce dermal remodeling without the obvious epidermal injury and the wound created with earlier ablative approaches.[8,38,39] The popularity of these new techniques lies significantly in the lack of wound care and down time as well as reduced costs. Experience with attempts to reduce thermal damage by using devices other than the CO_2 laser has led to the belief that induction of collagen and ECM is possible with less injury. This has led to the development of the 1319/1320 nm and 1450 nm and 1540 nm infrared lasers with cryogen-cooled epidermal protection and low fluence pulsed dye lasers, but these nonablative techniques remain thermal in nature. The new theory of photomodulation proposes that such improvements in skin appearance, structure and function may be achieved via a different nonthermal pathway thus accomplishing nonablative skin rejuvenation without the use of a thermal injury and thus without the traditional activation of the wound healing mechanism. Total nonablative rejuvenation, however, must also include reversal of some of the visible changes that occur from photoaging, not entirely relating to structural changes. These include reduction of superficial dyspigmentation (both dermal and epidermal), reduction of dermal telangiectasias and the appearance of an overall smoother texture and tone. The visible wavelength lasers and intense pulsed light are especially useful for these aspects of photoaging. Ongoing studies continue to delineate the role of lasers and light sources in the treatment of photoaging.

References

1. Butler PE, Gonzalez S, Randolph MA, Kim J, Kollias N, Yaremchuk MJ. Quantitative and qualitative effects of chemical peeling on photo-aged skin: an experimental study. Plast Reconstr Surg 2001; 107(1):222–8.
2. Dover JS, Hruza G. Lasers in skin resurfacing. Australas J Dermatol 2000; 41(2):72–85.

3. Alster TS. Clinical and histologic evaluation of six erbium:YAG lasers for cutaneous resurfacing. Lasers Surg Med 1999; 24(2):87–92.
4. Ross EV, Naseef GS, McKinlay JR, Barnette DJ, Skrobal M, Grevelink J, et al. Comparison of carbon dioxide laser, erbium:YAG laser, dermabrasion, and dermatome: a study of thermal damage, wound contraction, and wound healing in a live pig model: implications for skin resurfacing. J Am Acad Dermatol 2000; 42(1 Pt 1):92–105.
5. Goldberg DJ, Cutler KB. Nonablative treatment of rhytids with intense pulsed light. Lasers Surg Med 2000; 26(2):196–200.
6. Goldberg DJ. Nonablative resurfacing. Clin Plast Surg 2000; 27(2):287–92, xi.
7. Menaker GM, Wrone DA, Williams RM, Moy RL. Treatment of facial rhytids with a nonablative laser: a clinical and histologic study. Dermatol Surg 1999; 25(6):440–4.
8. Fatemi A, Weiss MA, Weiss RA. Short-term histologic effects of nonablative resurfacing: results with a dynamically cooled millisecond-domain 1320 nm Nd:YAG laser. Dermatol Surg 2002; 28(2):172–6.
9. Wong WR, Kossodo S, Kochevar IE. Influence of cytokines on matrix metalloproteinases produced by fibroblasts cultured in monolayer and collagen gels. J Formos Med Assoc 2001; 100(6):377–82.
10. Kondo S. The roles of cytokines in photoaging. J Dermatol Sci 2000; 23 Suppl 1:S30–S36.
11. Lee MW. Combination visible and infrared lasers for skin rejuvenation. Semin Cutan Med Surg 2002; 21(4):288–300.
12. Munavalli G, Weiss M, Beasley K et al. Intense pulsed light vs 10 mm spot 532 nm KTP green for photorejuvenation: a split face comparison pilot study. Laser Surg Med 2005; Suppl 17:21.
13. Lee MW. Combination visible and infrared lasers for skin rejuvenation. Semin Cutan Med Surg 2002; 21(4):288–300.
14. Hardaway CA, Ross EV. Nonablative laser skin remodeling. Dermatol Clin 2002; 20(1):97–111, ix.
15. Zelickson BD, Kilmer SL, Bernstein E, Chotzen VA, Dock J, Mehregan D, et al. Pulsed dye laser therapy for sun damaged skin. Lasers Surg Med 1999; 25(3):229–36.
16. Bjerring P, Clement M, Heickendorff L, Egevist H, Kiernan M. Selective nonablative wrinkle reduction by laser. J Cutan Laser Ther 2000; 2(1):9–15.
17. Omi T, Kawana S, Sato S, Honda M. Ultrastructural changes elicited by a nonablative wrinkle reduction laser. Lasers Surg Med 2003; 32(1):46–9.
18. Weiss RA, Goldman MP, Weiss MA. Treatment of poikiloderma of Civatte with an intense pulsed light source. Dermatol Surg 2000; 26(9):823–7.
19. Bitter PH. Noninvasive rejuvenation of photodamaged skin using serial, full-face intense pulsed light treatments. Dermatol Surg 2000; 26(9):835–42.
20. Hardaway CA, Ross EV. Nonablative laser skin remodeling. Dermatol Clin 2002; 20(1):97–111, ix.
21. Weiss RA, Weiss MA, Beasley KL. Rejuvenation of photoaged skin: 5 years results with intense pulsed light of the face, neck, and chest. Dermatol Surg 2002; 28(12):1115–19.
22. Sadick NS, exiades-Armenakas M, Bitter P, Jr., Hruza G, Mulholland RS. Enhanced full-face skin rejuvenation using synchronous intense pulsed optical and conducted bipolar radiofrequency energy (ELOS): introducing selective radiophotothermolysis. J Drugs Dermatol 2005; 4(2):181–6.
23. Weiss RA, McDaniel DH, Geronemus R, Weiss MA. Clinical trial of a novel non-thermal LED array for reversal of photoaging: clinical, histologic, and surface profilometric results. Lasers Surg Med 2005 (in press).
24. Weiss RA, Weiss MA. Early clinical results with a multiple synchronized pulse 1064 nm laser for leg telangiectasias and reticular veins. Dermatol Surg 1999; 25(5):399–402.
25. Dayan SH, Vartanian AJ, Menaker G, Mobley SR, Dayan AN. Nonablative laser resurfacing using the long-pulse (1064-nm) Nd:YAG laser. Arch Facial Plast Surg 2003; 5(4):310–5.
26. Goldberg DJ, Whitworth J. Laser skin resurfacing with the Q-switched Nd:YAG laser. Dermatol Surg 1997; 23(10):903–6.
27. Muccini JAJ, O'Donnell FEJ, Fuller T, Reinisch L. Laser treatment of solar elastosis with epithelial preservation. Lasers Surg Med 1998; 23(3):121–7.
28. Hussain M, Suwanchinda A, Charuwichtratana S, Goldberg D. A new long pulsed 940 nm diode laser used for hair removal in Asian skin types. J Cosmet Laser Ther 2003; 5(2):97–100.
29. Sadick NS, Trelles MA. A clinical, histological, and computer-based assessment of the Polaris LV, combination diode, and radiofrequency system, for leg vein treatment. Lasers Surg Med 2005; 36(2):98–104.
30. Hardaway CA, Ross EV. Nonablative laser skin remodeling. Dermatol Clin 2002; 20(1):97–111, ix.
31. Ross EV, Sajben FP, Hsia J, Barnette D, Miller CH, McKinlay JR. Nonablative skin remodeling: selective dermal heating with a mid-infrared laser and contact cooling combination. Lasers Surg Med 2000; 26(2):186–95.
32. Menaker GM, Wrone DA, Williams RM, Moy RL. Treatment of facial rhytids with a nonablative laser: a clinical and histologic Study. Dermatol Surg 1999; 25(6):440–4.
33. Nelson JS, Millner TD, Dave D, et al. Clinical study of nonablative laser treatment of facial rhytides. Lasers Surg Med 1998; 17(suppl 9):150.
34. Hardaway CA, Ross EV, Barnette DJ, Paithankar DY. Nonablative cutaneous remodeling with a 1.45 micron mid-infrared diode laser: phase I. J Cosmet Laser Ther 2002; 4(1):3–8.
35. Hardaway CA, Ross EV, Barnette DJ, Paithankar DY. Nonablative cutaneous remodeling with a 1.45 micron mid-infrared diode laser: phase I. J Cosmet Laser Ther 2002; 4(1): 3–8.
36. Levy JL, Besson R, Mordon S. Determination of optimal parameters for laser for nonablative remodeling with a 1.54 micron Er:glass laser: a dose-response study. Dermatol Surg 2002; 28(5):405–9.
37. Bellew SG, Weiss MA, Weiss RA. Safety of monopolar radiofrequency for skin tightening – 3 year experience. Dermatol Surg 2005 (in press).
38. Goldberg DJ. Nonablative resurfacing. Clin Plast Surg 2000; 27(2):287–92, xi.
39. Menaker GM, Wrone DA, Williams RM, Moy RL. Treatment of facial rhytids with a nonablative laser: a clinical and histologic study. Dermatol Surg 1999; 25(6):440–4.

Chapter 9

Laser Treatment of Leg Veins

Neil Sadick and Lian Sorhaindo

Introduction

Unsightly telangiectasis and venulectasias occur on the lower extremity in up to 41% of women and 15% of men in the United States. The pathology of leg veins can be subdivided into the following categories: superficial spider veins or telangiectasis, deeper reticular veins, and protuberant varicosities. Heredity, hormonal dysregulation, prolonged periods of standing, obesity, pregnancy, and aging may all play a role in the etiology of leg veins. Symptomatically, leg veins may cause fatigue, aching, swelling, throbbing, and pain. Although all of the aforementioned symptoms may be present, the patient with lower extremity veins typically seeks treatment solely for their unsightly aesthetic appearance.

The vasculature of the lower extremity consists of a complex, intertwined network of superficial and deep venous plexuses. The superficial veins of the leg lie directly underneath the skin; while the deep veins traverse the muscles of the leg. The flow patterns of these two networks are intertwined to such a great degree that superficial spider veins may be the direct result of increased hydrostatic pressure in the deep reticular or varicose veins.

The variety of sizes, depths, flow patterns, and vessel thickness make the treatment of leg veins more difficult than the treatment of facial veins. Presently, there is no single treatment for all leg veins, and lasers are frequently used as adjunctive therapy in patients receiving phlebectomy, sclerotherapy, or vein stripping. Laser and light source technology, driven by consumer demand, have been effective in treating vessels that are scleroresistant, that arise from prior surgical or sclerotherapy treatment (telangiectatic matting or angiogenic flushing), and in the needle-phobic patient (Box 9.1). Lasers have been particularly useful in the setting of spider veins or telangiectasias (<0.5 mm). Although sclerotherapy has, and continues to be, the gold standard for large spider and reticular veins, lasers may also be effective in the treatment of these vessels. This chapter deals specifically with laser surgery and its role in the treatment of leg veins; other modalities of treatment including sclerotherapy, ambulatory phlebectomy, and endovenous ablation are discussed in other chapters of this book.

Patient Selection

Previous studies have demonstrated that lasers are most effective in the treatment of small, superficial, red or blue veins. As mentioned previously, lasers have been an ideal treatment option for those patients who are prone to telangiectactic matting, are scleroresistant, and who are fearful of needles. The relative contraindications to the use of laser surgery include: tanned skin, pregnancy, the use of iron supplements or anticoagulation, history of photosensitivity disorder, or hypertrophic/keloidal scarring.

Expected Benefits

Laser therapy has become an effective treatment modality for the treatment of veins in the lower extremity. Typically at the time of treatment, small telangiectactic vessels disappear, giving both the patient and physician a visual record of success. In contrast, larger telangiectasias and reticular veins do not resolve at the time of treatment but gradually improve over the course of several months.

Table 9.1 *Comparison of the 1064 nm Nd:YAG, 810 nm diode, and 755 nm Alexandrite Lasers for Leg Veins 0.3–3 mm in Diameter*

Laser	Patients achieving 75% clearance at 3 months
1064 nm Nd:YAG	88%
810 nm diode	29%
755 nm alexandrite	33%

Data from ref. 3.

Table 9.2 *Vessel Thermal Relaxation Time*

Vein diameter	Time (seconds)
0.1	0.010
0.2	0.080
0.4	0.16
0.8	0.6
1.0	1.0
2.0	8.0

Box 9.1 *Indications for Laser Therapy Treatment of Leg Veins*

- Refractory noncannulizable vessels
- Telangiectatic matting
- Angiogenic flushing
- Scleroresistance
- Needle-phobic patients
- Vessel smaller than the diameter of a 30-gauge needle are present

Box 9.2 *Fundamental Properties of a Laser for Leg Veins*

- Must have a wavelength proportionately better absorbed by hemoglobin than the surrounding tissue.
- Penetration should reach the full depth of the target vessel.
- Sufficient energy must be delivered to damage the vessel without damaging the overlying skin.
- Energy must be delivered over an exposure time long enough to slowly coagulate the vessel without damaging surrounding tissue.

Moreover, selected vessels may clinically darken following treatment as the blood in the vessels coagulates.

In a recent study, patients with reticular and spider telangiectasis on their lower extremity were treated using the monomodal approach with the 1064 nm Nd:YAG laser and variable spot sizes and pulse width parameters. After three treatments administered after 1-month intervals, 20% of the treated vessels exhibited a 50% to 75% improvement. Over time, gradual improvements were observed, with 80% of vessels having greater than 75% clearing at 6 months follow up.[1,2]

In another study involving 22 women, the 1064 nm Nd:YAG, 810 nm diode, and 755 nm alexandrite lasers were used comparatively in the treatment of leg veins 0.3–3 mm in diameter. The study demonstrated that the Nd:YAG laser was the most effective treatment modality at three months follow up (Table 9.1). The side effect profile for the alexandrite laser included purpura and matting; while the results of the long pulsed diode were unpredictable.[3] To date, no long-term controlled studies have been done regarding the persistence of vessel clearance after laser treatment of leg veins.

Overview of Treatment Strategy

Major Principles and Determinants

The option of using lasers for treatment of leg veins is not entirely novel; the concept of selective photothermolysis was developed in the late 1980s. This theory states that selective damage to a tissue structure can be achieved by means of a wavelength of light preferentially absorbed by a chromophore in light-absorbing molecules and laser exposure time less than or equal to the object's thermal relaxation time (i.e. the time required for the object to lose 50% of its thermal energy.) The thermal relaxation times of leg veins vary according to vessel diameter (Table 9.2).

A major consideration for the physician involves the utility of laser and intense pulsed light (IPL) technologies versus that of sclerotherapy for the treatment of lower extremity vessels. The fundamental requirements for a laser or IPL source in the treatment of leg veins are delineated in Box 9.2.

The principle of laser technology and its role in leg vein reduction is centered on hemoglobin and its absorption spectrum, which has broad peaks at 410, 540, and 577 nm and smaller peaks at 920 and 940 nm. The spectra are different for oxy and deoxyhemoglobin, so that bluer veins will tend to respond to wavelengths targeting the deoxyspectrum; while red veins respond better to wavelengths targeting the oxyhemoglobin spectrum (Fig. 9.1). In general, any vessel that is less than 3 mm in diameter may be treated by laser and IPL technologies. However, sclerotherapy is a more efficient modality for eradicating cannulizable vessels and, when small, difficult-to-cannulate vessels are present, microsclerotherapy may be implemented. The use of microsclerotherapy, however, is associated with a greater number of adverse sequela, including needle puncture marks, increased incidence of bruising and pigment dyschromia, microulcerations and inconsistent results (Table 9.3). It is in this setting, that the use of lasers plays an important role in the management of cosmetic veins. It is important to realize, however, that lasers or IPL are not substitutes for sclerotherapy, primarily because hydrostatic pressure considerations are not

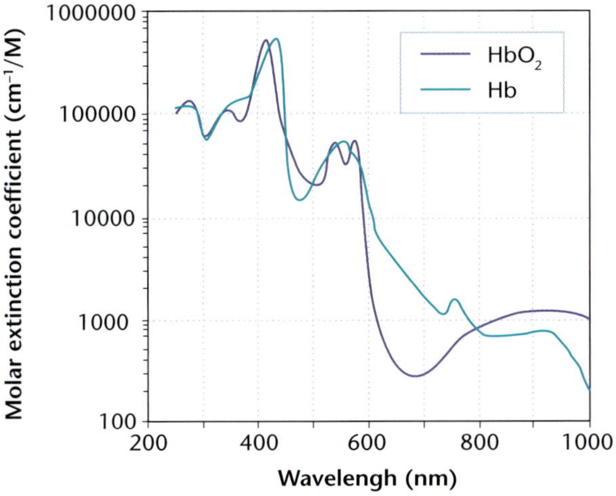

Figure 9.1 Absorption spectrum of hemoglobin/deoxyhemoglobin.

Table 9.3 *Microtelangiectasia <0.5 mm: Comparison of Microsclerotherapy and Laser Technology*

	Microsclerotherapy	Laser
Number of treatments	=	=
Bruising	–	+
Discomfort	–	+
Clinical efficiency	–	+
Purpura	+	–
Pigmentation	=	=
Ulceration	–	+
Cost	+	–
Patient satisfaction	–	+
Physician skill	=	=

addressed by light–endothelial interactions. With the use of noninvasive treatment modalities like laser technology, it is also inherently more difficult to have sufficient penetration of photons safely through the thick epidermal–dermal wall surrounding the lower-extremity vessels; the direct injection into the target chromophore is intuitively more efficient. Moreover, with the use of light one may observe an altered pattern of cytokine release with injury to the vessel that may lead to increased incidence of postinflammatory hyperpigmentation.

The major parameters selected to treat an individual vessel include wavelength, pulse duration, and spot size (Table 9.4).[4,5] In general, larger vessels respond best to longer wavelengths and the ratio of vessel to epidermal heating increases the probability of achieving complete vessel coagulation. Shorter wavelengths, in contrast, partially coagulate the vessel thereby increasing the incidence of treatment failures, and subsequent epidermal damage including hyperpigmentation. Thus, maximum efficiency of vessel clearing is obtained when the penetration depth of the beam most closely matches the vessel diameter.

Table 9.4 *Optimal Laser Parameters for the Treatment of Leg Veins*

Parameter	Value
Wavelength	530–1064 nm
Pulse duration	2–100 ms
Fluence*	30–150 J/cm^2
Spot size	3.0–10 mm

Adapted from refs 4 and 5.
*Depends on laser wavelength.

With regards to spot size selection, the spot size should be as large as possible, at least to the order of 4× the optical penetration depth. Selecting a sufficient spot size is significant in that it minimizes scattering losses while simultaneously maximizing beam penetration, which increases the probability that pan endothelial destruction will be achieved. Moreover, the use of larger spot sizes increases the level of pain and discomfort observed by the patient.

The parameters above have significantly influenced the development of a bimodal, dual-wavelength approach for the treatment of both red and blue lower extremity veins (Fig. 9.2). For the treatment of small, reddish telangiectasias with a high degree of oxyhemoglobin, short wavelengths (500–600 nm) were found to be most effective, whereas longer wavelengths (800–1100 nm) were found to be most effective for the treatment of deeper, blue telangiectasias and reticular veins.

With the advent of the monomodal approach, laser technology can now address variations in vessel size and depth with a single 1064 nm Nd:YAG laser (Table 9.5).[1,2] Delicate, red vessels <1 mm in diameter are typically superficial and have a high oxyhemoglobin saturation. As a result, they can be effectively treated with small spot sizes (<2 mm), higher fluences (350–600 J/cm^2), and short pulse durations (15–30 s). Larger blue vessels 1–4 mm in diameter are deeper and have a lower oxygenated hemoglobin component, that is they can be effectively treated with larger spot sizes (2–8 mm), moderate fluences (100–350 J/cm^2), and long pulse durations (30–50 ms). With the rising use of the Nd:YAG, the transition from a bimodal wavelength technique to a monomodal approach is inevitable.

Treatment Approach

Patients seeking treatment of leg veins should have a thorough physical examination to evaluate the type and size of the leg veins, and the presence/absence of reflux or incompetent valves. As part of the treatment algorithm, larger varicose veins with reflux should be treated first to avoid the unsuccessful treatment of smaller telangiectasias and potential complications such as dyspigmentation and telangiectatic matting.

Figure 9.3 illustrates a treatment algorithm for leg veins. Initially, treatment should begin with the surgical removal, i.e. ligation, stripping, or ambulatory phlebectomy of

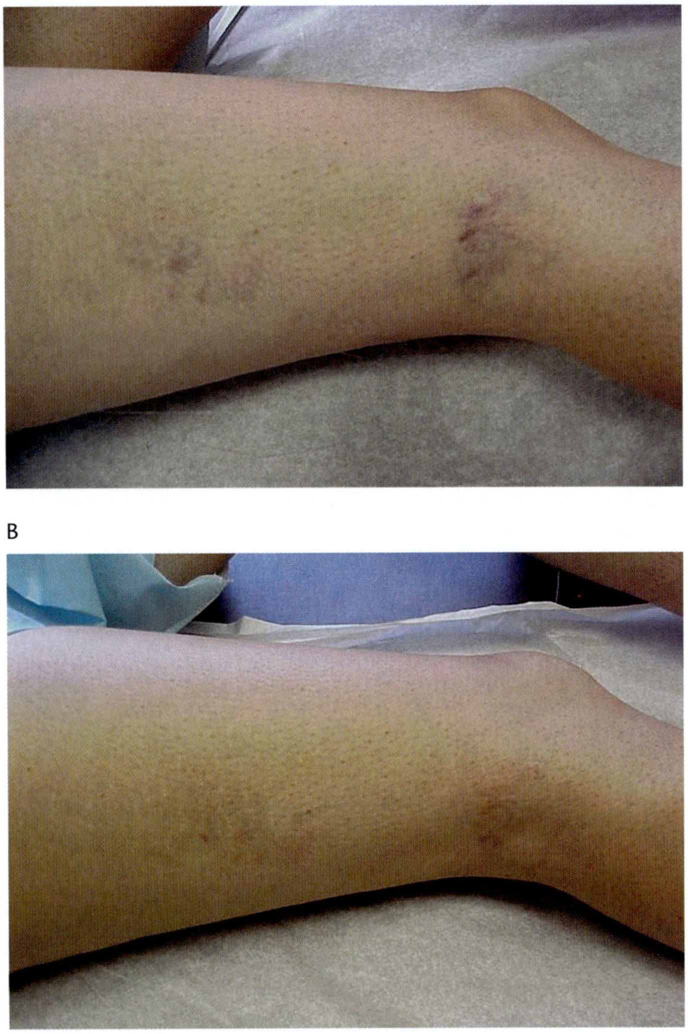

Figure 9.2 Pre- and postclinical pictures of lower extremity veins using biomodal technique.

Table 9.5 *Monomodal Approach to the Treatment of Leg Veins using the 1064 nm Nd:YAG Laser*

Vessel size	Spot size	Fluence	Pulse duration
<1 mm red	Small	High	Short
1–3 mm (blue)	Large	Moderate	Long

Adapted from refs 1 and 2.

varicosities and large feeder vessels. Then sclerotherapy should be performed proceeding from large to small vessels. This aspect of the treatment protocol will obliterate, on average, 80–90% of vessels in a single treatment. Moreover, laser and light therapy should be utilized in the treatment of any residual vessels including those that are too small in diameter to undergo sclerotherapy with a 30- to 32-gauge needle.

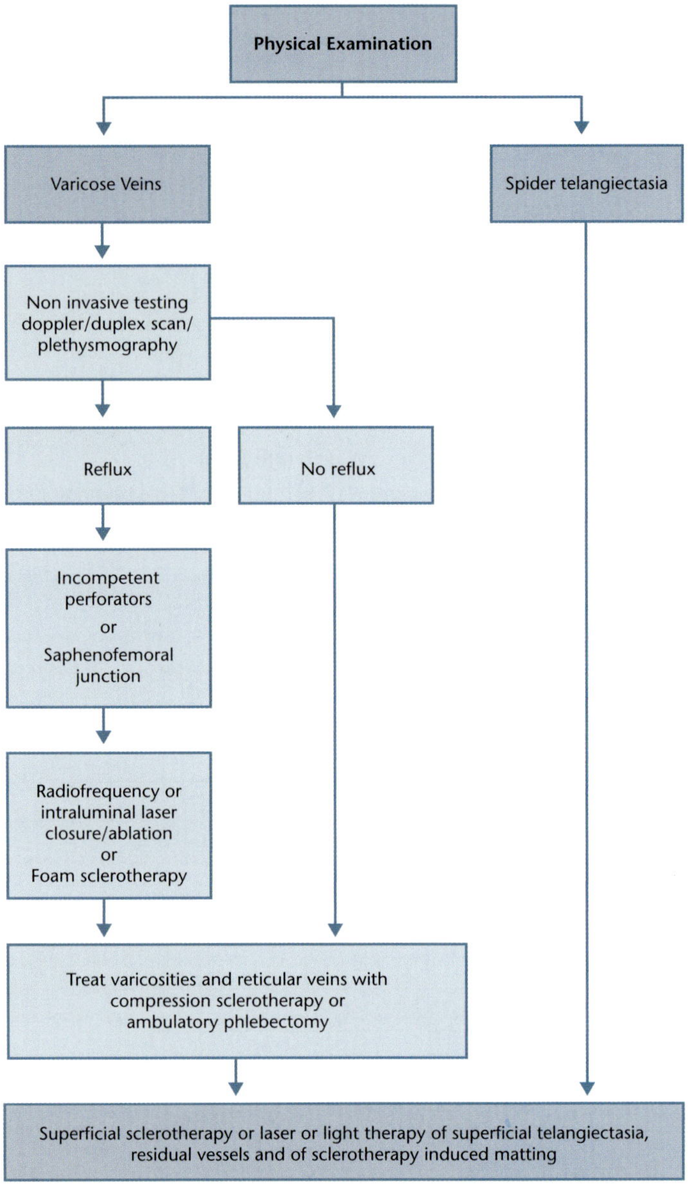

Figure 9.3 Systematic approach to the treatment of leg veins.

Patient Interviews

In addition to a thorough physical examination, making the diagnosis of spider or varicose veins warrants a detailed medical history including potential risk factors or etiologies for vascular pathology, such as hormones, prolonged standing associated with occupation, obesity, pregnancy, heredity, or aging. The physical examination should be conducted while the patient is standing erect, making note of epidermal pigmentation and the size and type of abnormal veins bilaterally. In addition, a hand held Doppler should be used to create a map of the venous network and to determine the direction of the blood flow. If the physician notes reflux as a result of venous valvular insufficiency, the patient must undergo further testing with a duplex ultrasound machine.

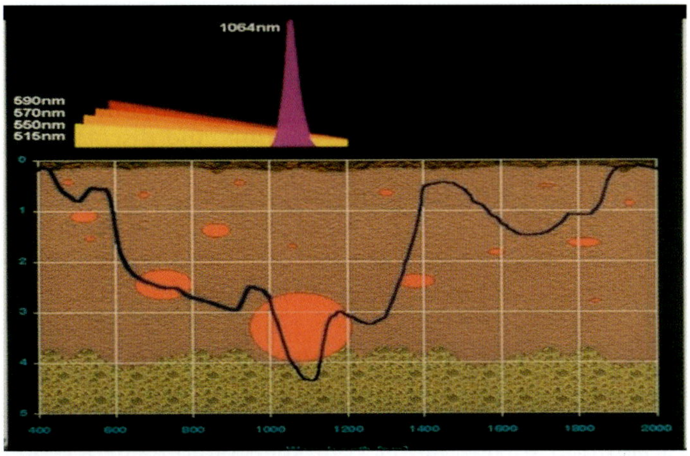

Figure 9.4 Wavelength and depth of penetration.

Table 9.6 *Lasers and Light Sources for the Treatment of Leg Veins*

Laser	Wavelength
Pulsed dye	585–605 nm
KTP	532 nm
Alexandrite	755 nm
Diode	810 nm
Nd:YAG	1064 nm
Intense pulsed light	515–1200 nm

Treatment Techniques

Patient Criteria

As previously mentioned laser therapy as opposed to sclerotherapy may be considered appropriate in patients who are: (1) fearful of needles; (2) cannot tolerate sclerotherapy; (3) have legs veins that are scleroresistant; or (4) are susceptible to telangiectatic matting (see Box 9.1). Ideally, candidates for laser treatment of leg veins have previously undergone appropriate surgery or sclerotherapy for the treatment of varicosities, incompetent perforators and reticular veins, as well as sclerotherapy to clear the majority of superficial vessels.

Equipment

A number of treatment systems are currently available. A compilation of laser and intense pulsed light sources utilized in this setting are presented in the following discussion and listed in Table 9.6. These devices utilize various wavelengths of light ranging form 515 nm to 1064 nm. As mentioned earlier, the longer the wavelength the greater the depth of penetration as illustrated in Fig. 9.4.

Pulsed Laser

In the 1980s, the pump pulsed dye laser was the first laser to achieve notable results in the treatment of leg veins. This treatment system employs short wavelength technology, utilizing a wavelength of 577 nm. Because of its short wavelength, relatively short pulse duration, and moderate energy fluence in general, this system is acceptable for treatment of leg vessels <1.0 mm, but cannot be recommended for treatment of blue vessels or red vessels >1.0 mm. Moreover, it is less effective than the long wavelength technologies and is associated with a number of side effects, including bruising and posttherapy hyperpigmentation.

With the recent development of longer wavelengths including the 1064 nm Nd:YAG, longer pulse duration lasers and light sources, there has been a great increase in treatment outcomes. Several long-pulse dye lasers are currently available, with variable pulse durations capable of deeper penetration into the skin and treatment of larger superficial telangiectasias. In addition, the development of cooling devices now provides epidermal bypass that protects the epidermis from damage, allowing delivery of higher fluences of energy. As a result, contact or dynamic cooling devices are incorporated into all devices currently manufactured. The increased utilization of extended pulse durations has also allowed delivery of greater amounts of energy in a more gentle fashion providing more consistent pan-endothelial destruction, translating into more consistent results with fewer treatments and lesser side effect. To date, the pulse duration most suited for the thermal destruction of leg telangiectasias appears to be 1–50 ms. Other advances including those made in gentle cavitation, captured pulse, and the regular use of large diameter beams have all lead to improvements in laser/IPL technology.

Pulsed Potassium-Titanyl-Phosphate Laser

The potassium-titanyl-phosphate (KTP) laser is effective for small telangiectatic leg veins in fair-skinned patients. With this treatment system, the most effective parameters include: spot size of 3–5 mm, pulse duration of 10–15 ms, and fluences of 14–20 J/cm^2. Side effects include, but are not limited to, temporary redness, superficial crusting, and purpura. Lower fluences must be utilized when administering this treatment modality to darker-skinned or tanned patients because the melanin in the skin also absorbs green light, posing a significantly increased risk of epidermal damage. Moreover, treatment failure is high in this select group of patients because the lower fluences may fall short of successfully coagulating the target vessel.

Alexandrite Lasers

Pulse alexandrite lasers constitute another treatment system utilized for both spider and reticular veins. The system uses an intermediate wavelength that allows slightly higher penetration of laser energy enabling treatment of reticular veins up to 4 mm in diameter. When compared to other available laser treatment systems, including the 1064 nm Nd:YAG laser and the superlong pulse diode, the alexandrite laser, 755 nm at a fluence of 60–70 J/cm^2, evoked a significant inflammatory response with concomitant purpura and matting. In a study conducted by Eremia et al,[3] it was concluded that the 755 nm wavelength utilized by the aforementioned system is limited to use in non-tanned patients with I–III skin types. Moreover, the most favorable treatment parameters for long-pulse alexandrite lasers appear to be 20 J/cm^3, double pulsed at a repetition rate of 1 Hz. Side effects include: purpura, matting, and long-term pigmentary alterations due to melanin absorption.

1064 nm Nd:YAG

The long pulsed Nd:YAG laser system has undoubtedly become the treatment of choice for spider and feeding reticular veins. The versatility of this particular treatment definitely accentuates its present success possessing the ability to treat both red, superficial vessels and deeper blue vessels with simple adjustments in spot sizes, fluences, and pulse durations. In addition, this system – via its utility of a longer wavelength and subsequent epidermal bypass – increases the ability to treat darker skin phenotypes. Issues stemming from the hydrostatic pressure of feeder and reticular veins can also be addressed because veins up to 3 mm can be treated, although patient's tolerance to pain may become an issue as pain increases with treatment of larger vessels. For superficial vessels less than 1 mm in diameter, the optimal parameters include: small spot sizes of <2 mm, short pulse durations of 15–30 ms, and high fluences of 350–600 J/cm^2. For reticular veins 1 to 4 mm in diameter, larger spot sizes (2–8 mm), longer pulse durations (30–60 ms) and moderate fluences (100–370 J/cm^2) should yield successful results. As a result, the Nd:YAG laser has been embraced by many clinicians world wide as the state of the art for laser treatment of lower extremity vessels.

Intense Pulsed Light (IPL)

Intense pulsed light sources (IPL), has been shown to have dual success in penetration of both superficial and deep tissues, in addition to absorption by both oxygenated and deoxygenated hemoglobin. The laser, unlike other treatment modalities, uses a non-coherent pulsed light source with wavelengths between 500 and 1200 nm, emitting a spectrum of light rather than a single wavelength in single, double or triple pulses. The results of this current system are variable. Schroter et al[6] reported immediate clearing in 73.6% of patients and in 84.3% of patients after four weeks. With respect to the immediate response, 82% clearing was seen in the group with veins up to 0–2 mm, 78.9% was seen in the group from 0.2 to 0.5 mm, and 59.7% was seen in the groups from 0.5 to 1.0 mm. Other investigators, in contrast, have found lesser success utilizing this technology for management of lower extremity spider veins. Results from a study done by Green[7] showed no improvement in 56% of patients, partial clearing in 25% of patients, and no improvement in 56% of telangiectasias. It is worth mentioning that this particular study was done at the incipient stages of the development of the IPL system. Associated side effects include blistering, crusting, and discoloration especially in darker skinned patients. With growing sophistication and use, however, IPL stands at the very forefront of laser vein technology, being the most effective for treating telangiectatic matting associated with diffuse erythema (see Chapter 2, Fig. 2.66, p. 78).

Combined Radiofrequency Pulsed Light Technologies

In addition to IPL, newer combined radiofrequency (RF) pulse light technologies are available, which employ the simultaneous use of a pulsed light source or a diode laser in conjunction with a bipolar RF delivery system. With utilization of this system, a high energy penetration depth (>2 mm) and a high energy density on the treated vein (>100 J/cm^2) can be achieved. The diode component allows strong absorption of energy by the hemoglobin and the RF allows protein denaturation of the blood vessel wall in conjunction with epidermal cooling.

Treatment Algorithm

In general, most patients whose leg veins are treated with laser surgery tolerate the procedure without difficulty. If a patient exhibits decreased tolerance to pain, or if larger telangiectatic or reticular veins are being treated, a topical anesthetic cream should be applied 1 hour prior to treatment and covered with a plastic wrap. When the patient and physician are ready for the treatment to be administered, the treatment area should be cleansed with alcohol. In addition, the physician, patient and any assistants throughout the treatment should wear protective eyewear.

When using the 532 nm KTP laser in the treatment of smaller telangiectasias, a spot size of 3–5 mm, fluence of 12–20 J/cm^2, and a pulse duration of 10–15 ms should be administered to receive the best results. Skin cooling, as discussed earlier, should be used before, during, and after treatment to prevent thermal damage to surrounding tissues and decrease patient discomfort. Laser pulses should then be applied individually, separated by at least 1–2 mm. Each laser pulse should be traced along the length of the vein with care not to overlap or double pulse. The physician should apply a minimal amount of pressure with the application device so as to not physically compress the selected target vessel. Ultimately, the treatment goal should be either vessel spasm with immediate clearance or thrombosis with darkening of the vessel. Although it is not rare to see complete clearance after just one treatment, typically patients require 2–3 treatment sessions with 6- to 12-week nontreatment intervals because of the intense cytokine release generated by the laser endothelial interaction for maximal results.

As previously mentioned, the long pulsed Nd:YAG laser is the treatment of choice for reticular or telangiectasias

>1 mm. The 1064 nm lasers possess the ability to vary spot sizes, pulse width parameters, resulting in a wide treatment range of leg veins including small telangiectasias. For superficial vessels less than 1 mm in diameter, the optimal parameters include: small spot sizes of <2 mm, short pulse durations of 15–30 ms, and high fluences of 350–600 J/cm^2. For reticular veins, 1 to 4 mm in diameter, larger spot sizes (2–8 mm), longer pulse durations (30–60 ms) and moderate fluences (100–370 J/cm^2) yield successful results. As with other laser modalities, cooling before, during, and after the pulse protect the patient's epidermal layer from damage when using higher fluences and also increase patient comfort. With application of this system, it is often useful to apply mild pressure with the hand piece when treating reticular veins to minimize the diameter and the amount of hemoglobin in the lumen. This allows greater vessel penetration with less total heat and reduced thermal damage to surrounding skin/tissue. After treatment with the Nd:YAG laser, small vessels experience immediate resolution; while larger telangiectasias and reticular veins experience no visual change during the treatment, but demonstrate improvement and ultimately clearance weeks to months following treatment.

After treatment with any laser system, patients may experience swelling, urtication, or erythema around the treated vessels. The application of ice packs or a topical steroid will speed the resolution of the above, in addition to decreasing the risk of postinflammatory hyperpigmentation. Although compression stockings are considered unnecessary after the treatment of small telangiectasias, they may improve results if worn 1 week after the treatment of larger telangiectasias and reticular veins by preventing vessel refilling.

Troubleshooting

A few common pitfalls must be addressed in the laser treatment of leg veins (Box 9.3). Physicians should avoid immediately retreating or double pulsing vessels when no instantaneous changes are present to avoid excessive thermal damage. Following treatment to a specific area with appropriate parameters, it can take several minutes for thermocoagulation to occur. When the physician retreats the area without allowing the layers of the skin and the surrounding tissue to cool, the patient is susceptible to excessive thermal injury, which may manifest as scarring and ulceration. Moreover, it is better to work on a distinctly separate treatment area and return to the resistant vessel in 5–10 minutes. It is also important to use the lowest possible fluence that will effectively treat a selected vessel to minimize complications. As a rule, the physician should always start at the lowest fluence and incrementally increase to higher energy levels as needed depending on the vessel response. Blanching of the skin is a sign of excessive thermal injury and should be avoided. Furthermore, the physician should take note of the lateral spread of the thermal energy into surrounding areas, particularly with the longer wavelength 1064 nm laser. Nontreated vessels connected to or adjacent to the desired treatment pulse area may receive enough thermal damage to unintentionally coagulate. As a result, all pulses should be ideally separated by 1–2 mm.

Box 9.3 *Common Pitfalls*

- Avoid immediately retreating or double pulsing vessels when no instantaneous changes are present
- Allow treated areas to cool before attempting a second pass
- Always use the lowest possible effective fluence
- Space adjacent laser pulses at least 1–2 mm apart to reduce excessive thermal damage

Box 9.4 *Side Effects*

- Transient hyperpigmentation
- Purpura
- Telangiectatic matting
- Pain
- Thrombosis
- Epidermal damage
- Incomplete clearance

Adverse Sequelae and Alternative Approaches

The complications for the laser treatment of leg veins include: epidermal damage, thrombosis, hyperpigmentation, matting, and incomplete clearance (Box 9.4). Patients typically complain of discomfort during the actual procedure but rarely feel uncomfortable postoperatively. For those patients who develop telangiectatic matting of incomplete vessel clearance, retreatment should be offered with either laser or sclerotherapy as deemed appropriate. Localized areas of thrombosis may resolve independently from treatment or can be easily expressed with an 18-gauge needle. Postprocedure hyperpigmentation is usually transient and has become less of an issue with the advent of the longer-wavelength technologies and improvement of epidermal cooling devices. Moreover, wound care should follow any procedure that results in epidermal damage, thereby decreasing the incidence of scarring.

Looking Forward

The future for laser treatment of leg veins is extremely bright as advances in laser, pulsed light and combined radiofrequency pulse light technologies continue at an amazing rate. The major advances that are in constant evolution center around the use and enhancement of longer-wavelength treatment systems, improved cooling technologies, varied spot size, pulse durations, and fluence-related monomodal approaches and combined lasers/radiofrequency. Moreover, with the introduction and continued sophistication of these light-based technologies for the treatment and management of lower extremity vessels, many patients now have available to them an array of safe, noninvasive treatment options with minimal side effects or complications.

References

1. Sadick N Laser treatment with 1064 nm laser for extremity class I–III veins employing variable spot sizes and pulse width diameters. Dermatol Surg 2003; 29:916–19.
2. Sadick N Updated laser approaches to the management of cosmetic leg veins. Phlebology 2003; 18:54–64.
3. Eremia S et al. A side-by-side comparative study of 1064 nm Nd : YAG, 810 nm diode and 755 nm alexandrite lasers for treatment of 0.3–3 mm leg veins. Dermatol Surg 2002; 28:224–30.
4. Sadick N Advances in laser surgery for leg veins. Bimodal wavelength approach to lower extremity vessels, new cooling techniques, and longer pulse durations. Dermatol Surg 2002; 28:16–20.
5. Sadick N A dual wavelength approach to laser/intense pulse light treatment of veins of the lower extremities. Cos Derm 2002;14:17–18.
6. Schroeter C et al. Clinical significance of an intense pulsed light source on leg telangiectasias of up to 1mm diameter. Eur J Dermatol 1997; 7:38–42.
7. Green D. Photothermal removal of telangiectases of the lower extremities with Photoderm VL. J Am Acad Dermatol 1998; 38(1):61–8.

Further reading

Apfelberg D. 1989 Study of three laser systems for treatment of superficial varicosities of the lower extremity. Lasers Surg Med 1989; 7:219–23.

Dover J et al. The role of lasers and light sources in the treatment of leg veins. Dermatol Surg 1999; 25:328–36.

Goldberg D. Nd : YAG laser treatment of spider veins. Scope Phlebol Lymphol 2001; 12:184–88.

Goldman M, Eckhouse S. Photothermal sclerosis of leg veins. Dermatol Surg 1996; 22:323–30.

Goldman MP, Bergan JB, Gvex JJ. Sclerotherapy Treatment of Varicose and Telangiectatic Leg Veins, 4th edn. Elsevier, London, 2006.

Kauvar A. The role of lasers in the treatment of leg veins. Sem Cutan Med Surg 2000; 19:245–52.

Sadick N. Long-term results with a multiple synchronized pulse 1064 nm Nd : YAG laser for the treatment of leg venulectasias and reticular veins. Dermatol Surg 2001; 27:365–9.

Sadick N, Weiss R. The utilization of yellow light laser (578nm) for the treatment of class I red telangiectasias of the lower extremity. Dermatol Surg 2002; 28:21–25.

Weiss R, Dover J. Laser surgery of leg veins. Dermatol Clin 2002; 20:19–36.

Chapter 10

Laser Scar Revision

Tina S. Alster and Divya Railan

Introduction

Over the past decade, refinements in laser technology as well as advances in laser techniques have enabled dermatologic surgeons to define the most appropriate lasers to use for different scar types without the adverse sequelae and recurrence rates noted with older surgical revision techniques and continuous wave laser systems.

Clinical technique

Scar Characteristics

Proper scar classification is important because differences in clinical scar characteristics determine the treatment protocol.[1] Scar color, texture, and morphology, as well as previously applied treatments, will affect the laser parameters and number of treatments required for optimal improvement (Table 10.1).[2,3]

Hypertrophic scars are raised, firm erythematous scars formed as the result of overzealous collagen synthesis coupled with limited collagen lysis during the remodeling phase of wound healing. The result is the formation of thick, hyalinized collagen bundles consisting of fibroblasts and fibrocytes. Despite the obvious tissue proliferation, hypertrophic scars remain within the confines of original integument injury and may regress with time.

Keloids are raised, reddish-purple, nodular scars that, on palpation, are firmer than hypertrophic scars. Keloids exhibit a prolonged, proliferative phase resulting in the appearance of thick hyalinized collagen bundles similar to those produced by hypertrophic scars, but extend beyond the borders of the inciting wound and do not regress over time. Although they can be seen in all skin types, keloids appear most frequently in patients with darker skin tones and are related to an inherited metabolic alteration in collagen.

Atrophic scars are dermal depressions most commonly caused by collagen destruction during the course of an inflammatory skin disease such as cystic acne or varicella. Scarring after inflammatory or cystic acne can manifest as atrophic, saucerized, ice pick, or boxcar scars.[4] While ice pick and boxcar scars respond best to dermal filler augmentation or punch excision, atrophic scars usually respond well to laser therapy.

Scar History

The duration of the scar and its developmental history should also be ascertained. Younger scars (<1 year old) are typically more erythematous than older scars. Although younger scars are quite amenable to pulsed dye laser irradiation, they may not necessitate laser treatment, as some spontaneous improvement is expected over the first 12 months. In patients whose scars continue to worsen, however, it is best to advise laser intervention to prevent further abnormal scar growth and to effect speedier improvement.

Whether a patient has received prior treatment to the scar is also important, as additional fibrosis may be present within the scar as a result of failed attempts to remove it, making it even more difficult to treat. Atrophic scars that have been treated with prior dermabrasion with resultant dermal thickening may not be vaporized as readily with CO_2 laser resurfacing, possibly reducing the final clinical response. However, individuals that have simply received intralesional injections of corticosteroids (for hypertrophic

Table 10.1 *Laser Selection for Different Skin Types*

Scar type	Clinical characteristics	Preferred laser choice
Hypertrophic	Raised, pink–red, limited to site of original trauma	585 nm PDL
Keloid	Raised, deep red–purple, extend beyond original traumatic border	585 nm PDL
Atrophic	Saucer-like or ice-pink indentations	CO_2 (10 600 nm) Er:YAG (2940 nm) Long pulse diode (1450 nm) Long pulse Nd:YAG (1320 nm)

scars and keloids, in particular) should not experience a significant reduction in response to subsequent pulsed dye laser treatment.

Laser Treatment for Hypertrophic Scars and Keloids

Progress in laser technology and refinements in technique have made laser therapy a preferred treatment choice for hypertrophic scars and keloids. Studies published using the 585 nm pulsed dye laser (PDL)[5–8] have demonstrated striking improvements in scar erythema, pliability, bulk, and dysesthesia with minimal side effects and treatment discomfort. These observations have been substantiated by skin surface textural analysis, erythema reflectance spectrometry readings, scar height measurements, and pliability scores. Patients with pruritic hypertrophic scars and keloids may require the use of oral antihistamines, but pulsed dye laser irradiation of these scars have also effected improvement in symptoms within one or two treatment sessions.

While significant improvement in hypertrophic scars is generally noted after PDL treatment, thick keloids may require the simultaneous use of intralesional corticosteroid or 5-fluorouracil injections to enhance clinical results.[9] The adjunctive use of intralesional corticosteroids does not significantly enhance the clinical improvement seen after PDL treatment in all but the most symptomatic or proliferative hypertrophic scars.[10]

Adjacent, non-overlapping laser pulses at fluences ranging 6.0–7.5 J/cm^2 (7 mm spot) or 4.5–5.5 J/cm^2 (10 mm spot) should be applied over the entire surface of the scar. Energy densities are decreased by 10% in patients with darker skin phototypes or for scars in delicate locations (e.g. anterior chest). With PDL irradiation, the patient experiences a snapping sensation similar to that of a rubber band. Posttreatment, a mild sunburn-like heating of the skin is experienced for 15–30 minutes. This is generally well-tolerated, although some patients may require application of an ice pack.

Laser Treatment for Atrophic Scars

Ablative Laser Skin Resurfacing

Cutaneous laser resurfacing of moderate atrophic scars with a high-energy pulsed carbon dioxide (CO_2) laser yields a mean improvement of 50–80%.[11–14] Collagen remodeling with further clinical scar effacement has been reported to occur for up to 12–18 months postoperatively,[14] so retreatment of residual scars should be postponed for at least 1 year to accurately gauge clinical improvements. The Er:YAG laser, although effective in the treatment of atrophic scars, does not typically offer the same amount of collagen remodeling as does the CO_2 laser, and should thus be reserved for sculpting of individual scar edges and in the treatment of mild acne scarring.[15,16]

Nonablative Laser Skin Remodeling

As a consequence of the risks associated with ablative laser resurfacing, great interest has been shown for less invasive methods to effectively treat atrophic facial scars. Several nonablative laser devices have demonstrated efficacy in the treatment of atrophic facial scars; however, the most popular and widely used are the 1320 nm neodymium:yttrium-aluminum-garnet (Nd:YAG) and 1450 nm diode lasers.[17,18] Each system combines epidermal surface cooling with deeply penetrating infrared wavelengths that selectively target water-containing tissue, thereby creating a discrete thermal injury in the dermis without damage to the epidermis. Protocols for treatment often include three consecutive monthly laser sessions with the greatest clinical improvement noted 3–6 months after the final laser procedure. Improvement of scars by 40–50% has been observed after 1320 nm Nd:YAG or 1450 nm diode laser treatment, with results being substantiated by clinical assessments, patient satisfaction surveys, histologic evaluation, and skin surface texture (profilometry) measurements.[17] Although a series of nonablative laser treatments can effect modest improvement in atrophic scars with minimal side effects, the degree of clinical improvement does not equal that of ablative laser resurfacing. Therefore, it is critical to identify those patients best suited for nonablative procedures to optimize patient satisfaction.

Case Reports

Case 1
Hypertrophic Scars

A 34-year-old man presented with hypertrophic scars at his popliteal fossae 2 years after knee surgery (Fig. 10.1A). No prior treatments had been obtained for the asymptomatic scars, but he was concerned about their obvious appearance and desired treatment.

Treatment plan included 585 nm pulsed dye laser treatments at 6- to 8-week time intervals at fluences ranging from 6.0 to 7.0 J/cm^2 (7 mm spot, 1.5 ms pulse duration). Nonoverlapping laser pulses were applied to the length of each scar. Two months after four PDL treatments, improvement of scars was evident (Fig. 10.1B).

Case 2
Keloid Scars

A 26-year-old woman presented with earlobe keloids that recurred within 1 month of two prior surgical scar excisions. Subsequent radiation treatments did little to reduce their size and symptoms (including pruritus). Intralesional corticosteroids had been used with mild and short-lived symptomatic relief, but no reduction of scar bulk or size was noted (Fig. 10.2A).

Treatment plan included 585 nm pulsed dye laser treatment of the keloids with concomitant intralesional corticosteroid injections at 4- to 6-week intervals. After four treatments at fluences ranging from 5.0 to 5.5 J/cm^2 (10 mm spot, 1.5 ms pulse), scars showed marked improvement in size, symptoms, and pliability (Fig. 10.2B).

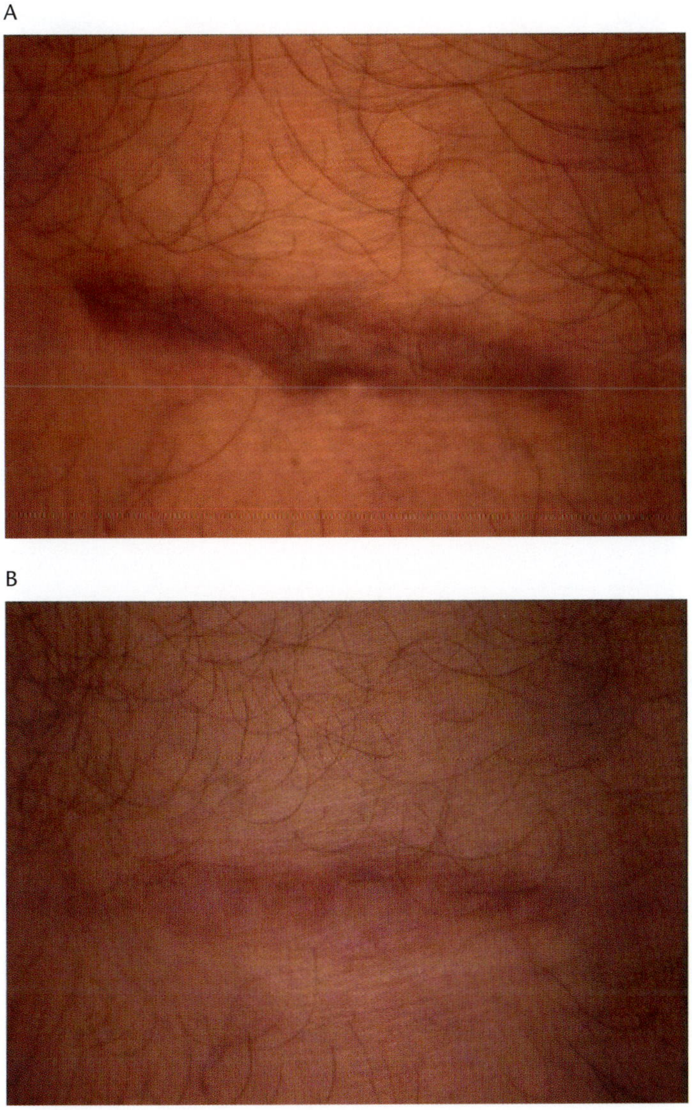

Figure 10.1

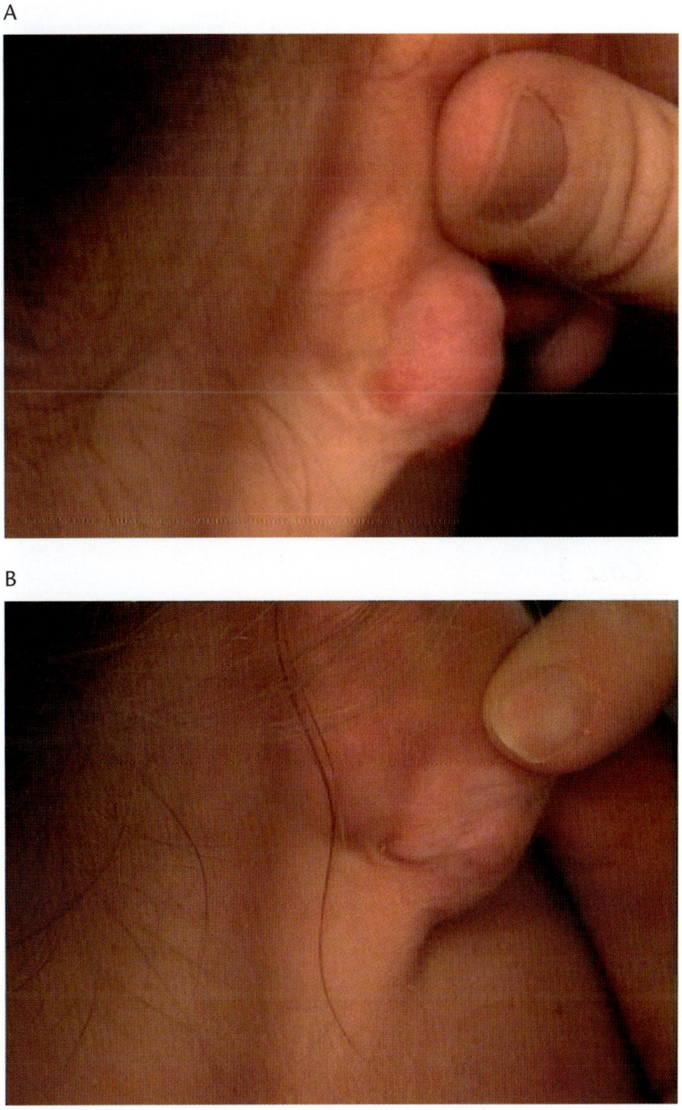

Figure 10.2

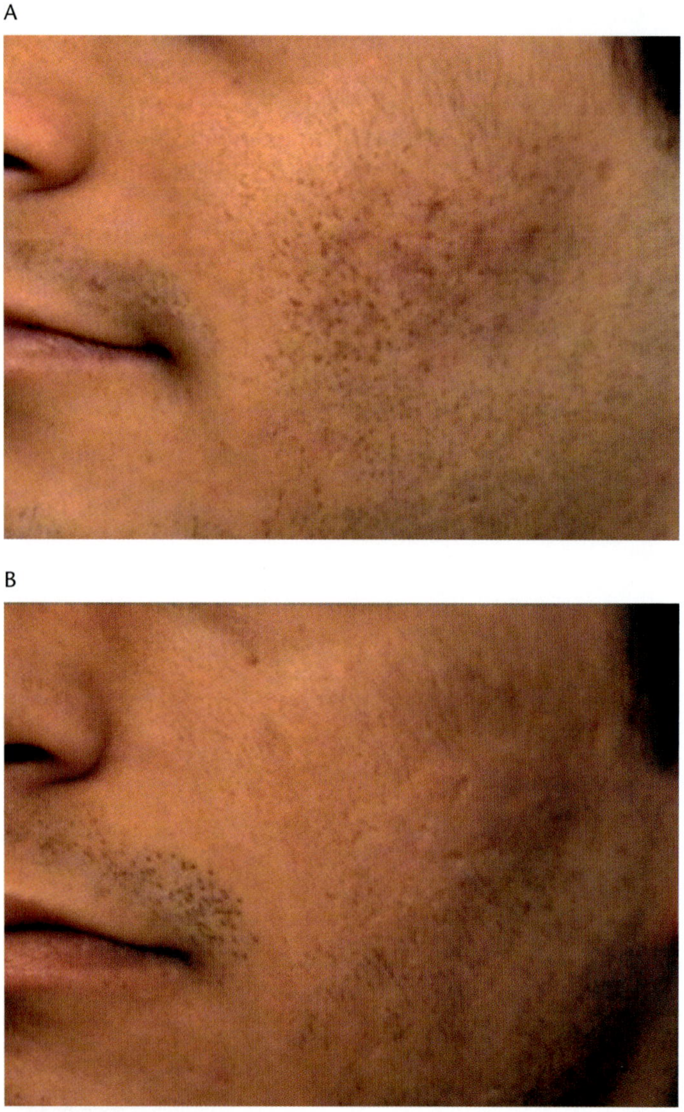

Figure 10.3

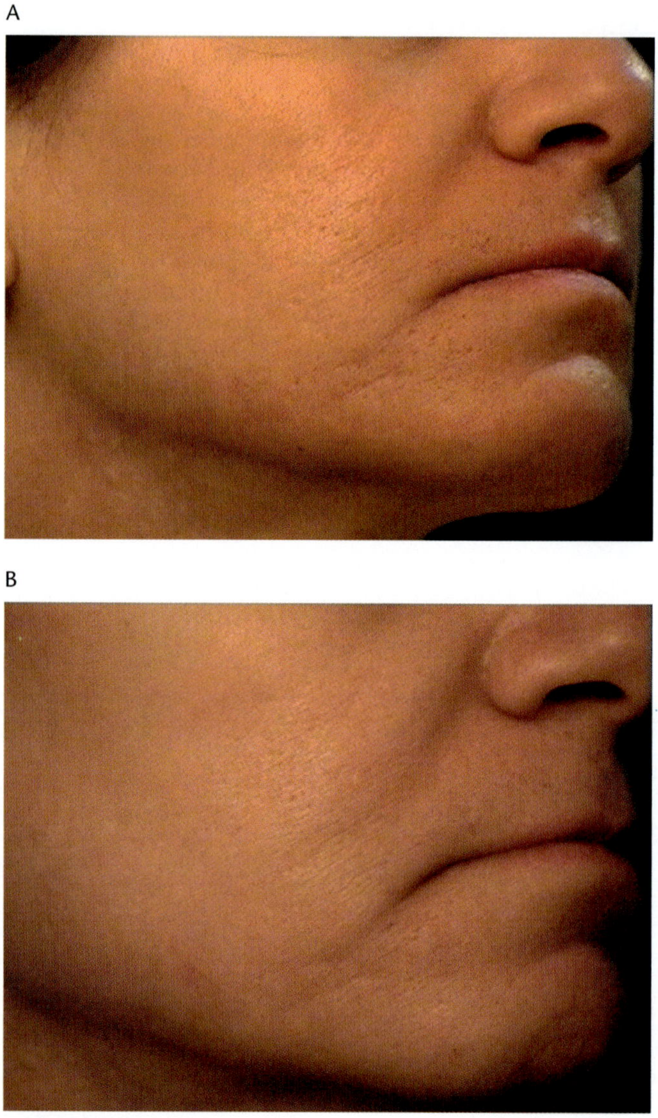

Figure 10.4

Case 3

Atrophic Scars

A 29-year-old man complained of extensive atrophic scarring on the cheeks and temples which resulted from severe cystic acne (Fig. 10.3A) His acne was treated successfully with isotretinoin 1 year prior to presentation.

Treatment plan included ablative erbium laser resurfacing, which resulted in improved skin tone and texture (Fig. 10.3B).

Case 4

Atrophic Facial Scars Secondary to Acne

A 52-year-old woman presented with atrophic facial scars secondary to acne which had required three separate courses of isotretinoin (the last course was more than 10 years prior to presentation) (Fig. 10.4A). She was not interested in undergoing a procedure that would require a prolonged recovery period and was willing to forego dramatic clinical improvement.

Treatment plan included a series of monthly nonablative long-pulsed 1450 nm diode laser treatments (12–14 J/cm^2, 6 mm spot). Improvement was evident 3 months after the third treatment (Fig. 10.4B).

Management of Complications

Pulsed Dye Laser

The most commonly experienced side effect of 585 nm PDL treatment is postoperative purpura, which can persist for several days. Swelling of treated skin may occur immediately after laser irradiation but generally subsides within 48 hours. Strict sun precautions should be practiced between treatment sessions to avoid stimulating pigment production in the treated areas. Subsequent laser sessions should be postponed until any excess pigment has resolved, so that the presence of epidermal melanin does not compromise the effectiveness of the laser. Topical bleaching agents may be applied to hasten pigment resolution. Treatments are typically delivered at 6- to 8-week intervals; however, longer treatment intervals may be necessary for adequate healing in patients with darker skin phototypes or in scars located in slower-healing areas (e.g. extremities) that have a higher tendency for postoperative hyperpigmentation.

Ablative Laser Skin Resurfacing

Side-effects and complications are potentially numerous after ablative laser resurfacing, even when proper protocols have been followed.[19–21] Expected side effects in the immediate postoperative recovery period include intense erythema, edema, and serous discharge. The degree of erythema is directly related to the number of laser passes delivered, but typically improves spontaneously over time without requiring specific treatment. Other possible complications include infection, acne or milia formation, and dyspigmentation. A significant side effect of treatment is transient hyperpigmentation. Although observed more frequently in patients with darker skin tones, hyperpigmentation may occur in any skin type. Transient hyperpigmentation is seen early in the postoperative course, occurring within 1 to 2 months of treatment. The process is self-limited, but resolution may be hastened with topical application of bleaching (e.g. hydroquinone) or acid (e.g. glycolic, retinoic, azelaic, ascorbic) preparations.

Hypopigmentation is a relatively late sequela of ablative laser resurfacing – typically observed 6 months or more postoperatively – and appears to be permanent. Fortunately, true hypopigmentation (with total loss of pigment) is rare. Rather, relative hypopigmentation is most frequently observed due to the obvious color difference seen when compared to adjacent nontreated (actinically bronzed) skin.

Infection is another postoperative concern after ablative laser resurfacing as reepithializing skin is vulnerable to bacterial, viral, and fungal infections. The incidence of infection is reduced with the appropriate use of prophylactic antibiotics, and more importantly, aggressive postoperative wound care.[22–24] Early diagnosis and treatment of suspected infection reduces patient discomfort and the risk of subsequent fibrosis.

Nonablative Laser Skin Remodeling

Side effects and complications of nonablative laser treatment of atrophic facial scars are generally mild. Transient posttreatment erythema is observed in almost all patients, resolving within 24 hours. Blistering, crusting, and scarring are rare and, although the risk of postinflammatory hyperpigmentation is substantially reduced with nonablative laser treatment (compared to ablative CO_2 or Er:YAG laser skin resurfacing), it is still possible – particularly in patients with darker skin phototypes. The postinflammatory hyperpigmentation observed, however, is typically mild and resolves more quickly than that seen after ablative laser procedures.

Adverse Sequelae

The most severe complications of laser scar revision may occur secondary to laser resurfacing and include hypertrophic scarring and ectropion formation, which are both due, in large part, to aggressive intraoperative laser technique. Hypertrophic burn scars can be treated effectively with 585 nm pulsed dye laser irradiation,[7] whereas ectropion typically requires surgical reconstruction.

Future Directions

Current laser technology permits successful treatment of various types of scars. It is not only imperative to properly classify the type of scar present, but to determine which laser system will provide optimum results. The 585 nm pulsed dye laser is best used to treat hypertrophic scars and keloids. Ablative CO_2 and Er:YAG laser systems effectively resurface atrophic scars, while nonablative infrared lasers (e.g. long-pulsed diode or Nd:YAG) can be used in treatment series to remodel scars through neocollagenesis. Future laser technologic advances as well as the concomitant use of other lasers and treatments may serve to further enhance clinical results.

The newest approach in the treatment of acne and atrophic scarring includes use of a nonablative radiofrequency device. Unlike a laser, which uses light energy to generate heat in targeted chromophores based on the theory of selective photothermolysis, radiofrequency technology produces an electric current that generates heat through resistance in the dermis and subcutaneous tissue, thus stimulating neocollagenesis and collagen remodeling. Preliminary studies demonstrate promise in the treatment of acne and, potentially, acne scarring.[25] Further investigation is warranted to determine the role of this novel device in the treatment of atrophic facial scars.

CLINICAL PEARLS

- Pulsed dye laser (585 nm) treatments for hypertrophic scars or keloids are best delivered at bimonthly (every 2 months) or longer time intervals in order for optimal tissue healing to occur.
- Use adjacent, non-overlapping laser pulses (the development of purpura is not necessary and thus should not be used as a treatment endpoint).
- Atrophic scars which are moderate to severe respond best to ablative (CO_2 or erbium) laser vaporization.
- Mild to moderate atrophic scars respond well to nonablative laser treatment.
- It often takes several months after a laser treatment or series of treatments for the final scar result to be realized.

References

1. Alster TS, Tanzi EL. Hypertrophic scars and keloids: etiology and management. Am J Clin Dermatol 2003; 4:235–43.
2. Lupton JR, Alster TS. Laser scar revision. Dermatol Clin 2002; 20:55–65.
3. Groover IJ, Alster TS. Laser scar revision of scars and striae. Dermatol Ther 2000; 13:50–9.
4. Jacob CI, Dover JS, Kaminer MS. Acne scarring: a classification system and review of treatment options. J Am Acad Dermatol 2001; 45:109–17.
5. Alster TS. Improvement of erythematous and hypertrophic scars by the 585 nm flashlamp-pumped pulsed dye laser. Ann Plast Surg 1994; 32:186–90.
6. Alster TS, Williams CM. Treatment of keloid sternotomy scars with 585 nm flashlamp pulsed dye laser. Lancet 1995; 345:1198–200.
7. Alster TS, Nanni CA. Pulsed dye laser treatment of hypertrophic burn scars. Plast Reconstr Surg 1998; 102:2190–5.
8. Dierickx C, Goldman MP, Fitzpatrick RE. Laser treatment of erythematous/hypertrophic and pigmented scars in 26 patients. Plast Reconstr Surg 1995; 95:84–90.
9. Fitzpatrick RE. Treatment of inflamed hypertrophic scars using intralesional 5-FU. Dermatol Surg 1999; 25: 224–32.
10. Alster TS. Laser scar revision: comparison study of 585 nm pulsed dye laser with and without intralesional corticosteroids. Dermatol Surg 2003; 29:25–9.
11. Alster TS, West TB. Resurfacing atrophic facial scars with a high-energy, pulsed carbon dioxide laser. Dermatol Surg 1996; 22:151–5.
12. Apfelberg DB. A critical appraisal of high-energy pulsed carbon dioxide laser resurfacing for acne scars. Ann Plast Surg 1997; 38:95–100.
13. Bernstein LJ, Kauvar ANB, Grossman MC, Geronemus RG. Scar resurfacing with high-energy, short-pulsed and flash scanning carbon dioxide lasers. Dermatol Surg 1998; 24: 101–107.
14. Walia S, Alster TS. Prolonged clinical and histological effects from CO_2 laser resurfacing of atrophic cars. Dermatol Surg 1999; 25:926–30.
15. Alster TS. Clinical and histological evaluation of six Er:YAG lasers for cutaneous resurfacing. Lasers Surg Med 1999; 24:87–92.
16. Tanzi EL, Alster TS. Treatment of atrophic facial acne scars with a dual-mode Er:YAG laser. Dermatol Surg 2002; 28: 551–5.
17. Tanzi EL, Alster TS. Comparison of a 1450 nm diode laser and a 1320 nm Nd:YAG laser in the treatment of atrophic facial scars: a prospective clinical and histological study. Dermatol Surg 2004; 30:152–7.
18. Rogachefsky AS, Hussain M, Goldberg DJ. Atrophic and mixed pattern of acne scars with a 1320 nm Nd:YAG laser. Dermatol Surg 2003; 29:904–8.
19. Nanni CA, Alster TS. Complications of CO_2 laser resurfacing: an evaluation of 500 patients. Dermatol Surg 1998; 24:315–20.
20. Bernstein LJ, Kauvar ANB, Grossman MC, Geronemus RG. The short and long-term side effects of carbon dioxide laser resurfacing. Dermatol Surg 1997; 23:519–25.
21. Tanzi EL, Alster TS. Side effects and complications of variable-pulsed erbium:yttrium-aluminum-garnet laser skin resurfacing: extended experience with 50 patients. Plast Reconstr Surg 2003; 111:1524–9.
22. Walia S, Alster TS. Cutaneous CO_2 laser resurfacing infection rate with and without prophylactic antibiotics. Dermatol Surg 1999; 25:857–61.
23. Alster TS, Nanni CA. Famciclovir prophylaxis of herpes simplex virus reactivation after cutaneous laser resurfacing. Dermatol Surg 1997; 25:242–6.
24. Sriprachya-Anunt S, Fitzpatrick RE, Goldman MP et al. Infections complicating pulsed carbon dioxide laser resurfacing for photoaged facial skin. Dermatol Surg 1997; 23:527–36.
25. Ruiz-Esparza J, Gomez JB. Nonablative radiofrequency for active acne vulgaris: the use of deep dermal heat in the treatment of moderate to severe active acne vulgaris (thermotherapy): a report in 22 patients. Dermatol Surg 2003; 29:333–9.

Chapter 11

Photodynamic Therapy

Michael H. Gold

Introduction

Photodynamic therapy (PDT), utilizing the topical administration of 20% 5-aminolevulinic acid (ALA), has become a very popular therapeutic option available for dermasurgeons and laser surgeons treating a variety of cosmetic and medical dermatologic concerns. This chapter will describe ALA-PDT and review the major literature regarding its use in dermatology. Clinical examples will also be presented and protocols described, all of which will demonstrate the usefulness and effectiveness of ALA-PDT as we move into the twenty-first century.

PDT can trace its origins back to 1900 when Rabb[1] found that *Paramecium caudatum* cells died faster when exposed to light in the presence of acridine orange. The term 'photodynamic effect' was described in 1904 when Von Tappeiner and Jodblauer[2] described an oxygen-consuming chemical reaction process with fluorescence in protozoa after the application of aniline dyes. In 1905, Jesionek and Von Tappeiner[3] utilized a topical 5% eosin as a photosensitizer along with artificial light to successfully treat human nonmelanoma skin cancers as well as other dermatologic entities, including condyloma lata and lupus vulgaris. Although these reports heralded a beginning for the use of PDT in research and science, its use was not very widespread and was not popularized again until 1948, when Figge and his colleagues[4] demonstrated that hematoporphyrin could be selectively concentrated into a variety of tissues, including neoplastic, embryonic, and traumatized skin. A purified synthetic hematoporphyrin derivative was then developed and became the standard for PDT at this time. In 1978, Dougherty and his collaborators[5] presented their data with the hematoporphyrin purified derivative and photo-activation with a red light source in the treatment of cutaneous and several other malignancies. Since that time, a number of investigators have reported on the use of PDT for a variety of malignancies[6–11] and other nononcologic conditions.[12–15] These medical uses are shown in Box 11.1.

Because of the unique nature of skin, and because of its accessibility to light and light sources, a great deal of research has been focused on the skin and its reaction processes in relation to ALA-PDT. Early on, it was established that by utilizing an appropriate skin photosensitizer or a precursor of the particular photosensitizer, there would be accumulation of the product predominantly in dystrophic/actinic cells and/or in the skin's pilosebaceous glands. With exposure of these areas of skin with an appropriate wavelength of light, the photosensitizing agent produces an activated oxygen species, known as singlet oxygen, that is capable of selectively destroying cells that contain the photosensitizing agent.[16,17]

The purified hematoporphyrin derivative served as the photosensitizer of choice until 1990, when Kennedy and his group[18] introduced 5-ALA as a new photosensitizing precursor agent. 5-ALA can penetrate the stratum corneum to accumulate in the dystrophic/actinic/cancer cells of the skin, as well as in the cells of the pilosebaceous units in the skin. Once in the appropriate skin cells, 5-ALA is transformed into a highly photoactive endogenous porphyrin derivative, protoporphyrin IX (PpIX). PpIX could then be activated by a variety of light sources to yield selective tissue destruction. The absorption spectrum for PpIX (Fig. 11.1) shows peak absorption bands in the blue and red light ranges of the absorption spectrum, but with a number of smaller peaks in between the blue and red, all of which have become important as we move into different applications for ALA-PDT in the twenty-first century.

In the United States, PDT therapy was first used as a treatment modality for nonhyperkeratotic actinic keratoses (AKs) of the face and scalp. AKs confront dermatologists on a daily basis in their clinical practices. The Actinic Keratosis Consensus Conference of 2001[19] reported that AKs are a marker for photodamage and that their etiology is ultraviolet (UV) light, specifically UVB light. The conference noted that AKs have DNA gene alterations that are associated with squamous cell carcinomas (SCCs), especially in alterations in the tumor-suppressing gene *p53*.

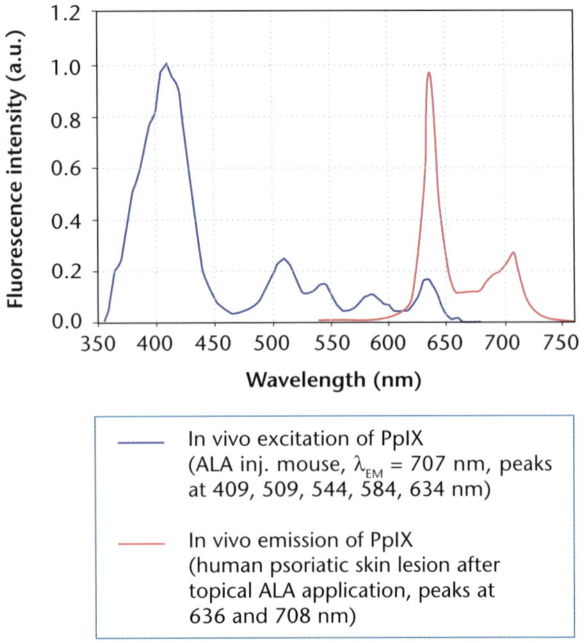

Figure 11.1 Absorption spectrum for protoporphyrin IX (PpIX).[67]

Box 11.1 *Medical Uses for Photodynamic Therapy*

- Malignancies:
  - lung
  - esophagus
  - colon
  - peritoneum
  - pleura
  - GI tract
  - brain
  - eye
  - skin
- Nononcologic conditions:
  - atherosclerosis
  - infectious diseases
  - rheumatoid arthritis.

Although the natural history of AKs was determined to be variable, in that some of the AKs will regress, some will remain stable and others will progress into SCCs, the conference concluded that AKs are a carcinoma in situ and that all AKs should be treated to prevent transformation into a cutaneous malignancy. In fact, the dermatologic literature has reports from 0.1% conversion to 20% conversion from AK to SCC. Treatment modalities, including both medical and surgical for AKs, are shown in Box 11.2.

In Europe, ALA-PDT research has centered not only on its ability to treat AKs but also on its potential for treating superficial nonmelanoma skin cancers. These have included its use in treating superficial SCCs, SCCs in situ (Bowen's disease), and to the treatment of superficial basal cell carcinoma (BCC). A number of peer-reviewed studies/reports have appeared in the medical literature over the past 20 or so years describing successes with ALA-PDT and AKs, Bowen's disease, SCCs, and BCCs.[20–22] These are summarized in Table 11.1.

Box 11.2 *Treatment Options for Actinic Keratoses*

- Medical:
  - 5-fluorouracil
  - imiquimod
  - topical retinoids
  - dicofenac
- Surgical:
  - cryosurgery
  - curettage
  - excisional surgery
  - diffuse destructive process:
    - chemical peels
    - dermabrasion
    - laser resurfacing
- ALA-PDT photodynamic therapy.

Box 11.3 *Dermatolgic Entities Treated with ALA-PDT*

- Cutaneous T-cell lymphoma
- Kaposi's sarcoma
- Malignant melanoma
- Keratoacanthoma
- Extramammary Paget's disease
- Acne vulgaris
- Sebaceous gland hyperplasia
- Hidradenitis suppurativa
- Psoriasis vulgaris
- Verrucae vulgaris
- Molluscum contagiosum
- Actinic chelitis
- Hirsutism
- Alopecia areata
- Photorejuvenation/photoaging.

Of note from the group of papers summarized in Table 11.1 is that a variety of light sources have been utilized over the years but the results have remained fairly constant. For AKs, response rates from 80% to 100% are routinely reported. For Bowen's disease, response rates of between 90 and 100% are common. For superficial BCCs and SCCs, response rates range from 67% to 100% clearance with ALA-PDT; slightly lower for more advanced/nodular lesions.[23,24] Treatment protocols varied amongst the authors presented in Table 11.1 but the majority utilized multiple treatment applications with sufficient follow-up time periods to document adequate response of ALA-PDT in treating these entities.

Other dermatologic entities, besides those already mentioned, that have been reported to be successfully treated with ALA-PDT are listed in Box 11.3.[21,22]

Two main photosensitizing agents are currently being utilized for PDT at this time: Levulan® Kerastick™ (Dusa Pharmaceuticals, Wilmington, MA) and Metvix® (PhotoCure ASA, Norway, with marketing rights by Galderma, Fort Worth, TX). The Levulan® is a 20% 5-ALA solution and the Metvix® is the methyl-ester cream derivative of 5-ALA. Both compounds have had extensive study over the past several years.

Table 11.1 *Peer-reviewed Medical Reports for ALA-PDT Utilizing 20% 5-ALA*[67]

Indication	Author(s)	Year(s)	Sensitizer/light source	Results
Actinic keratoses	Kennedy et al	1990	20% ALA/filtered slide projector	Complete response in 90%
	Wolf et al	1992, 1993	20% ALA/filtered slide projector	80–100% response
	Morton et al	1995	20% ALA/filtered slide projector	80–100% response
	Fijan et al	1995	20% ALA/filtered slide projector	80–100% response
	Calzavara-Pinton	1995	20% ALA/argon laser	100% response
	Calzavara-Pinton	1997	20% ALA/argon laser	84% response on F/U from 1995
	Jeffes et al	1997	10–30% ALA/argon laser	91% face/scalp; trunk/extremities 45%
	Pinzi et al	2000	20% ALA/incoherent light source	100% response
	Kurwa et al	1999	20% ALA/non-laser light	More rapid response than 5 FU/equivalent
	Fritsch et al	1997	20% ALA/green light	Results at 6 months Painless
Bowen's disease	Calzavara-Pinton et al	1997	20% ALA/argon laser	90–100% response
	Pinzi et al	2000	20% ALA/tungsten filament lamp	90–100% response
	Svamberg et al	1994	20% ALA/Nd:YAG dye laser	90–100% response
	Cairnduff et al	1994	20% ALA/CVDL	97% clearance at 2 months (35/36); 89% at 18 months
	Morton et al	1996	20% ALA/filtered xenon lamp	Superior to cryotherapy in 20 patients
	Morton et al	2000	20% ALA/non-laser light source	Red light more effective than green light
	Stables et al	1997	20% ALA/non-laser light source	Complete response in 3 patients
Basal cell carcinomas	Clzavara-Pinton et al	1997	20% ALA/argon laser	*The next 6 authors show following results*: superficial BCCs 87–100% response nodular BCCs 10–80% response
	Pinzi et al	2000	20% ALA/tungsten filament lamp	
	Thissen et al	2000	20% ALA/Versalight	
	Morton et al	1998	20% ALA/xenon lamp	
	Svamberg et al	1994	20% ALA/Nd:YAG-pumped dye laser	
	Wolf et al	1993	20% ALA/filtered slide projector	
	Kennedy et al	1990	20% ALA/filtered slide projector	*93.7% superficial BCC response; 19.4% recurrence rate;*
	Carinduff et al	1994	20% ALA/CVDL	
	McCaughan	1999	3.0 mg/kg ALA IV/2 argon laser	*88% superficial BCC response*
	Calzavara-Pinton	1993	20% ALA argon pumped dye laser	*100% response rate*
	Haller et al	2000	20% ALA/non-laser light source	*100% response rate*
	Itoh et al	2000	20% ALA/halogen lamp	*1 recurrence of 20 superfical BCCs; 16 months*
	Pennington et al	1998	5 mg/kg IV ALA/coherent light	*F/U* *16 pigment BCCs – good results* *100% response clinically; histological exam residual in 50%*
Squamous cell carcinomas	Kennedy et al	1990	20% ALA/filtered slide projector	*The next 5 authors show the following results*:
	Calzavara-Pinton	1997	20% ALA/argon laser	67–92% response for superficial SCCs
	Pinzi et al	2000	20% ALA/tungsten filament lamp	0–67% for nodular SCCs
	Calzavara-Pinton	1993	20% ALA argon pumped dye laser	High recurrence rates
	Wolf et al	1993	20% ALA/filtered slide projector	High recurrence rates
	Pennington et al	1988	5 mg/kg IV ALA/coherent light	10/10 response superficial SCCs; 50% nodular SCCs
	Fink-Puckes et al	1998	20% ALA/incoherent light source	
	Fritsch et al	1999	20% ALA ointment/Wood's lamp	

Metvix® is the main 5-ALA product currently being utilized in Europe. It has European Union (EU) approval for the treatment of nonhyperkeratotic AKs of the face and scalp and for the treatment of BCCs that are 'unsuitable' for conventional therapy. As of the time of this writing, Metvix® has US Food and Drug Administration (FDA) approval for the treatment of nonhyperkeratotic AKs of the face and scalp but it is not, at this time, being marketed or promoted in the US. The recommended treatment protocols describe the gentle scraping or curettage of the affected lesion prior to the application of the methyl 5-ALA cream. After the application of the cream, the area is occluded for 3 hours before the lesion is subjected to red light therapy.

Clinical studies/trials have recently shown the effectiveness of Metvix® in the treatment of AKs and BCCs. Freeman and colleagues[25] studied the methyl 5-ALA cream in 204 individuals with red light and compared their results to cryotherapy and placebo. The methyl 5-ALA group had better response rates as compared to cryotherapy and placebo as well as cosmetic improvements. Pariser et al[26] evaluated 80 patients with the methyl 5-ALA cream and AKs. Their study yielded an 89% response rate for the AKs and a 90% improvement in their cosmetic appearance; 72% preferred ALA-PDT over cryotherapy and 5-fluorouracil. Rhodes et al[27] reported on a prospective randomized study of 101 patients with BCCs either treated with methyl 5-ALA or surgery. After the first 3-month follow-up period there was a 98% complete response rate with surgery compared to a 91% response with the methyl 5-ALA. At 12 months, the response rate was 96% for surgery as compared to 83% for the methyl 5-ALA; the cosmetic appearance was noted to be better in the methyl 5-ALA group at this time period. At 24 months, one recurrence was noted in the surgical group; there were five in the methyl 5-ALA group. Recently, Wulf and Philipsen[28] reported a case of allergic contact dermatitis to the methyl 5-ALA that did not show an allergic response when repeated utilizing 5-ALA alone.

In the US, at the time of this writing, the only product currently available for use by physicians is the Levulan® Kerastick™. The Kerastick™ is shown in Figure 11.2. The Levulan® Kerastick™ is a 20% weight/volume 5-ALA solution with 48% ethanol. It has a dermatologic applicator attached at one of its ends, which allows for accurate application of the medication. The applicator tip is attached to a flexible glass tubing which contains two glass vials. One vial contains the 5-ALA in a powder form and the other glass vial contains the ethanol solvent. The vials are broken by light manual pressure to the tubing and then the contents are slowly mixed back and forth for several minutes by gentle rotation. The package insert recommendation is to rotate and mix the medicine in the tubing for three minutes prior to the application onto the skin.[29]

The patient requires preparation for the procedure as well. This will be covered in detail later (see p. 285). In brief, the skin is washed with a mild cleanser followed by one or two applications of the 5-ALA. Some clinicians recommend that all patients receive an acetone scrub or a microdermabrasion procedure prior to the application of the 5-ALA to enhance the penetration of the ALA into the skin. The drug is allowed to incubate on the skin for a certain time period which is determined by the physician and the entity being treated. Then the 5-ALA is washed off the skin with a gentle cleanser prior to the PDT treatment with an appropriate light source. Once the procedure is completed, care must be taken for the next 24–48 hours to avoid exposure to the sun and possibly creating a phototoxic response from this therapy.

The first clinical trial with Levulan® was reported by Jeffes et al in 2001.[30] In this Phase II FDA trial, 36 individuals with nonhyperkeratotic AKs of the face and scalp were evaluated for safety and efficacy of the product. The 5-ALA was prepared as previously described. The drug was placed on individual lesions and allowed to incubate on the skin/within the AKs for 14–18 hours without occlusion of the medication. The patients were then subjected to a low intensity blue light source for 16 minutes and 40 seconds (1000 seconds). The blue light source utilized for the trial was the BluU® (Dusa Pharmaceuticals, Wilmington, MA; Fig. 11.3). The BluU® has a wavelength distribution between 410 and 430 nm and provides a dose of $10\,J/cm^2$ to the affected areas.

The results from this initial clinical trial showed that nonhyperkeratotic AKs were effectively treated with this modality and the procedure was safe. Specifically, 66% of the treated AKs responded to one ALA-PDT treatment. For those AKs that did not respond ($n = 16$), a second treatment after 8 weeks improved the efficacy rate to 85% at

A B

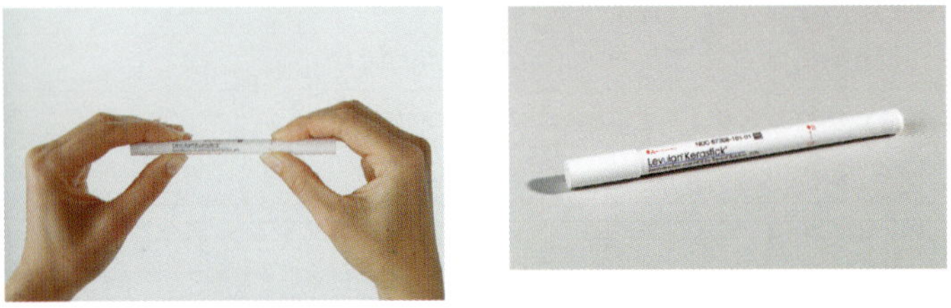

Figure 11.2 Levulan® Kerastick™. (Courtesy DUSA Pharmaceuticals, Inc.)

A B

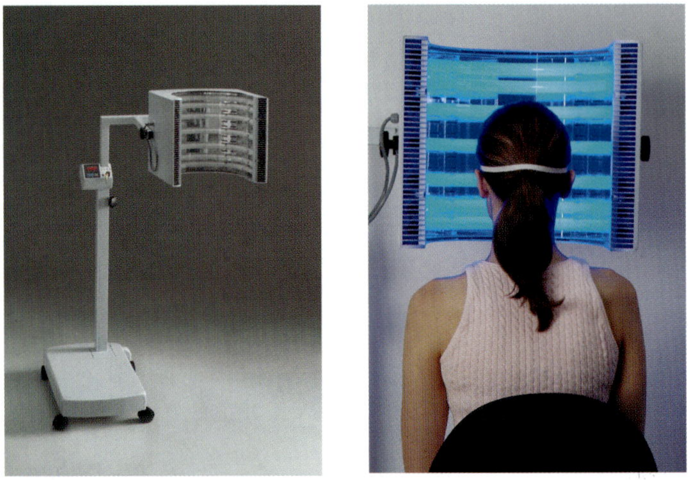

Figure 11.3 BlueU® light source. (Courtesy DUSA Pharmaceuticals, Inc.)

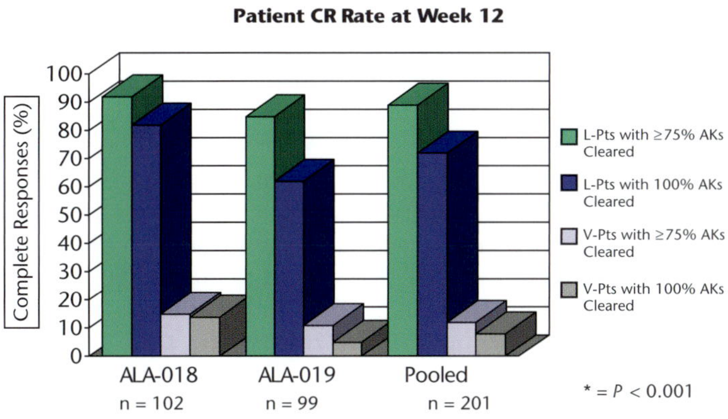

Figure 11.4 Levulan® Phase III efficacy data at 12 weeks. L, Levulan; V, vehicle (placebo). (Courtesy DUSA Pharmaceuticals, Inc.)

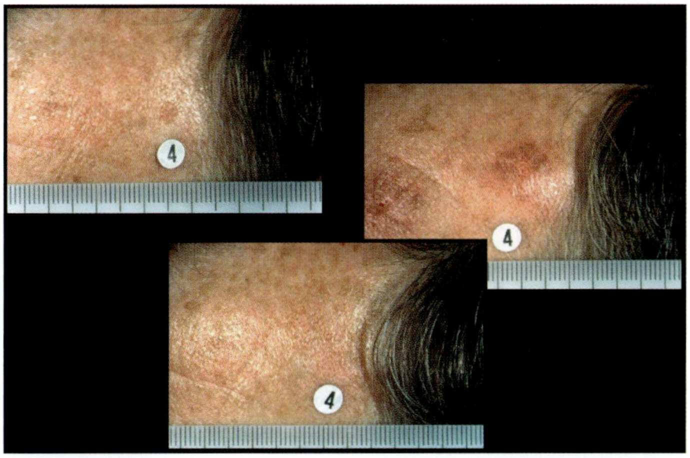

Figure 11.5 Clinical example from Levulan® Phase III Trial. Top: before; middle: 1 week post treatment; bottom: 1 month post treatment. (Courtesy DUSA Pharmaceuticals, Inc.)

week 16. All patients noted stinging and burning during their light therapy; facial erythema was noted in 96% of the patients; all resolved by the first four week follow-up time period.

A larger Phase III FDA pivotal trial was then conducted utilizing 243 individuals. Two applications of either the 5-ALA solution or a vehicle placebo solution were applied to individual AK lesions – nonhyperkeratotic AKs of the face and scalp. Patients had to have between 4 and 15 nonhyperkeratotic AKs to participate in this phase of the trial. Incubation times for the 5-ALA remained at 14–18 hours and patients once again received 16 minutes and 40 seconds of light therapy. Results from this Phase III trial showed statistical differences between active 5-ALA and placebo (Fig. 11.4). More than 70% of the lesions treated with active 5-ALA were reported clear at the end of a 12-week follow-up period. Lesions that had not cleared completely were retreated at 8 weeks. The results, at the conclusion of the trial, showed that 88% of the patients with active medicine had a greater than or equal to 75% response rate as compared to 20% in the vehicle/placebo solution group of patients.[31] A patient example is shown in Fig. 11.5. The treatments in this Phase III trial were well tolerated by the study participants. Adverse events, known as the PDT response or effect, included stinging, burning, itching, erythema, and edema. These were all local and transient responses with some patients requiring up to a one week 'healing' period; no noncutaneous responses were seen. An important secondary endpoint for this trial evaluated physician and patient assessments as to the improvement in the cosmetic appearance of the skin. A total of 94% of the patients and 92% of the physicians rated the cosmetic appearance as either good to excellent.

From these initial clinical trials, a group of clinical investigators began looking at alternatives to the previously described techniques to make the therapy more useful and more easily able to be utilized by colleagues in dermatology and laser medicine. Specifically, investigations began looking at drug incubation – both time and individual treatment. As photoaging and photodamage involve the entire face and not just the area where an AK is visible, studies looking at full-face 5-ALA drug applications began. Drug incubation times have also been looked at quite extensively; 14- to 18-hour drug incubation times are inconvenient to the majority of patients. Also, investigators began looking at the variety of lasers and light sources that fit into the two peaks seen in the PpIX absorption curves (see Fig. 11.1). Work with blue lights, intense pulsed lights (IPLs), and the vascular lasers have expanded the reach of ALA-PDT to include most physicians owning these devices. The newer lasers and light sources are faster procedures and have appropriate cooling devices which help make the procedures run smoother and as a result yield very little adverse events and associated downtime.

In a very important clinical trial, Touma et al[32] evaluated 18 patients with mild to moderate photodamage utilizing 1-, 2-, and 3-hour drug incubation versus traditional 14- to 18-hour drug incubation. A blue light source was used in this trial. The authors found no difference between one hour drug incubation and 14–18 hours. In fact, their patients noted improvement in the sallowness of the skin, fine wrinkling, and mottled hyperpigmentation with the short drug incubation times.

Ruiz-Rodriquez et al[33] studied short drug incubation (4 hours) and the use of an IPL in the treatment of photorejuvenation and associated AKs. Seventeen patients were evaluated with varying degrees of photodamage and AKs (n = 38). Two 5-ALA-PDT treatments utilizing the IPL yielded excellent cosmetic results and an 87% response – improvement in wrinkling, skin texture, pigmentation changes, and telangectasias, as well as improvement in 33 of the 38 AKs treated. They coined the term 'photodynamic photorejuvenation' for this type of treatment. Gold[34] has also reported findings utilizing short-contact, full-face ALA-PDT utilizing an IPL device in 10 patients. The patients received 3-monthly ALA-PDT IPL treatments with a 3-month follow-up period. Drug incubation was from 30–60 minutes. At the end of the follow-up time, 83% of the targeted AKs responded to the therapy; there was a 90% improvement in crow's feet appearance, 100% improvement in tactile skin roughness, 90% improvement in mottled hyperpigmentation, and 70% improvement if facial erythema.

Goldman et al[35] studied 32 patients with moderate photodamage and multiple AKs utilizing short-contact (1-

hour drug incubation), full-face ALA, and a blue light source (one session). At the end of the 6-month trial session, 90% of the targeted AKs responded to the therapy and photorejuvenation parameters improved as well (improvement in skin texture in 72% and skin pigmentation in 59%). Of interest, 62.5% of the patients in the study who had previous cryotherapy found the ALA-PDT treatment less painful. Avram et al[36] reported results with short-contact (1-hour drug incubation), full-face ALA-PDT utilizing an IPL device in 17 patients with photodamage and associated AKs. After one therapy, 69% of the targeted AKs responded to the ALA-PDT IPL and photorejuvenation results showed an improvement in telangectasias in 55%, pigment irregularities in 48%, and skin texture in 25%.

The vascular lasers, especially the pulsed dye lasers, have also been studied for their effects for use in ALA-PDT. Alexiades-Armenakas et al[37] evaluated both 3-hour and 14- to 18-hour drug incubation and found both successful in treating targeted AKs and in improving the parameters of photorejuvenation. Their group utilized a 595 nm pulsed dye laser, fluences of 4–7.5 J/cm^2, 10-ms pulse durations, 10-mm spot sizes, and 30-ms cryogen sprays. Their initial study evaluated 2561 face and scalp AKs with clearances of 99.9% at 10 days; 94.8% at 2 months; and 90.1% at 4 months. Torso lesions showed a 54.5% response at 10 days and 74.4% at 2 months. Recently, Alexiades-Armenakas et al[38] reported their use of a pulse dye laser system with ALA-PDT for the treatment of actinic chelitis. Nineteen patients were evaluated with a drug incubation period of 2–3 hours. Patients received up to three laser treatments. A 68% complete clearance rate was demonstrated at 12 months.

Two split-face ALA-PDT IPL trials have recently been reported. Bhatia et al[39] used three split-face treatments (IPL + ALA versus IPL alone) at 3-week intervals followed by two full face IPL treatments at 3-week intervals and a 4-week follow-up visit in 20 individuals. The global score for photoaging was 80% versus 50% (IPL +ALA versus IPL); 95% versus 65% for mottled hyperpigmentation; and 55% versus 20% for fine lines. Gold et al[40] used 3-monthly IPL + ALA versus IPL alone in a split-face technique in 13 patients. They found a 78% versus 53.6% difference in targeted AKs; a 55% versus 28.5% improvement in crow's feet appearance; a 55% versus 29.5% improvement in tactile skin roughness; a 60.3% versus 37.2% improvement in mottled hyperpigmentation; and an 84.6% versus 53.8% improvement in facial erythema.

The results outlined above show that a variety of lasers and light sources are useful for the treatment of photodamage/photoaging with concurrent AKs. The use of short-contact, full-face therapy with medical devices commonly seen in our offices makes this therapy very attractive to most clinicians. The results also indicate that with ALA-PDT one can shorten the expected number of treatments usually required for photorejuvenation, from an average of five or six total treatments to one to three treatments. As a result of our clinical experiments, it is also hoped that we are, perhaps, preventing or delaying the onset of a non-melanoma skin cancer and that perhaps this therapy is photo-protective in some manner. Researchers are evaluating this concept at this time.

Photodynamic therapy has also moved in other directions recently in the US. This has included investigations/studies for the management of moderate to severe inflammatory acne vulgaris, sebaceous gland hyperplasia, and hidradenitis suppurativa.

Acne vulgaris is one of the most common skin disorders seen, accounting for over 30% of all visits to the dermatologist. It is estimated that at least 80% of all individuals will suffer from acne vulgaris at some point in their lifetime.[41]

Acne vulgaris is a multifactorial disease. Genetics and hormonal factors that begin during puberty play an active role in the development of acne vulgaris. Acne is a disorder of the sebaceous glands, where hormonal activity causes dilatation and then obstruction of the glands themselves. The obstruction leads to the production and eventual proliferation of bacteria within the glands. The most common bacteria which are seen associated with acne vulgaris is *Propionobacterium acnes*. With this proliferation of *P. acnes*, acne lesions become inflammatory, with production of papules, pustules, and cysts.

Treatment options for acne vulgaris are myriad and varied; individualized treatment regimens assure the best possible chances for a successful therapeutic response. Both topical and systemic agents are available for the management of patients with acne vulgaris. However, recent reports have made warnings that we, as physicians, must be aware of, and help educate our patients, especially when we are dealing with those suffering from moderate to severe inflammatory acne vulgaris. Systemic drug resistance rates of up to 60% have been reported[41,42] and a study potentially linking long-term tetracycline (oral) use and the development of breast cancer has recently been published.[43] Teratogenic and potential psychiatric concerns with the oral retinoids at times hinder their regular use.

Exposure to natural and artificial UV light has been reported as successful in treating acne vulgaris over the years.[44] The exact mechanism is not fully understood but it is felt to be, in part, due to destruction of the *P. acnes* in the sebaceous unit. This is a natural endogenous PDT reaction but is precluded from regular use due to the known damaging effects of prolonged UV light including photodamage and the development of skin cancers.

During the growth cycle of *P. acnes*, there is a natural production of porphyrins in the bacteria. The porphyrins produced are predominately PpIX and coproporphyrin III, which have absorption spectra peaks in the near ultraviolet range of light, in the blue light range, with a peak absorption seen at 415 nm (see Fig. 11.1). The PDT reaction works through the photoactivation of the *P. acnes* porphyrins by exposure to an appropriate light source. Finally, destruction of the *P. acnes* will occur, with specific destruction of the inflammatory acne lesion, leaving surrounding structures and tissues alone.[45]

A variety of lasers and light sources have been used over the years to treat inflammatory acne vulgaris. These have included halogen, xenon, and tungsten light sources. More recently, investigations have focused primarily on blue and red light sources, and with the addition of 5-ALA, blue light, IPLs, and vascular lasers. These devices focus on destruction of the *P. acnes* and reduction of sebaceous gland output over time. Still other laser systems being studied focus on the destruction of the entire sebaceous gland and associated structures. These devices and clinical evaluations are summarized in Table 11.2.

As with the evaluations for photorejuvenation and associated AKs, a group of clinical investigators have begun to study ALA-PDT for those patients suffering from moderate to severe inflammatory acne vulgaris. The idea is to use short-contact, full-face therapy with 5-ALA and a variety of lasers and light sources to make them work better than has been previously described with the device alone. The first report describing the use of ALA for inflammatory acne vulgaris was in 2000 by Hongcharu et al,[53] who looked at a broad band light source (500–700 nm) using ALA with a 3-hour drug incubation in 22 patients with inflammatory acne vulgaris. The trial results showed significant clearance after four weeks which persisted for up to 20 weeks in those who had multiple treatments or 10 weeks in those who had one 5-ALA treatment. Adverse effects included a PDT effect of an acneform folliculitis, postinflammatory hyperpigmentation, superficial peeling, and crusting.

Itoh et al[54] reported the use of ALA and a 635 nm pulsed excimer dye laser in an 'intractable' case of inflammatory acne vulgaris on the face. After treatment the area remained clear for 8 months; a classic PDT reaction, however, was seen. A second study by Itoh et al[55] looked at single ALA treatments in 13 individuals utilizing a polychromatic visible light (600–700 nm, 17 mW/cm^2, and 13 J/cm^2). The inflammatory acne vulgaris lesions improved in all the patients and new lesion counts were reduced at 1, 3, and 6 months. From months 6–12, acne lesions and seborrhea recurred. Again, patients in this trial had a classic PDT effect with erythema, edema, and crusting.

Goldman[56] reported on his experience with short-contact (1-hour) drug incubation with 5-ALA and treatment with either the IPL or blue light source for the treatment of acne vulgaris and sebaceous gland hyperplasia. Treatments were noted to be pain free and were without adverse events. Relative clearing of the acne lesions occurred within 2–4 weeks. Gold[57] evaluated 10 patients with moderate to severe inflammatory acne vulgaris utilizing short-contact (30 minute ALA drug incubation) and a high intensity blue light source. Four-weekly treatments showed a response of approximately 60% (compared to 43% with blue light alone). The treatments were well tolerated with no PDT effect seen. Goldman et al[58] reported their experience with the blue light source with and without ALA in 22 individuals with inflammatory acne vulgaris. There was a greater response in the ALA-PDT/blue light group than blue light alone with no significant adverse effects and no PDT effect. Gold et al[59] recently reported a new IPL device used in conjunction with ALA-PDT in 12 patients. At the end of the trial, there was a 71.8% response seen in the inflammatory acne lesions. No significant adverse events were seen and, more importantly, no PDT effects seen.

From these clinical trials it appears that the use of short-contact, full-face 20% 5-ALA in conjunction with a variety of lasers and light sources provides a synergistic effect in the photodynamic process to effectively treat our patients suffering from moderate to severe inflammatory acne vulgaris. This combination therapy is safe with little downtime seen and appears to offer our patients a rapid response to this, at times, difficult problem. It also may eliminate the need for more intensive systemic therapies with potential adverse effects not acceptable to our patients.

As a caveat to the treatment of acne vulgaris, investigators have looked at treating lesions of sebaceous gland hyperplasia (SGH), often a difficult cosmetic problem to treat. Numerous therapies have been used, as outlined in Box 11.4.

Treatment with the pulsed dye laser (PDL) alone has shown promising results in patients with SGH.[60]

Horio et al[61] were the first to describe the use of 5-ALA in the treatment of SGH. Using a slide projector as a light source, they treated facial SGH lesions in a 61-year-old Japanese man three times at 1-week intervals. The drug incubation time was 4 hours. The lesions became smaller with each successive treatment and the reduced sizes per-

Table 11.2 *Acne Vulgaris: Lasers and Light Source Studies*

Source	Laser/light source	Percent response
Destruction of *P. acnes*		
Papageorgiou et al[46]	Blue light	63% response*
Kawada et al[47]	Blue light	65% response*
Elman et al[48]	Blue light	60–75% response*
Gold[49]	Blue light	43% response
Elman et al[48]	IPL	>50% response*
Gregory et al[50]	IPL	>50% response*
Destruction of sebaceous glands**		
Lloyd et al[51]		810 nm diode after ICG treatment
Paithanker et al[52]		1450 nm laser

*15–20% nonresponders eliminated from data.

**Both studies showed success in treating inflammatory acne lesions.

Box 11.4 *Treatment Modalities for Sebaceous Gland Hyperplasia*

- Cryotherapy
- Excision
- Electrodessication
- CO_2 laser surgery
- Oral isotretinoin
- Pulsed dye laser
- ALA-PDT with blue light, vascular lasers, IPLs.

sisted for 1 year. The treatments were well tolerated. Alster et al[62] reported on 10 patients with SGH using a 595 nm pulsed dye laser. The 20% 5-ALA was incubated on the lesions for 1 hour. Seven patients cleared with one treatment; three patients required two treatments. The ALA-PDT treated lesions were superior to pulsed dye laser treated only areas in this trial. Richey et al[63] used a blue light source and one hour drug incubation in treating 10 patients with SGH. Patients received 3–6 treatments at 1-week intervals and were followed for 6 months. A 70% clearance rate was seen with recurrences of 20% within 3–4 months following the final treatment. Gold et al[64] recently reported their results with SGH and both blue light and IPL. Six patients received short-contact (30–60 minutes), full-face ALA-PDT and blue light therapy monthly for four consecutive months; clearance rates of 55.3% were seen. Five patients received IPL therapy with clearance rates of 55.3%.

Finally, ALA-PDT has shown success in the treatment of recalcitrant hidradenitis suppurativa (HS), although this is typically thought of as an apocrine disorder. Gold et al[65] reported on the successful use of ALA-PDT and the high intensity blue light source in four individuals who had recalcitrant HS. Short-contact 20% 5-ALA was used for 30–60 minutes before exposure to a blue light source. Three to four sessions at 1- to 2-week intervals yielded between 75% and 100% improvements in all the patients treated. Further studies to verify these results need to be performed.

ALA-PDT has become an important therapeutic modality, finding new niches for its use in dermatology and laser medicine. The only approved indication for ALA-PDT is for the treatment of nonhyperkeratotic AKs of the face and scalp with a blue light source and with a drug incubation period of 14–18 hours. The clinical trials presented in this chapter for photorejuvenation, acne vulgaris, SGH, and HS are all off-label uses and the physician must inform patients of this. Physicians can use ALA-PDT in any fashion they feel it will benefit their patients and work is underway to expand the approved indications for its use.

Clinical Technique

Patient Selection

Candidates for ALA-PDT for photorejuvenation and associated AKs should have clinical signs of photodamage and AKs. Photodamage may be manifest by a patient having one or more of the following signs present on their facial skin: fine lines and wrinkles, irregular thinning of the epidermis, blotchy hyperpigmentation, and telangectasia formation. Fair-skinned individuals with photodamage and associated AKs of the face and scalp are the best candidates for photorejuvenation with ALA-PDT. It is of interest to note that in the Asian population, ALA-PDT is being used successfully for the treatment of melasma and other disorders of pigmentation.[66]

Those patients with acne vulgaris should present with moderate to severe inflammatory acne vulgaris lesions. Skin type is not as crucial here; skin types I–VI has been successfully treated with both blue light sources and the IPLs. Vascular lasers, if they are to be used, should be used only in more fairer-skinned individuals.

Choice of Lasers

The following lasers and light sources are currently being used for ALA-PDT and photorejuvenation with concurrent AKs:

1. IPL Quantum SR* (Lumenis Ltd., Yokneam, Israel):
   a. 560 nm filter
   b. double pulse (2.4/4.0 ms with 10-ms delay)
   c. single pass with no overlap
   d. 25–35 J/cm^2
2. Lumenis One* (Lumenis Ltd., Yokneam, Israel):
   a. 560 nm filter
   b. double pulse (4.0/4.0 ms with 20-ms delay)
   c. single pass with no overlap
   d. 15–25 J/cm^2
3. VascuLight SR* (Lumenis Ltd., Yokneam, Israel):
   a. 560 nm filter
   b. double pulse (3.0/6.0 ms with 10-ms delay)
   c. single pass with no overlap
   d. 30–35 J/cm^2
4. EsteLux Pulsed Light System* (Palomar Medical Technologies, Burlington, MA):
   a. 20 ms
   b. 19–30 J/cm^2
   c. single pass with no overlap
5. Photogenica V Star* (Cynosure Inc., Chelmsford, MA):
   a. 585 nm or 595 nm wavelength PDL
   b. 10-mm spot size
   c. 40-ms pulse width
   d. 7.5 J/cm^2
   e. two passes with 50% overlap
6. V Beam (Candela Corp., Wayland, MA):
   a. 595 nm PDL
   b. 10-mm spot size
   c. 6-ms pulse width
   d. 7.5 J/cm^2
   e. two 2 passes with 50% overlap
7. ClearLight* (Lumenis Ltd., Yokneam, Israel):
   a. 405–420 nm blue light
   b. 8–10 minutes under light
8. BluU* (Dusa Pharmaceuticals, Wilmington, MA):
   a. 417 nm ± 5 nm blue light
   b. 8–15 minutes under light
9. SkinStation* (Radiancy, Orangeburg, NY):
   a. 500–1200 nm pulsed light
   b. two passes
   c. 45 J/cm^2
10. Aurora (Syneron Medical Ltd., Yokneam, Israel):
    a. 580–980 nm
    b. optical energy of 16–22 J/cm^2; RF energy of 16–22 J/cm^2
    c. single pass
11. PhotoLight* (Cynosure Inc., Chelmsford, MA):
    a. 550 nm filter
    b. 8 J/cm^2
    c. 15–20 ms
    d. single pass

12. Sciton BBL* (Sciton Inc., Palo Alto, CA):
    a. 560 nm BBL filter
    b. 14 J/cm^2
    c. 12 ms
    d. single pass.

*Devices used by author; other settings from colleagues.

The following lasers and light sources are currently being used by the author for ALA-PDT treatments for acne vulgaris (other devices listed above are also able to be used) with similar parameters as listed above:

1. ClearLight
2. BluU
3. IPL Quantum
4. Lumenis One
5. VascuLight SR
6. SkinStation.

Treatment Protocol

There is no definitive treatment protocol which every clinician utilizes. Physicians must learn what works best in their clinical practice:

1. If there is a history of herpes simplex virus infection, it is recommended that the patient begins an oral antiviral either the day before the ALA-PDT therapy or on the day of treatment for 3–5 days. The choice of the antiviral is up to the treating physician.
2. The patient will gently wash their face with soap and water. Our patients routinely utilize Cetaphil® or Aquanil® soapless cleanser.
3. The skin is next prepped by either an acetone scrub or a microdermabrasion procedure. Acetone is used not only as an additional skin cleanser but also as a way to increase the penetration of the 20% 5-ALA into the skin. Microdermabrasion, with or without crystals, is another option for increasing the penetration of the 20% 5-ALA. Newer microdermabrasion devices are being promoted for increasing the penetration of topical medications.
4. The Levulan® Kerastick™ is prepared as has already been described in the text.
5. The Levulan®, now in liquid solution, is painted on to the area(s) of the skin you are going to treat. Two coats of the Levulan® are recommended to be applied and extra solution may be 'spot' treated to definitive AKs. It is important to get close to the eyes, as it will be apparent that the orbital skin will not be adequately treated otherwise. Care should be taken to avoid the eyelids, cornea, and ocular canthi.
6. The Levulan® is now allowed to incubate on the skin surface. Most authors recommend a drug incubation period of 1 hour (60 minutes) with the patient being kept indoors, away from direct or reflected light sources. Sun avoidance during this time is crucial, to avoid premature drug activation and the potential for phototoxic eruptions.
7. The face is washed once again with soap and water. This is done to remove any ALA remaining on the skin surface. If there is residual ALA on the skin, the potential for superficial skin burning is increased, as well as increased pain associated with the procedure.
8. The patient then receives his/her treatment with the appropriate light source. Appropriate patient and laser/light source operator protective eyewear and all other laser/light source safety guidelines are to be followed.
9. Following the treatment with 20% 5-ALA and an appropriate light source, various responses on the skin may be observed. Ideally, there will be minimal erythema and edema, which will respond very rapidly to cold compresses and/or ice packs. Swelling, if present, is most evident around the eye areas, and may not be evident for up to 24 hours:
    a. To reduce the potential of the PDT effect, it is recommended not to have the patient apply most topical agents to the skin, including high-potency corticosteroids, vitamin E products, aloe-containing products, and most moisturizers (most contain potential irritants, preservatives, and perfumes which may irritate the skin).
    b. Mild strength topical corticosteroids may be used to reduce potential inflammation, if needed.
    c. Moisturizers, such as Cetaphil® or Aquaphor®, are also regularly recommended.
    d. Analgesics, such as acetaminophen or ibuprofen, may be taken, as needed.
    e. Our office also recommends Avene™ Thermal Spring Water to be applied liberally for several days after the procedure. A new water gel is being evaluated to see how it fits into our treatment paradigm.
    f. Niadyne® skin cleanser and night-time moisturizer are recommended by some authors.
10. Patients must be advised to use proper sun protection for the first 24–48 hours after their light procedure. This is to avoid potential phototoxicity, perhaps the major adverse reaction now seen in our patients undergoing ALA-PDT treatments:
    a. The use of a sunscreen/block with an SPF of 30 or above.
    b. Outdoor exposure is to be limited.
    c. Reflected light, like that associated with light coming through a car window, must be protected against as this light can cause phototoxicity.
    d. Hats and scarves are also useful items to be used in the post-ALA-PDT treatment period.
11. It is important to remember that with the original 14- to 18-hour drug incubation protocol, a PDT effect with downtime and healing was common.
12. Several treatments may be needed for the desired effect to be achieved for each patient. For photorejuvenation and associated AKs, we recommend monthly treatments, as needed. For acne vulgaris treatments, weekly or every other week treatments may be used. The treatments must be individualized for each patient.

Figure 11.6 shows a sample PDT Patient Guide for Photorejuvenation and Associated AKs. Figure 11.7 shows a sample PDT Patient Guide for Acne Treatments. Figure 11.8 shows a sample Informed Consent for ALA-PDT treatments our office uses for all of these procedures. Figure 11.9 shows

THERAPY (PDT) PATIENT GUIDE

WHAT IS PHOTODYNAMIC THERAPY?

Photodynamic therapy (PDT) is a special treatment performed with a topical photosensitizing agent called Levulan (5-aminolevulinic acid or ALA) activated with the correct wavelength of light. This is also known as "ALA/PDT treatment". These treatments remove sun damaged pre-cancerous zones and spots called actinic keratoses. Sun damage, fine lines, and blotchy pigmentation are also improved because of the positive effect of Levulan and the light treatment. ALA/PDT treatment also has the unique ability to minimize pores and reduce oil glands, effectively treating stubborn acne vulgaris, acne rosacea, and improve the appearance of some acne scars.

HOW MUCH IMPROVEMENT CAN I EXPECT?

Patients with severe sun damaged skin manifested by actinic keratosis, texture, and tone changes including mottled pigmentation and skin laxity may see excellent results. You may also see improvement of large pores and pitted acne scars. Active acne can improve dramatically.

HOW MANY TREATMENTS WILL IT TAKE TO SEE THE "BEST RESULTS"?

To achieve maximum improvement of pre-cancerous (actinic keratoses) sun damage, skin tone and texture, a series of three treatments 2–4 weeks apart is the most effective. Some patients with only actinic keratoses are happy with just one treatment. More treatments can be done at periodic intervals in the future to maintain the rejuvenated appearance of the skin.

WHAT ARE THE DISADVANTAGES

Following PDT, the treated areas can appear red with some peeling for 2–7 days. Some patients have an exuberant response to PDT, and experience marked redness of their skin. Temporary swelling of the lips and around your eyes can occur for a few days. Darker pigmented patches called liver spots can become temporarily darker and then peel off leaving normal skin. (This usually occurs over seven to ten days.) Repeat treatments may be necessary as PDT medicine is not an exact science.

WHAT ARE THE ADVANTAGES

1. **Easier** for patients than repeated topical liquid nitrogen, Efudex (5-FU) or Aldara because the side effects are minimal, rapid, healing, and only 1–3 treatments required.
2. The ALA/PDT treatment at our clinic is **painless** verses liquid nitrogen, 5-FU and Aldara.
3. **Reduced scarring** and improved cosmetic outcome compared with cautery, surgery and Efudex. Liquid nitrogen can leave white spots on your skin.
4. **Levulan improves the whole facial area treated** creating one color, texture, and tone rather than just spot treating with liquid nitrogen, cautery and surgery.

In summary, PDT matches the **"Ideal Treatment" for actinic damage:**

- Well tolerated (essentially painless)
- Easily performed by a specialty clinic environment
- Non-invasive (no needles or surgery required)
- Excellent cosmetic outcome (particularly in cosmetic sensitive areas of the face)

TREATMENT STEPS

1. Patients who have a history of recurring cold sores (Herpes simplex type I) should start oral Valtrex 500 mg tablets, two tablets twice daily for three days – starting this prescription the morning of your PDT treatment. The prescription for this product will be ordered for you.
2. Make sure your skin is clean and free of all make-up, moisturizers, and sunscreens. Bring a hat, sunglasses, and scarf when appropriate to the clinic.
3. Photography will be done by the staff before the Levulan is applied.
4. You must sign a consent form.
5. An acetone scrub is performed. This will enhance the absorption of the Levulan and give much more even uptake. In some patients, microdermabrasion will also be performed immediately prior to the application of Levulan.
6. Levulan is applied topically to the whole area to be treated (such as the whole face, back of hands, extensor part of the forearms).
7. The Levulan is left on for 30–60 minutes before any treatment.
8. The Levulan is activated with the Blu-U. This unique spectrum of light activates the Levulan beginning with low energy levels.
9. Post-treatment instructions will be given to you to care for your improved skin.

Figure 11.6 Sample PDT patient guide for photorejuvenation and associated AKs.

PHOTODYNAMIC ACNE TREATMENT

A new procedure is now available that treats active acne as well as older acne scars leaving your skin smoother. The procedure is called Photodynamic Acne Treatment using Levulan.

Photodynamic Acne Treatment is a process by which a photosensitizing agent (Levulan) is applied to your skin. The Levulan is then activated with a specific wavelength of light, which "turns it on." Levulan has been used extensively for the treatment of a variety of different skin conditions, and it is approved by the FDA and Health and Welfare Canada for the treatment of sun damaged skin.

Levulan is a 20% solution of Aminolevulinic Acid (ALA). ALA is a natural substance found throughout your body, as it is a precursor for hemoglobin synthesis. You would be unable to make a red blood cell to carry oxygen without ALA in your body. Consequently, it is a "natural" product found in all humans.

Acne results from the obstruction and inflammation of the sebaceous glands, and it affects 80% of the human population. Acne typically begins in adolescence with hormonal changes. However, there are many older individuals who suffer from "adult acne."

There are several different presentations of acne ranging from comedonal (blackheads and whiteheads), papular, pustular, and cystic acne. In many cases, many of these presentations of acne can be present on an individual simultaneously.

Prior to Photodynamic Acne Treatment, the best available treatment option for cystic acne was Accutane. However, with Accutane there are many systemic side effects including birth defects, liver abnormalities, mood depression, and virtually all patients get dryness and night vision changes. PDT Acne treatment provides a viable alternative for all types of acne treatment.

Photodynamic Acne Treatment is done as follows: The Levulan is applied to your skin and left on for 30–60 minutes. Levulan is a clear solution and painless. Levulan is then activated with a specific wavelength of light called a BLU-U. This takes about 18–23 minutes. The Levulan targets active cells. Acne sebaceous glands are active cells. These cells preferentially absorb Levulan, and these cells are targeted by the Levulan once it is activated; hence the term, photodynamic therapy. The Levulan will also target sebaceous hyperplasia (which are those small (1–3 mm), benign, bumps on your skin) and the papules of acne rosacea. Skin oiliness is decreased, and the appearance of pores is minimized. The entire skin texture improves following a Photodynamic Acne Treatment.

The "downside" of Photodynamic treatment (PDT) is that you will be red and have some skin peeling (and crusting if you have skin cancers) for several days after the treatment.

The advantages of PDT are rapid treatment of acne lesions all over the face without scarring or surgical excision. The skin appears refreshed and younger following these treatments. We advise 2–3 treatments at 2–3 week intervals to obtain optimal results. There are no systemic side effects.

These ALA treatments can be combined with our regular Photorejuvenation treatments using IPL, which targets redness and brown spots, as well as stimulates formation of more collagen in the skin. There is normally no downtime for IPL treatments without Levulan. However, one can enhance and "boost" IPL photorejuvenation results by adding Levulan to the treatment process. This is termed an activated Fotofacial, or photodynamic skin rejuvenation when PDT is added to regular IPL photorejuvenation.

Naturally, you can use your topical acne lotions in between your Levulan treatments once the redness has settled down after a few days.

Figure 11.7 Sample PDT patient guide for acne treatments.

CLIENT CONSENT FOR LEVULAN PHOTODYNAMIC TREATMENT

Levulan (Aminolevulinic acid 20%) is a naturally occurring photosensitizing compound which has been approved by the FDA and Health and Welfare Canada to treat pre-cancerous skin lesions called actinic keratosis. Levulan is applied to the skin and subsequently "activated" by specific wavelengths of light. This process of activating Levulan with light is termed Photodynamic Therapy. The purpose of activating the Levulan is to improve the appearance and reduce acne rosacea, acne vulgaris, sebaceous hyperplasia, decrease oiliness of the skin, and improve texture and smoothness by minimizing pore size. Any pre-cancerous lesions are also simultaneously treated. The improvement of these skin conditions (other than actinic keratosis) is considered an "off-label" use of Levulan.

I understand that Levulan will be applied to my skin for 30–120 minutes. Subsequently, the area will be treated with a specific wavelength of light to activate the Levulan. Following my treatment, I must wash off any Levulan on my skin. I understand that I should avoid direct sunlight for 24 hours following the treatment due to photosensitivity. I understand that I am not pregnant.

Anticipated side effects of Levulan treatment include discomfort, burning, swelling, blistering, scarring, redness and possible skin peeling, especially in any areas of sun damaged skin and pre-cancers of the skin, as well as lightening or darkening of skin tone and spots, and possible hair removal. The peeling may last many days, and the redness for several weeks if I have an exuberant response to treatment.

I consent to the taking of photographs of my face before each treatment session. I understand that I may require several treatment sessions spaced 1–6 weeks apart to achieve optimal results. I understand that I am responsible for payment of this procedure, as it is not covered by health insurance.

I understand that medicine is not an exact science, and that there can be no guarantees of my results. I am aware that while some individuals have fabulous results, it is possible that these treatments will not work for me. I understand that alternative treatments include topical medications, oral medications, cryosurgery, excisional surgery, and doing nothing.

I have read the above information and understand it. My questions have been answered satisfactorily by the doctor and his staff. I accept the risks and complications of the procedure. By signing this consent form I agree to have one or more Levulan treatments.

____

Signature

____

Name

______________ ______________________

Date Witness

Figure 11.8 Sample informed consent for ALA-PDT treatments.

Home care instructions for patients following photodynamic skin rejuvenation

Day of Treatment:

1. If you have any discomfort, begin applying ice packs to the treated areas. This will help keep the area cool and alleviate any discomfort, as well as help keep down any swelling. Swelling will be most evident around the eyes and is usually more prominent in the morning.
2. Remain indoors and avoid direct sunlight.
3. Spray on Avène Thermal Spring Water often.
4. Apply Niadyne moisturizing cream.
5. Take analgesics such as Advil if necessary.

Days 2–7:

1. You may begin applying make-up once any crusting has healed. The area may be slightly red for 1–2 weeks. If make-up is important to you, please see one of our aestheticians for a complimentary consultation for Jane Iredale Mineral Make-up, which is all natural, inert, anti-inflammatory, and acts as a concealer with sunscreen. It is especially effective to mask redness.
2. The skin will feel dry and tightened. Niadyne moisturizer should be used daily.
3. Try to avoid direct sunlight for one week. Use a total block zinc oxide based sunscreen with a minimum SPF 30. We recommend Ti-Silc, Spa MD or Cool Clenz.

Figure 11.9 Sample home care instruction sheet.

A B

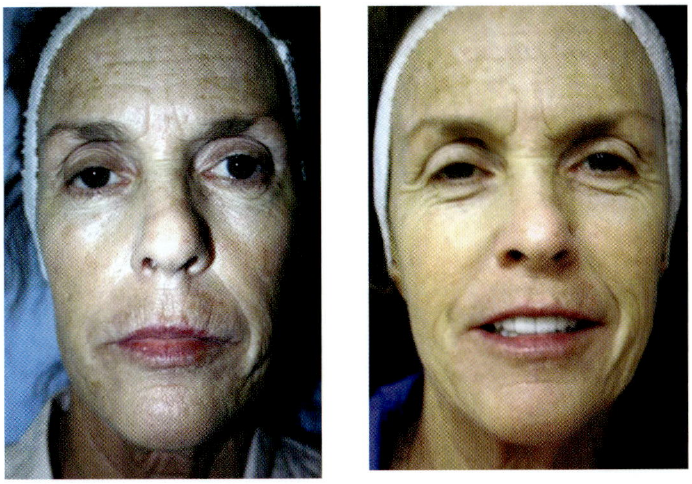

Figure 11.10 Case report 1. Before treatment (A) and 4 weeks after first treatment (B) (courtesy of Gold Skin Care Center).

a sample Home Care Instruction Sheet given to all patients following their ALA-PDT procedure.

Case Reports

Two case reports are presented below. The first case represents photorejuvenation utilizing ALA-PDT and an IPL device. The second case is a case of moderate to severe inflammatory acne vulgaris treated with ALA-PDT and an IPL device.

Case 1

Photorejuvenation with the Cynosure Inc. PhotoLight Pulsed Light System and Levulan®

1. Drug incubation: 60 minutes
2. 550 nm filter
3. 8 J/cm^2
4. 20 ms
5. rep. rate 5 ms

Photographs of case 1 before treatment and 4 weeks after the first treatment are shown in Fig. 11.10.

Case 2

Acne Vulgaris treated with Lumenis Ltd. IPL Quantum and Levulan®

1. Drug incubation: 30 minutes
2. 560 nm filter
3. 20 J/cm^2
4. Program one
5. Single pass

Photographs of case 2 before treatment and after three treatments (one every two weeks) are shown in Fig. 11.11.

Adverse Sequelae

The most common adverse reaction seen with ALA-PDT treatments is phototoxicity. This can be seen with any of the diseases/entities being treated with ALA-PDT. Most authorities feel that this phototoxic reaction is an exaggerated sunburn reaction. Patients may display an intense erythema and associated edema in the treatment areas with demarcation lines evident (Fig. 11.12). Pain and hyperesthesia may be associated with any phototoxic eruption.

A B

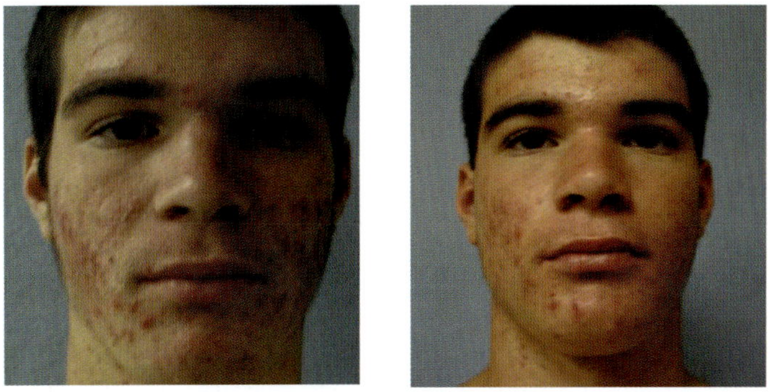

Figure 11.11 Case Report 2. Before treatment (A) and after 3 treatments (B) (courtesy of Gold Skin Care Center).

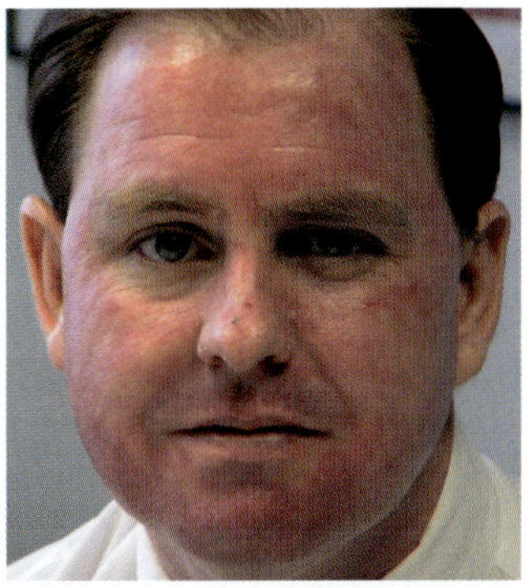

Figure 11.12 Phototoxic effect associated with ALA-PDT treatment (courtesy of DUSA Pharmaceuticals, Inc.).

Other adverse sequelae are rare but can include cutaneous viral and bacterial infections. Also, each machine carries the risk of potential adverse reactions. Most lasers and light sources can cause burning and skin blistering, hypo- and hyperpigmentation, and scarring. It is important that the operator/physician be very familiar with the device being used and that they are aware that they are adding a photosensitizer to the treatment algorithm, which may make the machine more 'sensitive' during the treatment process. In the US, different States have different 'rules' as to who can operate each device used for ALA-PDT; physicians need to know these rules and follow them appropriately.

When ALA-PDT was performed with a 14- to 18-hour drug incubation period and blue light therapy, most patients complained of a great deal of pain and discomfort during the light therapy itself. Stinging and burning routinely persisted for several hours in the postoperative period. Patients had erythema and edema, which would last several days. AK crusting and peeling, for up to a week, was common with this older technique. This, for the most part is now prevented utilizing the newer techniques described.

Management of Complications

As noted, phototoxicity is the principal adverse event seen with ALA-PDT treatments. The phototoxicity is minimized by adhering to the recommendations already described. This includes the shorter drug incubation periods, proper cleansing of the skin and removal of residual of 20% 5-ALA before and after the light treatments, and proper use of sunscreens and sun protection.

If a patient suffers a phototoxic reaction, several steps may be taken. These include:

- rest
- application of ice
- elevation of the area
- apply mild topical corticosteroids
- apply moisturizers regularly
- some recommend the use of an LED device for several days following the treatment, which may be useful in reducing any potential phototoxicity
- the proper use of sunscreens/sunblock.

Cutaneous viral and bacterial skin infections should be treated with the appropriate antiviral agents and antibacterial agents. Oral antiviral medications are usually more efficacious than their topical counterparts. Both topical and systemic antibiotics are useful if a bacterial infection develops. Laser and light source complications also must be treated early and aggressively, if they occur. All lasers and light sources can cause adverse events and physicians must be well versed in dealing with any untoward sequelae that may arise.

Future Directions

Photodynamic therapy, with a variety of lasers and light sources, is changing how many dermatologists and laser surgeons look at a variety of diseases/entities for which they are using the devices in their clinical practices. ALA-PDT has found its niche in the treatment of photorejuvenation and associated AKs, if present. It has also found its niche in the treatment of moderate to severe inflammatory acne vulgaris. Other entities, including sebaceous gland hyperplasia and recalcitrant hidradenitis suppurativa are also being treated successfully and routinely with ALA-PDT. Superficial skin cancers and Bowen's disease are also regularly treated with ALA-PDT. More and more entities will continue to be studied with ALA-PDT and its use expanded in the next several years. The future for this type of this therapy looks very bright.

References

1. Raab O. Ueber die Wirkung fluoreszierenden Stoffe auf Infusorien. Z Biol 1900; 39: 524–6.
2. Von Tappeiner H, Jodblauer A. Uber die wirkung der photodynamischen (fluorescierenden) staffe auf protozoen und enzyme. Dtsch Arch Klin Med 1904; 80:427–87.
3. Jesionek A, Von Tappeiner H. Behandlung der Hautcarcinome nut fluorescierenden Stoffen. Dtsch Arch Klin Med 1905; 85:223–7.
4. Figge FHJ, Weiland GS, Manganiello LDJ. Cancer detection and therapy: affinity of neoplastic embryonic and traumatized tissue for porphyrins and metalloporphyrins. Proc Soc Exp Biol Med 1948; 68:640.
5. Dougherty TJ, Kaufman JE, Goldfarb A et al. Photoradiation therapy for the treatment of malignant tumors. Cancer Res 1978; 38:2628–35.
6. Dougherty TJ, Gomer CJ, Henderson BW et al. Photodynamic therapy. J Natl Cancer Inst 1998; 90:889–905.
7. Gomer CJ, Rucker N, Ferrario A, Wong S. Properties and applications of photodynamic therapy. Radiat Res 1989; 100:1–18.
8. Dougherty TJ. Photodynamic therapy. Photochem Photobiol 1993; 58:895–900.
9. McCaughan JS Jr, Brown DG, Hawley PC. Photodynamic therapy: an eight year experience. In: Henderson BW, Dougherty TJ, eds. Photodynamic therapy: basic principles and clinical applications. New York: Dekker; 1992:323–31.
10. Pass HI, Delaney TF. Innovative photodynamic therapy at the National Cancer Institute: intraoperative intracavity treatment. In: Henderson BW, Dougherty TJ, eds. Photodynamic therapy: basic principles and clinical applications. New York: Dekker; 1992:287–301.
11. Rowe PM. Photodynamic therapy begins to shine. Lancet 1988; 351:1496.
12. Saito T, Hayashi J, Sato H, Kawabe H, Aizawa K. Scanning electron microscopic analysis of acute photodynamic therapy for atherosclerotic plaques of rabbit aorta using a pheophorbide derivative. J Clin Laser Med Surg 1996; 14:1–6.
13. Ben-Hur E, Oetjen J, Horowitz B. Silicon phthalocyanine Pc 4 and red light causes apoptosis in HIV-infected cells. Photochem Photobiol 1997; 65:456–60.
14. Ratkay LB, Chowdhary RK, Damaroon A et al. Amelioration of antigen-induced arthritis in rabbits by induction of apoptosis of inflammatory cells with local application of transdermal photodynamic therapy. Arthritis Rheum 1998; 41:525–43.
15. Hendrich C, Siebert WE. Photodynamic therapy for rheumatoid arthritis. J Lasers Surg Med 1997; 21:359–64.
16. Fritsch C, Lang K, Neuse W, Ruzicka T, Lehmann P. Photodynamic diagnosis and therapy in dermatology. Skin Pharmacol Appl Skin Physiol 1998; 11:358–73.
17. Stables GI. Photodynamic therapy in dermatology. J Dermatol Treat 1999; 10:213–19.
18. Kennedy JC, Pottier RH, Pross DC et al. Photodynamic therapy with endogenous protoporphyrin IX: basic principles and present clinical experience. J Photochem Photobiol B 1990; 6:143–8.
19. Lefell DJ. The scientific basis of skin cancer. J Am Acad Dermatol 2000; 42 (1pt2):18–22.
20. Lui H, Anderson RR. Photodynamic therapy in dermatology: recent developments. Dermatol Clinics 1993; 11:1–13.
21. McCaughan JS, Guy JT, Hicks W, Laufman L, Nims TA, Walker J. Photodynamic therapy for cutaneous and subcutaneous malignant neoplasms. Arch Surg 1989; 124:211–16.
22. Bissonette R, Lui H. Current status of photodynamic therapy in dermatology. Dermatol Clinics 1997; 15:507–19.
23. Cappugi P, Campolni P, Mavilio L, Prignano F, Rossi R. Topical 5-aminolevulinic acid and photodynamic therapy in dermatology: a minireview. J Chemother 2001; 13:494–9.
24. Kalka K, Merk H, Mukhtar H. Photodynamic therapy in dermatology. J Am Acad Dermatol 2000; 42:389–413.
25. Freeman M et al. A comparison of photodynamic therapy using topical methyl aminolevulinate (Metvix) with single cell cryotherapy in patients with actinic keratosis: a prospec-

tive, randomized study. J Dermatolog Treat 2003; 14:99–106.
26. Pariser DM et al. Photodynamic therapy with topical methyl aminolevulinate for actinic keratosis: results of a prospective randomized multicenter trial. J Am Acad Dermatol 2003; 48:227–232.
27. Rhodes LE et al. Photodynamic therapy using topical methyl aminolevulinate vs surgery for nodulus basal cell carcinoma. Arch Dermatol 2004; 140:17–23.
28. Wulf H, Philipsen P. Allergic contact dermatitis to 5-aminolevulinic acid methylester but not to 5-aminolevulinic acid after photodynamic therapy. Br J Dermatol 2004; 150:143–5.
29. Osmrod D, Jarvis A. Topical aminolevulinic acid HCl photodynamic therapy. Am J Clin Dermatol 2000; 1:133–9.
30. Jeffes E, McCullough J, Weinstein G et al. Photodynamic therapy of actinic keratoses with topical aminolevulinic acid hydrochloride and fluorescent blue light. J Am Acad Dermatol 2001; 45:96–104.
31. Jeffes E. Levulan®: the first approved topical photosensitizer for the treatment of actinic keratoses. J Dermatol Treat 2002; 13(S):19–23.
32. Touma D, Yaar M, Whitehead S et al. A trial of short incubation, broad-area photodynamic therapy for facial actinic keratoses and diffuse photodamage. Arch Dermatol 2004; 140:33–40.
33. Ruiz-Rodriquez R, Sanz-Sanchez T, Cordobo S. Photodynamic photorejuvenation. Dermatol Surg 2002; 28:742–4.
34. Gold MH. Intense pulsed light therapy for photorejuvenation enhanced with 20% aminolevulinic acid photodynamic therapy. J Lasers Med Surg 2003; 15(S):47.
35. Goldman MP, Atkin D, Kincad S. PDT/ALA in the treatment of actinic damage: real world experience. J Lasers Surg Med 2002; 14(S):24.
36. Avram D, Goldman MP. Effectiveness and safety of ALA-IPL in treating actinic keratoses and photodamage. J Drugs Dermatol 2004; 3(S):36–9.
37. Alexiades-Armenakas MR, Geronemus R. Laser mediated photodynamic therapy of actinic keratoses. Arch Dermatol 2003; 139:1313–20.
38. Alexiades-Armenakas MR, Geronemus RG. Laser-mediated photodynamic therapy of actinic chelitis. J Drugs Dermatol 2004; 3(5):548–51.
39. Bhatia AC, Dover JS et al. Adjunctive use of topical aminolevulinic acid with intense pulsed light in the treatment of photoaging. Presentation at Controversies and Conversations in Cutaneous Laser Surgery, Mt Tremblant, Canada, August 2004.
40. Gold MH, Bradshaw VL, Boring MM et al. A split-face comparison study of ALA-PDT with intense pulsed light versus intense pulsed light alone for photodamage/photorejuvenation. (Submitted for publication).
41. Leyden JJ. Therapy for acne vulgaris. N Engl J Med 1997; 336:1156–62.
42. Gollnick H et al. Management of acne: a report from a global alliance to improve outcomes in acne. J Am Acad Dermatol; 49(1Suppl):S1–S37.
43. Velicer CM et al. Antibiotic use in relation to the risk of breast cancer. JAMA 2004; 291:827–35.
44. Sigurdsson V et al. Phototherapy of acne vulgaris with visible light. Dermatology 1997; 194:256–60.
45. Touma DJ, Gilchrest BA. Topical photodynamic therapy: a new tool in cosmetic dermatology. Semin Cutan Med Surg 2003; 22:124–30.
46. Papageorgiou P et al. Phototherapy with blue (415 nm) and red (660 nm) light in the treatment of acne vulgaris. Br J Dermatol 2000; 142:973–8.
47. Kawada A et al. Acne phototherapy with a high-intensity, enhanced narrow-band, blue light source: an open study and *in vitro* investigation. J Dermatol Sci 2002; 30:129–35.
48. Elman M, Slatkine M, Harth Y. The effective treatment of acne vulgaris by a high-intensity, narrow band 405–420 nm light source. J Cosmet Laser Ther 2003; 5:111–17.
49. Gold MH. Photoclearing for acne vulgaris – a new approach in the management of mild to moderate inflammatory acne vulgaris. J Lasers Surg Med 18(S1), 44.
50. Gregory AN et al. A study on the use of a novel light and heat energy system to treat acne vulgaris. Cosmet Derm 2004; 17(5):287–300.
51. Lloyd JR, Mirkov M. Selective photothermolysis of the sebaceous glands for acne treatment. J Lasers Surg Med 2002; 31:115–20.
52. Paithankar DY et al. Acne treatment with a 1,450 nm wavelength laser and cryogen spray cooling. J Lasers Surg Med 2002; 31:106–14.
53. Hongcharu W et al. Topical ALA-photodynamic therapy for the treatment of acne vulgaris. J Invest Dermatol 2000; 115(2):183–92.
54. Itoh Y et al. Photodynamic therapy for acne vulgaris with topical 5-aminolevulinic acid. Arch Dermatol 2000; 136(9):1093–5.
55. Itoh Y et al. Photodynamic therapy of acne vulgaris with topical delta aminolevulinic acid and incoherent light in Japanese patients. Brit J Dermatol 2001; 144:575–9.
56. Goldman MP. Using 5-aminolevulinic acid to treat acne and sebaceous hyperplasia. Cosmet Dermatol 2003; 16:57–8.
57. Gold MH. The utilization of ALA-PDT and a new photoclearing device for the treatment of severe inflammatory acne vulgaris – results of an initial clinical trial. J Lasers Surg Med 2003; 15(S):46.
58. Goldman MP, Boyce S. A single-center study of aminolevulinic acid and 417 n, photodynamic therapy in the treatment of moderate to severe acne vulgaris. J Drugs Dermatol 2003; 2:393–6.
59. Gold MH, Bradshaw VL, Boring MM et al. The use of a novel intense pulsed light and heat source and ALA-PDT in the treatment of moderate to severe inflammatory acne vulgaris. J Drugs Dermatol 2004; 3(6):S14–18.
60. Schonermark MP et al. Treatment of sebaceous gland hyperplasia with the pulsed dye laser. J Lasers Surg Med 1997; 21:313–20.
61. Horio T et al. Photodynamic therapy of sebaceous gland hyperplasia with topical 5-aminolevulinic acid and slide projector. Br J Dermatol 2003; 148:1274–6.
62. Alster TS, Tanzi EL. Photodynamic therapy with topical aminolevulinic acid and pulsed dye laser irradiation for sebaceous hyperplasia. J Drugs Dermatol 2003; 2(S):501–4.
63. Richey DF, Hopson B. Treatment of sebaceous hyperplasia by photodynamic therapy. Cosmet Dermatol 2004; 17:525–9.
64. Gold MH, Bradshaw VL, Boring MM et al. Treatment of sebaceous gland hyperplasia by photodynamic therapy with 5-aminolevulinic acid and a blue light source or intense pulsed light source. J Drugs Dermatol 2004; 3(6):S5–8.
65. Gold MH et al. ALA-PDT and blue light therapy for hidradenitis suppurativa. J Drugs Dermatol 2004; 3(S):32–9.
66. Personal communication, Dr. Henry Chan, Hong Kong, 2004.
67. Gold MH, Goldman MP. 5-Aminolevulinic acid photodynamic therapy: where we have been and where we are going. Derm Surg 2004; 30:1077–84.

Chapter 12
Laser Safety: Risks and Hazards: Management and Control Measures

Jaggi Rao, Penny J. Smalley, Alim Devani and Mitchel P. Goldman

Introduction

Since the mid-1960s, lasers have proven to be one of the most powerful surgical tools. In North America today, almost every major hospital uses laser technology to perform certain procedures. As the devices become more available and less expensive, increasing numbers of hospitals will employ their use for many more important uses. Laser technology has already found its way into a broad range of medical specialties including dermatology, plastic surgery and cosmetic surgery.

The laser revolution in medicine has given practitioners new options in treatment but not without a price. Over the years, there has been a tremendous increase in the number of accidents and incidents related to laser use. Much of this can be attributed to the lack of training and safety procedures in terms of laser use. Facilities using lasers need to realize that standards and practice guidelines for laser use exist on both state and national levels and need to be instituted (Appendix 1). These standards provide the basis for establishing a laser safe environment for both patients and personnel which will be the focus of this chapter.

Regulators of Laser Safety in the United states

- American National Standards Institute
- Occupational Safety and Health Administration.

American National Standards Institute

The American National Standards Institute (ANSI) is a non-profit, voluntary organization responsible for developing, and maintaining over 10,000 safety standards in the United States. Although not regulatory, these standards are considered consensus documents and are frequently held up as the foundation for OSHA guidance, State law, and professional societies' recommended practices, as well as being considered the benchmark for practice in the medical-legal arena. ANSI represents the United States in international regulatory and standards setting bodies, such as ISO and IEC.

Healthcare laser standards are found in the ANSI Z136 series, including 136.1, and 136.3. The 136.1 is the parent standard, and contains technical information, applicable to all lasers in all use settings. 136.3 is the standard for the safe use of healthcare lasers, and applies to all healthcare practice settings including hospitals, clinics, private offices, mobile services, spas, and veterinary clinics. The committee that developed the standard is composed of members representing government and military agencies, industry, medical specialists, professional bodies, and individual experts. The document contains a glossary of terminology, hazard identification, control measures, and many examples of forms, and tools for individuals who are in the process of establishing a laser program. This standard includes engineering, procedural, and administrative controls necessary for the safety of patients and healthcare professionals. These controls are based on: evaluation of potential hazards from laser radiation; unique problems related to operating rooms, outpatient clinics, mobile laser units, and private medical and dental offices; and exposure risks to patients and professional staff.

In other sections, this document outlines the requirements for safety procedures in non-hospital environments, as equal to those in large institutions. It describes the need for safety policies and procedures, safety training, strict adherence, and auditing to ensure compliance. Of importance is the appointment of a laser safety officer (LSO), use of control measures, education and training, and assessing hazards which are all covered in this chapter.

The ANSI standards for laser safety contain control measures for all aspects of laser management, including: engineering, administrative, and procedural controls.

Occupational Safety and Health Administration (OSHA)

Occupational Safety and Health Administration (OSHA) is an agency of the United States Department of Labor with oversight of safety in the workplace. All OSHA investigations are in response to complaints or accidents; they are not random or scheduled. Audits are not done and compliance officers can examine any aspect of a facility they wish to once on site. Should laser use or safety come under scrutiny, OSHA officers use the directives under the general duty clause to issue any citations. There are no specific OSHA guidance documents applicable to the use of medical lasers. However, it is expected that facilities and users to comply with ANSI Z136.3 and, if they are found out of compliance, they may be issued with fines and other penalties, including halting practice and revoking licensure. Things OSHA may wish to examine in a laser facility include:

- established written safety policies and procedures
- identified criteria for selection of protective equipment (ANSI Z136.3)
- implemented adequate education and training for all personnel
- performed and documented periodic safety audits
- ensured surveillance of the safety programs.

OSHA should be viewed as an advocate for safe practice, offering education, assistance, advice, and resources to help the individual practice comply with standards and regulations. Everyone benefits, especially the patient, when laser users take advantage of these resources during the early phases of program planning, well before treating the first patient or making the decision to purchase or rent laser equipment.

Perioperative Safety Measures

- Laser hazard evaluation.
- Laser-beam-related hazards.
- Nonbeam-related hazards.

Laser Hazard Evaluation

A laser hazard evaluation is performed to identify all the hazards associated with a laser system and to help determine the necessary control measures. Laser hazards can be determined as either beam-related hazards or nonbeam-related hazards. The hazard evaluation takes into consideration many aspects, including the:

- potential of the laser to cause harm to personnel
- facility and environment the laser is being used in
- personnel who may use or be exposed to laser radiation.

When the evaluating process is complete and necessary safety measures are devised and implemented, it is necessary for the facility (LSO), or the principal operator, to develop what is referred to as the Standard Operating Procedure (SOP) manual. The SOP is required to give instruction for the operation, maintenance, and service activities of the laser. SOPs must be reviewed and signed by all laser personnel, updated periodically, and be posted in the area where the laser is located. SOPs must include the following (see Appendix 2):

- laser information
- supervisor information
- emergency contact information
- control measures
- personal protective equipment
- operation procedures
- beam and non-beam hazards
- emergency procedures
- other data pertinent to the safety of the laser.

Laser-Beam-Related Hazards

Lasers can produce an intense and highly directional beam of light and, with improper use, can be very dangerous. If the laser is directed or focused on an object it can cause irreversible damage. In particular, humans are quite prone to biological damage caused by lasers, which can range from mild skin burns to permanent damage to the eyes and skin. The biological damage caused by lasers is produced by three main mechanisms. These are:

- thermal effects
- photochemical effects
- mechanical effects.

Thermal effects are caused by the sudden rise in temperature when the laser's energy is absorbed. The damage to the tissue itself depends on factors including duration of exposure, wavelength of beam, and type of tissue exposed to the beam. Research has been conducted in the thermal effects of lasers and it is now widely accepted that the human eye is more vulnerable to injury than human skin.

Photochemical effects occur at short wavelengths of light, peaking at 550 nm, which can cause a photochemical injury similar to sunburn. This damage arises as a result of photons interacting with tissue cells and causing a change in cell chemistry. The effects of this type of damage are cumulative and result from long exposures (over 10–15 seconds).

Mechanical damage results from acoustic shock waves generated by very short pulses. Less is known about this mechanism but research is ongoing in this area.

Types of Beam Exposures

Exposure to the laser beam may be direct or indirect. The three types of beam exposure are:

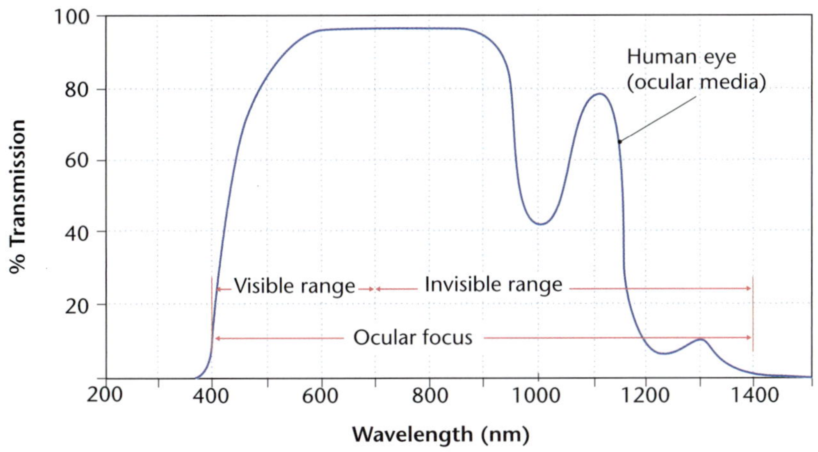

Figure 12.1 Transmission wavelengths of ocular media.

1. Intrabeam exposure: exposure occurs directly from the entire laser beam and involves the maximum possible irradiance.
2. Specular reflections: these are beam reflections from mirror-like surfaces. This type of exposure can be as damaging as intrabeam exposures, especially if the reflecting surface is flat.
3. Diffuse reflections: these occur when diffuse surfaces reflect the laser beam in many directions. These reflections are not as powerful, but may still be harmful in high-powered lasers.

Ocular Risk

The major dangers of lasers are due to their potential adverse effects to the human eye. The eye is the most sensitive organ to light. In the process of focusing light, just as a magnifying glass can magnify the light energy from the sun to burn paper, the human eye can focus incident light to burn the retina. The reason why the eye is vulnerable to damage relates to its anatomical structure. To understand how lasers damage the eye, it is important to understand its structure and function that may be compromised by laser radiation. Below is an illustration of the structure of the human eye.

Structure of the Human Eye

The cornea, which is the outer layer, is used as the main focusing element of the eye. Unlike skin, this layer does not have a dead layer of cells to help protect it from light. Damage to the upper corneal layer may be painful but is likely to heal. Unfortunately, damage to the deeper layers of the cornea can cause permanent damage. Within the eye, the lens focuses light to create an image on the retina. Over time, the lens becomes pliable and may also become cloudy making it more difficult to focus objects. The retina, another important layer, acts as a screen upon which light is focused from the outside world. The area of the retina involved in the highest visual acuity is known as the fovea centralis. This is is a very small area (3 to 4% of retina).

To see objects, light must be transparent to all the structures of the eye in its path from the outside world to the retina. These structures are referred to as the ocular media, and include the cornea, aqueous humor, lens, and vitreous humor. Figure 12.1 demonstrates that the ocular media are transparent to visible light only.

As illustrated, the range of wavelengths transmitted by the human eye to the retina ranges from 400 nm to 1400 nm (visible and near infrared). This range is known as the retinal hazard region. Figure 12.2 illustrates the absorption characteristics of the eye for different laser wavelengths. Lasers have the greatest potential for retinal injury in the visible and near-infrared regions of the spectrum, because the cornea and lens are transparent to those wavelengths. As a result, if the lens focuses laser with a high irradiance, damage to the retina may occur. The greatest concern for laser exposure is in the retinal hazard region between 400 nm (violet light) and 1400 nm (near-infrared). Argon and YAG lasers operate in this range, making them the most hazardous lasers with respect to eye injuries.

The risk of damage to the eye depends upon several factors, including:

- wavelength: determines energy of the light
- pulse duration: the shorter the pulse duration, the greater the chance of injury
- pupil size: the smaller the pupil size, the less chance of injury
- amount of pigmentation: the darker the pigment, the more heat is absorbed.

The spot size of a laser beam is also an important safety consideration for ocular risk. As defined by the law of the conservation of energy, the energy density of a laser beam (energy per unit area) increases as the diameter of the laser decreases. This means that the energy of a laser focusing on the retina can be magnified up to 100,000 times just by lens magnification.

For those who experience eye-associated laser damage, there are some associated symptoms. If the laser burn occurs on the fovea, where visual acuity is at its maximum, fine vision may be lost immediately. This is known as scotoma or blind spot in the fovea. If the burn occurs in the peripheral vision, it may produce little or no effect on fine vision. Other symptoms may include headache after

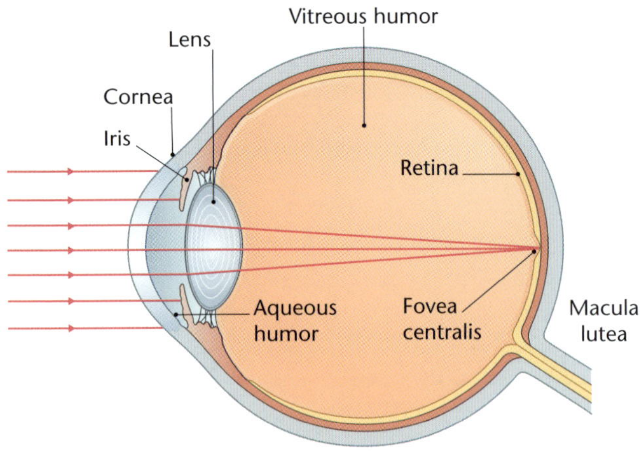

Visible and Near-infrared (400–1400 nm) radiation

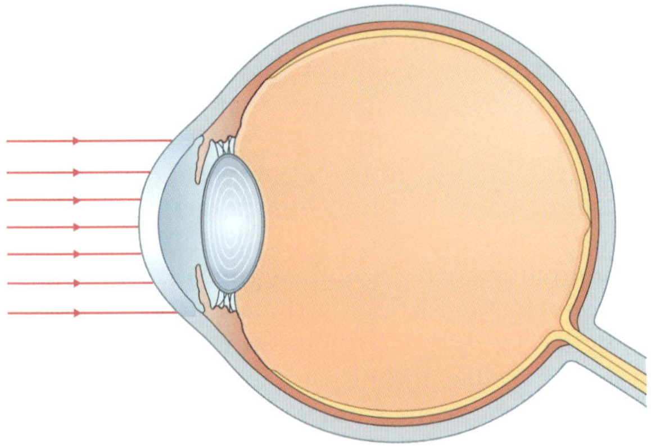

Mid-infrared and Far-infrared (1400 nm–1 mm)
Far-ultraviolet (180–315 nm) radiation

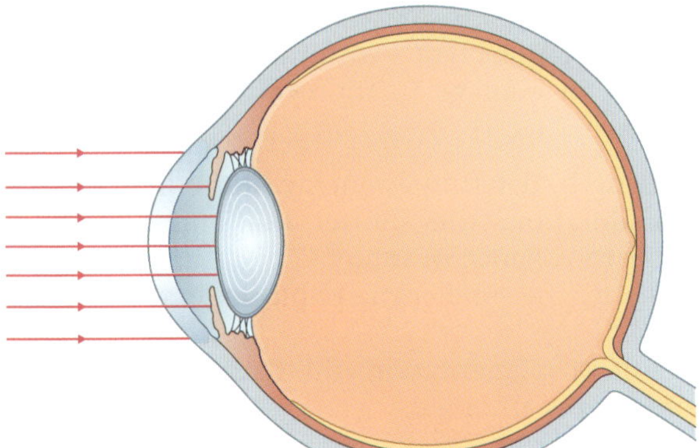

Near-ultraviolet (315–390 nm) radiation

Figure 12.2 Ocular absorption site versus wavelength.

exposure, watery eyes, and blurred vision. Associated corneal burns may cause a gritty feeling, often described as having sand in the eye.

There are also specific effects to the eye from particular lasers. These include:

- Exposure to a CO_2 laser beam can cause a burning pain on the cornea or sclera.

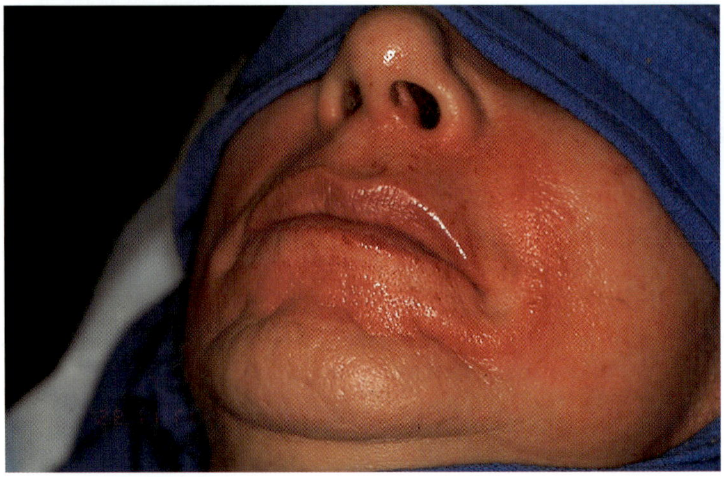

Figure 12.3 Only wet and/or nonflammable, nonreflective draping material is used to prevent fire hazards in the laser room.

Table 12.1 *Ocular Damage Caused by Different Wavelengths of Laser Radiation*

Light spectrum (wavelength)	Structure of eye	Disease
UV-C (200–280 nm)	Cornea	Photokeratitis
UV-B (280–315 nm)	Cornea	Photokeratitis
UV-A (315–400 nm)	Lens	Cataract
Visible (400–780 nm)	Retina	Retinal injury
IR-A (780–1400 nm)	Retina, lens	Retinal burn, cataract
IR-B (1400–3000 nm)	Cornea, lens	Corneal burn, cataract
IR-C (3000–1 000 000 nm)	Cornea	Corneal burn

- Exposure to a visible laser beam can be detected by a bright color flash of the emitted wavelength and an after-image of its complementary color.
- If the retina is damaged, there may be cone damage resulting in difficulty detecting blue or green. Funduscopy may demonstrate pigmentation of the retina.

The eyes have protective blink or aversion responses, which can react within a quarter of a second of being stimulated. Unfortunately, high-powered lasers can cause damage in less time than this. Thus, laser users must adopt preventative measures, including the use of properly labeled laser goggles (Fig. 12.3).

The following is a summary of ocular damage that may be caused by various wavelengths of laser radiation (Table 12.1).

Cutaneous Risk

Laser radiation can have profound effects to the skin. The mechanism by which this occurs is via photochemical and thermal burns. The skin layer is very thin and laser light

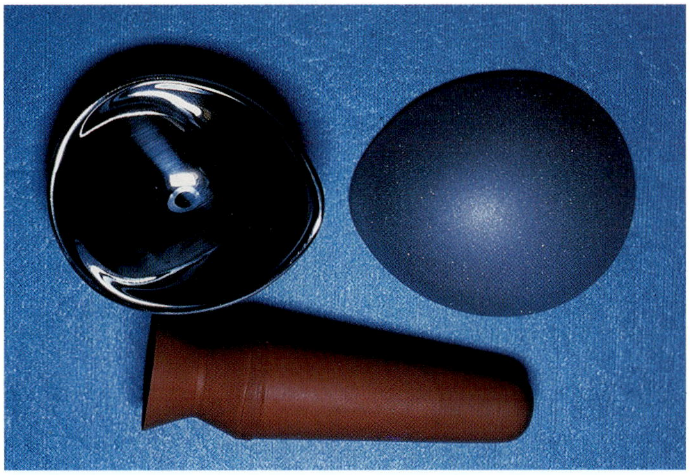

Figure 12.4 Eye shields offer protection from both transmitted light and heat. Left, Cox Stainless Ocular Laser Shield; right, Stefanovsky metallic eye shield; bottom, suction cup to place and remove eye shield.

Table 12.2 *Cutaneous Damage Caused by Different Wavelengths of Laser Radiation*

Light spectrum	Laser bioeffect
UV-C (200–280 nm)	Erythema, cancer, accelerated aging
UV-B (280–315 nm)	Erythema, increased pigmentation, cancer, accelerated aging
UV-A (315–400 nm)	Erythema, increased pigmentation, skin burn
Visible (400–780 nm)	Photosensitive reactions, skin burn
IR-A (780–1400 nm)	Skin burn
IR-B (1400–3000 nm)	Skin burn
IR-C (3000–1 000 000 nm)	Skin burn

has the potential to penetrate both the epidermis and dermis. The wavelength of light absorbed maximally by the epidermis is located in the mid- to far-ultraviolet range. With short-term exposure to this range of UV light, a sunburn-type reaction may occur (redness, edema and blistering). With increased exposure to UV light, there is an increased risk of both melanoma and non-melanoma skin cancers, and premature aging of the skin.

The skin is also at risk of developing thermal burns when exposed to laser light. Thermal burns to the skin occur less often than photochemical. The risk of thermal burns increases with the use of wavelengths that can penetrate deeply into the dermis. The resultant burn may be first degree (erythema only), second degree (blistering of skin) or third degree (full thickness with eschar formation) (Fig. 12.4).

Table 12.2 provides a summary of cutaneous damage that can be caused by various wavelengths of laser radiation.

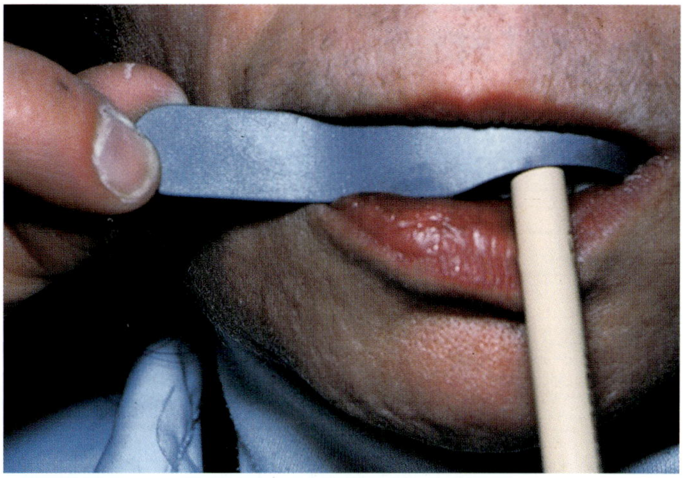

Figure 12.5 Covering teeth with specially designed protector can prevent such damage as cracking and discoloration to enamel veneers or dentures.

Dental Risk

When working in and around the oral cavity, care should be taken to avoid directly exposing the teeth to laser radiation. Many patients have enamel veneers or dentures that can be cracked or discolored if impacted by the laser beam. It is possible to protect the teeth by covering them with water-soaked gauze or other specially designed protectors that have undergone prior testing (Fig. 12.5).

Other Associated Hazards of Specific Laser Beams

Many other biological effects result from exposure to different wavelengths of energy. Table 12.3 provides a summary of the commonly used lasers and their associated hazards to various human tissues.

Non-Beam Hazards

In addition to the direct hazards to the human eye and skin, there are other hazards associated with laser use. These are referred to as non-beam hazards and in some cases, can be life threatening. The types of non-beam hazard included are:

- electrical hazards
- laser-generated air contaminants (LGAC)
- fire hazards
- chemical hazards.

Electrical Hazards

Electrical hazards are the most common non-beam hazards in terms of lasers. Currently, there have been more than a dozen electrocutions of individuals from laser-related activities in the United States. This total includes only the reported ones and not the dozens more that have gone unreported. The risk of electrical shock can occur during laser installation, maintenance and service, normal laser operation or anytime where protective covers are removed to access components of the laser system. The end effect of electric shock can range from minor injury to possible

Table 12.3 *Commonly Used Lasers and Their Associated Hazards to Various Human Tissues*

Laser	Wavelength (μm)	Bioeffect process	Tissue affected			
			Skin	Cornea	Lens	Retina
CO_2	10.6	Thermal	✓	✓		
HFl	2.7	Thermal	✓	✓		
Erbium:YAG	1.54	Thermal	✓	✓		
Nd:YAG	1.33	Thermal	✓	✓	✓	✓
Nd:YAG	1.06	Thermal	✓			✓
Gas (diode)	0.78–0.84	Thermal	✓			✓
HeNe	0.633	Thermal	✓			✓
Ar	0.488–0.514	Thermal/photochemical	✓			✓
XeFl	0.351	Photochemical	✓	✓		✓
XeCl	0.308	Photochemical	✓	✓		

electrocution and death. Accidents of this type are fully preventable with the use of a barrier system and common sense.

The following is a list of recommendations for preventing electrical shocks for lasers:

1. Install equipment according to regulations set by occupational health and safety or local government.
2. Perform visual checks of all power cords, fuses, circuit breakers, and plugs.
3. Before servicing a laser, ensure equipment is unplugged and not connected to any power source.
4. While working on laser systems, use tools with insulated handles.
5. Avoid working alone with laser systems.
6. Learn rescue procedures to help those who get electrocuted (i.e. discontinue circuit, CPR, emergency procedures).
7. Do not operate equipment when fatigued, stressed, intoxicated or using medications affecting mental status.
8. Avoid wearing rings, metallic watchbands or other metallic objects.
9. Never handle equipment on a wet floor or when hands, feet or body are wet.

Laser-generated Air Contaminants (LGAC)

Surgical smoke – its hazards and its management – has become a focus of infection control and has drawn the attention of government risk managers because of the interest in air-quality issues in health care. It has been determined that surgical smoke created from lasers can be contaminated with particles including carbon, blood, viruses, bacteria, and toxic gases. These contaminants are referred to by ANSI as laser-generated air contaminants (LGAC). LGAC may be produced with the use of specific lasers, especially the higher powered ones (i.e. CO_2).

Research has proven that thermal disruption of viable human cells results in the ejection of carbon particles, virus, bacteria, DNA, and a number of toxic gases. These hazardous particulates are found in all surgical smoke, regardless of the energy source used (laser, ESU, argon beam coagulator, ultrasonics) in similar distribution patterns, and in all types of surgical procedures.

This means that mutagenic material, aerosolized blood, blood-borne pathogens, and known hazardous gases such as benzene, formaldehyde, and acrolein, are forcefully ejected when the cell disrupts, and become airborne in the steam that comprises at least 80% of the smoke.

Forceful microexplosions of tissue, as in applications of the Q-switched Nd:YAG, or ruby lasers, as well as the tissue splatter associated with the erbium:YAG laser, also present airborne contamination hazards, often in excess of that resulting from thermal injury to tissues.

There is a global trend towards eliminating the hazards of smoke from our daily lives. The main focus has been on public smoking in confined areas, such as airplanes, restaurants, offices, and hotels. The hazards contained in smoke are well documented and governments around the world, such as America, Canada, United Kingdom, Australia, New Zealand, Germany, and Singapore, have taken action.

This same activity has now entered our healthcare workplaces, as we become more and more aware of the hazards associated with surgical smoke. Surgical smoke is more than an inconvenience and must be treated as an occupational hazard with a high level of risk. Effective removal results from both proper filtration equipment and good work practices, including appropriate capture (device positioned not further than 2 cm from the point of evolution of the smoke) systems, closed systems for laparoscopy, in-line filters for wall suction, patient protection during airway procedures, and evacuation systems now known as local exhaust ventilation systems (LEVs) (Fig. 12.6).

Smoke evacuation systems should be selected after careful evaluation of need and options available. Filters

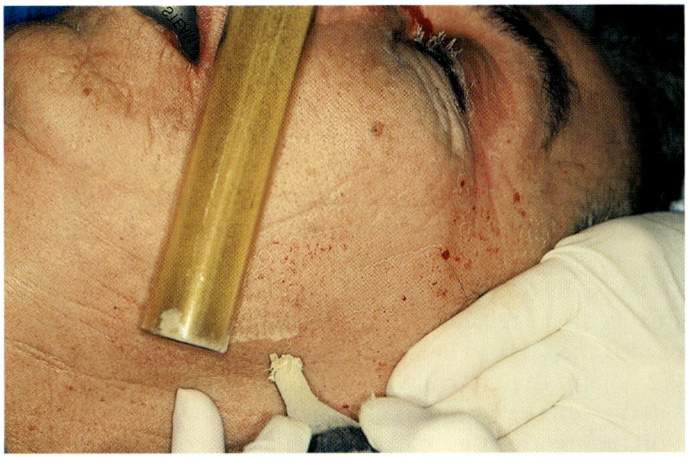

Figure 12.6 Risk of smoke inhalation is reduced when the collection tube/suction is held 1 cm from the point of laser impact.

must remove particulates to 0.1 micron, which is the mean average diameter of viral particulates found in surgical smoke. This requires an ULPA (ultra low particulate air) filter to eliminate the viral hazards, and should be rated to 99.999% efficiency to be effective. Filters should have a filter life monitor, indicating when to change the filters. Units should also be assessed for suction power measured in cubic feet per minute (CFM; suction should not be < 50 CFM), and for the noise factor (should not exceed recommended OH&S decibel levels).

HEPA (high efficiency particulate air) filters are *not* adequate, filtering only to particle sizes of 0.3 microns (mean average diameter of bacteria and not the area of greatest concern in medicine).

Masks are not meant to be a first-line protective device. According to current research, no mask on the market today is capable of filtering out all airborne contaminants. Furthermore, high filtration material works only when dry so, during a lengthy surgical case, the filtration medium stops working when the mask gets damp from breathing, defeating the purpose of the mask. Also a factor is fit and wearing technique. Masks must be fit tested for each employee, to be sure of a tight seal, and must be tied and worn properly at all times, if they are to be effective. If a facility is going to follow standard precautions (blood borne pathogens standard), then high filtration masks should be worn for all surgical smoke producing cases – about 97% of all procedures. This can be a costly and relatively ineffective control measure and it is recommended that infection control nurses work with facility managers to develop a reasonable policy and procedure for the use of protective face masks.

Wall suction lines should always be protected with in-line filters that are placed between the wall inlet and the floor canister. Although these filters may decrease suction strength, they will prevent the build-up of particulates and debris in suction lines in the wall, which often result in expensive repairs to the central vacuum system.

All materials used to collect and handle surgical smoke should be considered as biohazard, and disposed of according to infection control procedures. Staff must wear masks, goggles, and gloves, to change and handle filters, and should place all used materials in biohazard bags.

The following toxic chemical by-products can be released as LGAC from medical procedures:

- acetonitrile
- acetylene
- acrolein
- acrylonitrile
- alkyl benzenes
- benzene
- butadiene
- butene
- carbon
- carbon monoxide
- creosols
- ethane
- ethene
- ethylene
- formaldehyde
- free radicals
- hydrogen cyanide
- isobutene
- methane
- *p*-aminohippuric acid (PAH)
- phenol
- propylene
- pyridene
- styrene
- toulene
- xylene
- xylent.

Fire Hazards

The use of lasers can present a potential fire hazard. With the extreme heat generated by the laser, flammable materials are at risk of catching fire. These materials can include certain hair preparations (styling sprays, gels), nail polish, dry sponges, towels, alcohol-based cleansing solutions, methane gas, oxygen, plastics, benzene, and hemostatic agents. To help prevent these hazards, the operative site and path of the laser beam must be kept free of all flammable materials. There should also be safety equipment in the area including an open basin of water, a fire extinguisher, a fire blanket, and wet, nonflammable, nonreflective draping materials. Users of commercial lasers should obtain appropriate fire prevention information from the manufacturer. For this reason, fire fighting equipment should be provided to be used to extinguish or control small fires. If a fire starts, be sure to contact the proper authorities to minimize harm and damage.

Added precautions should also be taken when using CO_2 laser systems. When skin lesions are vaporized using the continuous wave CO_2 laser, a layer of carbon builds up on the skin. If this layer is not removed, the laser beam cannot penetrate the tissue and will be absorbed by the layer of carbon on the skin. This will allow superheating of the carbon film and heating of the surrounding tissue to extreme levels. As the carbon temperature reaches above

1000°C, the layer may cause a spark leading to fire, burn injury, and tissue damage. This hazard is easily prevented by irrigating the tissue with water when carbon buildup occurs on the skin.

Laser reflection is also a concern as it may result in fire or burns to personnel around the laser site. This can be prevented by keeping metallic objects away from the surgical site. Additionally, instruments used should be anodized to help decrease the chance of reflection. It is also important to roughen surfaces of metal to help cause diffuse reflections of the laser beam. Plastic accessories (mouth gags, eye shields) should never be used unless thoroughly tested for laser safety. The use of wet cloths to cover any unprotected metal surface is also encouraged.

Chemical Hazards

Common chemical hazards include the use of compressed gases and solvents in laser systems. Care should always be taken with tanks of compressed gas as they can cause severe physical harm. When using laser dyes or solvents, it is important to take safe precautions as these substances have been found to be toxic and carcinogenic. The use of gloves, protective masks, and working under a fume hood or ventilation are good protective measures.

Implementation of Laser Safety

- Safety standards.
- Laser hazard classification.
- Controlling laser hazards.
- Education and training.
- Warning signs and labels.
- Protective equipment.
- Personnel roles and responsibilities.

Safety Standards

Manufacturers of lasers are also held to strict standards and are regulated by the Center for Devices and Radiological Health (CDRH) as well as the Food and Drug Administration (FDA). The FDA's role is to regulate product performance and certify that all laser products meet safety standards. Each laser must then bear a label indicating that it complies with all safety standards and as part of this label, it is given a specific laser hazard classification. This classification is mainly used to place lasers into specific risk categories. As a result of this, laser users can adopt specific safety measures to reduce or eliminate accidents depending on the class of lasers being used.

Laser Hazard Classification

Lasers are classified according to the acuity of hazard to skin and eye should someone be exposed to the beam for a period of time longer than that beam's maximum permissible exposure (MPE). The MPE is then compared to the human aversion response (including movement of the head and eye blink). The aversion response is 0.25 s, and will protect against light exposure that occurs for longer than that time. If a light exposure can harm the eyes in less than 0.25 s, the aversion response cannot protect, and protective goggles must be worn. The International Electrotechnical Commission (IEC) established revised classifications in 2000, and these have been adopted by ANSI, and integrated into all US laser standards.

Class 1–3 laser systems have undergone numerous changes, and users of those types of systems must completely revise their operational procedures. However, Class 3b, and Class 4, which includes all healthcare laser systems, have not changed significantly. The reason for this is that, regardless of application, these lasers will exceed the MPE (in less time than the human eye can avert: 0.25 s) and therefore always require the protection of laser safety eyewear. Additionally, these two levels of classification require the user to implement all aspects of laser safety practice as described in the Z136.3, to be applied, including all administrative, engineering, and procedural controls. For further information, see ANSI Z136.1 and ANSI Z136.3.

Lasers can be grouped into four specific risk categories (classes 1 to 4) according to ANSI. The criteria used for classification are:

- beam output power and wavelength
- exposure duration
- cross-sectional area of laser beam
- maximum permissible exposure (MPE), which is the maximum safe exposure time allowed before possible damage may occur.

The basic approach to the ANSI Laser Classification System is to classify lasers based on their capability to produce injury. Subsequently, for each classification, a standard set of safety controls applies. The greater the classification number, the greater potential for the laser to cause harm. A brief description of each Hazard Class is described below.

Class 1: No Risk

Class 1 lasers, under normal working conditions, do not pose any appreciable health hazard. These lasers do not produce harmful levels of output radiation. They are referred to as 'no risk' because they emit radiation below the exposure limits for the human eye. A class 1 device does not permit access during its operation to levels of laser radiation in excess of accessible emission limits.

A standard office laser printer, compact disc player and geological surveying equipment are examples of class 1 laser devices.

Class 2: Low Power, Low Risk

Class 2 lasers are those which have low power and emit radiation in the visible range (400–700 nm wavelength), that could possibly cause damage to the human eye. If class 2 laser beams are directly viewed for long periods of time (e.g. greater than 15 minutes), optical damage could result.

Examples of class 2 laser devices include most laser pointers, aiming devices, range finding equipment, and code readers in grocery stores.

Class 3: Moderate Power, Moderate Risk

Class 3 lasers are moderately powered, continuous wave devices that generally do not cause harm to the human eye if viewed only momentarily (no longer than 0.25 s, corresponding with the eye's aversion reflex). Direct viewing of class 3 laser beams for even short periods longer than that of the aversion reflex can be hazardous. These lasers require strict control measures to prevent direct exposure to eyes or skin, and are often labeled with CAUTION or DANGER to warn users of potential hazards.

Class 3 lasers can be further categorized as either class 3a or class 3b. The output of class 3a devices can cause biological damage to the eyes if the beam is collected by an optical instrument and directed into the eye. In contrast, class 3b lasers can cause optical damage if viewed briefly, without need for external instrumentation.

Examples of class 3 lasers are the same as class 2 but with higher power. Most uses are in laser pointers and laser scanners.

Class 4: High Power, High Risk

Class 4 lasers are high powered lasers with outputs of greater than 500 milliwatts. These lasers present a 'high risk' of causing optical, cutaneous and dental injury, as well as igniting flammable materials. Hazards are produced not only from direct viewing, but also from diffuse reflections. Much greater controls are required to ensure the safe operation of this class of laser devices. Class 4 lasers require warning labels and the use of other protective measures. Very stringent control measures are required for this type of device.

Class 4 devices are now commonly used for surgery, research, drilling, cutting, welding, and micromachining.

Controlling Laser Hazards

Due to the inherent risk of danger with lasers, a system must be developed to ensure safety. As with other potentially hazardous operations, lasers can be used safely if certain guidelines are followed. These guidelines include the use of lasers in a proper facility, with proper equipment, and most importantly, with properly trained and experienced staff. Regulatory bodies like OSHA and ANSI have detailed outlines of control measures which can be put in place to protect against accidents.

Control measures used to help protect against accidents can be divided into the following categories:

- controls for specific classes of laser
- protective equipment controls
- administrative controls
- procedural controls
- engineering controls.

Controls for Specific Classes of Laser

Many of the controls for laser safety depend on the specific laser that is being used. Below, the safety control for each ANSI laser class will be described.

Class 1

Class 1 lasers do not require much control. Despite this, it is recommended that users post warning signs to ensure personnel are aware of lasers in use. In addition, persons should receive training on the hazards and controls for those particular lasers.

Class 2

Class 2 lasers require a few more controls than Class 1. With this class of lasers, it is mandatory to post the area with a WARNING sign. It is also important to use non-reflective tools and surface to minimize beam reflection.

Class 3

These types of lasers are the most commonly used and due to their hazards, posting signs with CAUTION or DANGER is mandatory (Fig. 12.7). Personnel using Class 3 lasers should also have a baseline eye exam from an ophthalmologist. The use of protective goggles is also mandatory. Other important controls include:

- ensuring users do not look directly at the beam
- permitting only experienced individuals to operate the laser
- not leaving active lasers unattended
- placing the laser in a restricted location
- eliminating any mirror like surface from the area.

A

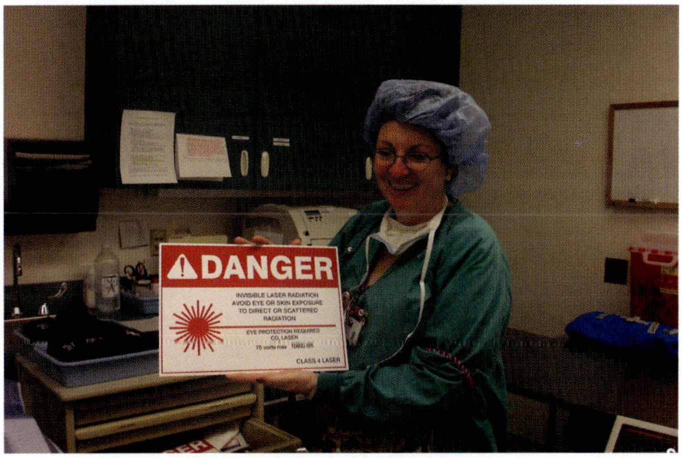

B

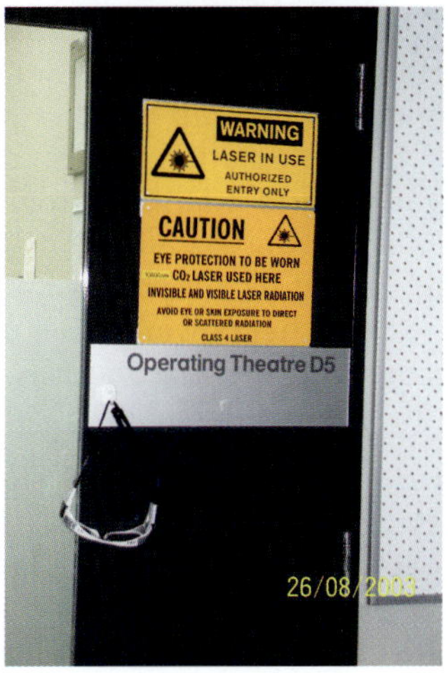

Figure 12.7 Typical laser danger and caution signs.

Class 4

These devices present the most serious of all laser hazards and controls should include:

- mandatory use of proper eye protection for all personnel in the active laser area
- due to fire hazard, a protective fire shield should be in place
- the use of fire resistant materials around the laser
- minimizing reflective material
- efficient ventilation system to control exposure to air contaminants
- only properly trained personnel to have access to laser.

In addition, it may be useful to develop a safety procedure manual for all users to read and sign. This manual can describe the laser's potential hazards and what controls have been put into place to reduce the risk of injury. It may also outline what to do in case of accidents, how to report incidents, and who to contact for more information. Each personnel should read, sign and date a form to ensure compliance with the aforementioned control standards.

Protective Equipment Controls

Protective equipment controls refer to items that are designed to protect personnel from incidental or accidental laser emission. These include window barriers, signs, labels, protective eyewear, fire extinguishers, nonflammable drapes, anodized instruments, beam stops, skin protection, masks, in-line suction filters, ventilation systems, and smoke evacuation systems.

Administrative Controls

The improper use of lasers can be a potential hazard to the user but also to other personnel including physicians, nurses, and patients. This is why it is important to institute administrative controls to assure that laser personnel are fully protected from potential hazards. The focus of these controls is to provide adequate education and training in safety and laser use. They are also used to teach procedures relating to the operation, maintenance, and service of lasers. Of all the administrative controls instituted, the most important is the appointment of the Laser Safety Officer (LSO). Other important administrative controls include monitoring of the safety program by a laser committee, development of written policies and procedures, development of documentation tools, development of mandatory education and training program, and lastly, development of a reporting system.

Safety training should be adopted for all types of lasers especially those with higher powers. Laser users should also be trained to recognize potential hazards. Factors important in recognizing hazards include:

- laser location
- access to lasers
- unprotected personnel around active laser
- potential beam paths
- presence of objects able to reflect laser near beam path.

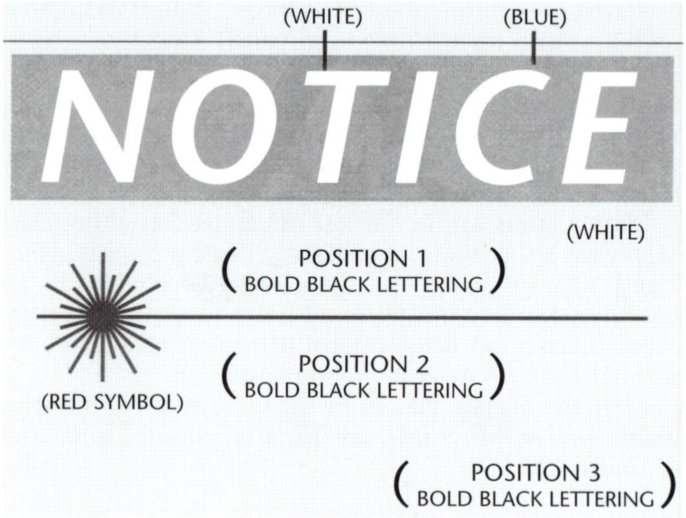

Figure 12.8 Laser warning sign template.

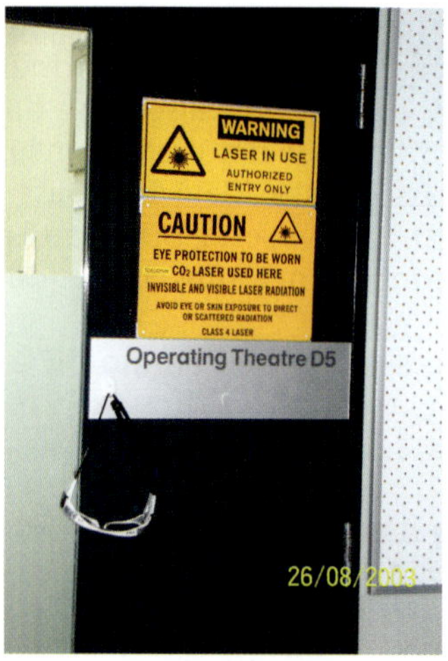
WARNING
LASER IN USE
AUTHORIZED
ENTRY ONLY
CAUTION
EYE PROTECTION TO BE WORN
INVISIBLE AND VISIBLE LASER RADIATION
Operating Theatre D5

Figure 12.9 Laser warning sign template.

Apart from training personnel in the dangers of lasers, it is also important to label working areas with warning labels and caution signs. These labels remind users of possible dangers and help to ensure that safe practices are being employed. They also warn unauthorized individuals of possible risk in the area (Figs 12.8–12.10).

When choosing the area within which lasers will be used, the controlled area should have:

- limited access to unauthorized personnel
- limited ability to cause diffuse and specular reflections
- eye protection for all personnel in close vicinity to laser.

In addition to the above, it is important that only trained individuals operate laser equipment.

Procedural Controls

Procedural controls are those perioperative or work practices expected of all personnel in a laser facility. Included

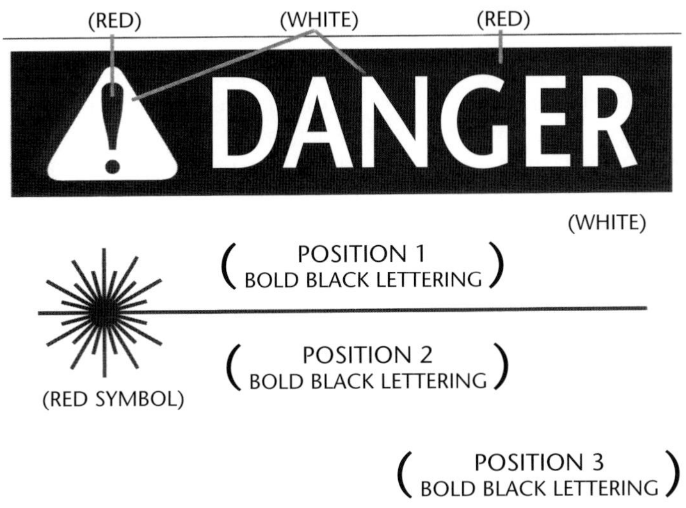

Figure 12.10 Laser danger sign template.

in these practices is the monitoring of controlled areas, preparing a laser safe operative site, elimination of laser generated air contaminants, ensuring properly trained individuals in treatment room, testing of laser equipment regularly, and providing patient advocacy.

Engineering Controls

Laser devices are complex, computerized and electronic devices that should be regularly inspected and maintained by expert technicians. Should a device fail to function adequately or appropriately, it is important that the laser operator and non-certified workers not tamper with the inner workings of the device itself. Unauthorized or experimental adjustments to the internal components of laser systems could result in serious injury and irreparable damage to the device itself. In the event of malfunction, the LSO should be contacted immediately. The LSO in turn should temporarily place the device 'out of order' and notify the laser manufacturer of the problem. This includes disconnecting the device from its electrical source and placing appropriate signs notifying personnel of the problem and not to touch the machine. The manufacturer may give specific instructions to assist with diagnosis and treatment of the malfunction, or more than likely, dispatch a trained service engineer to examine the problem on-site. In the interim, it is crucial that no facility employee attempt to utilize or repair the problem themselves. In fact, unauthorized interventions will often immediately void the facility's warranty with the laser manufacturer.

Regular service and maintenance checks should be arranged with the laser manufacturer along with cleaning schedules. It is important that lenses be periodically cleaned if non-disposable to prevent dust and debris from causing opacification and resultant diminishment of laser output. By ignoring seemingly simple cleaning rituals, the transmission of laser light may be compromised, sometimes causing reflectance back into the device and destruction of laser components and further safety risks to the operator.

Education and Training

In accordance with the standards set out by ANSI Z136.3, all personnel working with lasers require education and training including LSOs, clinicians, nurses, technicians, assistant staff and all other team members. Since there is no standard education program, each facility must establish its own educational criteria using guidelines set out by ANSI.

The education provided should be a combination of both didactic and practical components and cover topics including:

- basic laser science
- operation of lasers
- classification of lasers
- biological effects of lasers
- beam- and nonbeam-related hazards
- control measures and protection
- indications and contraindication.

This education and training should also be specific to the laser wavelength being used in the facility. It is also important that nurses and assistants be trained in perioperative safety and patient management. Further, laser instructors should be professionals who are trained and certified in the area of laser safety. With this education and training, workers can be confident in their techniques and provide a safe environment for their patients.

In many instances, physician courses do not teach safety to the same degree that nursing courses do and on the opposite scale, nursing courses do not discuss the clinical applications and techniques in great detail. These discrepancies lead to an information deficit and can create noncompliance. This makes it necessary for physicians and nursing staff to be trained and educated on similar topics to ensure compliance with safety standards.

Role of Nurses and Other Nonphysician Laser Operators

In many facilities in North America and abroad, nurses, technicians, assistants, and other nonmedical personnel are performing laser procedures. This mostly includes less invasive procedures such as laser hair removal. Although these procedures may not have mush risk or danger to patients, serious accidents have occurred and need to be recognized.

States have begun to pass legislation defining scope of practice for both users and operators of Class 3b and Class 4 healthcare laser systems. Each state is different in the extent of the law, the requirements for registration and licensure, and the individual's legal obligations to the state agency. As recently as February 2005, Arizona passed a new law requiring 40 hours of documented education and training by a state approved provider. Laws are in a state of flux, and it is necessary for each laser user or owner to check with their state agency (Board of Medical Records and the agency that regulates nonionizing radiation, e.g.

Radiation Safety or Nuclear Safety Agency) for current laws and titled codes.

As there is no recognized regulatory body in this area, many physicians have adopted this practice under the assumption they can train and vouch for their personnel. Physicians with this practice style should proceed with extreme caution and verify with local governing bodies if this is both legal and advisable. Nurses should clarify their roles with presiding medical and nursing boards. If the employee is an unlicensed assistant, the clinician must acquire information from their malpractice insurance carrier. If they ignore this information, physicians and/or nurses can face serious consequences in the event of an incident or accident. These consequences may include fines and loss of personal or facility licensure.

Before clinics allow nurses to perform procedures using lasers, it is important that they examine the following issues:

- Does the state have legislation governing ownership, installation, registration, and use, of lasers?
- Under which license (malpractice and liability) will the nurse practice?
- What position do the local governing boards of medicine and nursing have, on this issue?
- What documentation is required?
- What education and training must be documented?
- What supervision and control measures need to be adopted?
- Other important questions.

Warning Signs and Labels

Laser safety regulatory bodies mandate the appropriate labeling of all Class 2, 3, and 4 laser equipment. Information on the labels should include laser hazard classification, output energy and wavelength. It is also important that labels and warning signs be displayed in areas where they would best warn bystanders and other personnel of potential safety hazards. There are particular types of warning signs that are important and they will be outlined below.

Written Warning Signs

All locations using lasers are required to post a visible laser radiation label. For Class II lasers, the sign should be worded with CAUTION (see Fig. 12.7).

For Class III and Class IV, signs should be worded with DANGER (Figs 12.8, 12.9, 12.10).

Protective Equipment

In order to protect users from laser hazards, it is important understand the following concepts:

- maximum permissible exposure (MPE)
- optical density (OD)
- nominal hazard zones (NHZ)
- nominal ocular hazard distance (NOHD).

Maximum Permissible Exposure (MPE)

The MPE is a measure of the maximal amount of radiation exposure one can have without hazardous effect to tissue. The MPE is based on laser properties such as wavelength, energy, and duration of the exposure. The MPE is also important in determining the OD and NHZ, which are defined below.

Optical Density (OD)

The OD of the laser is important to determine the appropriate eye protection for the user. The OD of the eyewear is a measure of its capacity to filter light. In quantitative terms, the higher the OD, the lower amount of light that is transmitted to the eye. The OD employed is not to reduce vision significantly but is chosen to reduce the laser light below the MPE. The OD can be defined as the following ratio:

$$OD = \log_{10} [H_o/MPE]$$

H_o is defined as the worst case exposure conditions (watts/cm^2) and MPE has the same units. Optical density values of common lasers for various MPE times are shown in Table 12.4.

Nominal Hazard Zone (NHZ)

The NHZ is defined as the space in which the level of direct, reflected, or scattered radiation used during normal laser operation exceeds the applicable maximum permissible exposure. Exposure levels beyond the boundary of the NHZ should be below the MPE of the laser and control measures are not usually needed here. It is important that special eye and skin precautions be enforced when within the NHZ.

Nominal Ocular Hazard Distance (NOHD)

The NOHD is the distance along the axis of the direct laser beam to the human eye beyond which the MPE of the laser is not exceeded.

Protective Eyewear

Ocular injuries are preventable and regulatory bodies such as ANSI and OSHA mandate the use of protective eyewear for Class 3 and Class 4 lasers. When eye protection is employed, it is important that it is suitable for the specific wavelength and power of the corresponding laser.

Types of eye protection include goggles, face shields, or prescription eyewear with the goal of reducing exposure of the harmful beams to the eyes. Eyewear can also protect against other physical or chemical safety hazards.

To determine which eyewear is most suitable, the following factors should be considered:

- wavelength of laser
- mode of operation (continuous wave or pulsed)
- amount of radiation energy (maximum irradiance)
- maximum exposure duration
- maximum irradiance (W/cm^2) or fluence (J/cm^2)
- maximum permissible exposure (MPE)
- optical density (OD)
- side shield protectors

Table 12.4 *Optical Densities for Protective Eyewear for Various Laser Types*

Laser type/power	Wavelength (μm)	OD 0.25 for seconds	OD 10 for seconds	OD for 600 seconds	OD for 30,000 seconds
XeCl 50 watts	0.308[a]	–	6.2	8.0	9.7
XeFl 50 watts	0.351[a]	–	4.8	6.6	8.3
Argon 1.0 watt	0.514	3.0	3.4	5.2	6.4
Krypton 1.0 watt	0.530	3.0	3.4	5.2	6.4
Krypton 1.0 watt	0.568	3.0	3.4	4.9	6.1
HeNe 0.005 watt	0.633	0.7	1.1	1.7	2.9
Krypton 1.0 watt	0.647	3.0	3.4	3.9	5.0
GaAs 50 mW	0.840[c]	–	1.8	2.3	3.7
Nd:YAG 100 watt	1.064[a]	–	4.7	5.2	5.2
Nd:YAG (Q-switch)[b]	1.064[a]	–	4.5	5.0	5.4
Nd:YAG[c] 50 watts	1.33[a]	–	4.4	4.9	4.9
CO_2 1000 watts	10.6[a]	–	6.2	8.0	9.7

[a] Repetitively pulsed at 11 Hertz, 12 ns pulses, 20 mJ/pulse.
[b] OD for UV and FIR beams computed using 1 mm limiting aperture which presents a 'worst case scenario'. All visible/NIR computations assume a 7 mm limiting aperture.
[c] Nd:YAG operating at a less common 1.33 μm wavelength.
Note: All OD values were determined using MPE criteria of ANSI Z-136.1.

- type of protection needed (goggles or glasses)
- types of tasks being performed

The laser safety eyewear is chosen based on the level of protection needed to protect the eyes from the worst case scenario. If several products offer adequate protection, the following factors should be considered:

- cost
- effect on color vision
- fit and comfort
- prescription lenses
- field of view provided by the eyewear
- visible light transmission.

There are also different types of laser protection eyewear that one can choose from. The two most important ones include:

- Glass: this type is more expensive but it provides good visible light transmission. There are two types of glass eyewear to choose from: (i) those with absorptive glass, and (ii) those with reflective coatings.
- Polycarbonate: this type is very lightweight and less expensive, but allows less visible light transmission, and may not be as durable.

In accordance with the ANSI Z136.3 Guidelines 2000 each laser requires a specific type of protective eyewear, and one pair of eyewear may not be sufficient to protect you when working with different lasers. Be sure to check the label (OD and wavelength) on the eyewear to confirm protection from the laser being operated. It is also important to periodically inspect eye protection for cracking, discoloration, coating damage, and integrity to ensure full protection.

Other examples of protective equipment controls include the wearing of gloves during procedures, and the use of specialized clothing. This clothing can be fire resistant or of a disposable type.

Personnel Roles and Responsibilities

In locations where lasers are used, it is important that there be administrative controls to govern laser operations. This body includes the LSO, who will ensure that safety standards and regulations are properly followed. This body will also ensure those who work with lasers have received the proper training. The LSO has other important responsibilities including:

- Providing standard operating procedures (SOPs) regarding operation and maintenance of lasers in the workplace.
- A written laser safety manual, included in the SOPs or separate, describing the safety programs in detail. This should be regularly updated.
- Knowledge of the education and training requirements for laser safety.
- Knowing potential laser hazards, and control measures to reduce hazards.
- Reporting known accidents to the proper authorities.
- Maintaining service records of laser systems.
- Approving protective equipment.
- Training users in laser safety.
- Establishing and enforcing compliance with regulations established.
- Complying with all regulatory local, state, and national requirements.

- Ensuring effective interaction among medical staff and patient when laser is active.

The LSO must be available when lasers are in use and serves as the facility's point of contact for any investigation, audit, accreditation, or compliance review. The LSO must have adequate training and education to perform these duties and is vital to the safe operation of the laser. It is therefore the responsibility of the facility to establish its own criteria for LSO education and develop its own certification process.

Audit for Safety Program Monitoring

You can have an excellent safety program on paper but if you cannot validate compliance, it is not effective. The only way to prove compliance is to perform routine and comprehensive audits. The standards mandate this, as does OSHA, and it must be done annually or at frequencies determined by the LSO, based on the amount of use, and number of people involved.

A laser safety audit, for those who have not done one, is simply an assessment of staff compliance, equipment, supplies and documents involved in performing laser treatments in a facility (see Appendix 3). It can be performed by anyone familiar with the systems but must be supervised by the LSO, who is ultimately responsible. Audits help identify areas of deficit requiring further education and training, purchase of new equipment, or the need for additional control measures. Audits should always be done when new systems or procedures are initiated. Audit requires completing each of the following steps:

- inventory all equipment and develop a checklist
- inspect every item on the checklist, assessing its condition, placement, and handling
- interview staff working with the laser systems
- observe laser procedures (set up, testing, and intraoperative management)
- document results
- remedy deficiencies identified
- monitor outcomes and follow-up.

An inventory/checklist includes: laser unit, keys and storage system, delivery devices, signs, protective eyewear, window barriers, logs, tanks, supply carts, smoke evacuation systems, lens filters for microscopes and endoscopes, cleavers and strippers for fibers, operation manuals, adapters, and policy/procedure manuals. Include all lasers and all systems in all areas of the facility, including ophthalmology, clinics, hospital owned professional offices, emergency room, day surgery, cardiac catheter laboratory, dental unit, physiotherapy, or any other clinical or research area. If the facility operates a mobile service or satellite centers, all lasers in those areas must be included as well.

Questions to ask during an audit are:

1. Is it where it should be? (Stored, covered, cleaned)
2. Does it work properly? (Test all delivery systems and controls)
3. Is it being handled and used properly? (Observe staff, sign posting, eyewear etc.)
4. Is it safe? (All parts present and correct, policies present, etc.)
5. Is it intact?
6. Does it need repair or replacement?
7. Has it been misused or abused?

Results should be documented and reported to the program administrator, for action. The purpose of an audit is to identify potential hazards in equipment or work practices, and to lead to corrective actions. An example might be the discovery that the CO_2 laser arm is not replaced properly, potentially leading to damage and misalignment of the optics. If such an item is noted in the audit report, the resulting action could be to require every staff member to attend an inservice on handling the laser arm, and validate skill by performing a return demonstration for the LSO. Another audit result might be that glasses need to be replaced because they are scratched and have loose frames.

Audits should also include calibration and output testing, which can be delegated to biomedical engineering or the company laser technician. The LSO should keep a copy of audit reports in the laser program files, along with user credentials, equipment history, staff training validation, service agreements, logs, and other documentation.

Should there be an accident, incident, or occurrence, documentation of a current audit will help substantiate that the user maintained both safe systems, and staff compliance, in accordance with expectations of standards.

Safety is Everyone's Responsibility

Routine audit, troubleshooting, training, policy and procedure development, and compliance enforcement, are duties of the LSO, but case by case, day by day, patient by patient, laser safety depends on each and every healthcare professional's commitment and vigilance.

Lasers can offer patients a wonderful range of treatment options, from standard of care to experimental innovation. Laser users are constantly challenged to redefine who they are, what they do, and their scope of practice, with each new laser system or application. It must be remembered that every new system may demand a new look at safety policies and procedures, and that only through teamwork, communication, and respect for the technology, can we establish the foundation for a truly effective laser safety program.

Appendix 1
Summary of Settings for Laser Safety in the Workplace

A. Facilities where laser procedures are performed must develop a laser safety program:

1. Delegate responsibility for supervising laser safety to a laser safety officer (LSO).
2. Ensure laser safety officer conducts periodical audits of all lasers in facility.
3. Implement and enforce the safety recommendations and requirements outlined in safety manual.
4. Establish procedures regarding laser use in the facility.
5. Ensure only qualified personnel are permitted to operate laser.
6. Identify laser hazards and appropriate control measures.
7. Educate personnel on laser safety and use.
8. Notifying the authorities immediately in the event of an accident or incident.
9. Ensure all lasers in the facility are properly classified and labeled.
10. Register lasers with proper governing body and medical surveillance if available.

B. Educate personnel specific to laser systems used and procedures performed in facility:

1. Education programs should be in accordance with applicable federal, state, and local regulation.
2. Personnel should be required to demonstrate laser competency periodically.
3. Personnel should be re-trained when new equipment is brought into the practice environment.
4. Ensure laser operators follow established standard operating procedures.

C. Access to areas where lasers are used should be controlled:

1. Nominal hazard zone must be established.
2. Personnel with nominal hazard zone should be aware of hazards and precautions to prevent exposure.
3. Signs should be in place warning bystanders in facility of possible danger.
4. Lasers should be placed into restricted areas to minimize unauthorized access.

D. Persons in laser area should be protected from beam exposure:

1. Active lasers should never be left unattended.
2. Laser switches should be placed in location convenient to the operator.
3. Exposed tissues around the surgical site should be protected with saline-saturated or water-saturated materials.
4. People in nominal hazard area should wear appropriate eyewear which is specific to the wavelength and density of the laser being used. This includes laser operator, support staff and patient.
5. Refrain from wearing watches or reflective jewelry around live lasers.

E. Personnel in laser environment should protect themselves from air contaminants released from surgical process:

1. Operator, staff and patients should wear high-filtration surgical masks.
2. Laser-generated air contaminants should be removed by local ventilator. This collection device should be placed as close as possible to point where air contaminants are produced.

F. All people in laser area should be protected from electrical hazards associated with laser use:

1. Electrical hazards should be evaluated and minimized before using laser.
2. Regular maintenance and service should be performed on laser systems to ensure safety.

G. All people in laser area should be protected from fire hazards associated with laser use:

1. Fire hazards should be evaluated before and minimized before laser use.
2. Flammable liquids, combustible ointments, gases, paper, and other flammable materials should be properly placed before laser is used.
3. Fire extinguishers and water should be available in area of laser use.

Appendix 2
Sample: Standard Operating Procedure Form

Principal Investigator: .... Date: ....

Department: .... Location: ....

1. Laser safety contact information:

i. Principal investigator: phone: ....
ii. Laser safety officer: phone: ....
iii. Service contractor: phone: ....
iv. Emergency contact: phone: ....

2. Laser description:

Type: ....
Wavelength: ....
Classification: ....
Manufacturer: ....
Model: ....
Serial number: ....

3. Operating procedures:

i. Start up procedures
ii. Normal operating procedures
iii. Shut down procedures
iv. Special operating procedures
v. Emergency procedures

4. Control measures:

	Yes/No/Not Applicable	Comments
Administrative measures		
1. Lasers classified		
2. Standard operating procedures		
3. Laser users attended appropriate training		
Labeling		
1. Certification label present		
2. Class designation with warning label		
3. Radiation output on label		
4. Appropriate warning/danger sign posted		
5. Warning posted for invisible radiation		
Control measures		
1. Beam is enclosed as much as possible		
2. Beam not directed toward doors or windows		
3. Surfaces minimize specular reflections		
4. Controls are located so that the operator is not exposed to beam hazards		
Personal protective equipment		
1. Eye protection is appropriate for wavelength		
2. Eye protection has adequate OD		
Non-beam hazards		
1. High voltage equipment grounded		
2. High voltage equipment located away from wet surfaces or water sources		
3. High voltage warning label in place		

5. Additional comments:

....
....

6. Review by operators:

I have read and understood this document and its content.

Name: ....
Signature: ....
Date: ....

Appendix 3
Laser Program Audit Plan

Conducted by: Penny J. Smalley
Office: 773-262-2810
E-mail: pennyjs@aol.com

It is understood that the following is a flexible plan, and may change as needed during the site visit. Additional materials may be requested, and the facility is asked to supply the consultant with any contracts, waivers, or letters of agreement they may require, in order to assure access to needed materials, prior to the audit. It is also understood that should requested documents or materials be unavailable, either before or during the site visit, the audit results may be altered. It is essential that the audit address all laser use sites at all facilities within the corporate system, to assure compliance against national standards.

1. Administrative control

1. Materials needed: Membership roster for committee
2. Recent minutes
3. Points to be evaluated:
   i. Committee membership reviewed / leadership appropriate
   ii. Meetings well attended / agenda followed
   iii. Has the committee dealt effectively with issues

2. Laser safety officer (deputy laser safety officer)

1. Materials needed: Job Descriptions for LSO/DLSO
2. Statement of Authority from Management
3. Points to be evaluated:
   i. LSO/DLSO appointed – Statement of authority from administration
   ii. Training and qualifications documented
   iii. Time available for related duties
   iv. Continuing education plan
   v. LSO deals appropriately with problems and is available when needed
   vi. Safety audits and reporting completed

3. Equipment

1. Materials needed: I will need to go to wherever lasers and all associated delivery systems and accessory equipments are kept and I will be examining everything in their use areas.
2. Points evaluated are:
   i. Status and condition of equipment (history and documentation)
   ii. Physical plant (handling and moving, fire extinguishers, storage, etc.)
   iii. Proper handling, set-up, storage by staff

4. Continuing education

1. Materials needed: records of all inservice and training programs for nursing and technical staff
2. Credentialing criteria, forms, policies for medical staff
3. Notes, syllabus, materials from any courses attended
4. Points evaluated:
   i. Medical staff credentials (policies and forms) in order and current
   ii. Nursing staff training documented
   iii. New or additional staff orientation
   iv. Annual refresher and skills validation
   v. Conferences/workshops attended or planned
   vi. Learning needs assessment (current and future)

5. Documentation

1. Materials needed (copies I can keep) and points evaluated:
   i. Policies / procedures
   ii. Log sheets (review of current logs, and a copy of blank form)
   iii. Incident / Accident report forms and procedures for reporting
   iv. Problems identified (any QA reports or accidents that have occurred)
   v. Knowledge / presence of ANSI standards
   vi. Equipment inventory (biomed) with service contract information

6. Program development

1. No specific materials needed, unless identified by facility for any of the following points:
   i. New procedures / instrumentation to be acquired or initiated
   ii. Credentialing and training needs of new clinicians/ staff
   iii. Clinical research projects – industry partnerships
   iv. Alternative / additional practice sites or redesign/ expansion

v. Teaching program involvement (medical and/or nursing)

This audit will result in a written report that contains:

1. Executive Summary
2. Identification of areas of non-compliance with standards
3. Needs assessment
4. Recommendations for remedy of deficiencies
5. Long-term recommendations for growth of service

Further reading

American National Standards Institute. American National Standard for the Safe Use of Lasers: ANSI Z 136.1, 2000.

American National Standards Institute. American National Standard for the Safe Use of Lasers in the Health Care Environment: ANSI Z 136.3, 2005.

Food and Drug Administration. Performance standard for laser products, center for devices and radiological health, Food and Drug Administration (DHHS), 50 CFR 161: 33682–33702, 1985.

Laser Institute of America. Safety information on electrical hazards. Laser News, Laser Inst. America 1984; 6(5):8–14.

OSHA Instruction Pub 8-1.7. Guidelines for laser safety and hazard assessment. Occupational Safety and Health Administration. United States Department of Labor: Washington DC; 1991:29.

Chapter 13
Anesthesia for Cutaneous Laser Surgery

Nina Pabby, Anju Pabby and Mitchel P. Goldman

Children

Laser surgery can be uncomfortable, both for adults and for children. Some laser treatments can be accomplished without anesthesia, depending on the location, extent of the lesion, and the age and cooperation of the patient. Certain treatments are limited because of the pain experienced by the patient. This phenomenon is particularly evident in the treatment of vascular malformations in children, particularly port-wine stains (PWS), because children often complain of increased perception of pain with each subsequent treatment. The reason for this increased pain perception remains to be elucidated; however several potential explanations exist.

PWS have been shown to be derived from a progressive ectasia of the superficial vascular plexus. One hypothesis on the etiology of PWS stresses the importance of a near absence of sympathetic innervation, which modulates blood flow, possibly leading to defective maturation of the cutaneous sympathetic component and forming the basis for this progressive vascular ectasia.[1,2] One would assume that as the lesion lightens (losing its target vascularity), less laser energy would be absorbed, leading to less pain. However, as previously noted, patients often note that, as lesions lighten, successive treatments actually result in a slight increase in their perception of pain. This increased pain perception may occur because treating PWS reestablishes a normal vessel growth pattern leading to normalization of vessel innervation. Regardless of the exact reason for this phenomenon, treating vascular malformations with minimal pain in children is an important dilemma facing laser surgeons.

Nonetheless, the use of anesthetics in children undergoing cutaneous laser surgery remains a controversial issue, and its use is left to the discretion of the treating physician.[3–9] Painful laser treatments are made more tolerable by the use of different anesthetic techniques. Anesthesia may be delivered simply by precooling the lesion, applying a topical anesthetic such as LMX (Ferndale Laboratories, Inc., Ferndale, MI) or administering intralesional/block anesthesia using 1% lidocaine with or without epinephrine. Larger lesions in young children may be more effectively managed with the aid of general anesthesia or sedation. These anesthetic modalities along with their advantages and disadvantages are detailed below.

The surgeon must balance the advantages and disadvantages when deciding to use anesthesia. If the treating physician decides to use anesthesia, he/she must then decide which anesthetic modality to use. The list of criteria below will help discern physicians which anesthetic type would be most appropriate:[3,8]

1. patient's age
2. patient's medical history
3. patient and family preference
4. duration of procedure
5. skill and experience of anesthesiologist in different technique options
6. availability of appropriate monitoring equipment, medications, emergency equipment, and personnel
7. prevention of ignition by limiting ambient oxygen concentration near the laser.

The advantages of anesthesia in laser cutaneous surgery in children include less long-term emotional trauma because fewer details of treatments will be remembered, more treatment compliance, and more thorough treatments in each session (thereby decreasing the number of treatments required). In addition, it is particularly crucial that children are comfortable during a laser treatment, as erratic patient movement can result in excessive overlapping and double pulsing of laser impacts leading to possible adverse results. Furthermore, anesthesia serves to maintain a friendly rapport among the laser center staff, physician, patient, and family by making the patient feel comfortable.

Nonetheless, there are several disadvantages of anesthesia that must be considered. An exhaustive list of each complication of every anesthetic technique is beyond the scope of this chapter. However, the most significant complications from various anesthetic techniques include hypoxia from airway obstruction, bronchospasm, aspiration, hypoventilation, pulmonary edema, and laryngospasm. Allergic reactions to the anesthetic agent may also occur, with the rare possibility of malignant hyperthermia from inhalational anesthetic agents. Dysphoric and dystonic reactions, including emergence delirium, hallucinations, and flashbacks, may also occur with certain anesthetic agents (e.g. ketamine hydrochloride). In particular, with general anesthesia, children (especially those under 2 years of age) are at greater risk for hypoxia for a variety of reasons. These reasons include the propensity for airway obstruction from their relatively large tongue, a small functional residual lung capacity, high oxygen consumption, possibility of undiagnosed arterial cardiac shunts, possible patency of foramen ovale, and frequent upper respiratory tract infections, which result in prolonged hyperreactivity of airways.

Hypnosis 'Talkathesia'

All patients may benefit from soothing verbal and tactile reinforcement from both their doctors and families. This method uses hypnosis as an aid to improving a patient's tolerance level. The physician should coach the patient to relax and modify his or her own state of consciousness. One useful method is to have the patient concentrate on breathing. This simple maneuver is performed by having the patient take a slow, steady breath in to the count of 'one-two-three' and a slow, steady breath out to the count of 'one-two-three'. Timing the laser impact to a point in expiration appears to be less traumatic. Holding the patient's hand, with or without gentle stroking, is also a calming procedure. Adults sometimes wish to squeeze a nurse's hand. A complete discussion on formal hypnotic techniques is beyond the scope of this chapter. The reader is referred to an excellent text on this subject.[10]

Topical Cryothesia

Pretreatment application of ice bags and/or cryogen spray minimizes treatment pain and posttreatment tenderness. However, cooling the vessels to be treated will result in the need for a higher fluence to achieve effective treatment (see Chapters 1 and 2). For this reason, pretreatment ice application should be limited to a few seconds and repeated immediately after treatment. In addition, the ice bag is then moved over previously treated areas during the course of treatment. A decreased efficacy with this form of laser anesthesia has not been reported.

Topical Anesthetics

Lidocaine/Prilocaine (EMLA)

EMLA cream (Astra Pharmaceutical Products, Inc., Westborough, MA) is a 5% eutectic mixture of two local anesthetics, lidocaine (107 mmol/L = 25 mg/L) and prilocaine (113 mmol/L = 25 mg/L), with Arlatone 289 (emulgent), Carbopol 934 (thickener), and distilled water in 1 mL cream. The pH is adjusted to 9.4 with sodium hydroxide. One gram of cream is applied to a 10-cm^2 area.

EMLA cream has been found to be nontoxic, with plasma levels in the circulation measured at 100 times lower than those associated with toxicity.[11,12] In 22 infants, ranging in age from 3 to 12 months, 2 mL of EMLA was applied to 15 cm^2 of skin surface for 4 hours. In each case the plasma concentration of lidocaine and prilocaine was below toxic levels.[11]

The only adverse sequelae reported in the literature include mild local reactions, such as pallor, erythema, or edema, observed in treated skin areas.[11,13–19] Cutaneous blanching is thought to be secondary to vasoconstriction, which raises the possibility of decreasing the efficacy of laser treatment. Decreased efficacy was not found in one clinical study,[20] nor have we noted a decreased efficacy in our patients treated with EMLA.

EMLA is recommended to be applied thickly under occlusion with a polyurethane dressing (Tegaderm) for 60 minutes (Fig. 13.1). A maximum of 10 g should not be exceeded at any time in any patient. Below the age of 1 year the maximum application quantity is 2 g. A prospective double-blind randomized study assessing pain during laser treatment of PWS skin occluded with either Emla or placebo showed that pain scores for EMLA-treated sites were significantly lower ($p < 0.0001$).[21]

A study with the argon laser compared injectable lidocaine hydrochloride to Emla cream. Experimental subjects were adults with normal skin. The argon laser was used at a duration of 200 ms, beam diameter of 3 mm, and maximal intensity of 2.4 W. Interestingly, after 60 minutes of Emla application, pain blockade was obtained in nine of 12 subjects, with total sensory blockade in the remain-

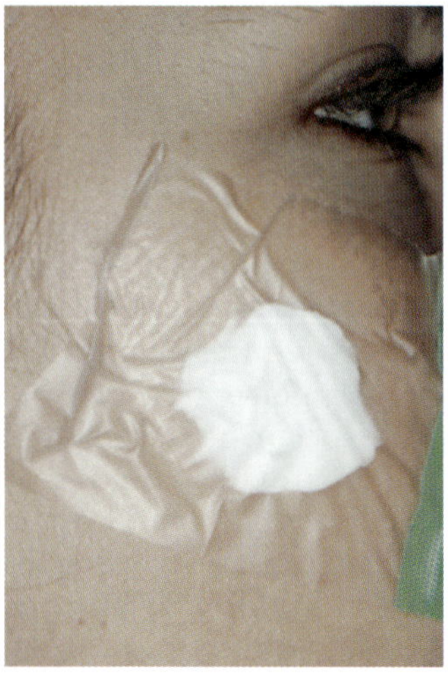

Figure 13.1 Appearance of EMLA under Tegaderm dressing. Note thickness of application.

ing three subjects. In addition, after a 60-minute application of Emla, analgesia did not immediately occur after removal of the cream, but reached a maximum extent 15 minutes after cream removal. The analgesic efficiency of EMLA cream increased with longer application time (60–120 minutes), approaching an analgesic state similar to conventional lidocaine infiltration. Lack of anesthetic effect of the EMLA returned to baseline 90 minutes after removal of the cream.[22]

Unfortunately, there has been some indication that experience with EMLA cream may be variable. Anecdotal evidence indicated that some patients will have excellent anesthetic results with an almost imperceptible reaction to laser pulses, while on another day the same patient may have absolutely no response to the cream. Therefore, it has been recommended by some to use Emla for small lesions but that it may not be useful for total, predictable anesthesia.

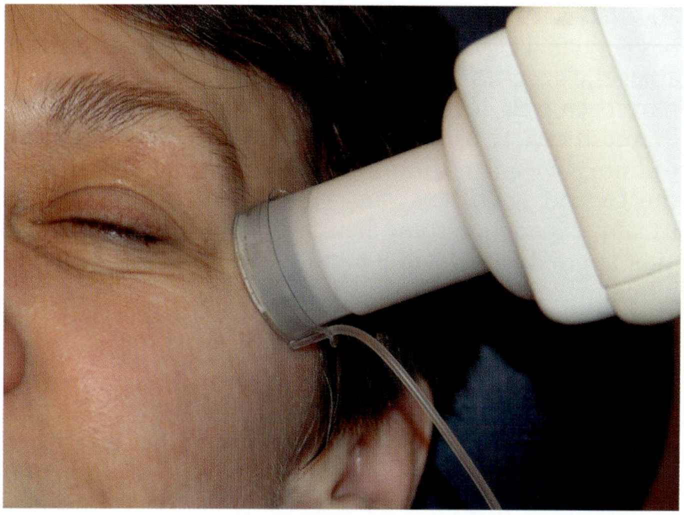

Figure 13.2 Iontophoresis. (Courtesy of Jaggi Rao, MD.)

Lidocaine/Tetracaine (LaserCaine)

Another topical anesthetic agent available for physician use within the office is LaserCaine (Unit Dose Pharmacy and Packaging, Phoenix, AZ). LaserCaine Compound contains 1% lidocaine and 3% or 4% tetracaine in a proprietary formulation. It is available in 2- and 3-oz sizes in two strengths, Classic, 3% tetracaine, and Forte, 4% tetracaine. It is intended for use on intact skin.

Preliminary observations indicate that LaserCaine has a 30% to 50% faster onset than Emla, produces little to minimal skin changes, and does not require the use of an occlusive dressing. It appears to have minimal toxicity. LaserCaine is rapidly metabolized in tissue through hydrolysis by serum cholinesterase. The half-life in serum is $1\frac{1}{2}$ to $2\frac{1}{2}$ minutes with a toxic blood level of 8 µg/mL, which is higher than the toxic level of lidocaine, 5 µg/mL. In addition, only 5% of tetracaine is present in the nonionized or active form at physiologic pH. However, patients with atypical plasma cholinesterase enzyme may be at increased risk for developing excessive plasma concentrations of local ester anesthetics because of absent or minimal hydrolysis. There have been reports of anaphylaxis with the use of tetracaine containing topical anesthetics.

Iontophoresis of Lidocaine

Iontophoresis describes the process of transporting charged ions across a membrane by means of an electric current. This technique can be used to deliver a large amount of medication into the skin, including local anesthetics.[23] Anesthesia induced by iontophoretic delivery of lidocaine is most effective when treating lesions within the epidermis and upper dermis.[4] The procedure entails adding 1.5 mL lidocaine hydrochloride 4% with epinephrine 1:50,000 to the polymer gel medication delivery electrode. Anesthesia is achieved with a minimum current delivered over 20 minutes. The duration of anesthetic effect with this mixture lasts between 60 and 90 minutes.[24,25] Two studies evaluating three[26] and eleven[27] patients respectively with PWS were conducted to test the efficacy of iontophoresis. Patients demonstrated significant decreases in discomfort of pulsed dye laser impulses with this iontophoretic mixture. In addition, no detrimental effect on flashlamp-pumped pulsed dye laser (FLPDL) ablation of PWS occurred despite significant decreases in perfusion, as measured by laser-Doppler velocimetry of the PWS receiving iontophoresis with the lidocaine/epinephrine mixture.[27]

The average time of iontophoresis is approximately 12 minutes. This usually yields a 30-minute anesthetic effect. The most common side effects to this treatment are prolonged erythema under the dispersive electrode and a burning sensation to underlying skin. A metallic taste has been noted by patients during some procedures when the electrode was placed on the face.[26,27] In a cooperative patient with a limited lesion, this modality may be useful (Fig. 13.2).

General Anesthesia

Use of general anesthesia is highly regulated by the Federal and State governments, and can only be administered in approved surgical centers that are meticulously monitored. Each surgical center must have specified updated equipment including anesthesia machines with appropriate vaporizers, intraoperative and postoperative monitoring systems, resuscitation equipment (defibrillator, oxygen delivery, intubation equipment, various intravenous drugs, etc.). A strict record-keeping system of the monitoring environment and procedures, as prescribed by the US Occupational Safety and Health Administration (OSHA), is also mandatory. Finally, specifically trained personnel are required. The physician is referred to the American Academy of Pediatrics (AAP) guidelines for the use of conscious sedation, deep sedation, and general anesthesia in pediatric patients for further information on this subject.[27] A complete discussion regarding these requirements is beyond the scope of this chapter.

Gaseous Anesthesia

Nitrous oxide (N_2O_2) is a sweet-smelling, nonexplosive gas with low anesthetic potency. It is administered with at least

30% oxygen (O_2) to prevent hypoxia. Nitrous oxide also has good analgesic properties and thus is useful as the sole analgesic agent for brief procedures. Its safety and efficacy have been well documented in numerous studies.[28,33]

Anesthesia is usually given initially at a flow rate of 6 L/min N_2O_2 and 6 L/min O_2. After approximately 1 minute the O_2 and N_2O_2 flows are reduced to 3 L/min. Patients usually experience some lightheadedness and relaxation after approximately 2 to 3 minutes. Patients usually report a tingling sensation of the toes or fingers. We typically use 'talkathesia' during N_2O_2 use to facilitate the anesthetic state. Nitrous oxide sedation is a helpful method for calming both children and adults and has been extremely safe in approximately 3000 pediatric procedures.[33]

Nitrous oxide is 35 times more soluble in blood than nitrogen. Therefore, at the end of the procedure, it is important to wash out all alveolar N_2O_2. To avoid diffusion hypoxia, we discontinue the N_2O_2 flow and ventilate the patient for 1 minute with 100% O_2 after the procedure has concluded.

Complications from N_2O_2 anesthesia use are limited. The most common adverse effect is postoperative nausea and vomiting occurring in up to 15% of patients.[34] A more serious complication from N_2O_2 use is fire. Gauze is capable of igniting when the FLPDL is used at 7 J/cm^2 in the presence of 100% O_2.[6] Hair has also been reported to ignite in room air when struck repeatedly at this laser energy or in the setting of 100% O_2.[6] Anecdotal report indicates one episode of ignition of a patient's eyebrow hair by the FLPDL during the use of nitrous oxide/oxygen. Therefore it is recommended to wet hair and gauze with saline and apply saline-soaked gauze to cover the exit ports of the nose inhalation piece.

Intravenous Sedation

Preoperative Preparation

A history and physical examination is recommended for each patient. The anesthetic plan should be discussed with parent(s) or guardian, and informed consent should be obtained. Families should be alerted to the possibility of unpleasant dreams and emergence phenomena for the patient. Such occurrences should be reported to modify future anesthesia.[35–40]

Routine laboratory tests are usually not required. Patients should be fasting overnight prior to administration of the anesthetic, with the exception of clear liquids, which are allowed 4 to 6 hours before the procedure. This regimen can probably be liberalized further based on recent studies.[41] In patients with acute, resolving, or recent respiratory infections the procedure should be postponed until symptoms, especially nasal secretions and cough, resolve.[42]

Premedication

Typically, no premedication is given for the first treatment. Subsequently, families are given the option of administering oral diazepam (Valium, 0.1–0.2 mg/kg) preoperatively if desired.

Induction/Maintenance/Emergence

The treatment room is prepared as follows. Oxygen E cylinder is checked and linked to a resuscitation bag. Suction equipment is assembled and readied with both a Yankauer suction and soft suction tip. An intravenous (IV) solution of lactated Ringer's with or without 5% glucose with microdrip system is prepared. Endotracheal tube and laryngoscope are readied. Medications are prepared, including ketamine, midazolam, fentanyl citrate hydrochloride, glycopyrrolate, atropine, succinylcholine chloride, droperidol, epinephrine, lidocaine, diphenhydramine hydrochloride, and others as needed. Monitors include precordial stethoscope, temperature monitor, Criticare #506 (contains noninvasive blood pressure measurement, pulse oximetry, electrocardiography), and backup manual blood pressure cuff with sphygmomanometer. Ohmeda 9000 continuous/bolus infusion pump is readied with diluted ketamine solution, usually with milligrams of ketamine 3 to 6 times patient weight in kilograms in a final volume of 20 mL (Fig. 13.3).

The patient and at least one family member are brought to the treatment room. Most patients allow IV placement with parental presence. Some patients are given an initial intramuscular (IM) dose of ketamine, 2 to 3 mg/kg of body weight with or without atropine, 0.02 mg/kg, as sedation for placing the IV catheter.

Once the IV 22-gauge catheter is secured, IV sedation is started. Initially, 0.01 mg/kg of glycopyrrolate (Robinul) is given, followed by small increments of midazolam (Versed) to induce amnesia and anxiolysis and prevent unpleasant dreaming and emergence phenomena from ketamine. Doses of midazolam vary with age, weight, and level of anxiety; for example, 0.25 mg for a 1-year-old versus 11 mg for a 10-year-old child. Ketamine is started, usually with a small bolus followed by an infusion. The typical initial bolus is usually up to about 1 to 3 mg/kg, sometimes in increments. This is followed by ketamine infusion titrated to effect. The dose range for infusion is typically between

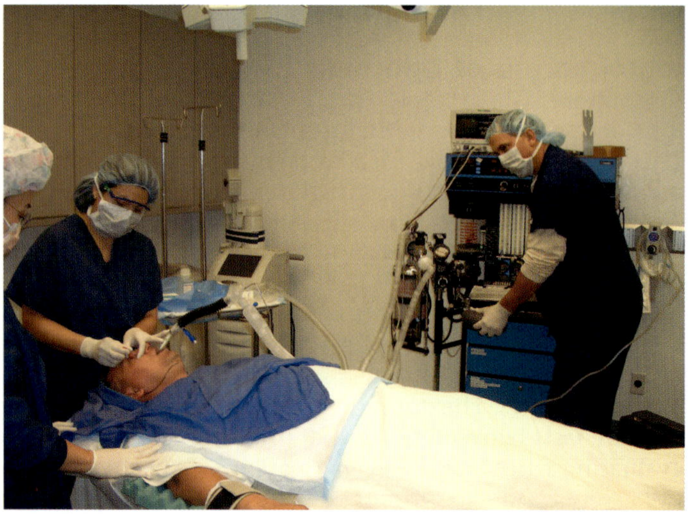

Figure 13.3 Typical laser operatory with monitoring, anesthesia, and emergency equipment readily available.

50 and 200 µg/kg/min, using higher rates initially and lower rates as the procedure progresses. The infusion is stopped shortly before or at the conclusion of the procedure. The level of sedation varies among patients, with most patients calm and quiet on this regimen.

Some patients talk and move during the procedure. If patients move excessively or begin to cry, the rate of ketamine infusion is increased or supplemented with other IV agents (usually, small doses of midazolam or fentanyl). Patients with a history of emesis during the procedure are often given prophylactic droperidol (Inapsine), 0.1 to 0.25 mL IV. Some patients also receive IV diphenhydramine at the beginning of the procedure to help limit erythematous flaring around the lesion, which at times obscures the margins for treatment.

At the conclusion of the procedure, the patient is closely observed and monitored until consciousness resumes. In particular, the patient is monitored for any problems with emergence, such as vomiting, delirium, and coughing. Most patients do very well with the above regimen; they maintain stable vital signs, tolerate the procedure well, and awake calmly. As with any technique, some problems are encountered, as follows:

- coughing during procedure
- coughing on emergence
- hiccups during procedure
- emesis during procedure
- emesis on emergence
- excitement on emergence
- irregular or decreased respiratory rate.

Each of these events occurs infrequently (less than 4% of procedures), and most are mild. Coughing responses are the most worrisome reactions because of the concern for potential laryngospasm.[43,44] Occasional respiratory rate irregularity or slowing is extremely mild and responds well to adjustment of ketamine infusion and avoidance of other IV agents. Emesis is usually mild; vomitus is gently suctioned if necessary and droperidol occasionally given. Hiccups rarely occur secondary to midazolam or possibly ketamine use.[39,43,45]

The use of ketamine in small boluses and infusion usually permits adequate spontaneous ventilation so that supplemental O_2 is not routinely required (although O_2 must always be available in case needed, and oximetry is critical). This lack of necessity of oxygen is desirable in laser procedures where ignition is always a risk, and also allows for avoidance of masks, which could restrict the field of the laser treatment for facial lesions. The continuous infusion of ketamine helps limit the total dose of the drug and allows flexible and delicate titration during the procedure. The recommended dosage range is well documented.[46–52] Glycopyrrolate prevents the excessive secretions that ketamine typically causes, and midazolam promotes tranquility and amnesia.

Furthermore, the disadvantages of intravenous sedation should be considered. Although ketamine usually permits adequate or even increased ventilation, hypoventilation can occur.[40,44,53–56] Coughing and laryngospasm, although rare, may also occur.[39,43,44] Excessive salivation with ketamine, although usually blocked with a drying agent, may predispose to coughing and laryngospasm.[39] Emergence phenomena can be a problem with ketamine, but midazolam seems to control this problem adequately.[35,36,40,56] Midazolam itself can cause hypoventilation, hiccups, excessive sedation, emesis, and emergence delirium; careful dosing and vigilance are critical.[39]

Propofol Anesthesia

Propofol (Diprivan) is an IV sedative-hypnotic agent that can be used for sedation, induction, and maintenance of general anesthesia. It is slightly soluble in water and is formulated as an emulsion containing the active agent 2,6-diisopropylphenol (10 mg/mL) along with soybean oil, egg lecithin, and glycerol. Propofol may be used as a single agent or in combination with other sedatives, narcotics, or inhaled anesthetics. Induction of anesthesia with propofol is smooth and rapid. Intermittent bolus injections or a continuous infusion can be used to maintain anesthesia.

Propofol may offer advantages over the other sedative-hypnotics because of its short duration of effect, rapid recovery, and minimal side effects.[57] Propofol is highly lipid soluble, so after an induction dose, rapid blood–brain equilibration occurs, resulting in rapid loss of consciousness. After a single bolus, blood concentrations fall rapidly because of extensive tissue redistribution and rapid elimination. Metabolic clearance is the highest of any IV hypnotic, even with impairment of renal and hepatic function. Propofol blood concentration and depth of sedation may be maintained by intermittent bolus or continuous infusion.

Numerous dosage guidelines for propofol are provided in the literature.[58–62] A dosage range of 2 to 3 mg/kg for induction followed by an initial infusion of 100 to 300 µg/kg/min is common. If the infusion rate is titrated to match the level of anesthesia to the level of surgical stimulation, excessive drug level and prolonged recovery may be avoided. Dosage requirements decrease with age and debility, as well as with adjuvant opiates and premedication. Maintenance of anesthesia should be administered by continuous infusion rather than intermittent boluses which may result in undesirable oscillations of the propofol blood concentrations and will vary the anesthetic depth. The infusion rate should be titrated to the level of desired central nervous system (CNS) depression and to the duration of the procedure.[58]

The major hemodynamic effect of propofol is arterial hypotension (up to 30%) with minimal change in heart rate. Both decreased systemic vascular resistance and direct myocardial depression have been implicated as important factors in producing hypotension after large bolus doses of propofol.[57] The cardiovascular effects are accentuated and may be significant in the presence of hypovolemia (excessive NPO status) and preexisting cardiovascular disease and in elderly patients. Most investigators seem to agree that the clinical significance of these changes in young, healthy, normovolemic patients is negligible.[63] Once again, dosage should be titrated for the individual patient and surgical procedure.

Propofol has a profound respiratory depressive effect including a decrease in tidal volume, minute ventilation, and a depressed ventilatory response to hypoxemia[64] and hypercarbia. Apnea (20–30 s) may occur after a large bolus, stressing the importance of infusion rate titration to allow spontaneous ventilation without supplemental oxygen. The expertise and equipment necessary to monitor and maintain the airway, including supplemental oxygen and ventilatory support, are implicit in the use of this drug.[65]

Several minor disadvantages accompany this technique. IV access must be established in small children with each treatment. With an uncooperative or very frightened child, low-dose IM ketamine, 2 to 3 mg/kg, with atropine, 0.02 mg/kg, is used as a pre-induction sedative to facilitate establishment of IV access. Pain on injection of propofol into a vein in the dorsum of the hand is common (30%–45%). The incidence of pain can be decreased (6%–12%) if injection is made into a large vein of the forearm or antecubital fossa.[61,65] The incidence of injection pain can be decreased with a dose of IV lidocaine, modified Bier block,[66] or addition of 1 mg/mL lidocaine to the propofol emulsion will significantly reduce the incidence of injection pain.

Nonetheless, the aforementioned emulsion formulation is capable of supporting rapid growth of bacteria if contaminated. Therefore, strict aseptic techniques must be maintained when handling propofol. In addition, it is recommended that unused drug be discarded at the end of the procedure or at 6 hours, whichever occurs sooner.

Overall, propofol is a desirable sedative agent because of its rapid induction, rapid re-distribution, rapid recovery with clear emergence and a low incidence of nausea and vomiting.[57] Studies also suggest that propofol can be used safely in malignant hyperthermia-susceptible patients.[67–69] For these reasons, propofol anesthesia is popular among children and their parents.

Inhalation Anesthesia

When general anesthesia has been selected as the anesthetic technique, no single approach will be effective for all children in all situations. Of the various routes of induction (rectal, IV, IM, and inhalation), halothane inhalation is the most commonly used technique in pediatric anesthesia. Inhalation induction of anesthesia may be preferred for small infants and children with abnormal airways. Halothane offers a rapid, smooth induction with rapid recovery for brief procedures. Nausea and vomiting may occur, but recovery is usually uneventful. Other inhalation anesthetic agents such as isoflurane and enflurane have a longer induction period and produce a higher incidence of coughing and breath holding.[70] Two new potent agents, sevoflurane and desflurane, are in clinical trials. Both appear to have significant advantages over present agents.[71] A detailed discussion is beyond the scope of this chapter.

Summary

A variety of anesthetic modalities can be employed when treating children with laser surgery depending upon the need and preferences of the physicians, the patient, and the families. The choice of agents and technique should be based on the needs of the individual child[72] and the surgical requirements while balancing the risks and benefits of the various techniques.

Adults

As with children, many laser treatments in adults can be painful and uncomfortable, although some treatments can be accomplished without anesthesia or with limited application of topical agents. Nonetheless, more painful procedures may require more invasive anesthetic techniques.[73,74] For example, facial laser resurfacing is a highly stimulating and often painful procedure requiring a combination of anesthetic modalities. Furthermore, the anesthetic goal during surgery is to render the patient insensitive to pain over the treated area, motionless during the procedure, and amnestic for the time spent in the operating suite. Specific pharmacologic agents are selected to meet these clinical objectives. Anxiolytics, hypnotics, dissociative agents, narcotics, and nonsteroidal antiinflammatory drugs (NSAIDs), as well as inhaled anesthetics, all may play a role in meeting anesthetic goals. The advantages and disadvantages of various techniques will be discussed below.

General Anesthesia

General anesthesia with endotracheal (ET) intubation may be administered quickly and is usually safe when proper monitoring occurs. General anesthesia ensures airway control and allows the administration of adequate narcotic analgesia without concern for respiratory depression. However, not all facilities are equipped to provide general anesthesia, and because of potential complications while the patient is unconscious, the patient or physician may be reluctant to use this technique.

Intravenous Anesthesia

Advances in anesthetic airway management, specifically the development of the laryngeal mask airway (LMA), has allows for increased flexibility in office-based practice. For example, LMA allows facial laser resurfacing to be safely performed using IV and or inhaled agents while maintaining spontaneous ventilation and airway control. If necessary, the technique of IV anesthesia combined with the use of an LMA can provide safe and effective anesthesia for laser facial resurfacing without the need for an anesthesia machine.

Although some surgeons have utilized a combination of local and regional anesthetic techniques, total intravenous anesthesia offers several advantages since infiltration of local anesthetics may often distort facial anatomy and increase post operative discomfort. In addition, any movement of the patient may alter the surgical result and increase the risk of complications. Given these risks, total intravenous anesthesia provides a cost-effective method to provide anesthesia with minimal risk to patients undergoing laser facial resurfacing. Sore throats, however, related to LMA use, are common.[75] Despite this minimal risk, proper patient monitoring and availability of airway management equipment, emergency airway and cardiac medications, and a defibrillator should be ensured. A potential intravenous anesthesia regimen is discussed below.

Often-times in laser resurfacing, propofol (Diprivan) is the primary IV sedative agent used because it provides rapid induction, easy maintenance, and quick termination. Analgesia is provided by fentanyl (Sublimaze) supplemented intermittently with ketamine (Ketalar). To counteract the potentially troublesome side effects of ketamine, as well as to provide sedation and amnesia, all patients receive midazolam (Versed) on initiation of IV access and the total dose of ketamine is limited to 1 mg/kg. This regimen decreases the risk of 'bad dreams' and adverse psychic experiences. In addition, Glycopyrrolate (Robinul) can be used as a drying agent to help keep the airway free of excess secretions.

After IV access has been secured, sedation is generally achieved with midazolam at a dose of 0.05 to 0.1 mg/kg. Glycopyrrolate 0.2 mg, and fentanyl, 50 to 100 μg are given, followed by an initial dose of propofol, 1 to 2 mg/kg, to facilitate the placement of the LMA. With the LMA in proper position and the patient breathing spontaneously, propofol is administered in a continuous infusion using an IV infusion pump in a dose of 4–8 mg/kg/h. Supplemental oxygen may be supplied from the circle system of an anesthetic machine or through tubing from an oxygen cylinder at 2–4 liters/min. If an anesthetic machine is being used, N_2O and anesthetic gases may also be used; however, their addition may lead to an increased incidence of postoperative nausea and vomiting. IV analgesia is provided as needed with small doses of ketamine, 10–20 mg, and/or fentanyl, 25–50 μg. Continuous electrocardiography (ECG), pulse oximetry, blood pressure at 5-minute intervals, and continuous end-tidal CO_2 volume are used to monitor the patient. At the conclusion of the laser resurfacing, the propofol infusion is discontinued, and the patient rapidly awakens. The LMA is removed when the patient is able to follow commands, usually within about 5 minutes.

The aforementioned anesthetic technique requires an EKG machine, blood pressure monitor, functional suction apparatus, pulse oximeter, supplemental oxygen source, LAM and IV infusion pump. Capnography, although optional, is desirable to monitor the adequacy of ventilation. Any facility administering narcotics or sedatives must have appropriately trained medical personnel, a fully stocked resuscitation cart, intubation equipment (laryngoscope, blades, ET tubes), a method for delivering positive-pressure ventilation (Ambubag or Jackson Rees circuit), and a charged and functional defibrillator. In addition, a recovery area staffed with qualified nursing personnel should have the capacity to monitor ECG, blood pressure, and pulse oximetry.

Even in a properly monitored environment, there has been some concern over the safety of using lasers in close proximity to oxygen. The use of opioids mandates the use of oxygen to maintain the pulse oximetry above 90%. Although modern inhaled anesthetics are nonflammable, CO_2 and N_2O_2 are combustible. Therefore, it is imperative that flammable liquids and prep solutions not be used in the facial preparation. The LMA and its pilot tube used to inflate the pharyngeal cuff are both very resistant to damage from inadvertent laser strikes, but green O_2 tubing is easily damaged by a few laser pulses. However, the oxygen flowing through the tube will not ignite. ET and LMA tubes can be fully protected by wrapping them with saline-soaked gauze or towels. With proper technique and caution preventing combustible liquids near operative areas, laser resurfacing in the presence of oxygen and an anesthetic delivery system such as an ET or LMA can be very safe.

Conscious Sedation without LMA

Conscious sedation is defined as a depressed level of consciousness during which a patient retains control over his protective reflexes and can respond to commands. This type of anesthesia is being used more frequently for outpatient dermatologic and cosmetic surgery, and is particularly relevant in laser rejuvenation. Sedation renders a patient less mobile than simply injecting a local anesthetic or using topically applied cream, thereby decreasing the risks of complications from the surgical procedure. A combination of propofol, a nonbarbiturate anesthetic, and fentanyl, an opioid agonist, is often used. The nonbarbituate anesthetic provides amnesia as well as mental detachment from the the procedure.

In a recent study, twenty patients received conscious sedation for procedures including dermabrasions, blepharoplasties, facelifts, CO_2 laser resurfacing, and liposuction. First, each patient was given 1 μm/kg IV of fentanyl. Then, the patient received an initial bolus of propofol of 0.5 mg/kg followed by a continuous infusion rate at 150 μg/kg/min to achieve conscious sedation. A total of 95% of the patients reported a lack of pain from the procedure; only two experienced nausea after the procedure. Other analgesic choices include ketorolac (up to a total 30 mg), phenoperidine, and pentazocine. Midazolam (up to maximum of 20 mg) has also been used as a short-acting powerful sedative. Although this technique is designed to maintain protective reflexes, it should be avoided in patients who are at high risk for airway incompetence during sedation. Basic monitoring should occur throughout the procedure, including pulse oximetry, blood pressure and EKG. Emergency drugs and equipment must be available. Pulse oximetry should be continued for about 20 minutes after the conclusion of the procedure. Generally, the patient can then be discharged after an hour with a responsible adult. Potential problems with conscious sedation include oversedation, undersedation, and drug reactions.[76,77]

Propofol–Ketamine Technique With Opioid Avoidance

Opioid use has been associated with an 8.3% incidence of postoperative nausea and vomiting when used with droperidol and ondansetron prophylaxis. A recent retrospective study using propofol–ketamine anesthetic technique with opioid avoidance, room air, and spontaneous ventilation indicates that this combination may be an excellent anesthetic alternative for full-face laser resurfacing. Patients in this study were given glycopyrrolate 0.2 mg at the onset. Some patients then received 2 or 4 mg of midazolam to reduce propofol requirements. Propofol was administered as a dilute (5 mg/mL) solution in a 50-mL bag connected via a 60 drops/mL IV set piggybacked into the most proximal main IV port. The patients were titrated to a loss of lid reflex and verbal response, and then given a 50 mg IV bolus of ketamine. Within 2 minutes, injection of local anesthetic could begin. The main branches of the trigeminal nerve were blocked with 2–5 mL of 2% lidocaine with 1:100,000 epinephrine (Fig. 13.4) One milliliter of this solution was also injected into the zygomaticotemporal and zygomaticofacial branches. Then, a field block of 1% lidocaine with 1:100,000 epinephrine was injected along the entire perimeter of the face, and sometimes this was followed by a fan injection in the cheek area with the 1% solution. A retrospective chart review of 95 consenting adults receiving this anesthesia regimen in an office-based setting indicates no evidence of hallucinations, postoperative nausea and vomiting, and no cardiovascular instability or seizures (signs of lidocaine toxicity). In addition, this technique allowed for an immobile, unconscious patient with adequate local anesthesia, without the increased equipment requirements and complication risk associated with general anesthesia.[78]

Iontophoresis

Iontophoresis, the introduction of various ions into the skin through the use of electricity, has been increasingly used by dermatologists to provide pain relief in outpatient procedures. Iontophoresis uses an electric current to overcome some of the barriers of the skin and assist the penetration through the movement of ions into the skin via sweat glands, hair follicles, and sebaceous glands. Generally, a constant direct current is used, although pulsed currents have also been shown to be effective. Constant direct current is generally limited to 10 to 15 minutes and 1 mA/cm^2 secondary to burns that can result from generated hydrogen and hydroxide ions. Ultimately, iontophoresis can be used to deliver chemicals to both superficial and deeper layers of the skin. The advantages of this technique are multifold: (1) it avoids the pain associated with injection and IV modalities; (2) it prevents the variation in absorption seen with oral medications; (3) it bypasses first-pass elimination; (4) drugs with short half-lives can be delivered directly to tissues; and (5) rapid termination can occur. Disadvantages to this technique include discomfort and erythema at the site of iontophoresis secondary to pH changes. There is also the potential for skin irritation and burns; however, these risks can be minimized by thoroughly cleansing the skin, using well-saturated pads for electrodes, and ensuring even skin contact.[79]

Iontophoresis of lidocaine diluted in distilled water has allowed for anesthesia to the depth of at least several millimeters. This mechanism allows for minimal systemic absorption of the drug and direct delivery of the drug to the tissues. The addition of epinephrine assists in penetration and increases the duration of anesthesia. According to the 'bottleneck theory' which states that there is a thresh-

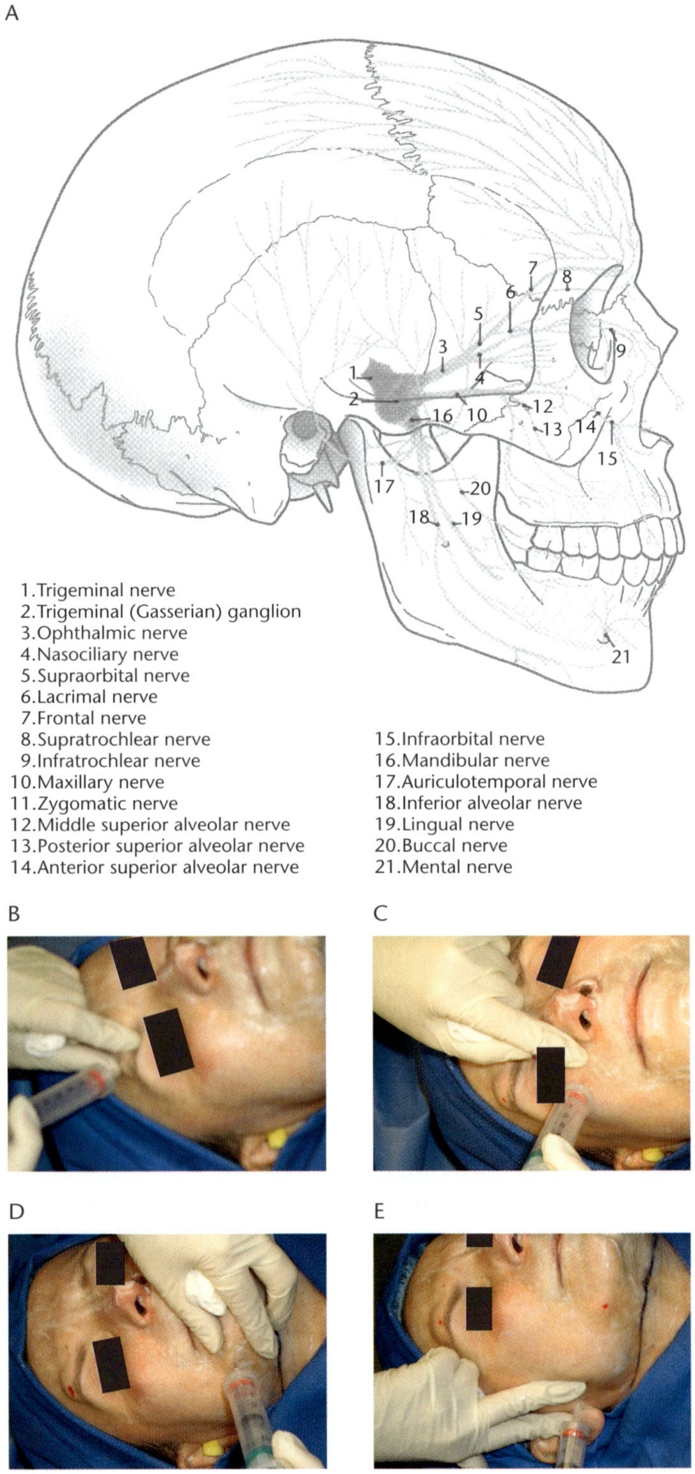

Figure 13.4 (A) Nerve blocks required for facial analgesia. (B) Supraorbital injection. (C) Maxillary nerve injection. (D) Mandibular nerve injection. (E) Auriculotemporal nerve injection.

old number of molecules able to penetrate the skin via iontophoresis, the duration of current flow and the amount of applied current predominantly determine drug penetration. Recent research has shown that iontophoresis of 4% lidocaine with epinephrine (1:50,000) using a mean total current of 3.4mA for an average of 8 minutes caused an 80–100% relief of pain from injections, dermabrasions, superficial laser surgery, and electrosurgery. Approximately 25% of patients experienced adverse effects including erythema, mild tingling, stinging, burning, and a transient metallic taste. Furthermore, a study conducted by Greenbaum and Bernstein comparing the efficacy of iontophoresis of a lidocaine solution for 30 minutes with topical EMLA applied for 30 to 60 minutes. Iontophoresis of lidocaine was found to be more anesthetizing to pinprick. Overall, it seems that iontophoresis may be very useful in superficial ablative procedures with lasers, electrosurgery, dermabrasion, scalpel, or scissors. For deeper procedures, this technique can allow for enough anesthesia to allow for painless infiltration with lidocaine.[79]

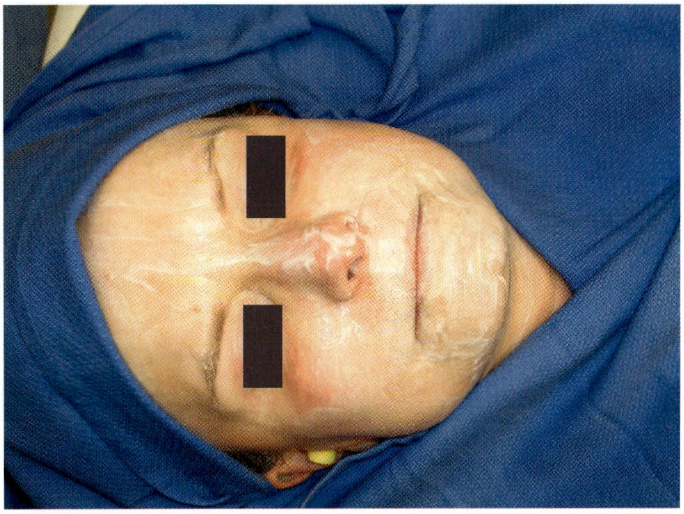

Figure 13.5 Application of LMX to full face prior to a one- or two-pass Er:YAG laser resurfacing.

Topical Anesthesia

In addition, to the aforementioned techniques, topical anesthesia continues to be used with laser and surgical techniques. Recently, the movement towards less aggressive laser resurfacing techniques (such as single-pass CO_2 laser ablation and nonablative laser remodeling) has increased the demand for adequate topical anesthetics to replace intravenous sedation. Generally, topical anesthetics function by inhibiting sodium channels, leading to a block of nerve impulse conduction.

As mentioned previously, EMLA cream is a 5% eutectic mixture of lidocaine and prilocaine, and remains the most widely used topical anesthetic. Several studies have indicated that EMLA is effective in reducing or eliminating pain associated with pulsed dye laser treatments after a 60-minute application period. EMLA has been shown to be effective on the face and thighs after 25 minutes. Potential side effects that must be considered include methemoglobinemia (rare), blanching, redness, pruritus, burning, and purpura. Caution must be exercised when EMLA is used near the eyes as it may cause chemical eye injuries, including but not limited to corneal abrasions and ulcerations.

LMX is another topical anesthetic consisting of 4% or 5% lidocaine in a liposomal delivery system. After a 60-minute application period under occlusion, 5% liposomal lidocaine was recently shown to be effective in producing anesthesia to laser induced pain stimuli. Its efficacy seems to be comparable to EMLA but superior to betacaine LA and tetracaine (see below). Its liposomal delivery system enhances its effects by facilitating penetration of the anesthetic into the skin and providing sustained release. A recent study evaluated the efficacy and onset of action of EMLA versus LMX using a high energy pulsed light source. Results of the study indicated that a maximum anesthestic effect was achieved 20 minutes after application of LMX, and that a similar maximum effect was achieved after 1.5 hours of EMLA under occlusion. Nonetheless, lidocaine toxicity may occur when LMX is used over large areas for more than 2 hours.[80–82] We use LMX routinely with or without nerve blocks to perform one- or two-pass Er:YAG laser resurfacing of the face (Fig. 13.5). We have found that a 20-minute application of LMX provides adequate anesthesia for the 20–40μm ablative effects of the Er:YAG laser at 1–2J/cm^2.

Betacaine-LA is another topical anesthetic consisting of lidocaine, prilocaine, and a vasoconstrictor. Some preliminary anecdotal reports indicate that this anesthetic may be more effective than EMLA, however more controlled research is necessary. Betacaine-LA is not approved by the FDA. In addition, Amethocaine 4.0% gel, which contains 4% tetracaine, has been used extensively in Europe. Studies have indicated that tetracaine may be significantly effective in reducing pain associated with pulse dye laser treatment. Potential side effects include local erythema, pruritus, and edema. Tetracaine gel is a compounded anesthetic containing 4% tetracaine in lecithin-gel base. This gel has not yet received FDA approval, however it may be beneficial. Another topical anesthetic agent is Topicaine, consisting of 4% lidocaine in gel microemulsion. Studies indicate that Topicaine has a very rapid onset of action with a long duration of effect. Topicaine is FDA approved with a recommended application time of 30 to 60 minutes with occlusion, and is gaining popularity in laser hair removal. Side effects include erythema, blanching, and edema.[80]

S-Caine Patch

The S-Caine local anesthetic patch (ZARS, Inc. Salt Lake City, UT), which utilizes a disposable, oxygen-activated heating element to assist in dermal penetration, contains a eutectic 1:1 mixture of lidocaine base and tetracaine base. After it dries, this peel becomes a flexible membrane that provides inherent occlusion, and is readily removed (Fig. 13.6). Studies have indicated that the S-Caine local patch has been effective in alleviating pain associated with shave biopsies, venipuncture, and vascular access procedures.

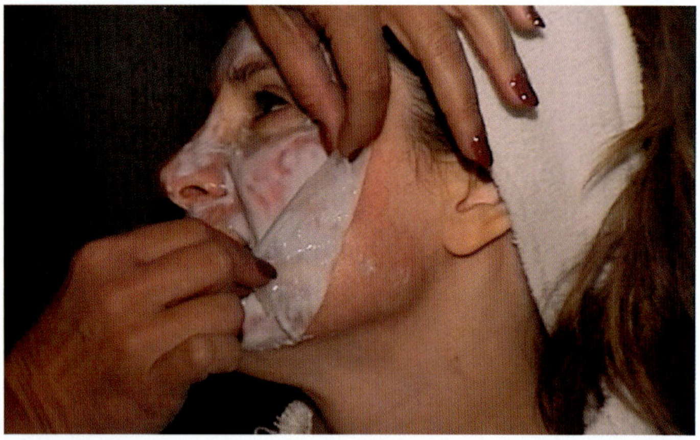

Figure 13.6 S-Caine peel anesthesia. (Courtesy of Tina Alster, MD.)

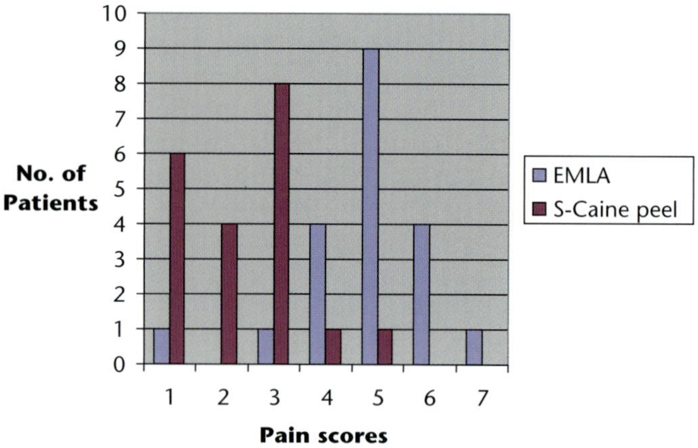

Figure 13.7 Emla versus S-Caine peel. (Reproduced from Alster T, Lupton J: Evaluation of a novel topical anesthetic agent for cutaneous laser resurfacing: a randomized comparison study. Dermatol Surg 28: 1004–1006, 2002.)

This peel is currently in FDA Phase III clinical trials, and its use for laser and surgical procedures is still being investigated. A recent randomized, double-blind, placebo controlled trial with the S-Caine peel for anesthesia prior to pulsed dye laser treatments indicates that a 60-minute application of the peel is more effective than placebo in pain relief for these procedures.

Alster has evaluated the efficacy of the S-Caine peel versus Emla cream in providing anesthesia prior to cutaneous laser resurfacing.[81] Twenty patients were enrolled in a double-blind institutional review board approved study in which a 4-cm × 4-cm patch of each cheek was randomized to receive either EMLA cream or S-Caine peel. The creams were applied for 30 minutes (previous studies indicate that the optimal application time for the S-Caine peel is 30 minutes) with EMLA cream being occluded under plastic. After removal of the creams, the area was evaluated for erythema, edema, and skin blanching. The patients then underwent single-pass CO_2 laser resurfacing to each area using the UltraPulse 5000C with an 8 mm^2 computer pattern generator scan at a density of 5. The laser has a pulse energy of 300 mJ, pulse power of 60 W, and pulse duration of 950 µs. After each area, patients evaluated their discomfort, pain relief, and side effects. The blinded investigator and independent assessor also evaluated the patients' level of discomfort. Results indicated that the pain scores were significantly lower using the S-Caine peel and side effects were limited to mild transient erythema and skin blanching (Fig. 13.7). In addition, 95% of patients reported adequate pain relief for the laser procedure on the side that had the S-Caine, compared to only 20% on the side with the EMLA cream. The investigator and independent observer had similar results regarding observed patient discomfort. The same study also makes reference to successful use of the S-Caine peel as a sole anesthetic in full-face ablative laser skin surgery (although some patients may require an additional local or nerve block in certain areas).

Others have also analyzed the efficacy of this peel as a topical anesthetic prior to pulsed dye laser treatment for vascular lesions of the face.[82–84] Results indicate that patients experienced significant pain reduction using the peel and that an application time of 20 or 30 minutes was as effective as 60 minutes. Another clinical trial evaluated the efficacy of the S-Caine peel for the induction of anesthesia after a 30-minute application period, and found that it provided effective dermal anesthesia for nonablative laser treatment with the 1450-nm diode laser.[85] In this study, twenty patients received concurrent 30-minute applications of the S-Caine peel and a placebo cream to either side of their face. After one pass of the 1450 nm diode laser, patients' pain levels were evaluated using a visual analog scale and through investigator and independent observer evaluation. The results indicated a statistically significant ($p < 0.001$) decrease in pain perception between the active and placebo sites. Also, a painless procedure was noted in 50% and 65% of the active sites by the independent observer and investigator respectively, while at the placebo sites a painless procedure was noted in 0% and 5% respectively. A study on pain relief with Q-switched laser tattoo demonstrated adequate pain relief in 50% of patients who applied the S-Caine peel versus 7% with placebo.[86] This study also showed that 70% of patients had less pain with the S-Caine peel, versus 10% with placebo cream. However, when the S-Caine was used as anesthesia in minor dermatologic procedures such as shave biopsy or superficial excision, there was no statistically significant difference than placebo.[87] Therefore, the depth of anesthetic effects of the S-Caine peel is fairly superficial.

The treatment of leg veins with the long-pulsed 1064 nm Nd:YAG laser can be quite painful (see Chapters 2 and 9). Topical application of S-Caine for 60–90 minutes has been shown to reduce pain associated with laser treatment of leg veins.[88,89] Ninety-minute application was demonstrated to be no better than a 60-minute application in both of these studies. Table 13.1 compares various topical anesthetics.

Full-face Laser Resurfacing and Supplemented Topical Anesthesia

Traditionally, full-face laser resurfacing, which removes the epidermis and upper portions of the dermis, has required

Table 13.1 *Topical Anesthetics*[a]

Anesthetic	Ingredients	Vehicle	Application dose	Occlusion required	FDA approved	Advantages	Disadvantages	Max dose/area
Betacaine-LA	Lidocaine, Prilocaine Dibucaine[b]	Vaseline ointment	60–90	No	No	Anecdotal reports of rapid onset	More clinical and safety trials needed	300 cm^2 – adults
LMX	4% Lidocaine	Liposomal	60	No	Yes	Liposomal delivery, long duration of action	Postapplication residue	100 cm^2 – children 600 cm^2 > 10 kg – adults + children
LMX 5	5% lidocaine	Liposomal	30	No	Yes	Rapid onset of action	More clinical trials needed	100 cm^2 – children 600 cm^2 > 10 kg – adults + children
EMLA	2.5% lidocaine: 2.5% prilocaine	Oil in water	60	Yes	Yes	Proven efficacy and safety profile	Long application, occlusion required	20 g/200 cm^2 – adults and children older than 7 and >20 kg
Tetracaine gel	4% tetracaine gel[b]	Lecithin gel	60–90	Yes	No	Anecdotal reports of rapid onset	More clinical and safety trials needed	None reported
Amethocaine	4% tetracaine		40–60	Yes	No	Rapid onset, prolonged effect	Ester anesthetic, avoid mucosal surfaces	50 mg – adults
Topicaine[b]	4% lidocaine	Microemulsion	30–60	Yes	Yes	Rapid onset, cost effective	More clinical trials needed	600 cm^2 – adults (children > 10 kg)
S-Caine	2.5% lidocaine, 2.5% tetracaine	Oil in water	30–60	No	Phase III clinical trails	Unique delivery system	Contains an ester anesthetic	To be determined

[a]Reproduced from Dermatologic Surgery: official publication for American Society for Dermatologic Surgery 2004; 30:1073–1076. With permission from Blackwell Ltd.[80]
[b]Over-the counter product.

general anesthesia or regional nerve blocks (with or without IV sedation and regional infiltration). The complications associated with general anesthesia were previously discussed. Regional nerve blocks often leave areas that are still sensitive to pain and require needle injections that increase patient discomfort. Recent research indicates that EMLA in a supplemented topical anesthesia protocol for full-face CO_2 laser resurfacing is safe, tolerable, and effective.[90] This protocol is as follows: After washing face, hot compresses are placed for 10 minutes. Then, 30 g of EMLA cream are applied to the face under occlusion. An hour-and-a-half later, the patient is given 1–2 tablets of 5 mg hyrocodone/500 mg acetaminophen PO, 5–10 mg of diazepam PO, and/or 30 to 60 mg ketorolac IM. Then, an additional 30 g of EMLA is applied under occlusion (anatomic areas are covered with individual pieces of plastic wrap). Approximately 1 hour later, laser resurfacing is performed by removing the plastic wrap from one area and wiping the area clean with a dry gauze. If possible, repeat passes are performed on the same area before moving to the next quadrant. This protocol was applied to 200 patients requiring full-face CO_2 laser resurfacing procedures. The procedure was tolerated with minimal pain, and only 5% required adjuvant anesthesia (nerve blocks or local infiltration). No adverse affects were seen in the study with topical EMLA. Patients generally reepithelialized by day 7. One year later, only one patient had hypopigmentation and scarring. In addition, EMLA treated skin and skin without EMLA treatment revealed similar depths of thermal damage as indicated through histological examination. It has been hypothesized that because CO_2 lasers target water, the hydrating effects of EMLA may contribute to the low rate of hypopigmentation and scarring seen in this study. In addition, research indicates that there is potential to use EMLA as a single agent since it has been shown to penetrate up to 5 mm 2.5 hours after application (the minimum required depth of anesthesia is general 100 μm).[90]

Lasers and Penetration of Topical Anesthetics

The skin forms a barrier to the penetration of topically applied anesthetics. Therefore, traditionally lidocaine has been administered either via subcutaneous injection (which is often painful), iontophoresis-aided delivery (which may cause irritation and burning), topical application after repeated tape stripping of the skin (which is inconvenient and uncomfortable), or topical application with occlusion (which is time consuming). The Er:YAG laser is used in superficial skin resurfacing, and is readily absorbed by the epidermis. Recent research indicates that a single pass of the Er:YAG (wavelength 2940 nm) laser enhanced the absorption and penetration of lidocaine, by disrupting the stratum corneum.[91] With this method, anesthesia can be induced in just 5 minutes compared to the 60 minutes required if lidocaine were applied under occlusion. Data from recent clinical trials evaluating pain associated with hypodermic needle insertion indicates that there is a 62% pain reduction with laser pretreatment plus lidocaine compared with laser pretreatment plus placebo, and a 61% pain reduction with laser pretreatment plus lidocaine, compared with lidocaine alone. Although this technique may not be adequate for invasive procedures, it may minimize pain and discomfort for more superficial cutaneous procedures, such as hypodermic needle insertion.

Despite these advances in safety in the office-based setting, patients with severe medical problems such as poorly controlled hypertension, congestive heart failure, severe/easily triggered asthma, orthopnea, morbid obesity, and other significant conditions are better treated in a hospital or outpatient surgery center setting. Nonetheless, with proper preoperative screening, appropriate patient selection, and careful monitoring, the anesthetic techniques described can readily be adapted to meet the specific needs of practitioners and patients in a variety of clinical settings.

References

1. Rosen S, Smoller BR. Port-wine stains: a new hypothesis. J Am Acad Dermatol 1987; 17:164.
2. Smoller BR, Rosen S. Port-wine stains: a disease of altered neural modulation of blood vessels? Arch Dermatol 1986; 132:177.
3. Lowe NJ, Burgess P, Borden H. Flash pump dye laser fire during general anesthesia oxygenation: case report. J Clin Laser Med Surg 1990; 8:39.
4. Garden JM, Polla LL, Tan OT. The treatment of port-wine stains by the pulsed dye laser. Arch Dermatol 1988; 124:889.
5. Tan OT, Sherwood K, Gilchrest BA. Treatment of children with port-wine stains using the flashlamp-pulsed tunable dye laser. N Engl J Med 1989; 320:416.
6. Tan OT, Stafford TJ. Treatment of port-wine stains at 577 nm: clinical results. Med Instru 1987; 21:218.
7. Garden JM, Burton CS, Geronemus R. Dye-laser treatment of children with port-wine stains. N Engl J Med 1989; 321:901 (letter).
8. Epstein RH, Brummett RR, Lask GP. Incendiary potential of the flash-lamp pumped 585 nm tunable dye laser. Anesth Analg 1990; 71:171.
9. Rabinowitz LG, Esterly NB. Anesthesia and/or sedation for pulsed dye laser therapy: special symposium. Pediatr Dermatol 1992; 9:132.
10. Spiegel H, Spiegel D. Trance and treatment clinical uses of hypnosis. New York: Basic Books; 1978.
11. Juhlin L, Hagglund G, Evers H. Absorption of lidocaine and prilocaine after application of a eutectic mixture of local anesthetics (Emla) on normal and diseased skin. Acta Derm Venerol 1989; 69:18.
12. Engberg G, Danielson K, Henneberg S et al. Plasma concentrations of prilocaine and lidocaine and methaemoglobin formation of infants after epicutaneous application of a 5% lidocaine-prilocaine (Emla). Acta Anaesthesiol Scand 1987; 31:624.
13. Hallen B, Olsson GL, Uppfeldt A. Pain-free venipuncture: effect of timing of application of local anaesthetic cream. Anaesthesia 1984; 39:969.
14. Moller C. A lidoocaine-prilocaine cream reduces venipuncture pain. Upps J Med Sci 1985; 90:293.
15. Ohlsen L, Englesson S, Evers H. An anaesthetic lidocaine/prilocaine cream (Emla) for epicutaneous application tested for cutting split skin grafts. Scand J Plast Reconstr Surg 1985; 19:201.
16. Rosdahl I, Edmar B, Gisslen H et al. Curettage of molluscum contagiosum in children: analgesia by topical application of a lidocaine/prilocaine cream (Emla). Acta Derm Venerol 1988; 68:149.
17. Ehrenstrom-Reiz GM, Reiz SL. Emla – a eutectic mixture of local anaesthetics for topical anaesthesia. Acta Anaesthesiol Scand 1982; 26:596.
18. Ehrenstrom-Reiz G, Reiz S, Stockmar O. Topical anaesthesia with Emla, a new lidocaine-prilocaine cream and the Cresum technique for detection of minimal application time. Acta Anaesthesiol Scand 1983; 27:510.
19. Evers H, von Dardel O, Juhlim L et al. Dermal effects of composition based on the eutectic mixture of lidocaine and prilocaine (Emla): studies in volunteers. Br J Anaesth 1985; 57:997.
20. Ashinoff R, Geronemus RG. Effect of the topical anesthetic Emla on the efficacy of pulsed dye laser treatment of port-wine stains. J Dermatol Surg Oncol 1990; 16:1008.
21. Tan OT, Stafford TJ. Emla for laser treatment of port-wine stains in children. Lasers Surg Med 1992; 12:543.
22. Arendt-Nielsen L, Bjerring P. Laser-induced pain for evaluation of local analgesia: a comparison of topical application (Emla) and local injection (lidocaine). Anesth Analg 1988; 67: 115.
23. Gangarosa LP, Park NH, Fong BC et al. Conductivity of the drugs used by iontophoresis. J Pharm Sci 1978; 67:1439.
24. Bezzant JL, Stephen RL, Petelenz TJ. Painless cauterization of spider veins with the use of iontophoretic local anesthesia. J Am Acad Dermatol 1988; 19:869.
25. Kennard CD, Whitaker DC. Iontophoresis of lidocaine for anesthesia during pulsed dye laser treatment of port-wine stains. J Dermatol Surg Oncol 1992; 18:287.
26. Maloney JM, Bezzant JL, Stephen RL et al. Iontophoretic administration of lidocaine anesthesia in office practice: an appraisal. J Dermatol Surg Oncol 1992; 18:937.
27. Committee on Drugs, Section on Anesthesiology, American Academy of Pediatrics. Guidelines for elective use of contra

sedation, deep sedation, and general anesthesia in pediatric patients. Pediatrics 1985; 75:317.
28. Ruben H. Nitrous oxide analgesia in dentistry: its use during 15 years in Denmark. Br Dent J 1982; 132:195.
29. Langa H. Relative analgesia in dental practice. Philadelphia: WB Saunders; 1976.
30. Langa H. Nitrous oxide–oxygen analgesia for modern dentistry. Dent Dig 1960; 66:126.
31. Allen GD. Nitrous oxide–oxygen sedation machines and devices. J Am Dent Assoc 1984; 88:611.
32. Stuebner EA. Nitrous oxide – analgesia or anesthesia? Dent Clin North Am 1983; 17:235.
33. Griffin GC, Campbell VD, Jones R. Nitrous oxide–oxygen sedation for minor surgery. JAMA 1981; 245:2411.
34. American Medical Association. AMA drug evaluations: nitrous oxide. Chicago: AMA; 1983.
35. Mattila MAK, Larni HM, Nummi SE et al. Effect of diazepam on emergence from ketamine anaesthesia. Anaesthesia 1979; 28:20.
36. Cartwright PD, Pingel SM. Midazolam and diazepam in ketamine anaesthesia. Anaesthesia 1984; 39:439.
37. Miller RD, ed. Anesthesia, 2nd edn. New York: Churchill Livingstone; 1986.
38. Gregory GA et al. Pediatric anesthesia. New York: Churchill Livingstone; 1983.
39. Physicians' Desk Reference, 47th edn. Montvale, NJ: Medical Economics; 1993.
40. Brown TCK, Cole WHJ, Murray GH. Ketamine: a new anaesthetic agent. Aust NZ Surg 1970; 39:305.
41. Schreiner MS, Triebwasser A, Keon TP. Ingestion of liquids compared with preoperative fasting in pediatric outpatients. Anesthesiology 1990; 72:593.
42. Cohen MM, Cameron CB. Should you cancel the operation when a child has an upper respiratory tract infection? Anesth Analg 1991; 72:282.
43. Dundee JW, Wyatt GM. Dissociative anaesthesia. In: Dundee JW, ed. Intravenous anaesthesia. Boston, MA: Little Brown; 1964.
44. Coppel DL, Dundee JW. Ketamine anaesthesia for cardiac catheterization. Anaesthesia 1972; 27:25.
45. Bailey PL, Pace NL, Ashburn MA et al. Frequent hypoxemia and apnea after sedation with midazolam and fentanyl. Anesthesiology 1990; 73:826.
46. Scarborough DA, Bisaccia E, Swensen RD. Anesthesia for outpatient dermatologic cosmetic surgery: midazolam-low-dosage ketamine anesthesia. J Dermatol Surg Oncol 1989; 15:658.
47. Pandit SK, Kothary SP, Kumar SM. Low dose intravenous infusion technique with ketamine. Anaesthesia 1980; 35:669.
48. Lilburn JK, Dundee JW, Moore J. Ketamine infusions. Anaesthesia 1978; 33:315.
49. Sher MH. Slow dose ketamine – a new technique. Anaesth Intens Care 1980; 8:359.
50. White PF. Use of continuous infusion versus intermittent bolus administration of fentanyl or ketamine during outpatient anesthesia. Anesthesiology 1983; 59:294.
51. Jastak JT, Goretta C. Ketamine HCl as a continuous-drip anesthetic for outpatients. Anesth Analg 1983; 52:341.
52. Ackerly JA. Ketamine anesthesia in burn patients. In: Anesthesiology Forum, vol IV. Ketamine anesthesia in open heart and burn patients. Presented in part at the Ketalar Roundtable, New Orleans, 13 October 1984. Morris Plains, NJ: Parke-Davis; 1984.
53. Virtue RW, Alanis JM, Mori M et al. An anesthetic agent: 2-orthochlorophenyl, 2-methylamino cyclohexanone HCl (CI-581). Anesthesiology 1967; 28:823.
54. Wilson RD, Traber DL, McCoy NR. Cardiopulmonary effects of CI-581: the new dissociative anesthetic. South Med J 1968; 61:692.
55. Kelly RW, Wilson RD, Traber DL et al. Effects of two new dissociative anesthetic agents, ketamine and CL-1848C, on the respiratory response to carbon dioxide. Anesth Analg 1971; 50:262.
56. Corssen G, Domino EF. Dissociative anesthesia: further pharmacologic studies and first clinical experience with the phencyclidine derivative CI-581. Anesth Analg 1966; 45:29.
57. Van Hemelrijck J, Gonzales JM, White PF. Pharmacology of intravenous anesthetic agents. In: Rogers MC et al, ed. Principles and practice of anesthesiology. St Louis: Mosby; 1993.
58. Stanski DR, Shafer SL. New intravenous anesthetics (no. 274). Presented at 41st Annual Refresher Course Lectures and Clinical Update Program, Park Ridge, IL, 1990. Park Ridge: ASA Inc.; 1990.
59. Fragen RJ, ed. Drug infusions in anesthesiology. New York: Raven; 1991.
60. Bloomfield EL, Masaryk TJ, Caplan A et al. Intravenous sedatives for MR imaging of the brain and spine in children: pentobarbital versus propofol. Radiology 1993; 186:93.
61. Cauldwell CB, Fisher DM. Sedating pediatric patients: is propofol a panacea? Radiology 1993; 186:9.
62. Patel DK, Keeling PA, Newman BG. Induction dose of propofol in children. Anaesthesia 1988; 43:949.
63. Apfelbaum JL. Outpatient anesthesia for adult patients (no. 412). Presented at 43rd Annual Refresher Course Lectures, Park Ridge, IL, 1992. Park Ridge: ASA Inc.; 1992.
64. Blouin RT, Seifert HA, Conrad PF et al. Propofol significantly depresses hypoxic ventilatory drive during conscious sedation. Anesthesiology 1992; 77.
65. Valtonen M, Iisalo E, Kanto J et al. Propofol as an induction agent in children: pain on injection and pharmacokinetics. Acta Anaesthesiol Scand 1989; 33:152.
66. Holak E, Mangar D. Modified Bier block abolishes local pain associated with propofol injection. Anesthesiology 1991; 75.
67. Raff M, Harrison GG. The screening of propofol in MHS swine. Anesth Analg 1989; 68:750.
68. Denborough M, Hopkinson KC. Propofol and malignant hyperpyrexia. Lancet 1988; 1:191.
69. Verburg MP, DeGrood PMRM. Safety of propofol in malignant hyperthermia: preliminary results. Anaesthesia 1988; 43(suppl):121.
70. Steward DJ. Anesthesia for pediatric outpatients. In: White PF, ed. Outpatient anesthesia. New York: Churchill Livingstone; 1990.
71. Eger EI. New inhalational anesthetic agents (no. 245). Presented at 43rd Annual Refresher Course Lectures, Park Ridge, IL, 1992. Park Ridge: ASA Inc.; 1992.
72. Hannallah RS. Anesthesia for pediatric outpatients (no. 133). Presented at 43rd Annual Refresher Course Lectures, 1992, Park Ridge, IL. Park Ridge: ASA Inc.; 1992.
73. Stafford TJ, Crocker D. Role of anesthesia in laser therapy. In: Tan OT, ed. Management and treatment of benign cutaneous vascular lesions. Philadelphia: Lea & Febiger; 1992.
74. Anesthesia Patient Safety Foundation Newsletter 5:4, 1990–1991.
75. Trytko R, Werschler W. Total intravenous anesthesia for office-based laser facial resurfacing. Lasers Surg Med 1999; 25:126–130.
76. Balance J. Sedational anaesthesia for laser skin therapy. J Cutan Laser Ther 1999; 1:57–9.

77. Friedberg BL. Facial resurfacing with the propofol–ketamine technique: room air, spontaneous ventilation anesthesia. Dermatol Surg 1999; 25:569–72.
78. Abeles G, Sequeira M, Swensen R et al. The combined use of propofol and fentanyl for outpatient intravenous conscious sedation. Dermatol Surg 1999; 25:559–62.
79. Greenbaum SS. Iontophoresis as a tool for anesthesia in dermatologic surgery: an overview. Dermatol Surg 2001; 27:1027–30.
80. Friedman PM., Mafong E, Friedman E et al. Topical anesthetics update: Emla and beyond. Dermatol Surg 2001; 27:1019–26.
81. Alster T, Lupton J. Evaluation of a novel topical anesthetic agent for cutaneous laser resurfacing: a randomized comparison study. Dermatol Surg 2002; 28:1004–6.
82. Wahlgren CF, Quiding H. Depth of cutaneous analgesia after application of a eutectic mixture of the local anesthetics lidocaine and prilocaine (Emla cream). J Am Acad Dermatol 2000; 42(4):584–8.
83. Altman D, Gildenberg S. High-energy pulsed light source hair removal device used to evaluate the onset of action of a new topical anesthetic. Dermatol Surg 1999; 25:816–18.
84. Bryan H, Alster T. The S-Caine peel: a novel topical anesthetic for cutaneous laser surgery. Dermatol Surg 2002; 28:999–1003.
85. Doshi S, Friedman P, Marquez D et al. Thirty-minute application of the S-Caine peel prior to nonablative laser treatment. Dermatol Surg 2003; 29:1008–11.
86. Chen ZSJ, Jacobson LG, Bakus AD, et al. Evaluation of the S-Caine peel for induction of local anesthesia for laser-assisted tattoo removal: Randomized, double-blind, placebo-controlled, multicenter study. Dermatol Surg 2005; 31:281–6.
87. Schecter AK, Pariser DM, Pariser RJ, et al. Randomized, double-blind, placebo-controlled study evaluating the lidocaine/tetracaine patch for induction of local anesthesia prior to minor dermatologic procedures in geriatric patients. Dermatol Surg 2005; 31:287–91.
88. Jih MH, Friedman PM, Sadick N, et al. 60-minute application of S-Caine peel prior to 1,064nm long-pulsed Nd:YAG laser treatment of leg veins. Lasers Surg Med 2004; 34:446–50.
89. Chen JZS, Alexiades-Armenakas MR, Bernstein LJ, et al. Two randomized, double-blind, placebo-controlled studies evaluating the S-Caine peel for induction of local anesthesia before long-pulsed Nd:YAG laser therapy for leg veins. Dermatol Surg 2003; 29:1012–18.
90. Kilmer S, Chotzen V, Zelickson B et al. Full-face laser resurfacing using a supplemental topical anesthesia protocol. Arch Dermatol 2003; 139:1279–83.
91. Baron Elma, Harris Lisbeth, Redpath William S et al. Laser-assisted penetration of topical anesthetic in adults. Arch Dermatol 2003; 139:1288–90.

Chapter 14

Noninvasive Skin Tightening Induced by Radiofrequency and Infrared Light Devices

Javier Ruiz-Esparza

Introduction

In the course of the early clinical testing of a new medical device (ThermaCool by Thermage, Hayward CA), it was first noticed that elevation of the eyebrows had occurred. Application of radiofrequency on the skin of the frontal and temporal hairline was done out of caution in those early cases. The skin along the hairline can be easily excised if a burn leading to a scar were to occur. Instead, this linear area of forehead and temporal skin contracted, leading to a lifting effect distally, which elevated the eyebrow. This observation by the author in early 2001 led to the first application for nonsurgical skin tightening: eyebrow lifting.[1,2] A multicentric study later corroborated that statistically significant brow elevation was a reproducible clinical effect of contracting the forehead skin with this new technology.[3]

Nonablative radiofrequency originally aimed to elicit dermal remodeling and tightening using the same principle as nonablative lasers (i.e. thermal energy delivered to the dermis through an epidermis protected by cold, as first demonstrated by the 1320 nm CoolTouch Laser; CoolTouch, Rosemont, CA) and to benefit periorbital rhytids by this approach in a more substantial way than nonablative lasers could. Radiofrequency being electricity lent itself to a more intense and sustained energy delivery to the target than that possible with any nonablative laser source. Nevertheless, whereas nonablative lasers were effective in treating rhytids, nonablative radiofrequency often produced exacerbation of the wrinkle lines when it was applied directly on them, perhaps from the tightening that occurred in the underlying dermis; this was called the 'napkin' or 'sausage' effect. In contrast, skin tightening was a significant new addition to the noninvasive procedure list. For the first time, without having to ablate the skin through aggressive resurfacing, skin tightening was possible.

The ThermaCool TC device consists of a high-frequency, 330-watt radiofrequency generator and a cooling unit (Figs 14.1 and 14.2).The radiofrequency generator produces a 6-megahertz signal. It has an internal computer that registers vital information in real time, including handpiece position, usable electrode life, application force, and uniformity of skin contact. The control panel displays energy settings, impedance, radiofrequency pulse width and error messages upon undue malfunction. A handpiece holds the electrode during treatment (Fig. 14.3). Radiofrequency is delivered through a capacitive membrane that lines the application surface of the electrode (Fig. 14.4). These electrodes are disposable, single-use consumable pieces needed for the operation of the device. They have factory-set parameters such as radiofrequency pulse and cooling times. Electrodes are hollow and house a nozzle that emits a spray of cryogen fluid immediately before, during and immediately after the radiofrequency energy pulse. This ingenious and highly precise method of cooling allows the spray to function from the inside of the hollow electrode and against the back of the electrode membrane, without the actual spray ever touching the skin of the patient directly. The timing is electronically controlled with utmost precision. The safety of each pulse against producing a burn depends in no small measure on the precision of this heat–cold combination. The treating surface of the electrode is covered by a dielectric membrane, which is sandwiched between an electric conductor: the electrode metal and a semi-conductor: the patient's skin. This forms a capacitor. It is this capacitive property that is believed to deliver the radiofrequency energy in a uniform manner

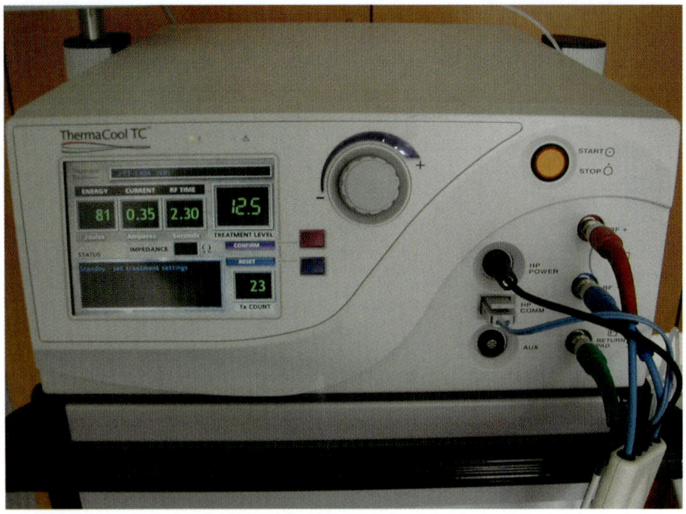

Figure 14.1 ThermaCool TCIII radiofrequency generator. A panel displays real-time information including energy (in joules), current (in amperes), and on times (in seconds). All these will automatically adjust to the selected treatment level, also shown in the display. It has a single dial; it is used to increase or decrease treatment levels. It also displays impedance during each firing (in ohms) and a counter of firings. If a malfunction occurs, an error message will appear in the status window.

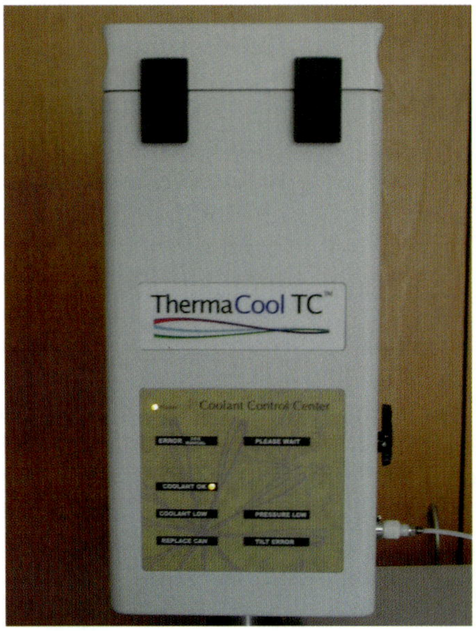

Figure 14.2 Cooling unit. This is the other basic component of this device. It holds a canister of environmentally safe cryogen. Warning lights alert the operator of the need to replace the canisters.

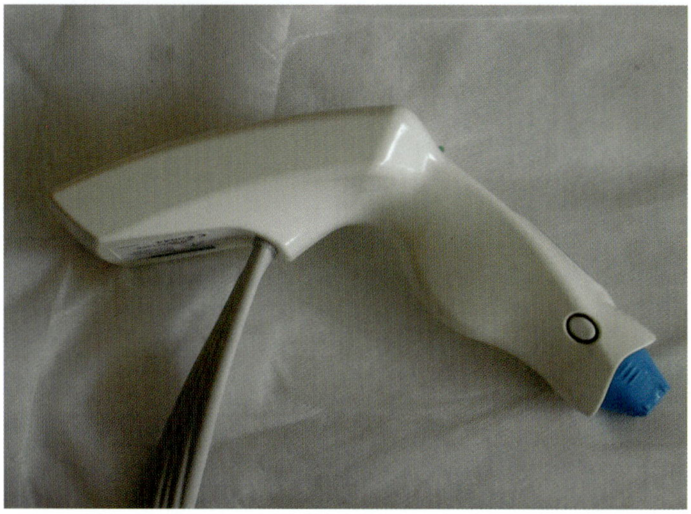

Figure 14.3 Handpiece. This has an ergonomic design. It holds the treatment tips (blue) and it has an activating button that fires the machine by digital pressure from the operator when desired.

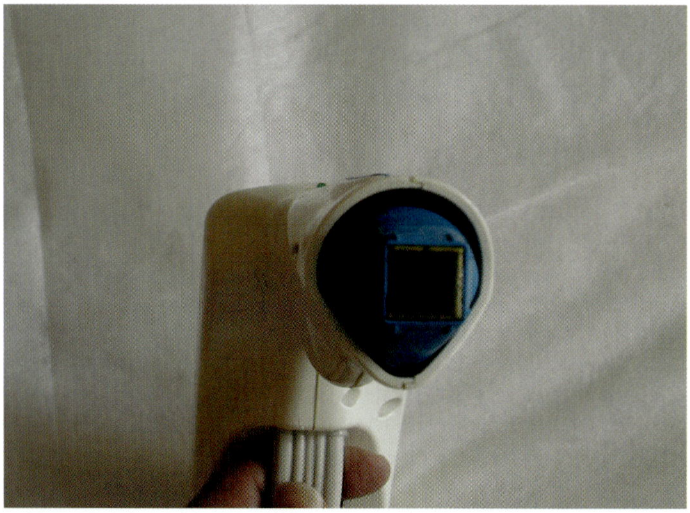

Figure 14.4 Disposable treatment tips. They contain the active electrode lined by a black dielectric membrane. In addition to an EPROM chip, it has four thermisters or pressure sensors to ensure full skin contact. The cryogen is sprayed in the inside of this hollow piece.

throughout the entire surface of the electrode, without 'hot spots.'

Radiofrequency delivered from a raw metal surface onto human skin would tend to concentrate in the perimeter of the treatment area, leading to an uneven distribution and very possibly a burn. Deterioration or otherwise damage of the capacitive membrane can similarly lead to a burn. Each electrode has a finite safe life, counted in a set number of pulses. They need to be discarded after a single use for this reason. Heat is produced by the semi-conductor nature of tissue, which offers a partial natural resistance to the flow of electrons; called impedance. The local impedance varies between anatomical areas and even within an anatomical area in the same patient. The machine will compensate for this variation by generating different levels of current within safe limits. But even within a single target spot, the impedance of the different skin components will vary. For example, the uppermost layers, which have been protected by the emission of cryogen prior to the energy pulse, will have less resistance or impedance than the deep layers, which are not affected by the superficial cooling. In addition, fat in the subcutaneous tissue has a natural high resistance to the flow of electricity. This high impedance may lead to an unwanted heat accumulation and injury to this tissue, which results in a depressed or deeply dented subcutaneous scar. Radiofrequency can be delivered in a monopolar or in a bipolar mode. In a monopolar configuration the energy travels from the active electrode, through the body and into the return or passive electrode or grounding plate. In a bipolar configuration, the energy travels superficially from one edge of the electrode into another, making the energy travel horizontally in a very superficial plane.

Although the possibility of nonsurgically producing eyebrow lifting by contracting the skin of the forehead was quite significant, the application that was found to be the most rewarding for patients, and which rapidly became the most widely used aspect of this technology, was skin lifting of the lower face and neck. The observation that this was possible was also made by serendipity: In the earliest cases in which we were applying the radiofrequency energy very carefully, only the preauricular skin was being treated in other patients, out of caution. A retrospective review by the author revealed that when this preauricular skin contracted, the effect was seen distally, again, on the nasolabial fold, producing lifting of the skin of the cheek and jowl as well as softening of the nasolabial fold.

This was found retrospectively to have occurred in 14 of the first 15 patients treated in this manner and repeated prospectively in 10 other patients.[4] Interestingly enough, 13 of those 15 patients were treated with bipolar treatment tips, and only two with monopolar ones. The device used for the treatment of the patients in the initial report was a prototype machine, which had different parameters from those in the device that was released commercially later on, including a longer radiofrequency pulse width. The pulse duration was shortened in the commercially available machine, and I was never able to duplicate the results from the initial cases using the new device. Lately, the pulse duration has been shortened even more, in the interest of having a 'fast tip'. In my hands, the new tips have not had the same degree of efficacy as the conventional 'slow 1 cm tips' and I have stopped using them altogether. Because of a shorter pulse, the pain produced is greater, and the risk for a burn is also increased in my experience. As mentioned in the original manuscript, the best results were seen with the lowest fluences used. Multiple passes at low fluences were suggested in the original paper as the safest and most effective approach.[5] This observation was repeated again when we reported our results on breast lifting using this technology.[6] Our early work in this area prompted an ever-increasing interest in the technology and has resulted in numerous reports by different authors as well. Iyer et al reported significant improvement in 70% of their patients 3 months after a single radiofrequency treatment,[7] although other authors reported a lesser degree of satisfactory results.[8,9] A low incidence of satisfactory results marred the procedure as it was being done by most practitioners and as recommended by the manufacturer. The recommendation was to use a high fluence, often as high as the pain tolerance of the given patient would allow, in a single and even in multiple passes. A 'therapeutic level' of energy was aimed for. In spite of using high energies, the average outcome remained modest and results were inconsistent. In addition, side effects started to appear. The most important, perhaps, was focal indentations from subcutaneous burns, areas of so called fat atrophy. High energies never translated into a higher success rate in our early clinical work. Low energy and multiple passes as mentioned in our original article[5] provided the best results. Therefore we proposed multiple passes as low settings since the publication of that article, treating only focal areas which, upon contraction produce a distal effect as seen in our original cases. In this manner, the procedure was faster, safer and less painful.[9] Not a single case of subcutaneous scar ('fat atrophy') in over 1500 treatments in a span of 4 years (unpublished data). Recently, Zelickson et al demonstrated more significant collagen changes with multiple passes at lower fluences than with a single pass at high energy[10] and this has now become the recommended approach by the manufacturer.

Although nonablative radiofrequency remains the gold standard for achieving noninvasive skin tightening, it is still a very painful procedure, even when using the lowest possible settings. Pain control is limited by the fact that only topical anesthesia is recommended. Injectable anesthetics change the impedance of tissues and this may lead to unexpected burns. In addition, deep sedation is not recommended because the pain sensation feedback is lost. The latter is an important warning sign in identifying burns early. Pain can be an important deterrent to prospective patients considering the procedure and in patients considering having a repeat treatment.

A new device, powered by a lamp that generates broadband infrared light in the 1100 to 1800 nm wavelength has also demonstrated the ability to produce significant skin tightening. In contrast to the 'flash heating' produced by the radiofrequency device (high peaks in very short pulses), the infrared machine delivers heat in a multisecond pulse, which accounts for a gentler and more sustained heating. This appears to be more effective in producing immediate skin contraction, as well as being virtually painless. Our early experience with the device in our first 60 patients has produced immediate skin contraction, sustained over the ensuing days, weeks and up to 7 months in up to 90% of the cases (submitted for publication). In addition, the procedure, which is done at much lower fluences than those possible with the radiofrequency apparatus, is virtually painless and needs no anesthesia. Painless immediate skin contraction seems to be now possible.

This new machine is called Titan (Cutera, Brisbane, CA). This device also has pre-, parallel and postcooling and delivers up to 50 J/cm^3 in pulse duration of up to 8.1 seconds. It has a consistent control of energy delivery through closed loop photometry. It has a delivery area of 10 by 15 mm (spot size), which provides contact cooling through a sapphire window driven by four Peltier (electric) cooling devices. The target chromophore is water. The device controls allow the operator to increase or decrease the exposure time and simultaneously the total energy delivered per pulse. At settings below 30 J/cm^3 these pulses are painless. No anesthetic is needed. At this power levels, the patient develops no erythema or postoperative swelling, nevertheless, immediate skin contraction is evident in the vast majority of cases.

True immediate collagen contraction has not been previously documented in the literature. It must be differentiated from postoperative edema. Aggressive treatment with either device using multiple passes at high fluences will result in transient edema that will give the illusion of skin contraction, however, it will be gone within 2–3 days. True contraction will persist throughout the ensuing days, weeks and months after the treatment.

Collagen is a family of structural proteins composed of a triple helix with hydrogen bonds that link the chains and give it a helical shaped structure. Breakage of these bonds results in the uncoiling of the chains with a structural change in the shape of the molecule, resulting in a shortened, amorphous, stable form.[11] Collagen contraction occurs between 57 and 61°C; higher temperatures may lead to irreversible denaturation. Collagen contraction, however, is a process characterized by the Arrhenius equation:

$$K = A \star \exp^{(-E_a/R \star T)}$$

where K is the rate, E_a is the activation energy for the process and T is the temperature. Based on assumed parameters for collagen in general, this equation shows that for every 5°C decrease in temperature, a 10-fold increase in time is needed to achieve a similar amount of collagen contraction.[12] Thus, no single shrinkage temperature exists and the amount of collagen contraction is determined by a combination of the time and temperature. Studies suggest that for millisecond domain exposures, the shrinkage temperature is above 85°C, whereas for relatively long exposures of several seconds, the shrinkage temperature is in the range of 60 to 65°C.[12,13] This suggests that at a longer exposure, immediate contraction is possible at even lower temperatures. If this is true, it would explain why we see skin contraction following the very long exposures at low energies (20 to 30 J/cm^3) possible only with this device. Furthermore, it opens a whole new avenue of possibilities for future devices with an even higher ability to contract tissue painlessly.

Clinical Technique

Perhaps the most critical point after making sure that the patient has realistic expectations is making sure that adequate preoperative photographs have been obtained. The patient must be informed that the changes obtained with these procedures are subtle and do not compare with those from a surgical procedure. On the other hand, they are much more natural and overcorrection is almost never seen. There are no scars to hide or recovery period from the procedure. No time is lost from work or social activities, and for the majority of patients, if treated at low to mid energy settings, there are no telltale signs that a procedure was done even shortly thereafter. The patient can then schedule his or her normal social or work activities without interruption. For most patients this is a most welcome possibility. A preoperative review of photographs showing the patient a gamut of possible results is advisable. It should also be noted that, in some cases, there are no results at all – in spite of our best efforts – for reasons that are not clearly understood. In the case of nonablative radiofrequency, the results are most often seen after 3 to 6 months from the procedure. Immediate changes are generally the result of edema from multiple passes, and fluences high enough to produce important pain from heat. Naturally, some degree of edema follows, but this is rarely an indicator of a positive eventual result in my experience.

Preoperative and follow-up photographs must be taken without make-up, using the same camera, in the same room, with the same head and body positions, at the same distance and height, with the same lighting and preferably by the same person. It is a good idea to display the preoperative photos on a computer monitor when the follow-up pictures are being taken. This will ensure the best match of position, perspective, distance, etc., enabling comparable pictures. This is an invaluable tool for evaluating and later demonstrating results to the patient.

Nonablative Radiofrequency

We ask patients to wash their face thoroughly three times while in our office. This will ensure removal of make-up and other cosmetic residues, which can interfere with the cooling or modify the local impedance.

We identify those critical areas which upon contraction will elicit a pull or lifting effect distally, the concept of anchoring points as described in our original paper.[5] These areas will vary from patient to patient, depending on their own individual characteristics such as bony structure, degree of laxity, eyebrow shape, depth and length of unwanted skin folds, etc.

The anchoring points are identified situating ourselves in front of the patient and using our thumbs to assess skin mobility (Figs 14.5–14.7). They are located in the perimeter of the face, along the frontal hairline and the preauricular areas. Our thumbs can ascertain that the skin next to the hairline is barely movable, the same as the skin of the preauricular sulcus. However, as one advances towards the center of the face, the skin becomes movable. It is at the junction of the nonmovable and the movable skin that the line of treatment is drawn. Any nonmovable skin up to that line is included in the treatment for anchoring purposes but it is the treatment of the freely movable edge that really matters for the desired effect. Upon moving our thumbs over that area we can observe the lifting of the eyebrow or the softening of the nasolabial fold. We can actually choose if we want to lift the medial or the lateral part of the eyebrow, or its entire length, by treating over the medial upper forehead or the lateral temporal areas. This is important in eyebrow enhancement, rather than plain eyebrow lifting. Elevation of the tails of the eyebrows will feminize the eyebrow. For men, it is always advisable to treat across the forehead rather than only over the temples. The areas to be treated are then marked with an eyebrow pencil (Fig. 14.8).

Lower eyelid laxity can be treated by one of two ways: (1) using the principle of anchoring points, one can treat the skin lateral to the eyelid as described previously;[15,16] or (2) by treating directly over the eyelid skin. Treating the

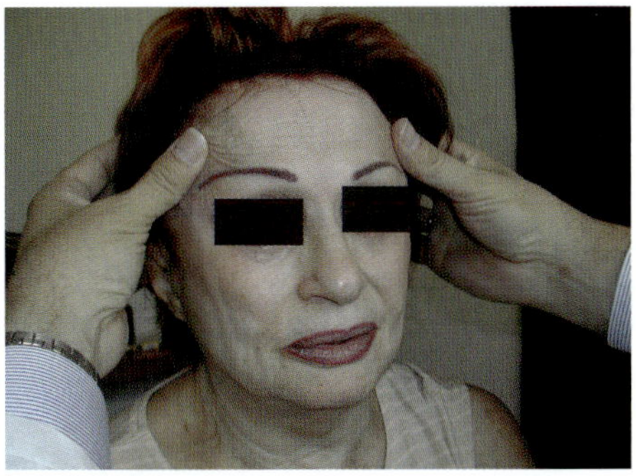
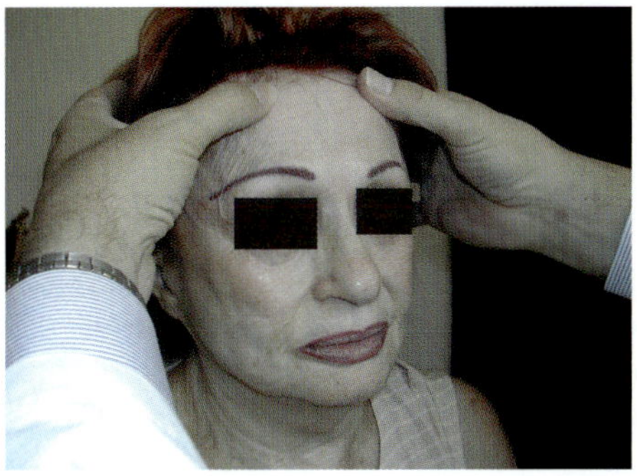
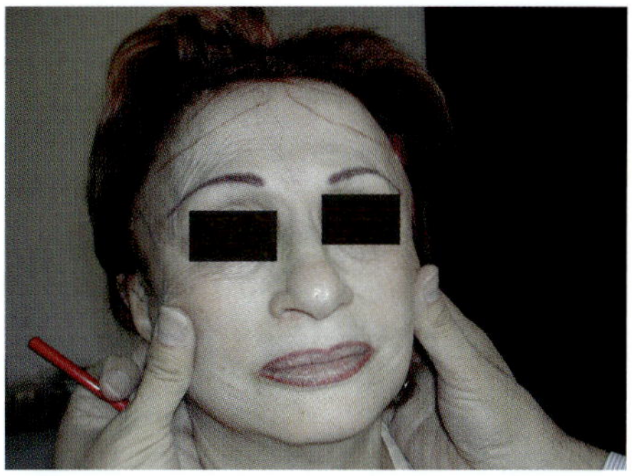

Figures 14.5, 14.6, 14.7 Anchoring points are identified by gentle lateral movement of thumbs over skin. The junction of nonmovable and freely movable skin is sought.

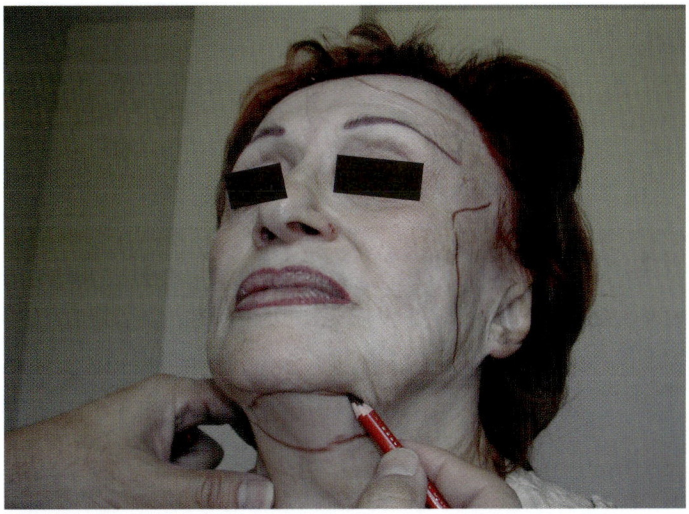

Figure 14.8 The anchoring points are delineated using eyebrow pencil. The flaccid area of submental skin is marked as well and treated directly.

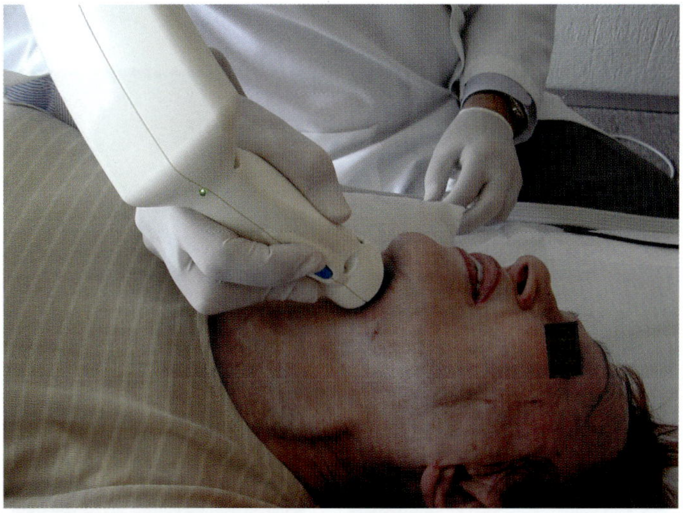

Figure 14.9 During treatment, the handpiece should be kept perpendicular to the skin and in a horizontal plane. This is sometimes difficult to achieve in areas such as the submentum.

skin lateral to the lower eyelids, over the zygoma or malar areas is by far the safest. One needs two or three passes at 12.5 using the conventional tip. We are talking about two squares of 1 cm^2 each, so the interval between pulses is very short and therefore higher fluences are risky and not recommended. The drawback of this approach is that only skin laxity can be corrected. Eyelid bags may have other anatomical components, such as excessive fluid, orbicularis muscle hypertrophy, and herniated fat. All of these will remain unchanged with this approach, only skin laxity will improve.

Treating directly over eyelid skin with the 1 cm conventional slow tip, is very rewarding when fat herniation is present but the appropriate technique must be strictly followed to avoid a disastrous burn on the eyeball. First, we palpate the orbital rim, if the bag of herniated fat extends up to the rim then the upper part cannot be treated. In most cases, however, the bulk of the fat is below the orbital rim. The skin is then pulled down and in a lateral direction, so that the entire fat prominence is against the orbital bone. The patient is instructed that they will feel a hot sensation but no significant pain, and to let us know if undue pain is felt by lifting a hand. If that occurs, the activating button is released instantly. If not, the machine is fired in two adjacent spots at settings of 11.5 for three to five consecutive passes; 12.5 can be used but only for up to two passes, when laxity rather than fat herniation is the problem. If we treat despite pain, there is the risk of a serious burn. If this happens, postoperative edema the following day may be significant and the results will be suboptimal. Visual control by the operator is a must to make sure that the eyeball is avoided. One-to-one training is recommended before attempting this advanced technique. The depth of penetration of the heat by these tips is 2.5 to 5 mm. The thickness of the eyelid is only 2–3 mm that is why extreme caution must prevail. New bipolar tips with shallow penetration are being tested by the company for a safer application.

For lifting the cheek skin, effacing or rather softening the nasolabial folds, one must treat in the preauricular areas. The upper part, extended anteriorly to the zygomatic area will help the upper part of the fold, while treating the skin in front of the earlobe will benefit the marionette lines and jowls. Sharpening of the mandibular line will often result.

The neck can be improved by treating directly over the submental skin (Fig. 14.9), which should always be done above the level of the thyroid cartilage. Care should be taken in patients with early platysmal bands. I have seen exacerbation of these bands as a result of tightening with radiofrequency (unpublished observation) (Figs 14.10 and 14.11). For patients with early bands, it is preferable to treat the inframandibular skin lateral to the bands. A very important area to treat is the mastoid skin and the skin along the lateral posterior hairline. Treatment of other neck areas is extremely sensitive and patients often do not tolerate the pain. Improvement of the neck can be seen by treating these peripheral areas, which again follows the principle of anchoring points.

By treating only over the anchoring points one can limit the total time of the procedure as well as the patient's pain, and have a better result, in my experience, than treating over the entire surface of the facial skin (Figs 14.12–14.27). When these areas contract, vectors of tissue movement are created. This is different than trying to treat over 'vector areas.' Or doing passes so that the axis '*x*' or axis '*y*' contract. I find the concept of predicting the dynamics of contraction extremely complex.

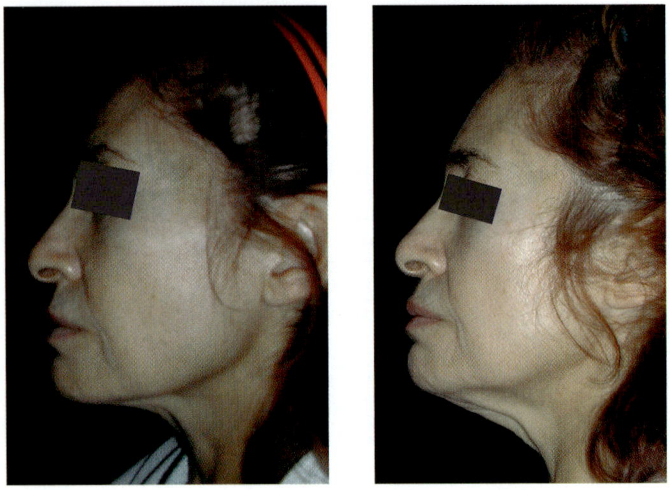

Figures 14.10 and 14.11 60-year-old woman. Preoperative view and showing how radiofrequency treatment of submental area worsened platysmal bands; 1-year follow-up.

One must first consider that if the radiofrequency energy penetrates the tissue evenly, as we assume it does, it will be in a cube of tissue directly under the square electrode. The depth of penetration will depend on the geometry and size of the electrode, whether it is monopolar or bipolar, and lastly the energy and length of exposure. If, indeed, we can heat a cube of tissue uniformly enough and at the right temperature to produce immediate contraction, the direction of this contraction will most likely follow the disposition of the collagen fibers. Each fiber will become shorter. Now, what is the disposition of the collagen fibers in the dermis? The answer is: random. Coiled and twisted on each other like worms in a can. More importantly, what direction the contraction of this cube of tissue will follow? Centripetal is the most likely answer. A compaction rather than a contraction of the cube will occur. If we consider that we treat numerous adjacent cubes of tissue, we can see how predicting the ultimate axis of contraction becomes very difficult. The reason is the likely interaction of many other factors such as: skin tension in a given area and in a given axis versus its opposing forces such as skin weight, degree of redundancy, shape and angles of the underlying bony framework, etc. Only the interaction of all these factors will determine the ultimate direction of tissue contraction.

Collagen fiber disposition in dermis is random. The dermis is part of the nonorganized connective tissues. Only in organized connective tissue (tendons, capsules, aponeuroses, etc.) are collagen fibers aligned parallel to each other

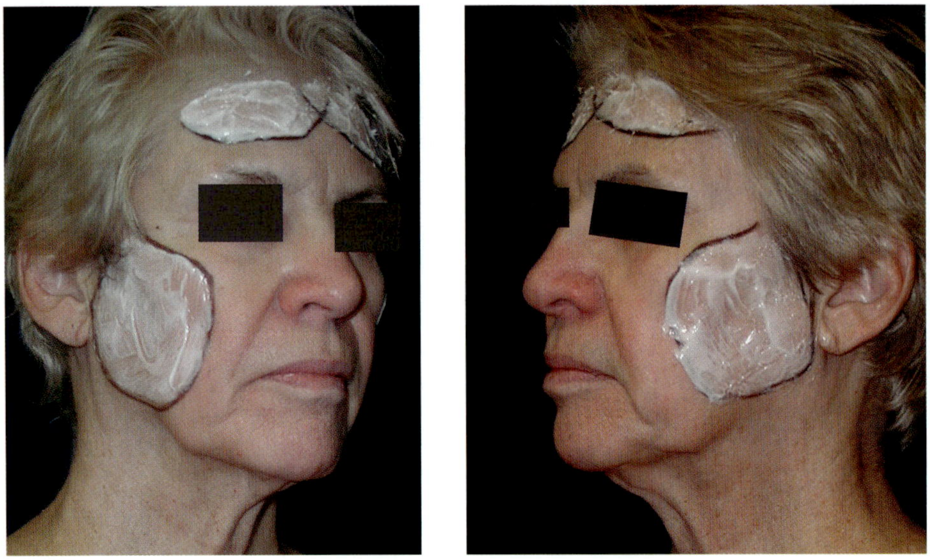

Figures 14.12, 14.13 Anchoring points on forehead and cheeks have been drawn in this 70-year-old woman, and a thick coat of topical anesthetic applied. ThermaCool: Single pass. Forehead: 14.0; Cheeks: 14.5 (anchoring points only).

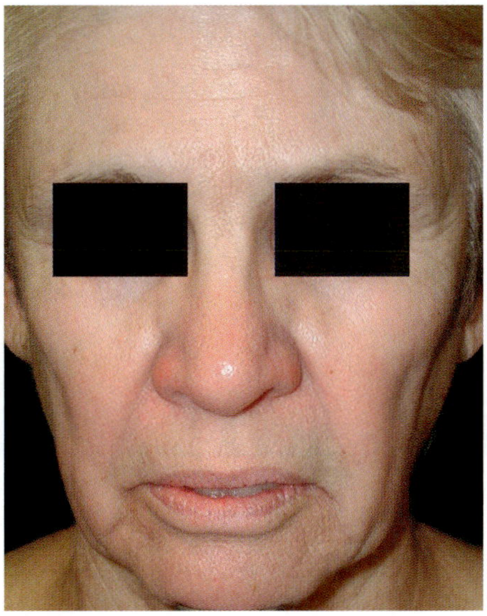

Figure 14.14 Preoperative.

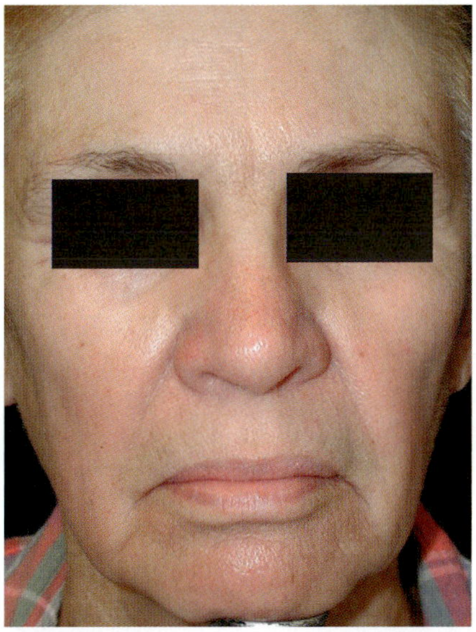

Figure 14.15 6 months postoperatively. Notice improvement in skin flaccidity on cheeks.

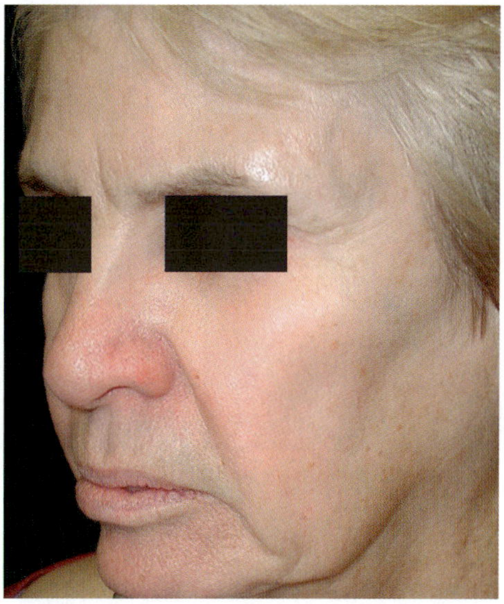

Figure 14.16 Preoperative.

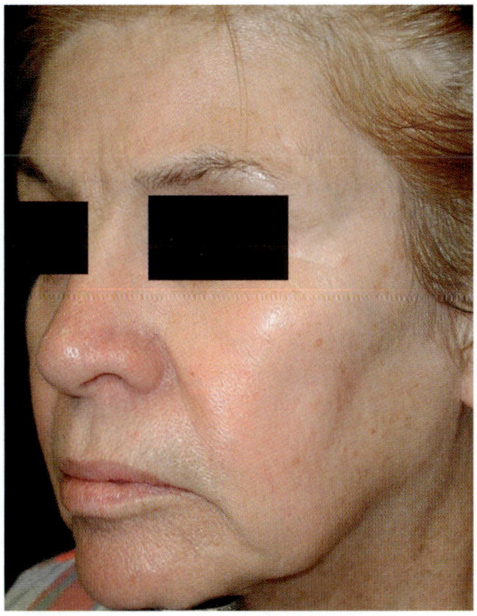

Figure 14.17 On lateral view, improvement of nasolablial fold, jowl area and mandibular line can be appreciated. This example demonstrates that thick skin can also respond well to radiofrequency treatment.

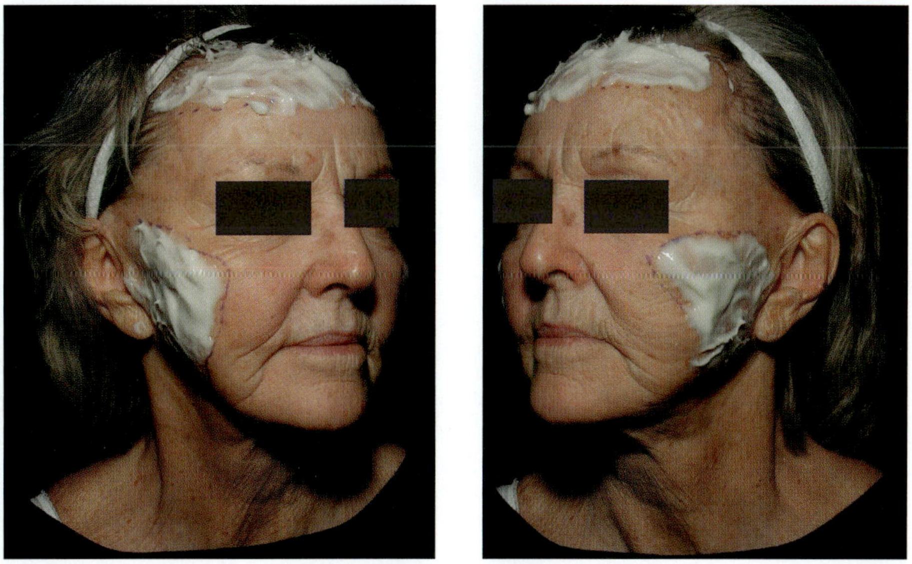

Figures 14.18, 14.19 Anchoring points in a 76-year-old woman. ThermaCool: three passes over anchoring points only; 14.5 to 13.5.

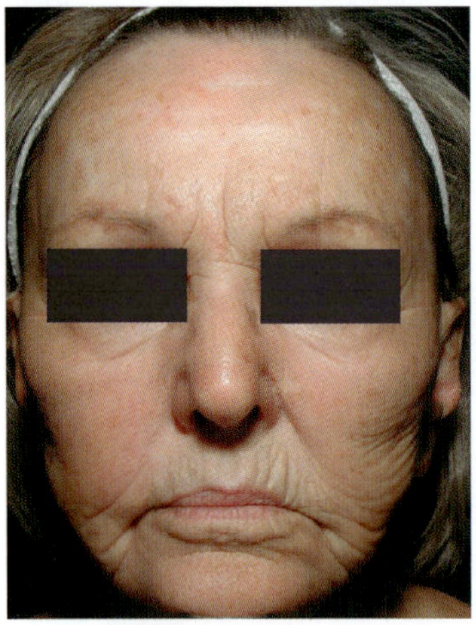

Figure 14.20 Preoperative view.

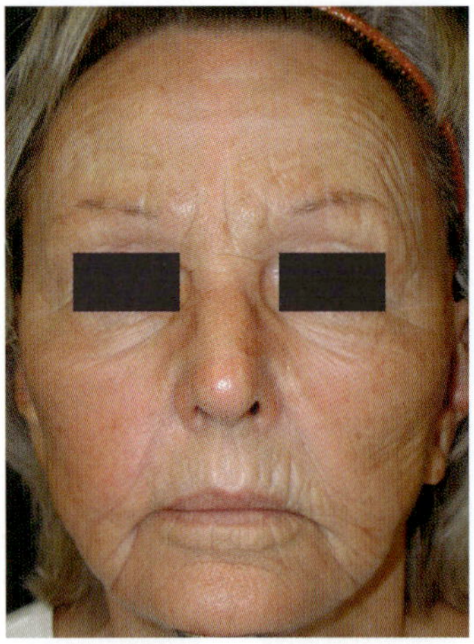

Figure 14.21 13 months after a single radiofrequency treatment.

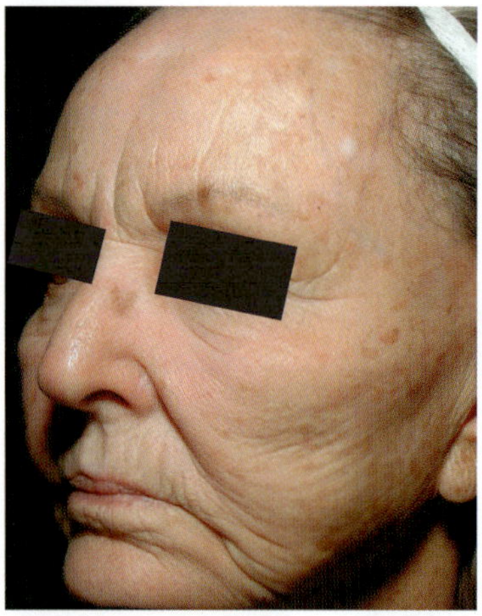

Figure 14.22 Preoperative view.

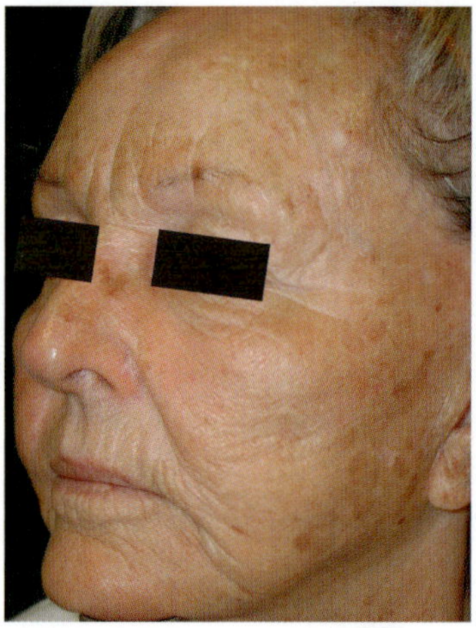

Figure 14.23 13-month follow-up. This case illustrates that age is not a good outcome predictor. Excellent results can be seen in older patients.

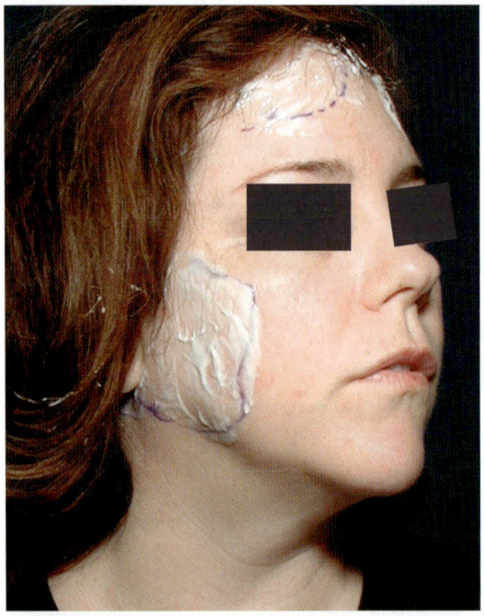

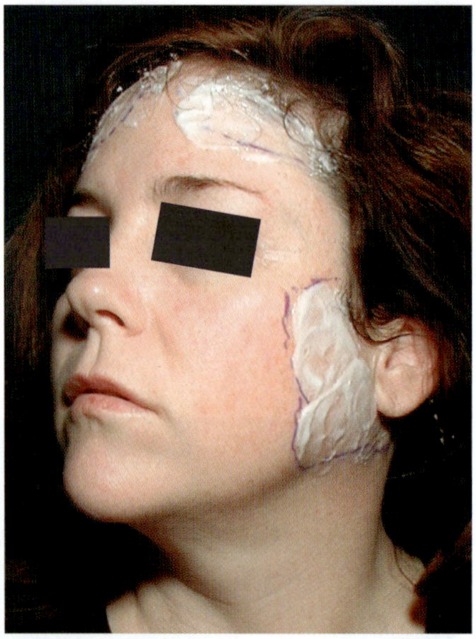

Figure 14.24, 14.25 41-year-old woman. ThermaCool: 13.5 two passes. Anchoring points for eyebrow lifting, cheek and neck improvement. Notice absence of treatment on the neck except for mastoid areas.

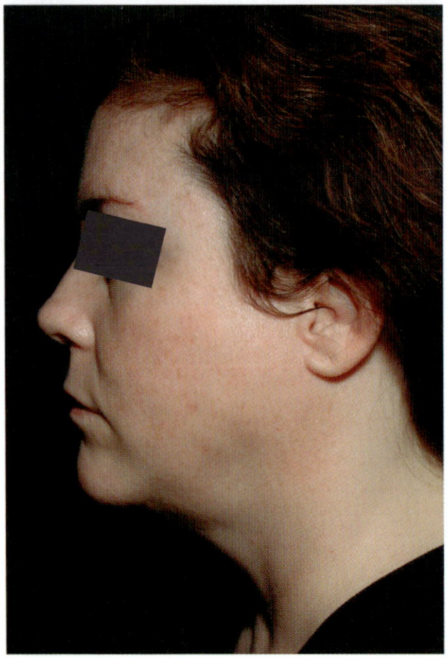

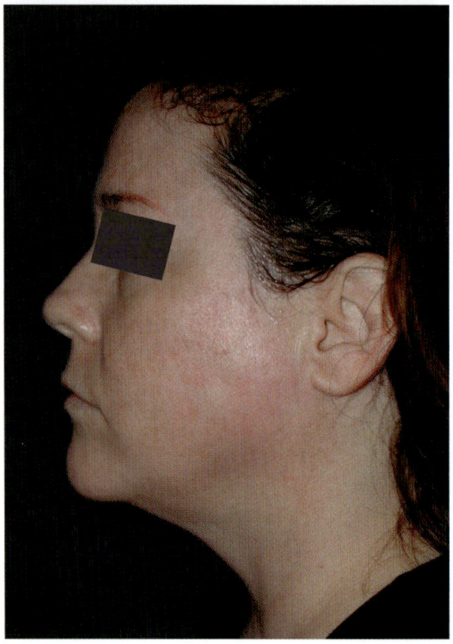

Figure 14.26 Preoperative.

Figure 14.27 6-month follow-up. Notice neck improvement without actually treating the neck. The eyelid profile is better as well.

and, therefore, contraction has a common and predictable axis. Where in the face is there organized connective tissue so that contraction will follow a predictable axis? Perhaps only at the areas of facial ligaments or muscle insertion points; if these areas are treated, perhaps we can expect to have longitudinal contraction rather than compaction.

Once the anchoring points have been identified and the areas to be treated outlined, we proceed to assess the need to treat the anterior cheeks. Treating the redundant skin lateral to the nasolabial fold can be rewarding. This will improve the contour beyond what can be expected from just pulling laterally from the preauricular areas.

A topical anesthetic is then applied. We prefer LMX 4% (Ferndale Laboratories, Ferndale, MI). We prefer this to the 5% product by the same manufacturer because it is easier to remove before the procedure and the level of efficacy is about the same for this use. Anesthetics with an ointment base may alter the impedance and lead to burns. They can also act as a physical barrier and prevent adequate cooling during the procedure. The anesthetic is left in situ for at least 1 hour. We do not reapply it in this interim and although the anesthetic cream seems to vanish after a few minutes, wetting the skin will make the cream white and visible again, revealing that the anesthetic is still there and that only the optical characteristics of the cream have changed. We sometimes use a hand-held iontophoresis machine (Ion Sonic, MS-JMA II, Tokyo, Japan) if we want to shorten the waiting period. If the iontophoresis massage is started at the time of application, only 15 to 20 minutes are needed before starting the procedure, with comparable levels of anesthesia (unpublished observation).

After the anesthetic waiting period is over, we put the patient in a supine position. All jewelry and other metal articles are removed from his or her attire. The nonactive electrode is placed on the lower back. The anesthetic is then removed with gauze moistened with normal saline. We have found that the proprietary coupling fluid from Thermage is an excellent solvent for the anesthetic cream and makes its removal extremely easy. We then proceed to calibrate the machine as per the manufacturer's recommendations. We use exclusively the conventional 1 cm slow tips, as explained earlier.

We then begin the treatment of the marked areas. We have found that a setting of 12.5 is a good and safe setting. Most patients will tolerate it well, although it is in reality quite painful. We rarely need to go to the next upper setting of 13.0 and we almost never now go any higher than 13.5.

Multiple passes of the small areas are done: two to four; rarely more, except when contouring of a fatty area such as the submentum or the jowls is the goal. In these cases, five or six passes are done. One must remember that there is heat build-up with all passes after the first one. The patient often will describe each pass as increasingly painful. We should lower the setting if this occurs (usually by one full setting, for example, 12.5 to 11.5 or even 10.5). I truly believe that what matters is not how intense the heat is but how long the tissue remains heated. So as a rule of thumb, multiple passes at low settings are better than one or two at higher ones. We have seen response to settings as low as 10.5, with multiple treatments (Figs 14.28 and 14.29).

The patient's pain perception is a key guiding factor throughout the treatment. I ask patients to grade their pain in a scale of 0 to 4, where zero is no pain, 1 is mild, 2 is moderate, 3 is strong and 4 is intolerable. I ask my patients to let me know if they feel a 4. I try to stay between a 2 and a 3 and definitely avoid 4s. Reaching a 4 makes me reluctant to go back to the same spot for a second or third pass, it also makes me ask the patient if any residual burning sensation remains. If it does, I immediately apply an ice cube wrapped in a piece of gauze until the burning sensation stops. Having ice cubes readily available during the procedure can prevent burns.

When a patient cannot tolerate a setting of 12.5, I will do the procedure at a lower level, 11.5. I might do an

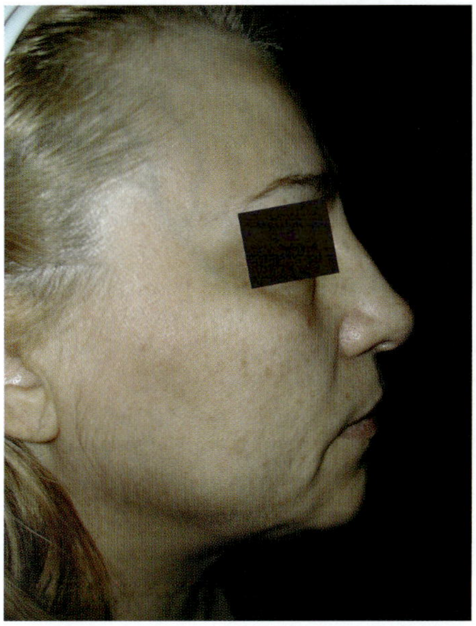

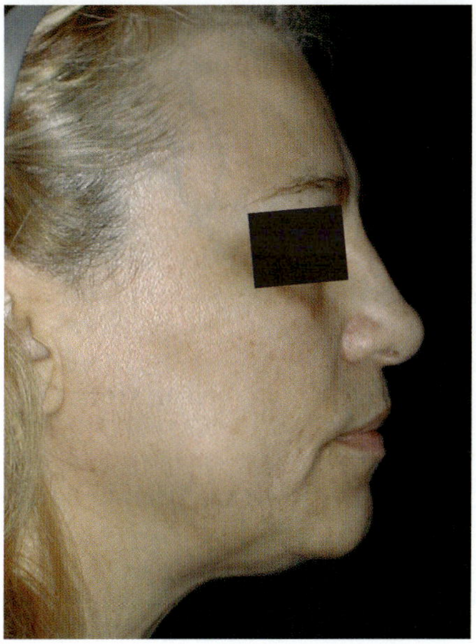

Figure 14.28 52-year-old woman with extremely low tolerance to pain, shown preoperatively.

Figure 14.29 Same patient after five radiofrequency treatments at the lowest settings possible with the ThermaCool device 10.5 using the conventional 1-cm slow tips. This is an example of response to hereby unprecedented low settings, demonstrating that repetition rather than high energy may be more important for obtaining a clinical response.

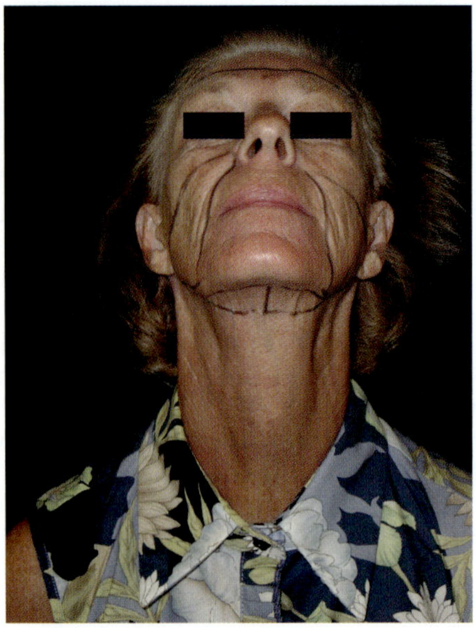

Figure 14.30 68-year-old woman. Titan: 180 pulses at 30 J/cm^3 Painless infrared treatment. Single session.

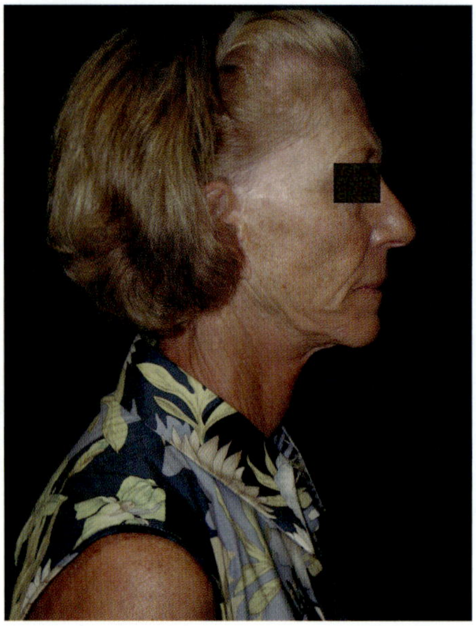

Figure 14.31 Preoperative view.

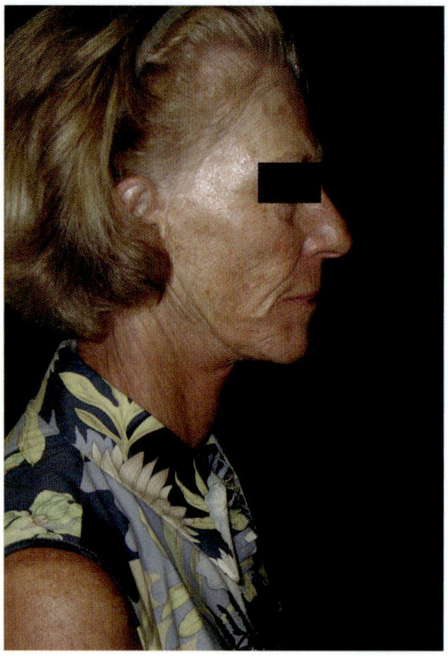

Figure 14.32 Immediate contraction in jowl and neck areas.

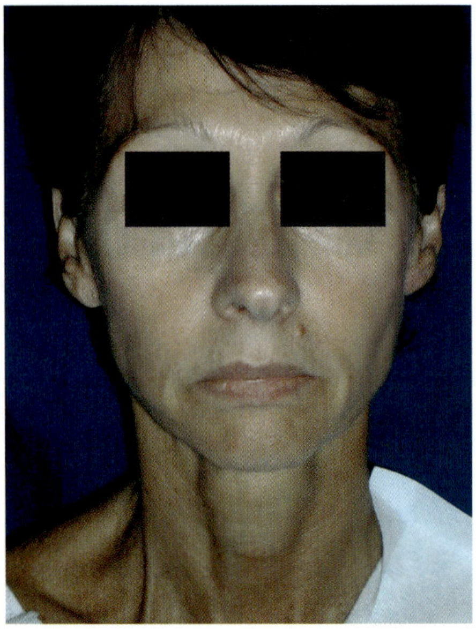

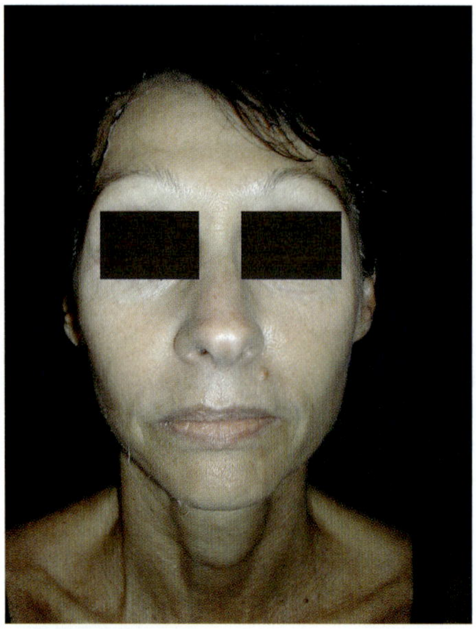

Figure 14.33 62-year-old woman. Titan: Infrared light. Preoperative view. Single session.

Figure 14.34 Immediate eyebrow lifting. Edema is highly unlikely to produce this change.

additional pass to compensate but only if tolerated by the patient. In my opinion, when the patient says the procedure is too painful it is best to stop. Normally the vast majority of patients will tolerate one to three passes at settings of 12.5 to 11.5 even if their pain tolerance is very low.

Infrared Light

After the patient washes his or her face thoroughly, the areas are marked with an eyebrow pencil. The skin needs no other preparation. No topical anesthesia if the fluences to be used are 30 J/cm^3 and below. The patient is positioned lying flat on his or her back and the areas are treated by activating the machine through a pedal for each firing.

The areas treated include the anchoring points as previously described and also any areas of skin flaccidity. These areas are treated directly including the jowls extending the treatment to the skin under the mandibular ridge and into the lateral neck (Fig. 14.30). Immediate contraction can be seen in most cases (Figs 14.31–14.34).

The total number of passes will vary but for treating the anchoring points of the forehead and temples, the anchoring points of the cheeks and the neck as well as the flaccid areas of the jowls a total of between 200 and 300 pulses are given.

Again, each pass will feel progressively hotter. One must stop if definite pain is perceived. If one does not stop, immediate changes may not be seen. The explanation for this is not clear. One may hypothesize that after a certain point there is a breakdown or total denaturation of protein, a meltdown of contractile proteins. This is not to say that eventual improvement will not be seen, but it will be a time-mediated phenomenon and may take months to appear.

Case Reports

Case 1

A 48-year-old woman treated with the Titan device at 30 J/cm^3 (Fig. 14.35). No anesthetic was needed. Immediate eyebrow lifting was seen. At 1 month, the eyebrows continue elevated, the arch of the eyebrows are enhanced. There is softening of the nasolablial folds as well.

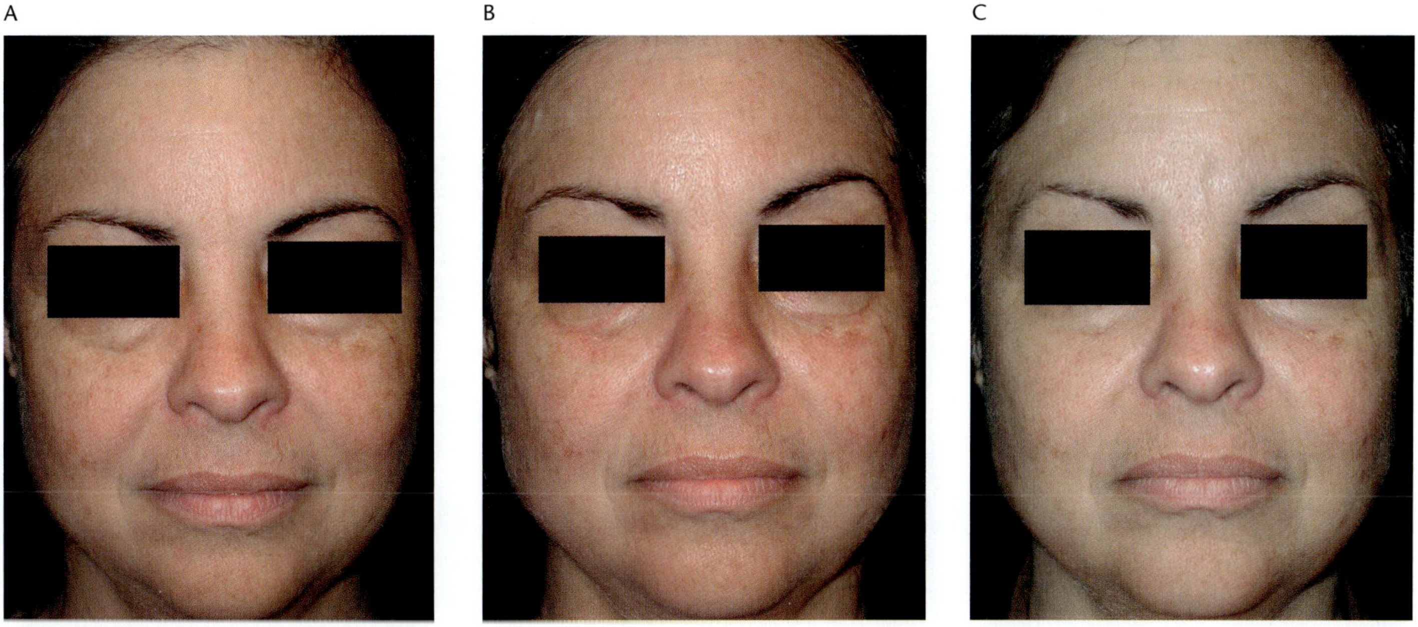

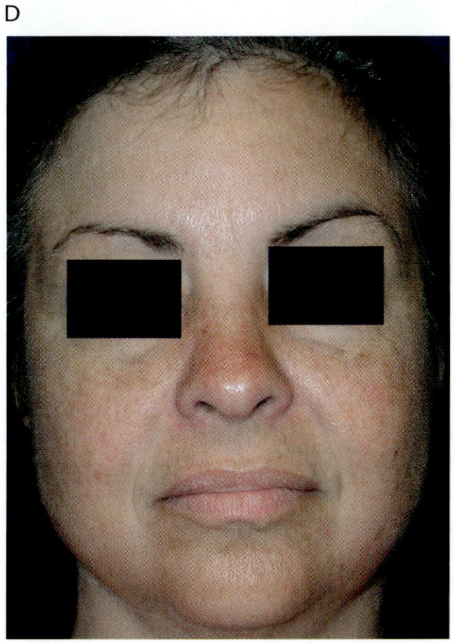

Figure 14.35 (A) Before; (B) immediately after, (C) after 1 month, (D) after 6 months.

Case 2

A 59-year-old woman who had two Thermage treatments prior to treatment with Titan (Fig. 14.36). Immediate changes after only one session with Titan are superior to the changes after two Thermage treatments. The jowl, cheek, mandibular line and neck areas improved immediately. The improvement is maintained at 7 months. Titan settings: 30 J/cm^3 166 pulses.

Case 3

A 53-year-old woman who had Titan treatment (160 pulses at 30 J/cm^3) (Fig. 14.37). Note eyebrow lifting and cheek flaccidity improvement starting immediately after treatment and sustained at 2 months.

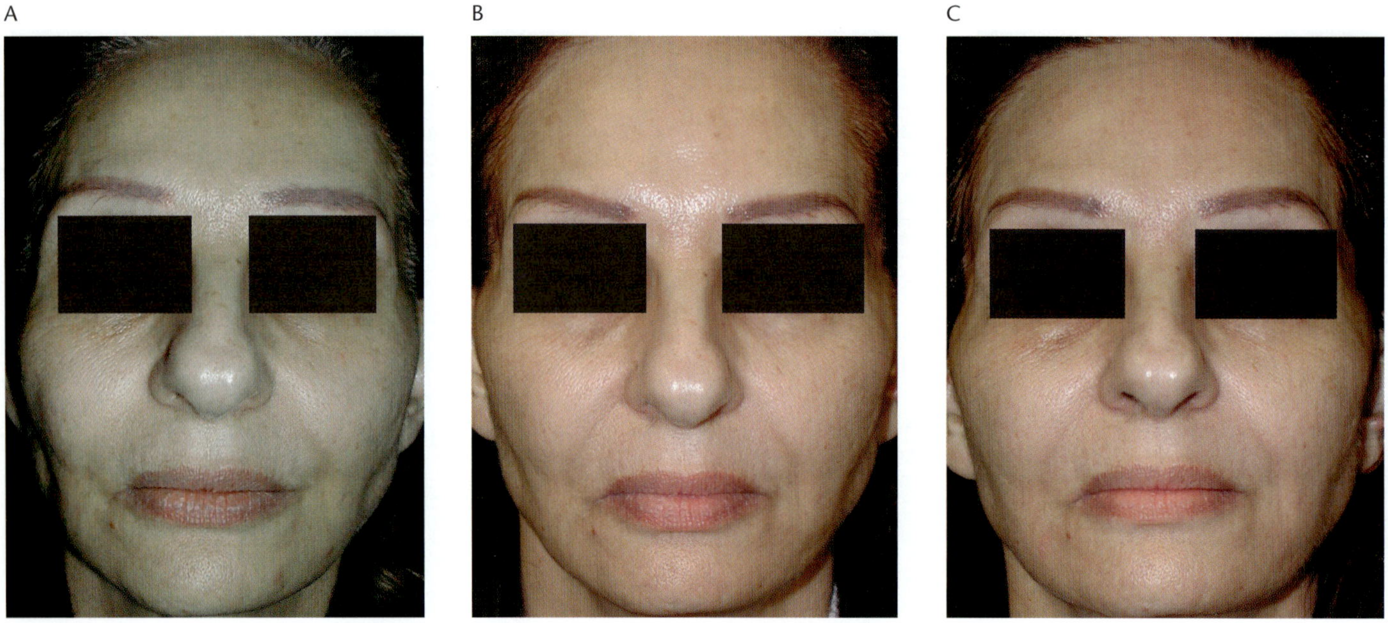

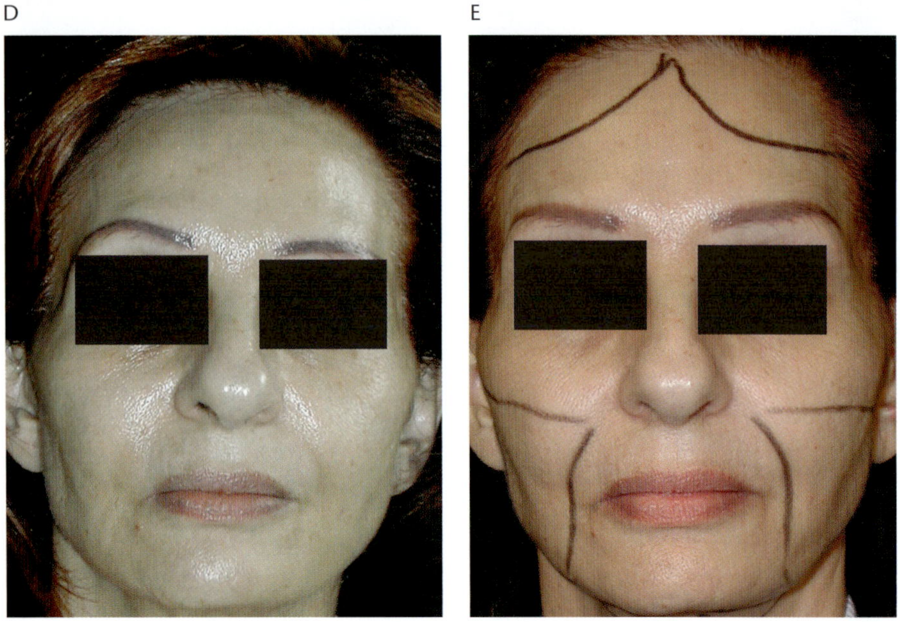

Figure 14.36 (A) Pre-Thermage, (B) After two Thermage treatments, (C) after Titan, (D) 7 months after Titan, (E) treatment areas.

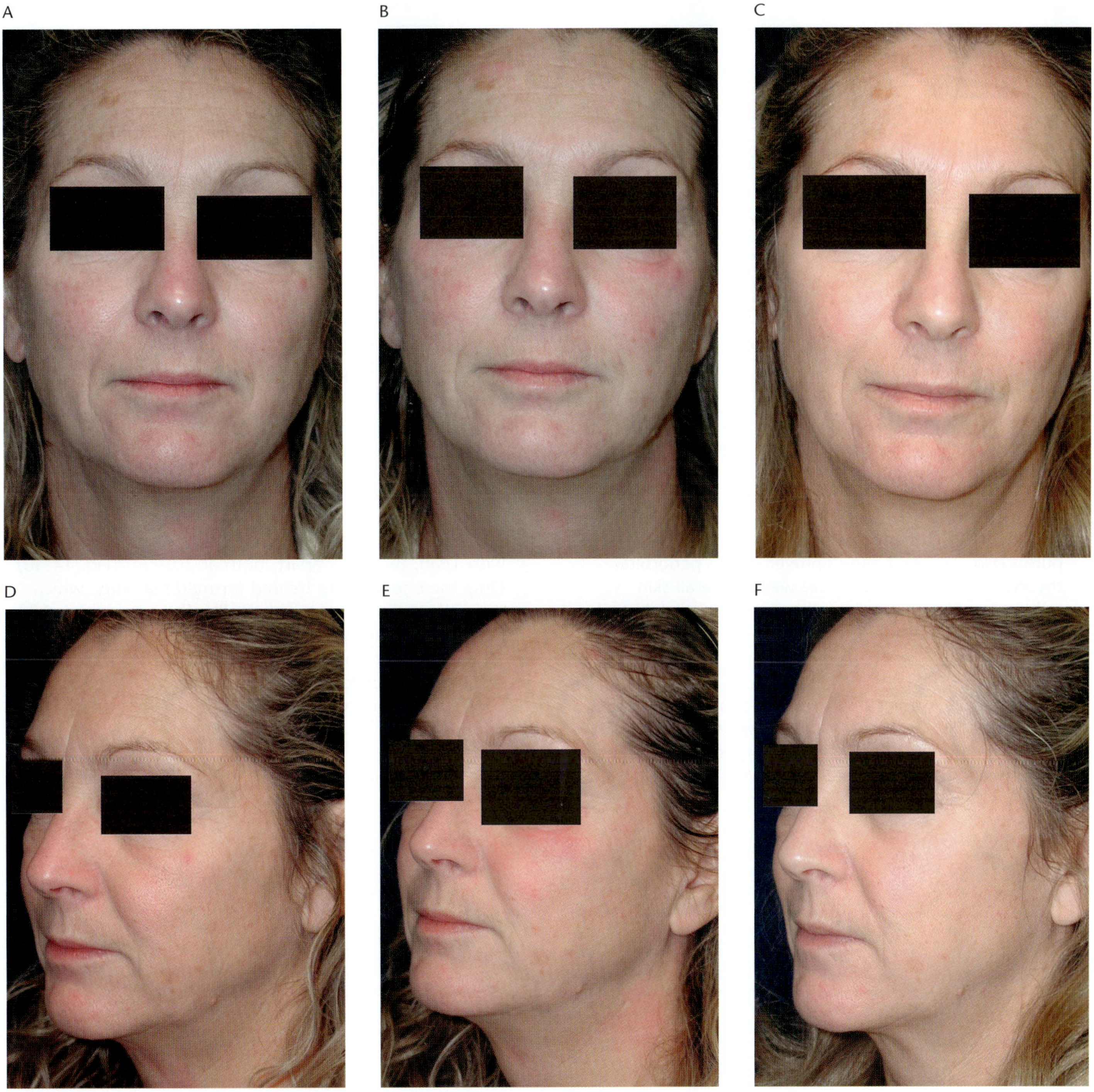

Figure 14.37 (A) Pre-Titan, (B) Immediate, (C) 2 months, (D) pre-Titan, (E) Immediate, (F) 2 months.

G H

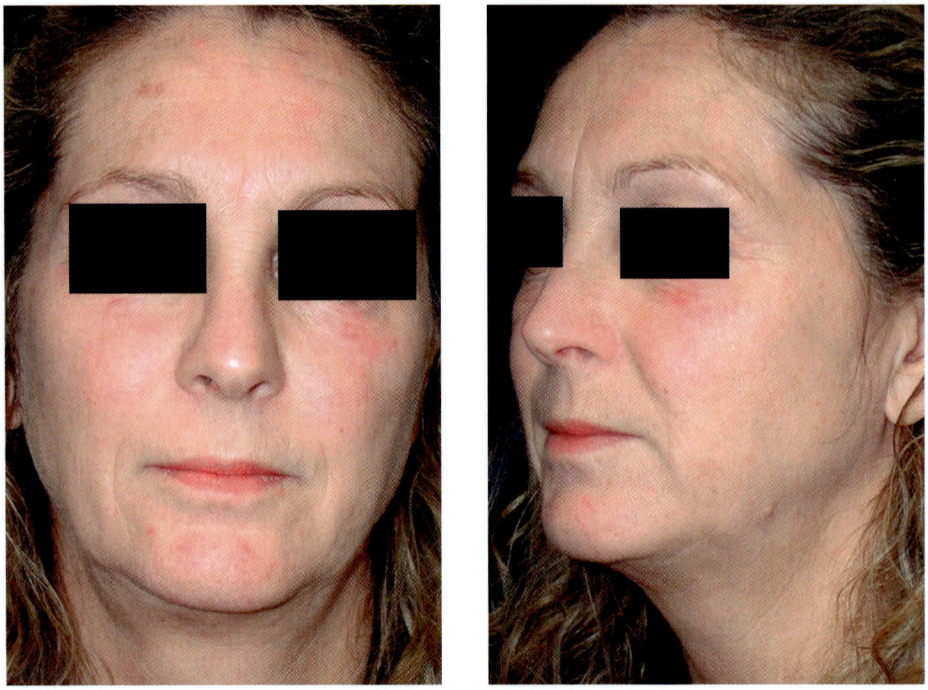

Figure 14.37, continued (G) and (H) same patient after 6 months.

Case 4

A 61-year-old woman treated with Titan at 30 J/cm^3 224 pulses (Fig. 14.38). Note improvement in periorbital rhytids, jowl and neck areas as well as overall skin tightening. The changes can be seen immediately and progress in the ensuing 3 months.

Case 5

A 59-year-old woman treated with Titan (Fig. 14.39). Immediate improvement of upper eyelid hooding, skin flaccidity and depth of rhytids. The improvement is maintained after 3 weeks. 20 to 35 J/cm^3 205 pulses.

Case 6

A 47-year-old woman who had two treatment sessions with Titan, two days apart, both at 30 J/cm^3 (Fig. 14.40). Only the cheeks were treated for mild flaccidity, which the patient disliked very much. The first session was 100 pulses long. Immediate changes were seen, maintained at 48 hours, when the patient returned for her second session. 158 pulses were given the second time. She continued to improve throughout her 7 month follow-up.

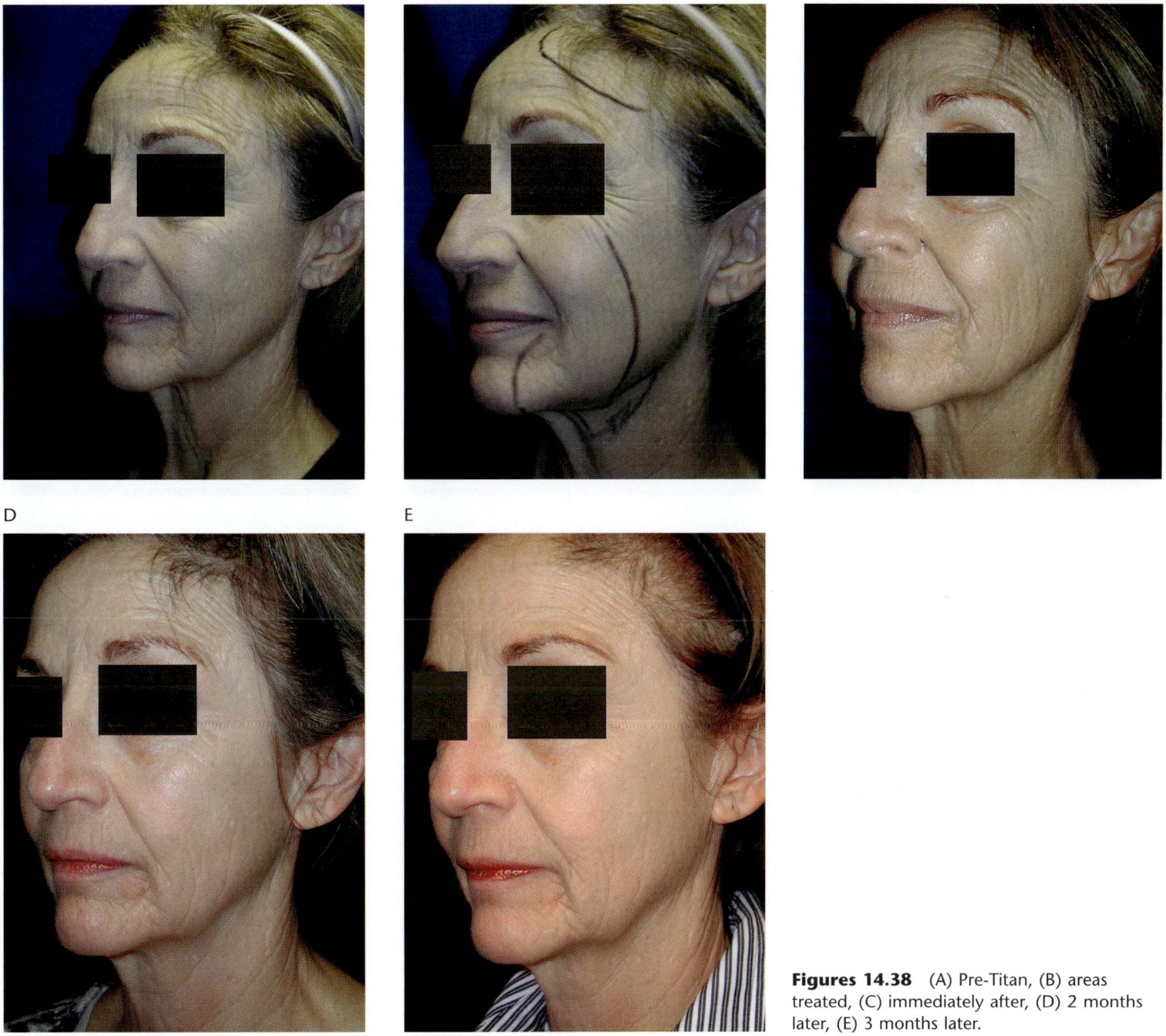

Figures 14.38 (A) Pre-Titan, (B) areas treated, (C) immediately after, (D) 2 months later, (E) 3 months later.

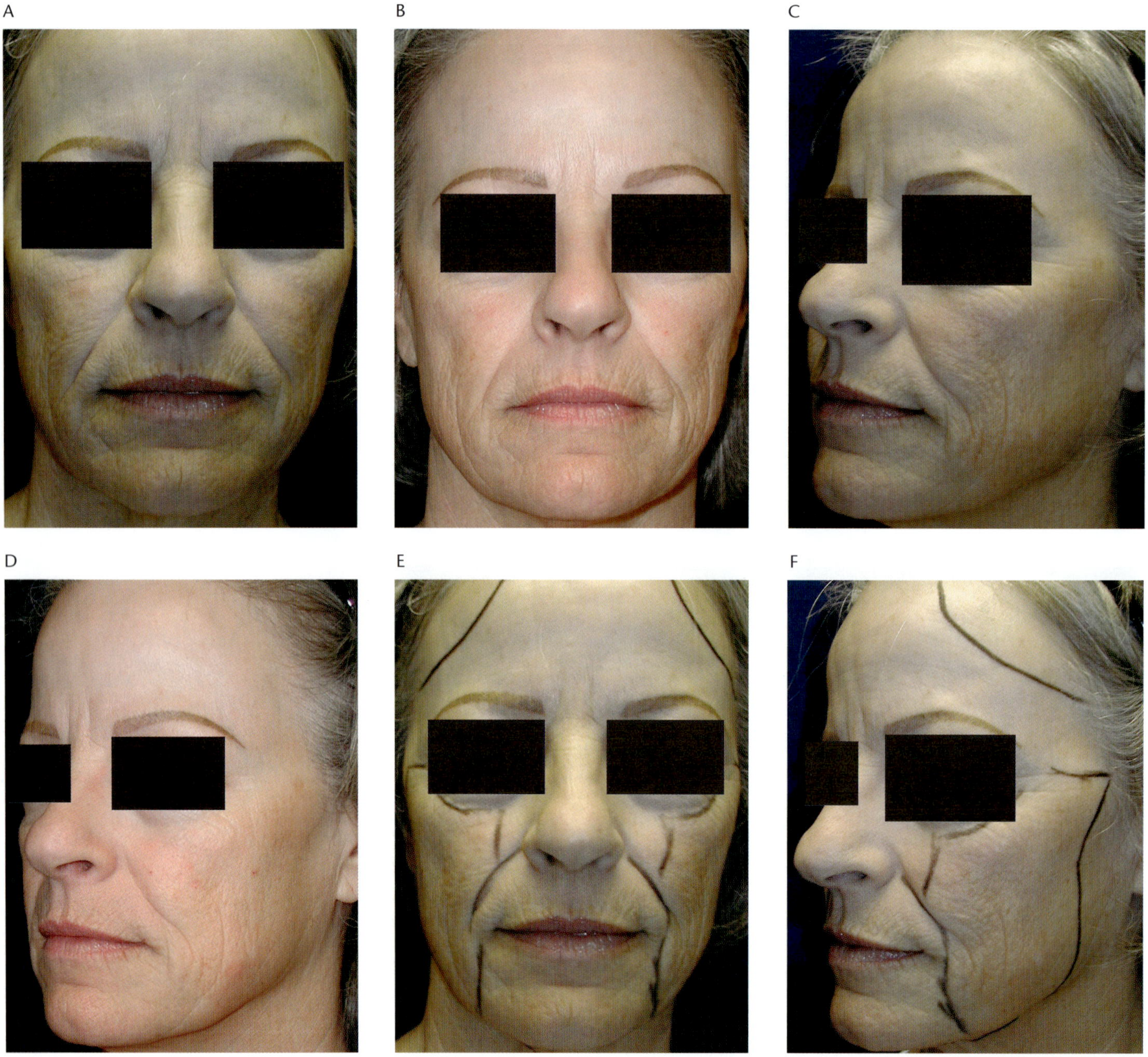

Figure 14.39 (A) Pre-Titan, (B) 3 weeks post-treatment, (C) pre-Titan, (D) 3 weeks post-treatment, (E) treatment sites (F) treatment sites.

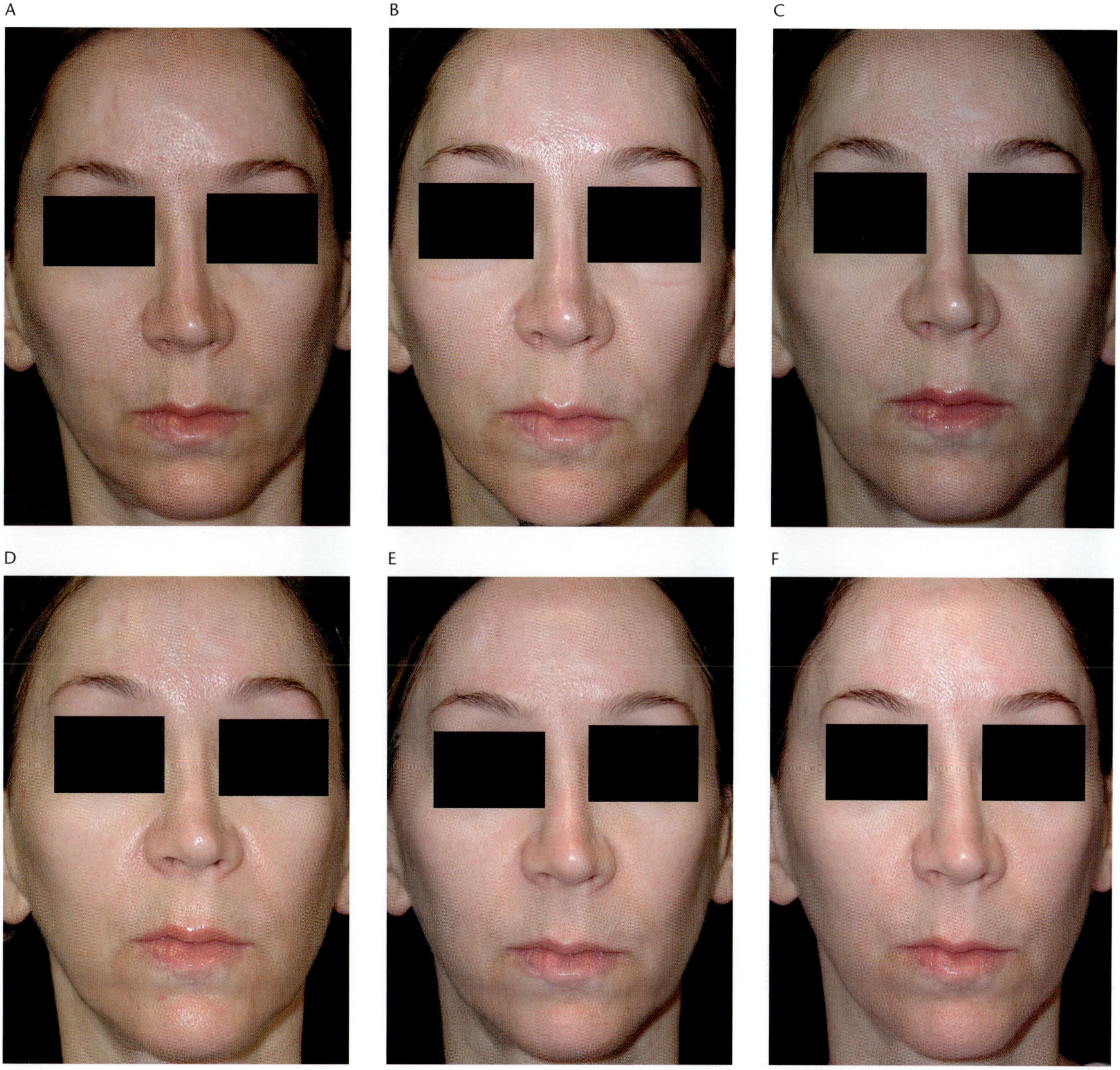

Figure 14.40 (A) Pre-Titan, (B) immediately after first session, (C) at 48 hours after first session, (D) after 1 week, (E) after 4 months, (F) after 7 months.

Case 7

A 63-year-old woman treated with Titan one time at settings of 30 J/cm^3, 217 pulses (Fig. 14.41). Note improvement in lower face and neck skin redundancy which can be appreciated immediately after treatment and improves substantially after four weeks.

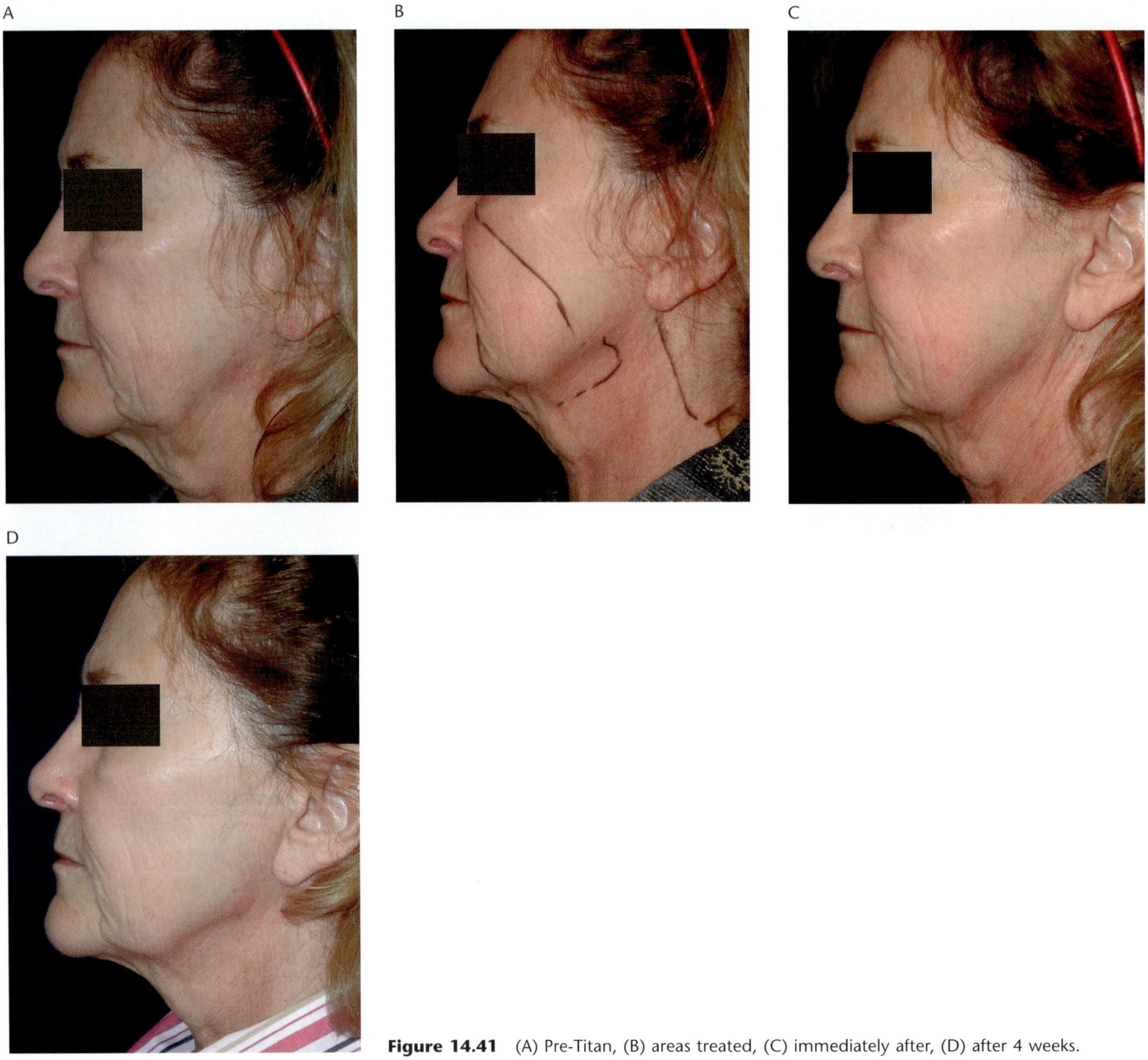

Figure 14.41 (A) Pre-Titan, (B) areas treated, (C) immediately after, (D) after 4 weeks.

Case 8

A 45-year-old woman treated with Titan between 15 and 30 J/cm^3, 146 pulses (Fig. 14.42). Single treatment. Immediate eyebrow lifting and neck tightening maintained at 13 days excluding edema as artifact.

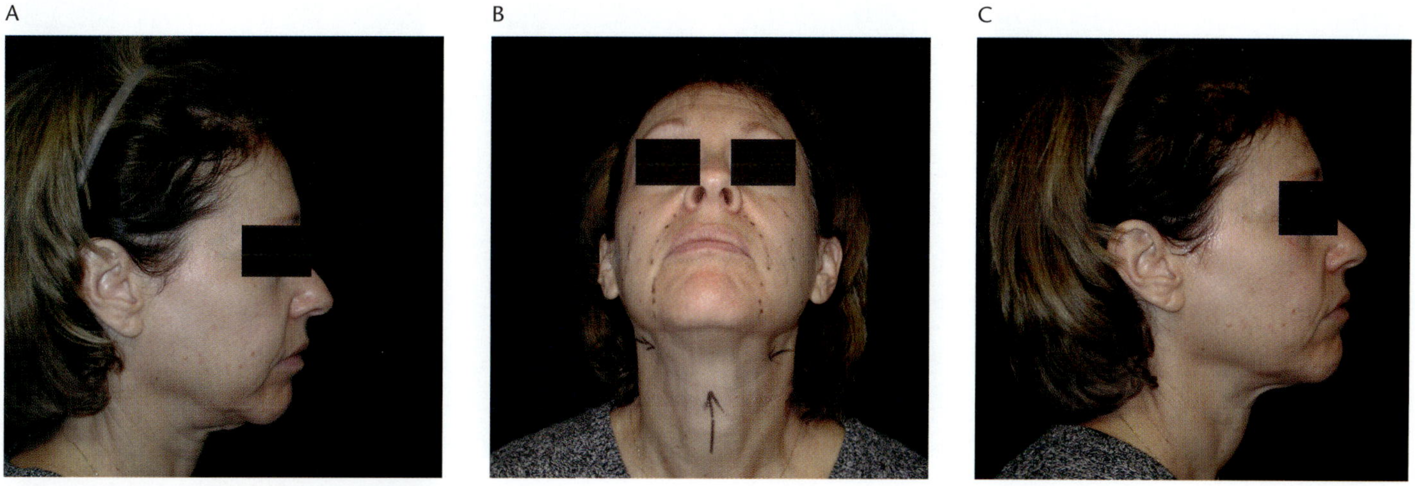

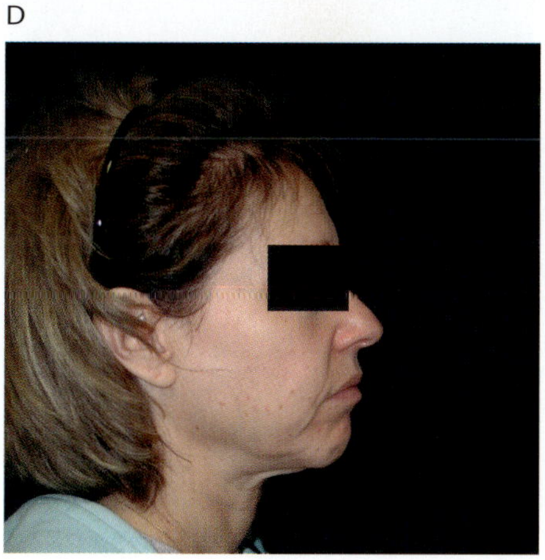

Figure 14.42 (A) Pre-Titan, (B) areas treated, (C) immediately after, (D) 13 days after.

Case 9

A 74-year-old woman who had a single treatment with Titan, using 30 to 40 J/cm^3, 224 pulses (Fig. 14.43). Notice the improvement of cheek and neck, starting immediately and continuing at 3 months.

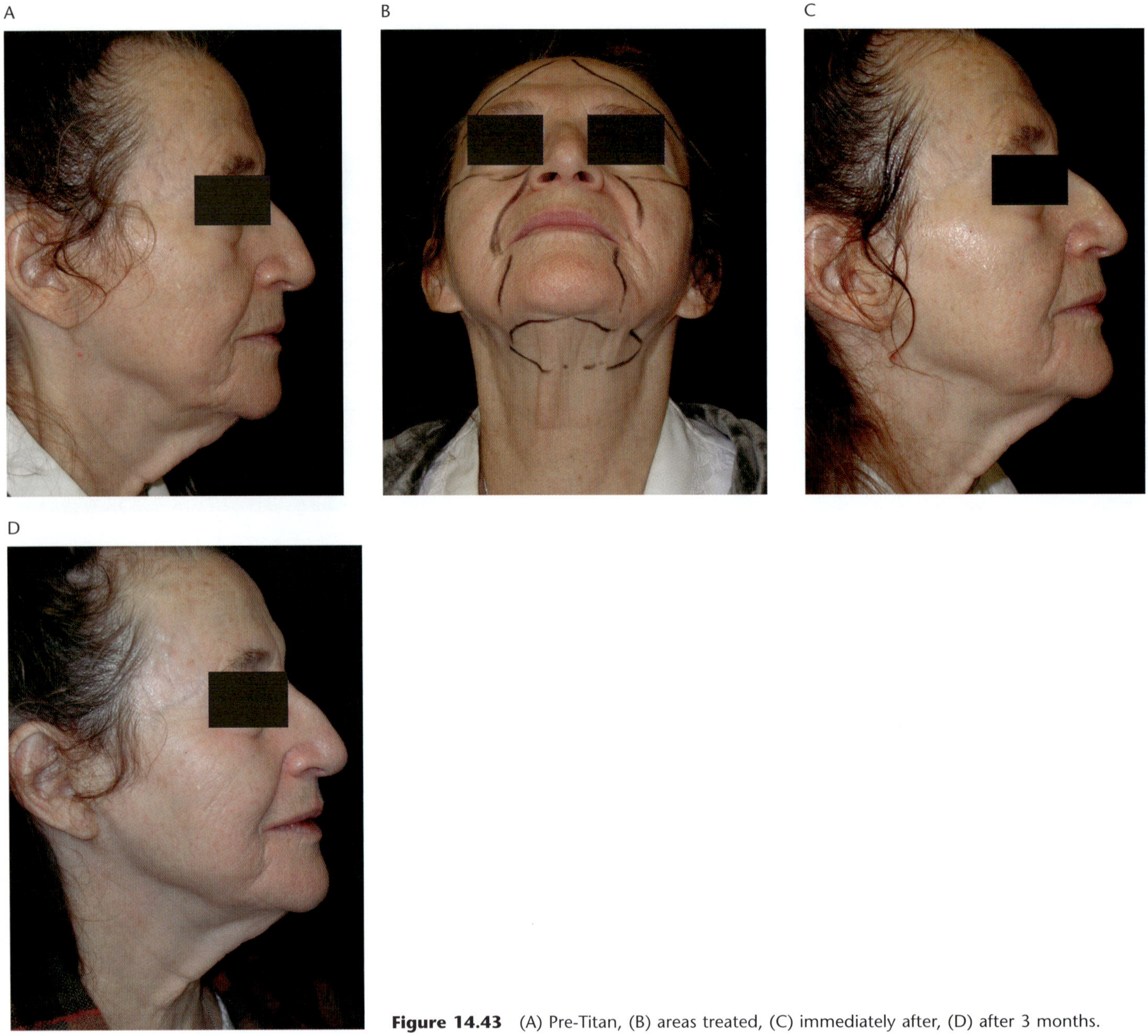

Figure 14.43 (A) Pre-Titan, (B) areas treated, (C) immediately after, (D) after 3 months.

Management of Complications

Radiofrequency

The most significant complication is the so-called fat atrophy. These are areas where too much heat was delivered to a spot, which resulted in one or multiple indentations, usually over the skin of the cheeks or temples. The true incidence of this complication is not known. Many cases probably go unreported; many others are reported only to the manufacturer. But it is not uncommon. It stems from early recommendations to utilize high fluences for treatment. It was wrongly assumed that higher energies would lead to more collagen denaturation and better clinical results. Extensive early clinical work had failed to show that this was true. Despite this, high fluences were recommended. As a result, excessive heat in the subcutaneous fat caused subcutaneous burns that healed with depressed subcutaneous scars. The treatment for these is through clinical observation in the early phases to see if spontaneous recovery will occur. Unfortunately, extensive damage to lipocytes and subcutaneous septi tends to heal with a permanent scar. Lipocytes can be replaced by new lipocytes from pluripotential mesenchymal cells but the repair process is slow and incomplete, and imperfect in terms of ultimate cosmesis. Permanent filler substances should be employed in those cases. Avoiding this complication is perhaps the best alternative. Low to mid fluences are highly effective. Multiple passes must always take into account the interval between these passes. In other words, has the tissue had enough time to cool off from the last pass? If this is overlooked, undue heat accumulation in the subcutaneous layer may occur leading to injury to fat cells and septi. Innervation in this layer is rather poor, so pain perception may not be a reliable warning sign.

Perhaps the most common complication is that of epidermal burns. They usually arise from faulty technique. Full-skin contact with the electrode, as well as sufficient amounts of coupling fluid, is needed to avoid burns. The treatment tips have sensors in each corner of the treating surface that detect incomplete skin contact and the machine will automatically prevent firing under those conditions. The treatment tip must be in a horizontal position rather than at an angle during treatment. Bony prominences such as the zygomatic arch, the mandibular angle, the temporal bone ridge, make the skin over them more susceptible to burns even at medium fluences that would not cause burns elsewhere. Pain is key to detecting when energy is excessive in these areas. When a burn occurs, the earliest clinical sign is intense pain. The patients often describe it as 'matchstick pain'. When this occurs, it is advisable to immediate apply ice wrapped in gauze over the area, particularly if the burning sensation remains after the electrode has been lifted from that spot. Then, the area turns gray. By then, a burn is almost unavoidable. Burns are usually superficial second-degree burns of the size of the electrode. They form a clear vesicle within 24 hours and then heal with or without a crust. Avoiding picking and other manipulation is key to preventing a scar. Simple wound care, with twice-a-day soap and water washing and the local application of an antibiotic ointment will suffice to heal uneventfully. Pink areas usually resolve without treatment in a matter of 1 hour. They are commonly seen in Fitzpatrick's type I skin individuals. Application of ice speeds recovery. Wheals are sometimes seen, at scattered areas over certain treatment spots. They also resolve spontaneously and without sequelae.

Dysesthesia is very rare. It may last for several weeks. I have had only one patient with it; spontaneous resolution followed.

Infrared Light

The only complication I have seen from this technology is vesicles in isolated scattered areas that heal without a scar. They happen in about 5% of cases and need no treatment. Superficial second-degree burns as seen with radiofrequency can also be seen with infrared light and have a similar incidence and management. Fat atrophy has never been seen with this technology.

Adverse Sequelae

Permanent sequelae have only been seen with radiofrequency. 'Foot printing' or 'waffling' indentations appearing from damage to the subcutaneous fat. Permanent fillers or fat injections are needed for correction in these cases. No other adverse sequelae have been reported.

CLINICAL PEARLS

1. **Make sure that the patient has realistic expectations.** The patient must be informed that the changes obtained with these procedures are subtle and do not compare with those from a surgical procedure. A preoperative review of photographs showing the patient a gamut of possible results is advisable. It should also be noted that in some cases, there are no results at all, in spite of our best efforts, for reasons that are not clearly understood.
2. **Secure standardized preoperative pictures before starting the treatment.** Preoperative and follow-up photographs must be taken without make-up, using the same camera, in the same room, with the same head and body positions, at the same distance and height, with the same lighting and preferably by the same person. It is a good idea to display the pre-operative photos in a computer monitor while the follow-up pictures are being taken. This will ensure the best match of position, perspective, distance, etc. leading to obtaining comparable pictures. This is an invaluable tool for evaluating and later demonstrating results to the patient.
3. **Patients must wash their face thoroughly three times while in the office.** This will ensure removal of make-up and other cosmetic residues which can interfere with the cooling or modify the local impedance.
4. **Make each treatment efficient.** Concentrate your heat in important key targeted areas. These areas will, upon contraction, produce the desired lifting effect distally. We can actually choose if we want to lift the medial or the lateral part of the eyebrow, or its entire length, by treating over the medial upper forehead or the lateral temporal areas. This for example, is important in eyebrow enhancement, rather than plain eyebrow lifting.
5. **Lower eyelid laxity can be treated by one of two ways.** (1) Using the principle of anchoring points, one can treat the skin lateral to the eyelid as described previously; or (2) it can be treated directly over the eyelid skin. One-to-one training is recommended prior to attempting this advanced technique.
6. **For lifting the cheek skin, effacing or rather softening the nasolabial folds, one must concentrate heat in the preauricular areas.**
7. **Avoid treating over early platysmal bands.** I have seen exacerbation from RF treatment.
8. **Consider iontophoresis to shorten anesthetic time.** We sometimes use a handheld iontophoresis machine (Ion Sonic, MS-JMA II, Tokyo, Japan) if we want to shorten the waiting period. If the iontophoresis massage is started at the time of application, only 15–20 minutes are needed before starting the procedure, with comparable levels of anesthesia (unpublished observation).
9. **LMX 4% is easier to remove prior to treatment than LMX 5%.** Incomplete removal can result in superficial burns. We have found that the proprietary coupling fluid from Thermage is an excellent solvent for the anesthetic cream and makes its removal extremely easy.
10. **A very important key factor is interval time.** That is, the time between two pulses in the same area. One must remember that there is heat build-up with all passes after the first one. The patient often will describe each pass as increasingly painful. We should lower the setting if this occurs (usually by one full setting, e.g. 12.5 to 11.5 or even 10.5). I truly believe that what matters is not how intense the heat is but how long the tissue remains heated. So, as a rule of thumb, multiple passes at low settings are better than one or two at higher ones.
11. **'Matchstick pain' is usually the first evidence of a burn.** Apply ice immediately. Reaching a 4 makes me reluctant to go back to the same spot in a second or third pass. Ask the patient for areas of residual lingering pain after the procedure. If there are any, I immediately apply an ice cube wrapped in a piece of gauze until the burning sensation stops. Having ice cubes readily available during the procedure can prevent burns.
12. **The most common complication is that of epidermal burns.** These usually arise from faulty technique. Full skin contact with the electrode as well as sufficient amounts of coupling fluid is needed to avoid burns.

Future Directions

Although predicting the future is always risky, I would like to think that both of these technologies are here to stay. I believe that both will further refine the application of energy in ways that are safer and more effective. Thermage will finally realize the importance of a slow rate of delivery of radiofrequency, a slow pulse. The resulting clinical effect will be substantially different and considerably less painful. The validity of needing precooling and post-cooling will be put in question. Exploring alternative cooling–heating combinations will be exciting and rewarding. The machine unfortunately is inflexible. Parameters of this nature are set at the factory and built into the electrodes. The operator can only vary the intensity of the energy. This is done in the interest of safety but it limits exploration into the clinical effects of varying the parameters. New electrode sizes, much larger than the current ones, are needed to treat areas such as the abdomen, the buttocks and the limbs. There is a large demand from our patients for skin laxity correction in those areas. The most urgently needed correction at present is decreasing the pain. The procedure is still very painful and patients do not like that.

The Infrared device by Cutera is already there. One can produce painless, predictable contraction with it. The fluences needed are surprisingly low. Much lower than the lowest capabilities of the current radiofrequency machine.

We are exploring new heat–cold combinations trying to improve results. The earliest indications are most encouraging that in the near future the procedures will be shorter and more clinically rewarding.

Noninvasive fat melting through heat remains the next frontier. Radiofrequency seems the logical choice for it. Fat has high impedance, which makes radiofrequency target it preferentially. Thus far, however, when fat melting occurs the results are disastrous. It is an accident, it is uneven, it creates a clinical skin depression and it is most unsightly. The reason is not, in my opinion, the energy used but the way it was delivered. A fresh look at the importance of this aspect will no doubt permit the development of new treatment tips that will make fat melting predictable, controllable and clinically useful. Or another company will develop the necessary machine, but the future holds a big promise in this area.

Acknowledgment

The author wishes to thank Gregg Spooner and Robert Shine for their contribution to the technical aspects in this chapter.

References

1. Ruiz-Esparza J. Volumetric heating of skin using radiofrequency: preliminary findings. In: Novel approaches to skin rejuvenation (excluding photo rejuvenation). Presented at the Controversies and Conversations in Laser Surgery. Beaver Creek. Vail, CO. August 2001.
2. Ruiz-Esparza J. Volumetric heating of skin using radiofrequency: preliminary findings. In: Arndt K, Dover J, eds. Controversies and conversations in cutaneous laser surgery. Washington, DC: American Medical Association Press; 2002:101–110.
3. Fitzpatrick RE, Geronemus R, Goldberg D, Kaminer M, Kilmer S, Ruiz-Esparza J. First multi-center study of a new non-ablative radiofrequency device to tighten facial tissue. Lasers Surg Med 2003; Suppl 15:114.
4. Ruiz-Esparza J, Barba-Gomez J. Non-ablative radiofrequency tissue tightening of facial skin: the medical face lift: a report of 25 patients. Lasers Surg Med 2003; Suppl 15:36.
5. Ruiz-Esparza J, Barba-Gomez J. The medical face-lift: a non-invasive, non-surgical approach to tissue tightening in facial skin using non-ablative radiofrequency. Dermatol Surg 2003; 29(4):325–32.
6. Ruiz-Esparza J, Barba-Gomez J. The non-invasive, non-surgical breast lift radiothermopexy: tissue tightening via non-ablative radiofrequency. Lasers Surg Med 2002; Suppl 15:36.
7. Iyer S, Suthamjariya K, Fitzpatrick RE. Using a radiofrequency energy device to treat the lower face: a treatment paradigm for a nonsurgical facelift. Cosm Dermatol 2003; 16(2):37–40.
8. Hsu TS, Kaminer MS. The use of non-ablative radiofrequency technology to tighten the lower face and neck. Semin Cutan Med Surg 2003; 22:115–23.
9. Alster TS, Tanzi E. Improvement of neck and cheek laxity with a non-ablative radiofrequency device: a lifting experience. Dermatol Surg 2004; 30:503–507.
10. Ruiz-Esparza J. A less painful, faster and safer application of non-ablative radiofrequency. Lasers Surg Med 2004; Suppl 16:28.
11. Zelickson B, Counters J, Kist D. Histological evaluation of the Thermage RF treatment. Lasers Surg Med 2004; Suppl 6:3.
12. Lennox FG. Shrinkage of collagen. Biochim Biophys Acta 1949; 3:170–87.
13. Ross VE, McKinlay JR, Anderson RR. Why does carbon dioxide resurfacing work?: a review. Arch Dermatol 1999; 135(4):444–54.
14. Zweig A, Meieirhofer B, Muller O. Lateral thermal damage along pulsed laser incisions. Lasers Surg Med 1990; 10:262–74.
15. Ruiz-Esparza J. Non-invasive, non-surgical correction of lower eyelid bags via non-ablative radiofrequency. Lasers Surg Med 2004; Suppl 16:73.
16. Ruiz-Esparza J. Noninvasive lower eyelid blepharoplasty: a new technique using nonablative radiofrequency on periorbital skin. Dermatol Surg 2004; 30:125–29.

Chapter 15

Use of Lasers on Asian Skin

Woraphong Manuskiatti and Mitchel P. Goldman

Introduction

The approximately 3.8 billion Asians in China, India, Japan, the Middle East, South-east Asia, and elsewhere represent the majority of the world's population. Racial differences in skin pathophysiology have been well documented.[1,2] The high risk of pigmentary alterations and scarring following any procedure that produces inflammation of the skin continues to influence physicians to exercise caution with this group of patients. This caution also applies to laser therapy. Even with the highly selective characteristic of current laser therapy, when results are expected to be similar between the races, they are not. Both genetic background and environmental factors are involved in these differences.

Skin laser surgery for Asians is different from that for Caucasians in several important characteristics. Asian skin is often more pigmented than Caucasian skin, resulting in interference by epidermal melanin when using lasers to treat dermal lesions. Consequently, adverse pigmentary reactions, especially postinflammatory hyperpigmentation, are more likely to develop following laser surgery. Another important issue is the differences in the biological behavior of melanocytes among patients from different genetic backgrounds. A controversial deleterious effect of laser exposure is malignant transformation. Unlike the Caucasian population, melanoma is uncommon among Asians and differences in skin types are uncertain to be the main explanation. Therefore, the risk of using laser for the removal of nevomelanocytic lesions in Asians differs from that of Caucasians.

Race is also a critical factor in the response of the skin to inflammation. Asians are far more likely than Caucasians to develop keloids. Some conditions such as nevus of Ota or acquired bilateral nevus of Ota-like macules (ABNOMs, Hori's nevus) are more commonly seen in Asians. Furthermore, photoaging in Asians tends to occur at a later age and has more pigmentary problems but less wrinkling than that in Caucasians.[3]

Differences between Pigmented and White Skin

The surgeon who considers performing laser surgical procedures in non-Caucasian patients should have an understanding of the morphologic differences between white and nonwhite skin, especially in patients of Asian and black descent. The major determinant of differences in skin color between nonwhite and white skin is the amount of epidermal melanin. Although there is no difference in the quantity of melanocytes between the two groups, the larger and more melanized melanosomes in nonwhite skin compared with white skin have been well documented.[4] In addition, the degradation rate of melanosomes within the keratinocytes of dark skin is slower than that of white skin. The larger and more melanized melanosomes of black skin absorb and scatter more energy, thus providing higher photoprotection. Conversely, the melanocytes and mesenchyma in darker skin seem to be more vulnerable to trauma and inflammatory conditions than those in white skin.[5]

The majority of cutaneous laser wavelengths have significant overlap with the absorption spectrum of melanin (see Chapter 1). Therefore, nonwhite skin presents a significant challenge because of greater absorption of laser energy resulting in damage to melanin-laden cells,

Box 15.1 *Fitzpatrick Classification of Skin Type*

I. Always burns, never tans
II. Burns easily, tans minimally with difficulty
III. Burns moderately, tans moderately and uniformly
IV. Burns minimally, tans moderately and easily
V. Rarely burns, tans profusely
VI. Never burns, tans profusely

increasing the risk of adverse complications including hypopigmentation, hyperpigmentation, and depigmentation. Interestingly, alterations in pigmentation may not be apparent for several months after laser therapy. Thus, when treating nonwhite skin, test sites and long-term follow-up should be considered.

Asian and black skins have a thicker dermis than white skin, the thickness being proportional to the intensity of pigmentation. This increased dermal thickness, along with photoprotection from an increase in the size and number of melanosomes, may account for a lower incidence of facial rhytides in Asians and blacks. Increased mesenchymal reactivity may result in hypertrophic scars and keloids. Like black skin, Asian skin has a greater tendency toward hypertrophic scarring. Asians may also have a greater tendency toward prolonged redness during scar maturation than whites do.[6]

Fitzpatrick developed the classification of skin phototypes based on response to ultraviolet irradiation of the Caucasian population (Box 15.1).[7]

However, it has often been found that a patient with skin phototype I or II may have genetic origins of skin phototypes III, IV, V and VI. Given the same clinical expertise in a specific cosmetically sensitive procedure such as laser surgery, the result would be significantly different in clinically similar patients if one had considered more distant ancestry. Lancer proposed the so-called 'Lancer Ethnicity Scale' (LES) (Table 15.1), factoring in this additional historical information to provide a method to presurgically skin type the patients and more clearly predict outcome.[8,9]

Recently, Goldman proposed a 'universal classification of skin type' that considers genetic racial heritage in the response of melanocytes to both ultraviolet light as well as inflammation (Box 15.2).[10]

Box 15.2 *World Classification of Skin Type*

1. European/Caucasian: white:
   a. Pale, cannot tan, burns easily, no postinflammatory pigmentation
   b. Tan, rarely burns, rarely develops postinflammatory pigmentation
   c. Deep tan, never burns, develops postinflammatory pigmentation
2. Arabic/Mediterranean/Hispanic: light brown:
   a. Pale, cannot tan, burns easily, no postinflammatory pigmentation
   b. Tan, rarely burns, rarely develops postinflammatory pigmentation
   c. Deep tan, never burns, develops postinflammatory pigmentation
3. Asian: yellow:
   a. Pale, cannot tan, burns easily, no postinflammatory pigmentation
   b. Tan, rarely burns, rarely develops postinflammatory pigmentation
   c. Deep tan, never burns, develops postinflammatory pigmentation
4. Indian: brown:
   a. Pale, cannot tan, burns easily, no postinflammatory pigmentation
   b. Tan, rarely burns, rarely develops postinflammatory pigmentation
   c. Deep tan, never burns, develops postinflammatory pigmentation
5. African: black:
   a. Pale, cannot tan, burns easily, no postinflammatory pigmentation
   b. Tan, rarely burns, rarely develops postinflammatory pigmentation
   c. Deep tan, never burns, develops postinflammatory pigmentation

Clinical Applications

Current laser or light-source systems can be classified according to the desired target of destruction (see Chapter 1). Like those clinical applications on white complexions, the indications of laser therapy in Asian skin include vascular-specific lasers, laser treatment for hypertrophic scars, keloids and striae, pigment-specific lasers, laser hair removal, ablative laser systems, and nonablative laser systems.[11] The increase in epidermal melanin in Asian skin compared to that of white skin has been claimed to be a limiting factor for obtaining beneficial results and to be a critical factor for developing adverse sequelae in dermatological laser treatment. Patients with nonwhite skin are generally less responsive to treatment because of competition from epidermal melanin for the laser energy.

Vascular-Specific Lasers

The indications for laser treatment of microvascular lesions are similar in Asians and Caucasians. Oxyhemoglobin, with its major absorption peaks at 418, 542 and 577 nm is the major chromophore in cutaneous microvessels.[12] Various lasers and intense-pulsed light systems are available, producing a spectrum of wavelengths that can be selectively absorbed by oxyhemoglobin. These include argon laser (488 and 514 nm), copper vapor laser (511 and 578 nm), potassium titanyl phosphate (KTP) laser (532 nm), variable pulse width frequency doubled Nd:YAG 532 nm (VP 532) laser, tunable dye lasers (577, 585, 595 and 600 nm), long-pulsed neodynium: yttrium-aluminum-garnet laser (1064 nm) and intense pulsed light system (>515 nm). In Asian skin, melanin competes strongly for laser light absorption. Melanin has strong absorption in

Table 15.1 *Lancer Ethnicity Scale (LES)8*		
LES skin type	**Fitzpatrick skin phototype**	**Background geography**
		European
LES type 3	Type II	Ashkenazi Jewish
LES type 1	Type I	Celtic
LES type 2	Type III	Central, Eastern European
LES type 1	Type I–II	Nordic
LES type 1–2	Type I	Northern European (general)
LES type 3–4	Type III	Southern European, Mediterranean North American
LES type 3	Type II	Native American (including Inuit)
		Asian
LES type 4	Type IV	Chinese, Korean, Japanese, Thai, Vietnamese
LES type 4	Type IV	Filipino, Polynesian
		Latin/Central/South American
LES type 4	Type IV	Central, South American Indian
		African
LES type 5	Type V	Central, East, West African
LES type 5	Type V	Eritrean and Ethiopian
LES type 5	Type V	North African, Middle East Arabic
LES type 4	Type III	Sephardic Jewish

To calculate an individual's skin on the LES, find the LES skin type numbers for each of his or her four grandparents. Add the numbers together and divide this total by four. The lower LES skin type, the better skin healing should be after laser surgery and the less risk there is of scarring, keloids, erythema, discoloration and uneven pigmentation.

Risk factors:

LES type 1 = very low risk
LES type 2 = low risk
LES type 3 = moderate risk
LES type 4 = significant risk
LES type 5 = considerable risk

the 350–1200 nm wavelength regions, being strongest in the ultraviolet range and decreasing exponentially through visible and into near-infrared wavelengths. In dark-skinned individuals the abundance of this chromophore in relation to oxyhemoglobin in cutaneous blood vessels acts as a total barrier to light from microvascular lasers and intense-pulsed light system.[13] Epidermal pigmentation is perhaps the most fundamental limitation, because it diminishes laser light reaching the dermis and causes unwanted thermal damage to the epidermis.[14–16]

Port-Wine Stain

A study on the treatment of port-wine stains (PWS) using a 585-nm flashlamp-pumped pulsed dye laser (PDL, SPTL-1; Candela Laser Corp., Wayland, MA) has shown that patients with skin type IV and V responded to treatment more slowly and required more treatment sessions to reach the same degree of clearing than patients with skin types I–III.[17] In addition, patients with skin types IV to V had a higher overall percentage of none to poor, and slight responders than those of the skin type I to III group (30% versus 16%). In contrast, when using the 585-nm PDL to treat facial telangiectasia, the same investigators found that skin type had no measurable influence on treatment response.

The influence of preoperative skin pigmentation on adverse effects following treatment with copper vapor laser (CVL), argon laser (AL), and 585 nm flashlamp-pumped pulsed dye laser (PDL) has been well documented.[18–20] Studies have shown that the risk of inducing clinically visible pigmentary alterations and textural changes increases with higher preoperative skin pigmentation, and with the application of increasing laser energy. However, pigmentary alteration (hyper- and hypopigmentation) was found to occur at a significantly lower intensity level than scarring (texture change, atrophy, hypertrophy and skin shrinkage). Darkly pigmented individuals obtained more severe wounding than fair-skinned subjects from AL and CVL treatment.[21] In addition, the immediate histological outcome after these laser treatments has been found to depend on the pretreatment pigmentation content.[15,16]

Side effects after laser treatment of vascular malformations are theoretically due to three different mechanisms, all of which result in nonspecific energy deposition: (1) direct and competitive absorption by epidermal melanin; (2) thermal diffusion away from the absorbing chromophores, primarily melanin and hemoglobin; and (3) scattering effects that indirectly increase epidermal and dermal nonspecific injury.[13,19]

Asian patients with PWS are less responsive to PDL and VP 532 laser treatment with higher risk for adverse effects such as vesiculation and pigmentary alterations (Fig. 15.1). However, dark-skinned patients should not be excluded from PDL therapy, provided that treatment expectation and risks are fully discussed.[22–24] A retrospective study evaluating the results of a VP 532 laser, coupled with a cooling tip in the treatment of PWS in Chinese patients, found that this laser was only partially effective.[24] Potential limitations of 532-nm light sources are that (although selective absorption of light by hemoglobin is equal to 585 nm) the shorter wavelength penetrates less deeply and is, therefore, less effective for deeper targets. Furthermore, melanin absorption is increased, making this wavelength suboptimal for Asian and darker skin types and also increasing the risk of hypopigmentation.

The development of a longer wavelength (595 nm), adjustable pulse width (0.45–40 milliseconds) with a cooling device, is an alternative vascular-specific laser for dark-skinned patients. The laser operating at a longer wavelength of 595 nm is less absorbed by epidermal melanin. Therefore, it causes less non-specific injury to the pigmented epidermis, compared to that of the 585-nm PDL. The adjustable pulse width and longer wavelength also enables the pulsed light to target larger caliber and more deeply situated vessels in the skin. However, the conventional 585-nm PDL has demonstrated a significantly greater clearance rate than it did at the same setting of 595-nm PDL. In addition, the former also caused higher incidence of adverse effects including pain, postoperative purpura, crusting, and transient hyperpigmentation.[25,26] The higher incidence of complications is more likely due to the slightly higher absorption by epidermal melanin at the 585-nm wavelength.

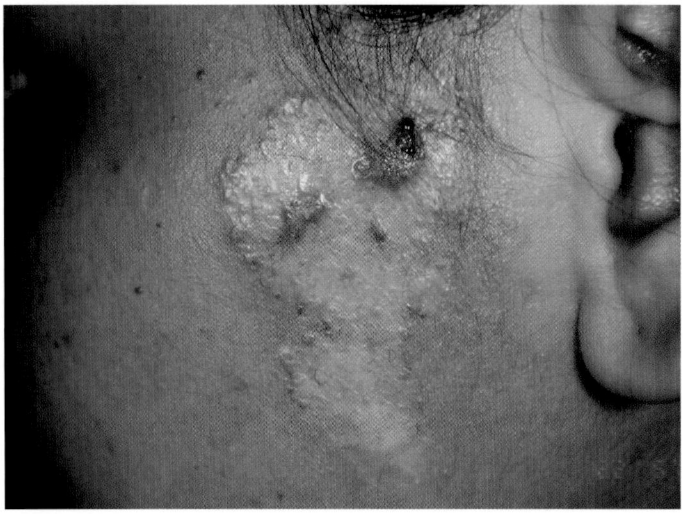

Figure 15.1 Atrophic scar and persistent hypopigmentation at six months after two, 585-nm PDL treatments at an average fluence of 7 J/cm^2 using a 7-mm spot size without epidermal cooling device.

The epidermal cooling device has been demonstrated to reduce adverse complications and improve the clinical efficacy of pulsed dye laser for the treatment of PWS in Chinese patients.[27,28] The use of cryogen spray cooling improves clinical efficacy and a higher fluence can be used without an increase in complications such as permanent scarring or dyspigmentation. As a result, pulsed dye lasers equipped with an epidermal cooling device of some type are considered to be the optimal lasers for treatment of PWS in Asians (Fig. 15.2).

Recently, Ho et al[29] studied the use of an intense pulsed light (IPL) for the treatment of PWS in Chinese patients. The clearing rate was reported to be better than that of PDL without cooling with fewer long-term complications. However, the authors pointed out that IPL could be effective in the treatment of PWS only when used by an experienced operator.

The introduction of long-pulsed 1064-mm lasers with epidermal cooling has also allowed for the treatment of

A B C

D E

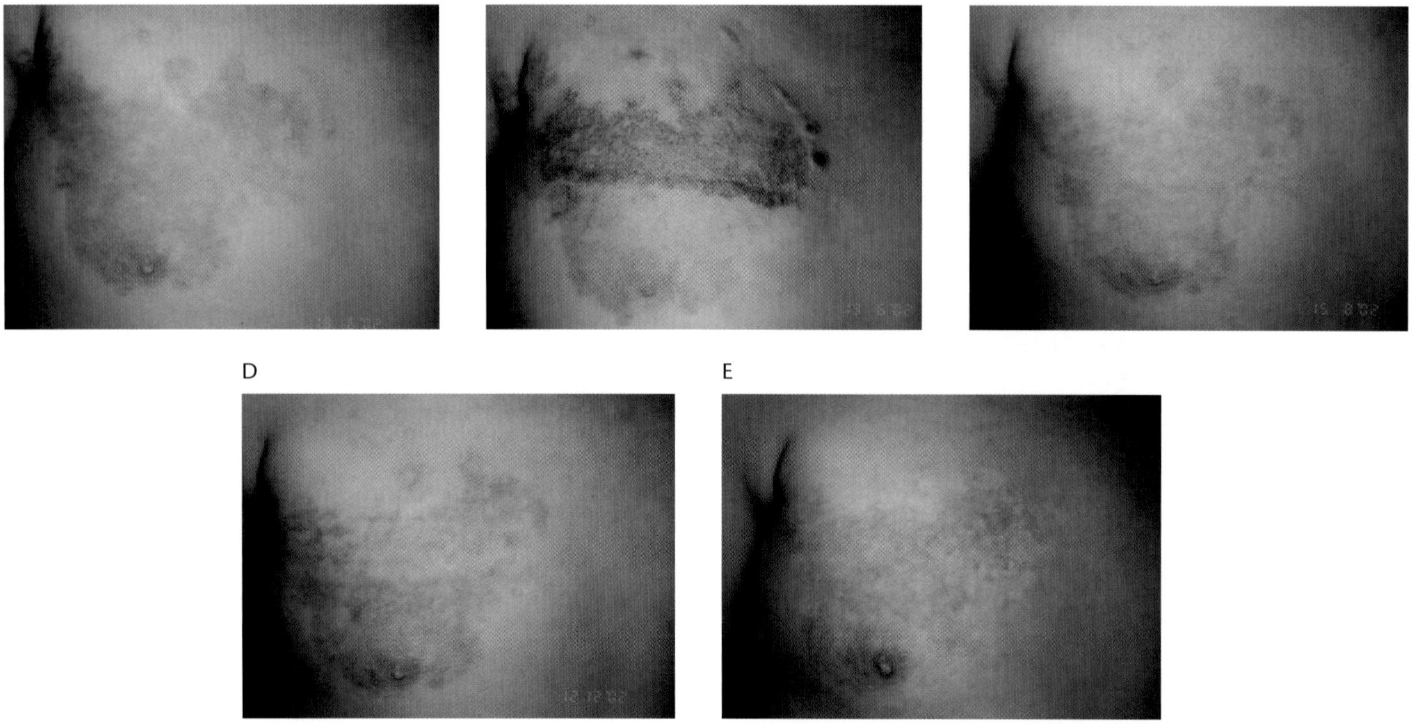

Figure 15.2 A 9-year-old Thai girl with port-wine stain (A) before and (B) immediately after a 595-nm pulsed dye laser treatment with a dynamic cooling device (DCD), treatments were performed using a 7-mm spot size and a cryogen spurt duration of 80 ms, and a delay of 30 ms between spurt termination and onset of the laser pulse. The upper half treated with a fluence of 8 J/cm^2 and a 0.45-ms pulse duration, whereas the lower half treated with a fluence of 15 J/cm^2 and a 40-ms pulse duration. (C) 2 months after one treatment, the clearance rate corresponded to the extent of the postoperative purpura. (D) 2 months after three treatments with the same parameter. (E) 2 months after the thirteenth treatment. During the fourth to the sixth treatments, the whole lesion was treated at a fluence of 8 J/cm^2 and a 0.45-ms pulse duration, whereas the seventh to the thirteenth treatments were performed at a fluence of 15 J/cm^2 and a 20-ms pulse duration. The DCD was set using the same parameters.

vascular lesions in darkly pigmented skin. We have found that telangiectasias, both on the face as well as other body areas, can be successfully treated using a 1064-nm laser with a pulse duration of 25 ms, a 3.5-mm spot size and fluences of between 200 and 250 J/cm^2. This is usually given in combination with dynamic cooling where a 30 ms cooling spray is given coincident with the laser pulse. Utilizing these parameters, we have not found epidermal hypopigmentation to occur. These millisecond-domain 1064-nm lasers also offer a feasible treatment option for vascular birthmarks and deep cutaneous vascular lesions in patients with darker skin phototypes.[30,31] As with the treatment of unwanted hair (as discussed later in this chapter), the long pulsed, 1064-nm laser with epidermal cooling has become the laser of choice for the treatment of darkly pigmented skin.

Laser Treatment of Hypertrophic Scars, Keloids and Striae

The 585-nm PDL has also been used as a treatment of choice for hypertrophic scars and keloids in fair-skinned individuals.[32,33] The efficacy of the PDL in treatment of scars in darker-skinned patients is not as good as that of white-skinned patients and the risk of pigmentary alterations is also higher. A study on the efficacy of the PDL performed in 20 patients with skin phototypes I to VI demonstrated no improvement of the hypertrophic scars on the laser-treated sites compared with untreated control. Eight of the 20 patients had skin phototype VI and two had type V. The effect of melanin was thought to be a factor of treatment failure.[34] Similarly, our previous study[35] noted that clinical improvement of scars in skin types IV to VI patients following multiple treatment sessions with the PDL had a lower response rate, and a higher incidence of epidermal damage, compared to those of the fair-skinned patients (Fig. 15.3). A recent study of PDL in the treatment and prevention of hypertrophic scars in Chinese patients also found that there was no signicant objective improvement in terms of scar thickness and viscoelasticity compared to the controls.[36] Our ongoing study on the effect of pulse width of the PDL on the treatment response of hypertrophic scars noted a lesser efficacy in Thai and Chinese patients with skin types III to V as well.

Treatment of stretch marks is another application of the 585-nm PDL that improves the appearance of these lesions.[37,38] An increase in dermal elastin noted following PDL treatment was speculated to be the mechanism of improvement. In contrast, several studies by other investigators noted no clinical improvement of striae and no increase in dermal elastin content histologically.[39,40] A study on the treatment of striae in skin types IV and VI patients has demonstrated no noticeable clinical improvement, with a higher risk of pigmentary alterations.[40] In our experience, we also found that PDL provides a very minimal beneficial effect on the treatment of striae in Asian skin.

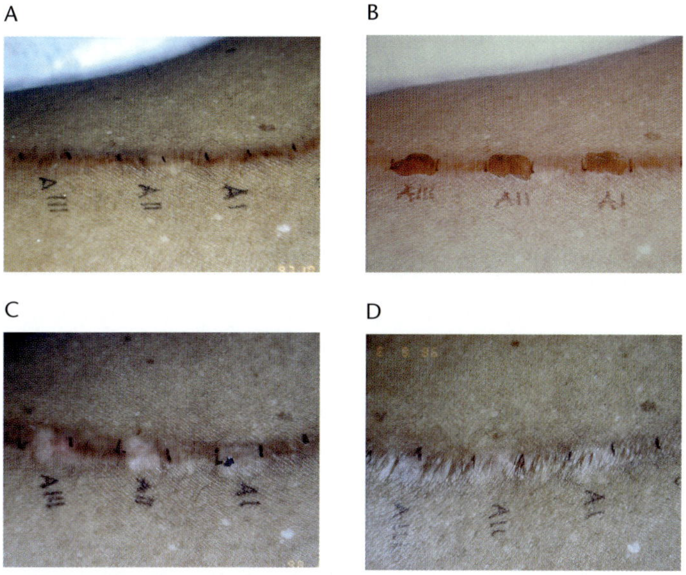

Figure 15.3 (A) Linear hypertrophic scar on the thigh in an Indian patient with skin phototype V, before treatment. (B) 1 week following the first treatment with a 585-nm PDL using a 5-mm spot size without epidermal cooling device; A I, treated with 3 J/cm^2; A II, treated with 5 J/cm^2; A III, treated with 7 J/cm^2. Epidermal necrosis is noted over all laser-irradiated segments. (C) 4 weeks following the second treatment, erythema and hypopigmentation was seen on the laser treated areas. (D) 12 weeks after the sixth treatment, flattening of the scar without dyspigmentation was demonstrated.

Clinical Technique

Patient Selection

- Patients with lesions amenable to vascular-specific laser treatment (see Chapter 2).
- Patients who understand treatment protocol and risks.
- Patients with realistic expectations of treatment.
- Patients who will comply with advised postoperative skin care and follow-up.
- Patients with suntanned skin should be avoided.

Choice of Laser

- A 585- or 595-nm pulsed dye laser coupled with an epidermal cooling device is a preferable option for most vascular lesions.
- The long-pulsed 1064-nm Nd:YAG and VP 532 lasers and intense pulsed light may be alternative light sources to treat resistant vascular lesions.
- Do not use an IPL if you do not have experience with it.

Actual Technique

- Treatment technique and parameters for vascular-specific lasers in Asian skin are similar to those of white skin (see Chapter 2) but more care is taken in selecting an appropriate energy and in determining proper treatment intervals. Because all laser-induced pigmentary alterations should be completely resolved before the delivery of additional laser treatment to effect the

optimal result from each session, longer intervals may be necessary between laser treatments.
- Nothing surpasses individualized protocols based on a patient's clinical examination, history and tissue responses.
- For treatment of PWS and hemangioma in untanned Asian skin, a combination of high fluence (15 J/cm^2), large spot size (e.g. 7 mm) at a longer wavelength (595 nm) can be used only when the epidermis is properly cooled with application of a cold pack or ice cube just before and immediately after treatment, and cryogen spray cooling (CSC) up to 70- to 100-ms spray duration.
- For treatment of facial telangiectasia and hypertrophic scars, similar parameters are applied with a lower fluence of 7 to 10 J/cm^2, depending on the skin types of individual patients. Epidermal cooling is also an essential maneuver.

CLINICAL PEARLS

- Pulse overlapping and stacking can be performed only when the epidermis is well preserved with a cooling device. Cautious stacking of not more than two pulses given 5 to 10 seconds apart may be employed before purpura develops. As a rule, the degree of lesion clearance corresponds to the extent of the postoperative purpura. However, severe purpura and any persistent whitening immediately after laser irradiation seems to correlate with side effects such as hypopigmetation or atrophic changes of the epidermis.
- For treatment of PWS and hemangioma, maneuvers such as gently stretching the skin to reduce dermal thickness, and subtle diascopy with a transparent plastic spoon or glass slide to compress superficial vessels at the time of laser exposure are used to enhance treatment efficacy.

In summary, treatment with hemoglobin-targeting lasers and intense-pulsed light systems in Asian patients should be performed with great caution. Because melanin acts as a competing chromophore for vascular-specific lasers, to be effective the starting energy density has to be higher than that used on fair Caucasian skin. However, the improvement following this procedure seems to be less effective and with a higher incidence of epidermal damage than those seen in white-skinned patients.

Pigment-specific Lasers

Selective destruction of melanosomes has been well demonstrated by exposing skin to submicrosecond, Q-switched, laser pulses.[41,42] A wide range of these is available, including a pulsed dye laser (510 nm), Q-switched frequency-double Nd:YAG laser (532 and 1,064 nm), Q-switched ruby laser (694 nm), and Q-switched alexandrite laser (755 nm). All of these Q-switched lasers are useful for treating superficial epidermal lesions such as lentigines and ephelides, café-au-lait macules (CALMs), seborrheic keratosis and dermal pigmented lesions such as blue nevus, nevus of Ota/Ito, acquired bilateral nevus of Ota-like macules (ABNOMs or Hori's nevus), infraorbital hyperpigmentation, drug-induced hyperpigmentaiton, and congenital melanocytic nevi.

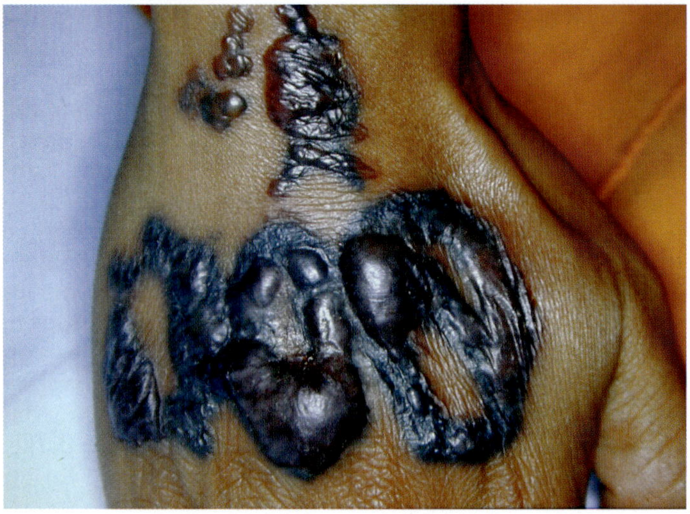

Figure 15.4 Blistering secondary to tattoo removal with the Q-switched ruby laser in a skin phototype IV Thai patient using a fluence of 6.5 J/cm^2 with a 5-mm spot size. (Courtesy C. Vibhagool, Bangkok, Thailand.)

Melanin absorption is stronger at shorter wavelengths, whereas longer wavelengths penetrate better into the skin.[13] Several factors are involved in using Q-switched lasers for treating benign pigmented lesions in Asian individuals.

First, the greater amount of epidermal melanin results in greater damage to lesions and adjacent normal skin pigment during laser irradiation. This increased absorption may lead to posttreatment blistering (Fig. 15.4), hyperpigmentation (Fig. 15.5), hypopigmentation (Fig. 15.6), depigmentation and even scarring.

Second, larger amounts of epidermal melanin in persons with dark skin tones act as a competing chromophore for laser light while using these Q-switched lasers for treating dermal pigmented lesions. Thus, a larger number of sequential treatments are required for complete clearing compared to those of white-complected persons. In addition, the adverse effects resulting from injury to epidermal melanin and the melanocytes responsible for producing normal skin color should be anticipated.

Benign Epidermal Pigmented Lesions

Benign epidermal pigmented lesions include lentigines, ephelides, café-au-lait macules, and seborrheic keratosis. In dark-skinned patients, these pigmented lesions have been successfully treated with the argon (488 and 515 nm, continuous wave [CW]) laser,[43] 510-nm short pulsed dye laser,[44] copper vapor (511 nm, CW) laser,[45] Q-switched frequency doubled Nd:YAG (532 nm) laser,[46,47] Q-switched ruby laser,[43,48–50] Q-switched alexandrite laser (755 nm)[51],

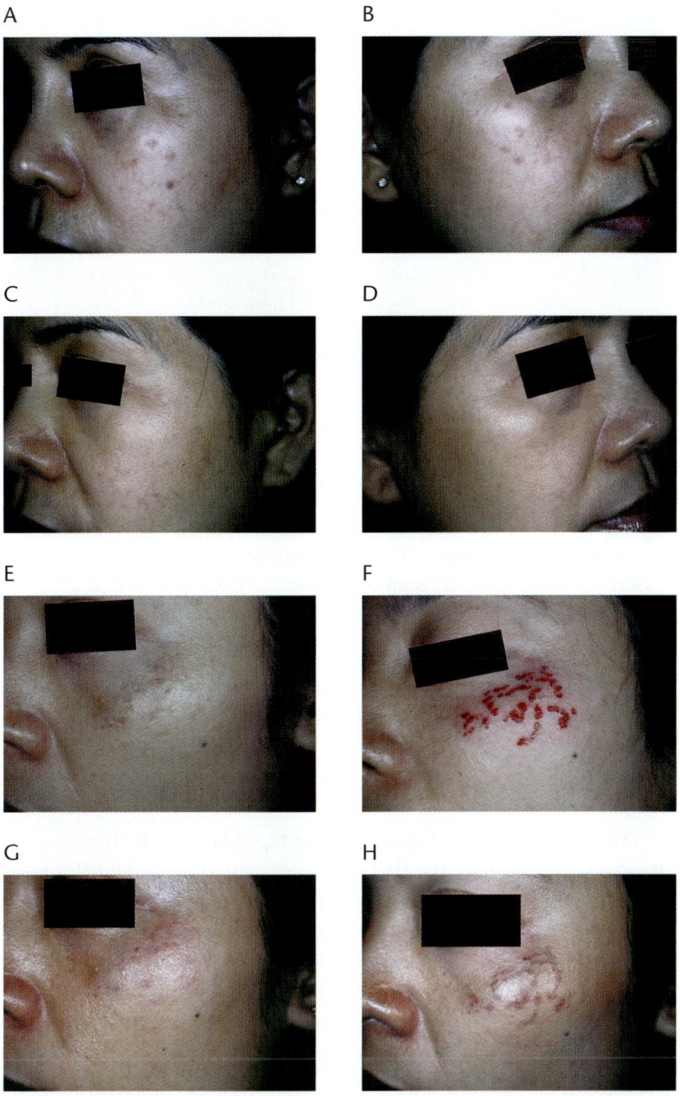

Figure 15.5 (A) A 36-year-old Thai woman with acquired bilateral nevus of Ota-like macules (ABNOMs, Hori's nevus), before treatment (left) (B) Before treatment (right). (C) Complete clearance of pigmented lesions after four 1064-nm QS Nd: YAG laser treatments at an average fluence of 7 J/cm^2 using a 3-mm spot size (left). (D) After four treatment sessions (right). (E) ABNOMs in another Thai woman with skin phototype IV, before treatment with 1064-nm QS Nd: YAG laser. (F) Immediately after laser treatment. Note the presence of pinpoint bleeding following fast-resolving ash-white tissue response. (G) One week following laser treatment. (H) Postinflammatory hyperpigmentation (PIH) occurred on day 14 postoperatively. This condition resolved with the use of topical hydroquinone for 1–2 months.

the low-fluence CO_2 (10,600 nm, CW) laser,[52] and intense pulsed light (IPL).[53] All of these lasers and light sources carry a small risk of depigmentation, hypopigmentation and hyperpigmentation. However, when treating darkly pigmented skin, pulsed lasers with appropriate energy density provide a more selective destruction with a lower incidence of hyperpigmentation and scarring as compared to continuous wave lasers.[54] The nonspecific injury to adjacent normal skin caused from CW lasers may result in 'laser tanning', which has been hypothesized to result from feedback inhibition of melanogenesis, stimulation of tyrosinase activity and/or release of intracellular or extracellular melanocyte-stimulating factors.[55] This phenomenon is independent of postinflammatory hyperpigmentation which constitutes another effect of the nonspecific damage caused from CW laser energy.

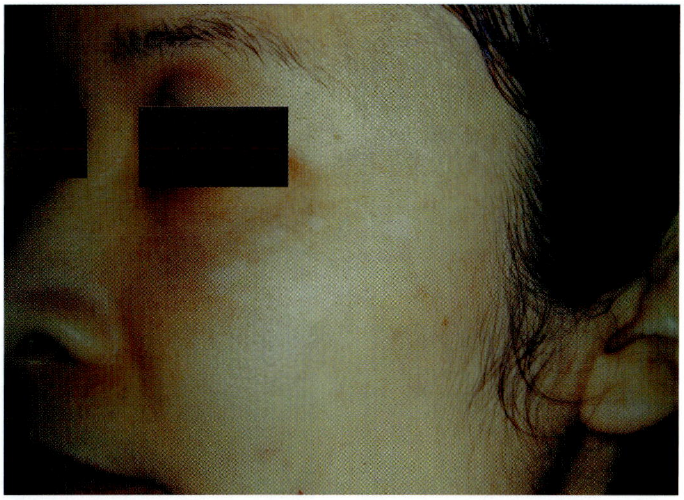

Figure 15.6 Hypopigmentation secondary to the Q-switched ruby laser treatment for Hori's nevus in a 30-year old Thai woman using a fluence of 6 J/cm^2 with a 5-mm spot size. (Courtesy C. Vibhagool, Bangkok, Thailand.)

Lentigines

Lentigines are a common sign of photoaging in Asians. This epidermal pigmented lesion has shown excellent response to Q-switched (QS)[46] and long-pulsed Nd: YAG (532 nm) laser,[56] Q-switched ruby laser (QSRL) (694 nm),[48,50] Q-switched alexandrite (QS alex) (755 nm)[51] and low-fluence carbon dioxide (CO_2 laser).[52] Our experience in treating Asian patients showed that the pulsed dye (510 nm) laser, QS Nd: YAG laser (532 nm, 5–10 ns) laser, QSRL and QS alex laser provided excellent results, usually with a single treatment (Fig. 15.7).

The clinical endpoint is defined as the lowest fluence that can achieve immediate whitening (Fig. 15.8, see video 1). This parameter is about 2.0–2.5 J/cm^2 for the 532-nm QS Nd: YAG laser (10 ns, 3-mm spot diameter)[46], and about 7.0 J/cm^2 for the QS alex (100 ns pulse width, 3-mm spot diameter).[51] For the long-pulsed 532 nm ND:YAG laser the clinical endpoint, defined as a slate gray appearance, is usually about 3.2 J/cm^2 (2–50 ms pulse width, 2-mm spot diameter).[56]

Recent studies on the use of IPL sources for skin rejuvenation[57] and for the treatment of facial freckles in Asians[53] have demonstrated satisfactory outcome on facial pigmentation. Negishi et al[57] addressed the use of the IPL device with integrated contact cooling for skin rejuvenation in Asian patients. A series of five or more treatments performed at 3- to 4-week intervals was given, using double-pulsing mode with a 560-nm cutoff filter and fluence of 23–27 J/cm^2. For patients with skin type III, the first and second pulse widths were set at 2.8 and 6.0 ms, respectively, at pulse intervals of 20 ms, whereas patients with skin types IV–V, the first and second pulse widths

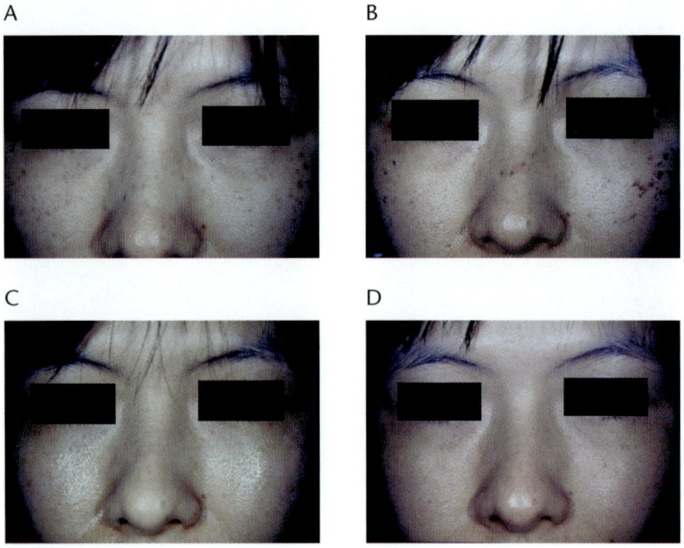

Figure 15.7 (A) Lentigines in a 30-year-old Thai-Chinese woman, before treatment. (B) Five days after one treatment with a 532-nm Q-switched Nd:YAG laser at a fluence of 2.0 J/cm^2 using a 3-mm spot size. Scabs developed on the laser-treated skin. (C) One week after treatment. The laser-treated areas were initially hypopigmented after the scabs resolved. (D) One month after treatment. The hypopigmentation spontaneously disappeared.

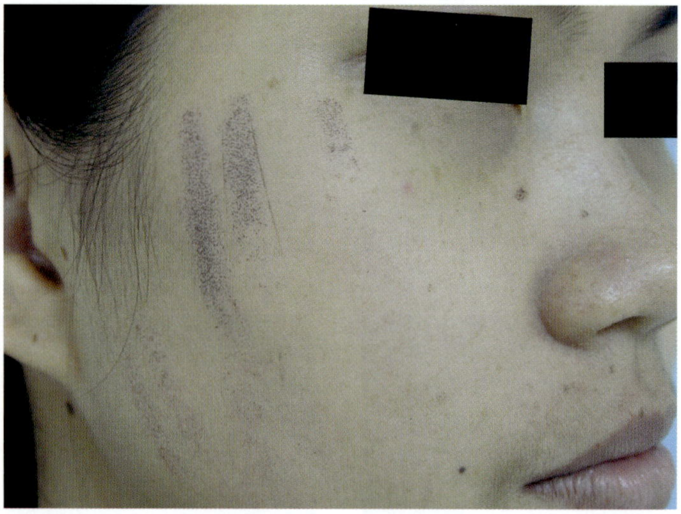

Figure 15.9 Barlike scabs in a 28-year-old Thai woman with skin phototype III, 1 day after a full-face photorejuvenation with intense pulsed light equipped with an active skin cooling system delivered through a 560-nm cutoff filter using a fluence of 22 J/cm^2 by double pulsing (the first and second pulse widths were set at 3.2 and 6.0 milliseconds, respectively at pulse interval of 20 milliseconds). A chilled, colorless ultrasonic gel was applied directly to the filter surface prior to application to the skin.

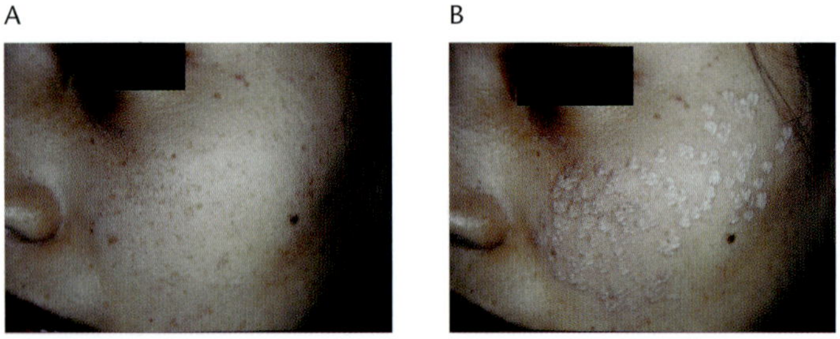

Figure 15.8 (A) A 21-year-old Thai woman with multiple lentigines on her cheek, before treatment. (B) An ash-white tissue response immediately after a treatment with a 532-nm QS Nd:YAG laser at a fluence of 2.0 J/cm^2 using a 3-mm spot size.

were adjusted to 3.2 and 6.0, respectively, at the same pulse interval. Greater than 60% improvement in pigmentation was noted in 81% of the 73 patients. Minor and transitory erythema with burning sensation was reported in 2.7% of those patients.

In our experience with Asian patients with skin types III–V, a longer-wavelength cutoff filter (590- or 640-nm) was used to minimize epidermal injury. A more conservative parameter using a longer pulse width, lower fluence and proper epidermal cooling is recommended. The most common adverse complication was epidermal damage resulting in rectangular scale-crusts, matching the footprint of the IPL crystal, which came off in 1–2 weeks, followed by a rectangular hypopigmentation that spontaneously resolved in 4–16 weeks (Fig. 15.9). Of interest is that we found much lower incidence of postinflammatory hyperpigmentation, compared with that of pigment-specific lasers.

When treating Asian patients, transient hyper- or hypopigmentation are the most common adverse effects of these pigment specific lasers. However, the QSRL can cause long-term or permanent hypopigmentation, especially in dark-pigmented Asians (see Fig. 15.6). The QS Nd:YAG laser is associated with purpura and more erythema, secondary to its increased absorption by oxyhemoglobin. A low fluence CO_2 laser has been successfully used to remove lentigines in fair-skinned patients without posttreatment hyper- and hypopigmentation.[52] In contrast, when treating lentigines in Chinese and Thai patients with dark complexion using the high energy, pulsed CO_2 laser, transient posttreatment hyperpigmentation was the most common adverse sequelae noted in as much as 50% of the patients.

Café-Au-Lait Macules (CALMs)

Alster and Williams[44] successfully treated a boy with type V skin presented with a CALM, with six 510-nm short pulsed dye laser treatment at an energy fluence of 2.5 J/cm^2, at 2-month intervals. Hypopigmentation or textural changes did not occur. No lesion recurrence was noted at a 2-year follow-up period.

Treatment of café-au-lait macules with a copper vapor (511 nm) laser also provided favorable results in Thai patients (skin type V).[45] With a mean follow-up period of 22 months after one treatment, nine of 16 (60%) patients achieved 90–100% clearance, whereas the remainder of the 16 improved 40–80%. Repigmentation to normal skin color was complete within 1–2 months with slight hyperpigmentation at the periphery of the treated area, which responded favorably to topical hydroquinone. Transient hypopigmentation recovery after 2–3 months was observed in most cases. A hypertrophic scar developed in one of the 16 patients in the study. In essence, CALMs variably respond to laser treatments and may recur within a few weeks and up to years after complete clearance. Retreatment often results in rapid clearing.[54] Studies on treatment of CALMs with lasers in white[58,59] and Asian[47,50] populations demonstrated a similar variable degree of repigmentation following a long-term follow-up period of up to 50%. This variable behavior of treated lesions implies a subset of lesions with unique biologic behavior.

Mixed Epidermal and Dermal Pigmented Lesions

Postinflammatory Hyperpigmentation and Melasma

Mixed epidermal and dermal lesions such as post inflammatory hyperpigmentation or melasma respond variably and unpredictably to Q-switched lasers[60–62] and intense pulsed light.[63,64] It is possible that not all pigment-producing structures are affected following a single irradiation. Therefore, residing melanocytes may cause additional pigmentation in patients tending to post-lesional hyperpigmentation or melasma. In addition, melasma tends to recur, often fairly soon, without ongoing topical bleaching medications. In our current practice, sunscreen use is mandatory.

The use of resurfacing lasers alone[65,66] or combined with a pigment-specific laser[67,68] have shown favorable results in the treatment of melasma. However, postinflammatory hyperpigmentation (PIH) commonly develops and can last for 3–6 months. This temporary worsening of the pigmentation may result from an inflammatory dermal reaction that stimulates the activity of melanocytes in the melasma-irradiated skin. Our own experience has found that PIH occurs in nearly 100% of the patients with skin type III and IV who underwent CO_2 laser resurfacing for treatment of melasma. Segmental hypopigmentation or pseudohypopigmentation is another common complication that develops when only the melasma area is resurfaced (Fig. 15.10). Pseudohypopigmentation, the situation in which the resurfaced area has a relatively light skin color, is similar in color to the pigmentation of non-sun-exposed skin but contrasts distinctively with the more darkly pigmented photodamaged adjacent skin.

The etiology of melasma remains unknown. The idea behind such an aggressive approach is that melasma may be caused by an abnormal epidermis, not abnormal melanocytes. This idea is supported by a finding from a recent study showing that keratinocytes play a role in regulating distribution patterns of recipient melanosomes.[69] Taking into consideration expense and the risk of adverse effects, the use laser resurfacing alone or combined techniques should be preserved for those refractory melasma that do not respond to conventional treatments.

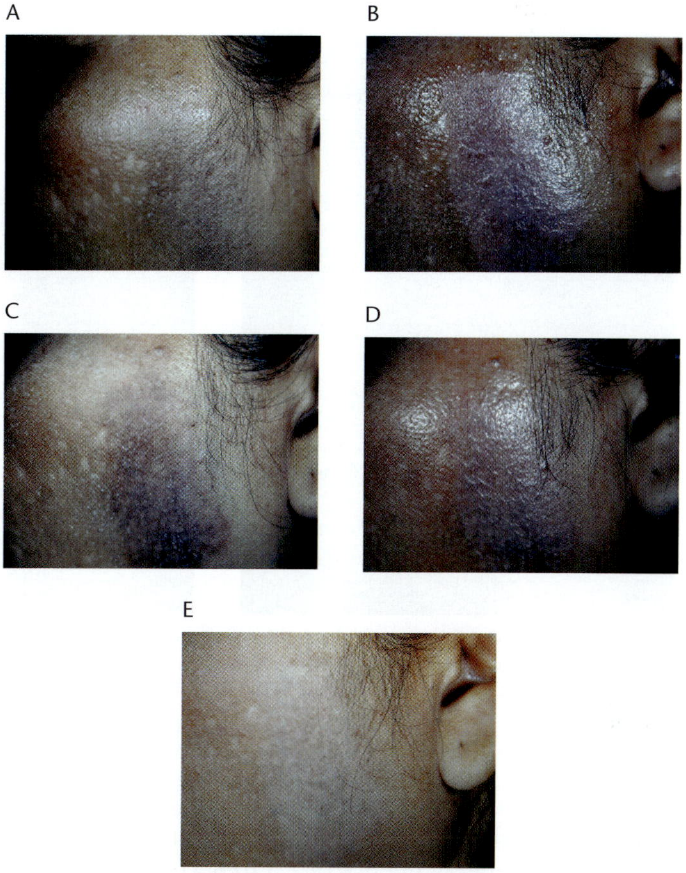

Figure 15.10 (A) A 55-year-old Thai woman with melasma, before treatment. (B) Erythema was noted 1 week after two-pass CO_2 laser resurfacing. (C) Post inflammatory hyperpigmentation developed 4 weeks after treatment. (D) Again 4 weeks after treated with hydroquinone 4% cream twice daily, hyperpigmentation had faded. (E) Pseudohypopigmentation without recurrence of melasma on the resurfaced area 4 years after treatment. She received no further topical bleaching agent but used only a SPF 30, broad-spectrum sunscreen.

Dermal Pigmented Lesions

Nevus of Ota

Nevus of Ota, a dendritic melanocytosis of the papillary and upper reticular dermis involving the eye and surrounding skin innervated by the first and second branches of the trigeminal nerve, is a cosmetic problem commonly found in Asians but is also seen in blacks and whites. An incidence of 0.6% has been noted in the Japanese.[70] Malignant degeneration has occasionally been reported.[71,72] Studies in fair- and dark-skinned populations have demonstrated that red (Q-switched ruby),[73–75] near infrared (Q-switched alexandrite),[76–78] and Q-switched Nd:YAG[79,80] lasers are very useful for treating nevus of Ota with fading over several months following each treatment session.

The 'threshold' radiant exposure response defined as immediate whitening of pigmented lesions after short pulse laser exposure is a useful clinical end point with any Q-switched laser because the whitening correlates directly with melanosome rupture and pigment cell injury. Geronemus[73] treated nevus of Ota in 15 patients of skin phototype II to V with a Q-switched ruby laser and noted that

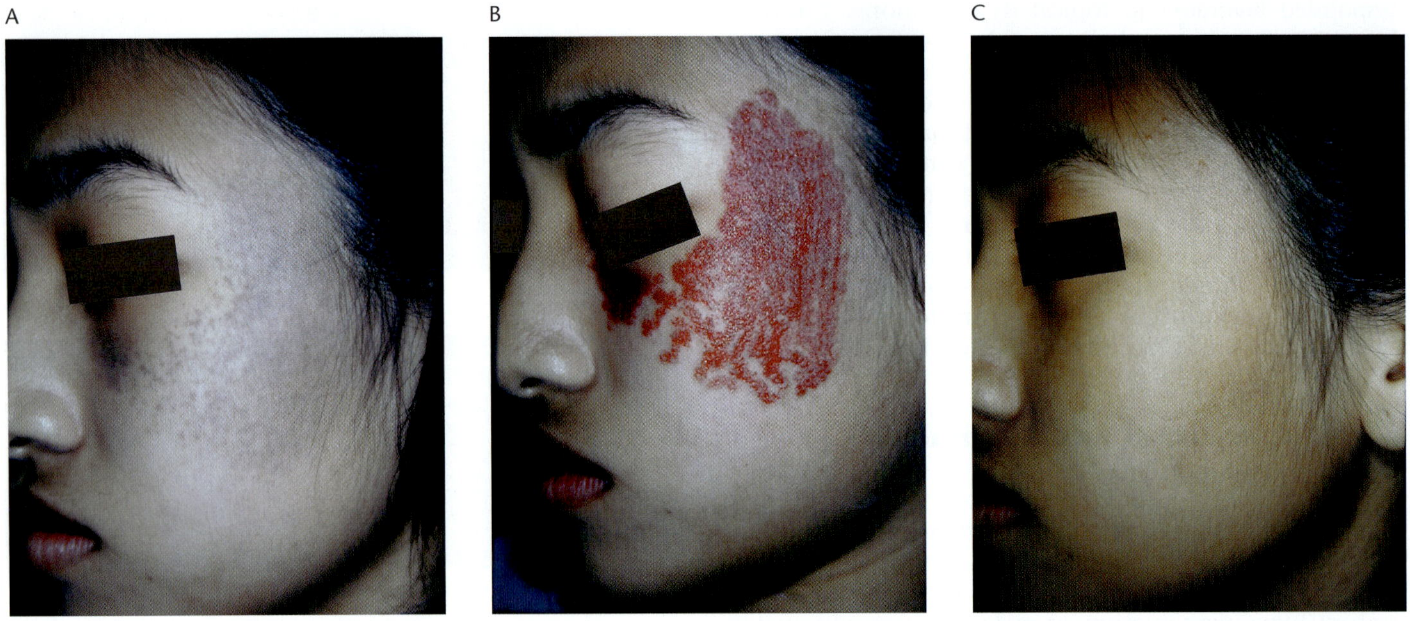

Figure 15.11 (A) A 16-year-old Thai girl with a nevus of Ota, before treatment. (B) Pinpoint bleeding was demonstrated after disappearance of the immediate whitening of the pigmented lesion following a 1064-nm QS Nd:YAG laser treatment using a fluence of 7 J/cm^2 through a 3-mm spot size. (C) 6 months after the fourth treatment. Slight hypopigmentation was noted on the laser treated skin.

this threshold response was based on the patients' skin phototype. Asian patients (skin types IV–V) required slightly lower energy fluence of 7.5 to 8.5 J/cm^2 to achieve immediate whitening compared with white and Hispanic patients (skin type II to IV) (8.5 to 10 J/cm^2).

When treating nevus of Ota with Q-switched lasers, lightening of the lesion is noted after the first session with additional clinical improvement noted after every session. Multiple, sequential treatments appear to increase the response rate and may be required for complete clearing of the lesion (Fig. 15.11, see video 2). The response of nevus of Ota to Q-switched laser treatment also appears to depend on the color of the lesion. The maximum response rate is found in the brown color, and gradually decreases in the brown–violet, violet–blue and blue–green colors, respectively. In average, brown lesions can be cleared by three laser treatments, brown–violet lesions by four sessions, violet–blue lesions can be eliminated after five sessions, and blue–green lesions require at least six treatment sessions for complete clearance.[81]

Studies comparing the use of QS alex and QS Nd:YAG lasers showed that most patients more easily tolerated the former.[79] However, the QS Nd:YAG laser was found to be more effective than the QS alex in the lightening of nevus of Ota after three or more laser treatment sessions.[80] In terms of adverse effects, hypopigmentation is the most common adverse effect after treatment with QS lasers[82] and can be permanent, especially among those treated with QSRL.[83] Transient hyperpigmentation can be found especially after the first treatment session. The incidence of textural changes and scarring are minimal.

Recurrence of original pigmentation could occur after complete laser-induced clearing. The rate of recurrence is estimated to be 0.6–1.2%.[83] Laser treatment of nevus of Ota in children demonstrated a better response and a lower risk of adverse effects than in adults.[84] Early treatment, leading to complete clearance before school, may mean avoiding the childhood psychological trauma associated with the cosmetic disfigurement of the birthmark. This advantage must now be weighed against the risk of recurrence and the stress and cost associated with multiple sessions of laser treatment.

In our current practice, patients are treated with a 1064-nm QS Nd:YAG laser every 6–8 weeks. In a review of 98 patients 1 to 4 years postoperatively, we found that longer duration between treatments provides a decrease in the total number of treatments necessary over time (unpublished data, 2004). We encourage the parents and/or the patients to start the treatment as early as possible. Parents and patients are advised of the risks of complications, including hyperpigmentation and hypopigmentation, and are informed of the chance of recurrence after complete eradication. Ocular involvement including elevated intraocular pressure with or without glaucoma occurred in 10.3% of the patients; as a result, ophthalmologic assessment is necessary.[85]

Acquired Bilateral Nevus of Ota-like Macules (ABNOMs, Hori's Nevus)

Acquired bilateral nevus of Ota-like macules (ABNOMs, Hori's nevus) is a common condition that affects about 0.8% of the population with a marked female preponderance (a male:female ratio of 1:6).[86] Clinically, ABNOMs present as speckles or confluent blue-brown or slate gray pigmentation that usually affects the bilateral malar areas. Other involved sites include the temples, the root of the nose, the alae nasi, the eyelids and the forehead. Unlike in nevus of Ota, the pigmentation in ABNOMs occurs in a symmetric bilateral distribution, has a late onset in adulthood, and does not involve mucosa. Histologically, lesions of ABNOMs demonstrate diffuse upper dermal melanocytosis and differ from nevus of Ota, in which dermal melanocytes occur not only in the upper dermis but also in the deep reticular dermis.

Pigment-specific lasers, including QSRL,[87,88] QS alex,[89] and QS Nd:YAG[90–92] lasers have been proven effective in the treatment of ABNOMs. The treatment responses have been noted to be less effective than those of the nevus of Ota, and multiple sequential treatments are also required to achieve the desired improvement (see Fig. 15.5 and video 3). A total treatment of two to five sessions is usually required for complete clearance of the lesions. The treatment interval is controversial. Some groups[87,89] retreat the patients as soon as the wounds have healed, usually within 2–4 weeks. The rational for early retreatment is to treat prior and to prevent epithelial repigmentation so that more laser energy can reach the dermal target. However, a greater rate of complications, especially persistent hypopigmentation, can occur. Polnikorn et al[91] and our group[88] usually retreat the patients every 8–12 weeks, depending on the clearance of postinflammatory hyperpigmentation. In fact, we noted the benefit of delayed treatment as significant lightening can sometimes be seen many months after the initial treatment session.

Postinflammatory hyperpigmentation (PIH) is more common than that of nevus of Ota, occurring in 50–73% of Asian patients (see Fig. 15.5).[91] The benefit of using topical bleaching agents to prevent or to treat PIH in ABNOMS is also controversial. A previous study noted PIH in 73% of the 66 patients who underwent the treatment with a QS Nd:YAG laser despite the use of topical hydroquinone,[91] whereas another series of 70 patients who developed PIH following the laser treatment responded readily to topical hydroquinone within a few days to weeks of application.[90] In our experience, there is little beneficial effect in using topical bleaching agents preoperatively to decrease the rate of PIH. PIH usually persists for 2–3 months even with prompt postoperative treatment with hypopigmenting topical medications, sun avoidance and a broad-spectrum sunscreen with a SPF of at least 30.

As red (Q-switched ruby) and near-infrared (Q-switched alexandrite and Q-switched Nd:YAG) wavelengths can be selectively absorbed by dermal pigment, the use of these lasers in the treatment of other melanocytic processes with dermal involvement, including nevus of Ito,[54] Becker's nevus,[93] nevus spilus,[94] blue nevus[95] and congenital melanocytic nevus,[96–99] may be effective. The café-au-lait background of nevus spilus and Becker's nevus frequently recurs after treatment.[54] The short pulse width and low energy fluence of these Q-switched lasers are probably not able to damage clusters or nests of nevomelanocytic components. The development of dermal-pigment targeting lasers[100–102] and intense pulsed light systems[103] with long pulse widths shows encouraging results on the treatment of these pigmented lesions.

As described previously, multiple, sequential treatments are typically required for desired cosmetic results of the dermal pigmented lesions. Attempts to accelerate treatment response of dermal pigmentation have been employed including the use of multiple lasers on the same treatment session[88,104,105] and the application of bleaching agents prior to laser treatment.[106]

Epidermal ablation with a resurfacing laser may enhance the effectiveness of the laser for removing dermal pigmentation by eliminating competing epidermal melanin and melanocytes, and removing the epidermis itself, thereby reducing a scattering of the beam and physically placing it closer to the dermal target. Thus, a higher delivered energy fluence will impact on the target-dermal melanin.

To improve the response rate of treating dermal pigmented lesions, we developed a technique using a combination of scanned CO_2 and Q-switched ruby laser (QSRL) to treat ABNOMs in a series of 13 Thai women. A significantly higher percentage of clearing was noted on the sides treated with a combination of CO_2 and Q-switched ruby lasers, compared with those treated with Q-switched ruby laser alone (Fig. 15.12).[88] By combining laser resurfacing and QSRL, a retrospective study in Korean patients with nevus of Ota and congenital nevus showed that the treatment period had been reduced by 2–3 months, and the number of treatments had been reduced two- to threefold.[105] However, the use of this combined laser technique to nonfacial areas is yet to be fully evaluated. The risk of delayed healing time and adverse effects may be higher because of the decreased vascularity and the sparse adnexal structures relative to the face.

Elimination of epidermal melanin by using topical bleaching agents has also been used to pretreat the skin 6–8 weeks prior to QSRL for acquired dermal melanosis (ADM) in Japanese patients. This combined therapy appeared to treat ADM consistently with a low occurrence rate of PIH and lessen the number of laser treatment sessions.[106]

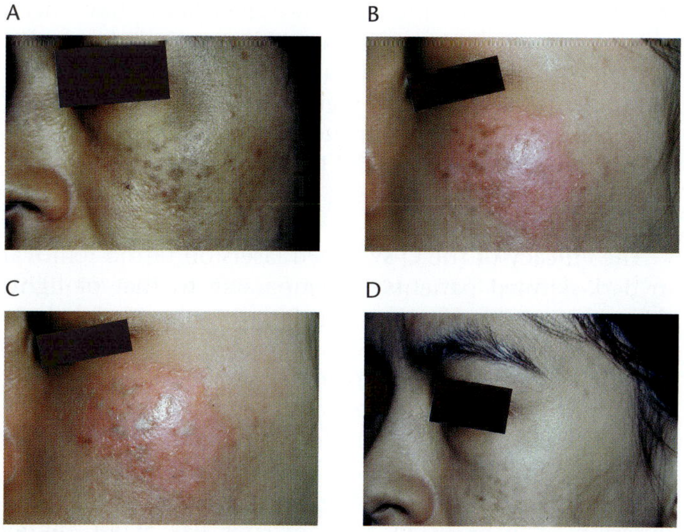

Figure 15.12 (A) ABNOMs in a 40-year-old Thai woman, before treatment. (B) just after epidermal ablation with carbon-dioxide laser. (C) immediately after Q-switched ruby laser irradiation on dermal pigmented lesions. (D) 4 months after a combined laser treatment. (From Manuskiatti W, Sivayathorn A J Am Acad Dermatol 2003; 48:586.)

Nevomelanocytic Nevi

The treatment of congenital and acquired melanocytic nevi with laser irradiation is a very controversial issue. This concern has already been discussed in detail (see Chapter 3). In Asian populations, melanocytic nevi are common and are often removed for cosmetic and superstitious concerns. The normal-mode ruby laser (NMRL) alone,[43,100,101] or together with QSRL or QS alex, have been employed to remove melanocytic nevi in Asians with good cosmetic results following multiple treatment sessions.[107–109]

In spite of clinical improvement, complete histologic clearance can not be achieved. Long-term histologic follow-up of congenital melanocytic nevi after NMRL treatment demonstrated that the subtle microscopic scar about 1 mm thick was required to mask the underlying residual pigmentation for good cosmetic results. The long-term follow-up for at least 8 years showed no histologic or clinical evidence of the development of malignant change in the laser irradiated areas.[101] A NMRL appears to provide a more effective clearing on the basis that a longer pulse duration induces more melanocytic destruction to the clusters of nevus cells, and hence better clears pigmentation.[97,100]

In our current practice, a CO_2 laser is commonly used to vaporize benign melanocytic nevi with promising outcomes and low risk of side effects (see also ablative laser system). Importantly for Asians, laser treatment to remove melanocytic nevi is avoided if there is any risk of melanoma, including previous history or family history of melanoma, and clinical evidence of atypia. Although melanoma is uncommon in Asians, laser for the removal of nevomelanocytic nevus should be avoided if the lesion is located in the acral area which is a common region of melanoma in Asian populations.

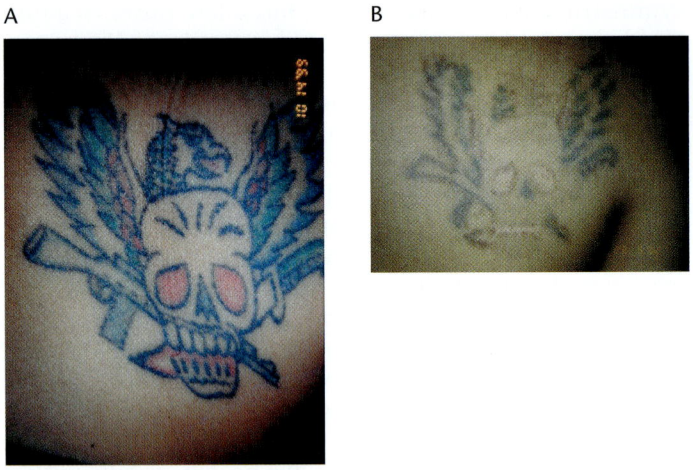

Figure 15.13 (A) Multicolored professional tattoo on the shoulder of a 20-year-old Thai woman, before treatment. (B) Four months after the last treatment with the QS Nd:YAG laser. The dark blue and green inks received eight 1064-nm laser treatments, whereas the red ink got two 532-nm laser treatments. The green ink was incompletely eliminated. Hypertrophic scars developed on the previous red-ink portions.

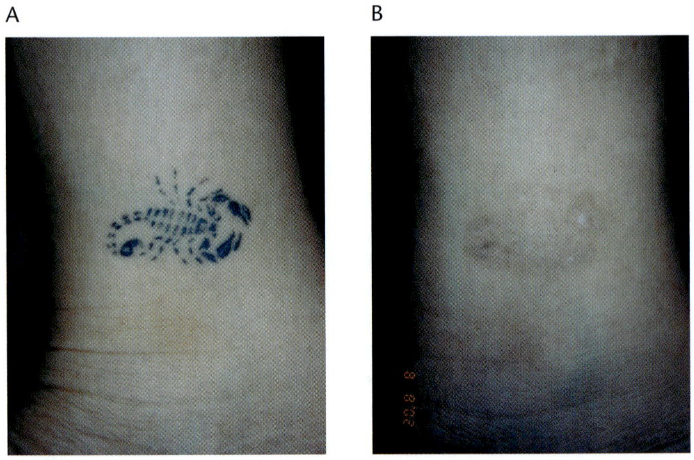

Figure 15.14 (A) A professional tattoo with blue ink on the ankle of a 18-year old Thai woman, before. (B) Persistence of skin dyspigmentation, 12 weeks after five 1064-nm QS Nd:YAG laser treatments.

Tattoo Removal

In fair-skinned individuals, Q-switched lasers have been proven effective in removing pigmented lesions and tattoos with minimal risk of adverse sequelae.[110–113] Laser tattoo removal in darkly pigmented patients has often been presumed to have a greater risk of complication such as hypertrophic scar (Fig. 15.13) and keloid formation, and pigmentary alterations (Fig. 15.14), as compared with fair-skinned patients.

The efficacy of the Q-switched lasers on tattoo removal in dark-skinned patients is comparable to that of light-skinned patients. Studies on tattoo removal in dark-complexioned patients (skin phototypes III–VI) with Q-switched lasers have shown favorable results without scarring or significant permanent pigment changes.[114–120]

Grevelink et al[116] determined the efficacy and side effects of Q-switched lasers on a small series of skin phototypes V and VI patients. A QSRL at 694 nm, with a pulse duration of 20 ns using a 5-mm spot size at an energy fluence ranging from 4.5 to $6.0 J/cm^2$, and a QS Nd:YAG laser at 1064 nm, with a pulse duration of 10 ns using a 3-mm spot size at an energy fluence ranging from 4.5 to $7.3 J/cm^2$, were used to treat four of five patients presented with charcoal-injected tattoos on the face or neck, and one of five patients with a multi-colored tattoo on the mid-chest region. Two of five patients (40%) cleared by more than 90% after six treatments. Lesions of the other three patients were 50% and 60% cleared after four to eight treatments, respectively. A similar study on laser treatment of tattoos in skin phototype VI patients using a QS Nd:YAG laser demonstrated that after three to four treatments at 8-week intervals, eight of 15 (53%) tattoos were 75%–95% cleared, five of 15 (33%) were 50% cleared, and two of 15 (13%) were only 25% cleared.[117] Compared to a study on light-skinned patients using a QS Nd:YAG laser for tattoo removal,[115] 77% of patients' lesions cleared by more than 75% in four treatments, and in 28% of patients lesions cleared by more than 95% in four treatments. The Q-switched alexandrite (755 nm, 100 ns) laser has also been proven effective in removal of various traumatic tattoos in Asian (skin phototypes III to V)[119, 120] and Spanish (skin phototypes III to IV)[121] skin.

Multiple treatments are necessary. On average, 8 to 12 sessions may be required, with a minimum of 6–8 weeks between treatments with longer durations acceptable. Amateur tattoos require a fewer number of treatments than professional tattoos. There is rarely 100% clearing. Most tattoos clear to a point of being cosmetically acceptable.

When treating patients with dark skin types, pigmentary changes are the most common encountered side effect. Scarring can occur but is very rare when appropriate laser energy (the energy that produces nonexplosive effects on the skin) is selected.[116–121] However, transient textural alterations associated with the healing response can occur during multiple treatments. The lack of clinical scarring noted with Q-switched lasers, even when epidermal damage is noted, is most likely due to the lack of thermal injury to collagen, as evidenced by the absence of histologic fibrosis in areas treated multiple times with both the QSRL[114] and QS Nd:YAG laser.[115]

Transient pigmentary changes including hypopigmentation and hyperpigmentation, have been noted in the early healing phase but are commonly resolved in 6–8 weeks. As with treatment of all other pigmented lesions in pigmented races, the incidence of hypopigmentation appears to be a wavelength-dependent phenomenon; the shorter the wavelength, the greater the incidence of hypopigmentation. The incidence of hyperpigmentation is comparable between QSRL and QS Nd:YAG laser, which is mostly transient, and has been reported only in darker-skinned patients (skin phototypes II–V).[114,115] A dose–response study on the treatment of tattoos by QSRL noted hypopigmentation at all doses greater than 1.5 J/cm^2. This persistent hypopigmentation was apparent in four of ten tattoos followed-up 1 year after treatment.[114] In contrast, hyperpigmentation was seen in only one of 13 skin phototype V patients. The QSRL treatment typically results in blistering at the dermoepidermal junction (see Fig. 15.4),[55] transient hypopigmentation and, less frequently, hyperpigmentation.[122]

As previously noted by others,[114–117] we found that when treating tattoos in Asian patients, the QSRL commonly causes hypopigmentation, whereas the QS Nd:YAG laser at appropriate fluences has a very low incidence of hypopigmentation. At the wavelength of 1064 nm, the QS Nd:YAG laser light penetrates deeper and therefore might provide less injury to the unintentionally targeted melanosomes.[123] We therefore agree with the recommendation of others[110,116] that the longer wavelength (1064 nm) QS Nd:YAG laser is preferable to the QSRL and QS alex in the treatment of deeper dermal and blue/black tattoo pigments in dark-skinned patients.

Clinical Technique

Patient Selection

- Patients with lesions amenable to pigment-specific laser treatment (see Chapter 3).
- Patients who understand treatment protocol and risks.
- Patients with realistic expectations of treatment.
- Patients who will comply with advised postoperative skin care and follow-up.
- Patients with suntanned skin should be avoided.
- Patients with lesions that are less responsive or show unpredictability to pigment-specific lasers such as post inflammatory hyperpigmentation or melasma should be avoided.

Choice of Lasers

- Epidermal pigmented lesions: 532-nm QS Nd:YAG laser, QS ruby laser
- Dermal pigmented lesions: QS alexandrite and 1064-nm QS Nd:YAG lasers (avoid using QS ruby laser)
- Tattoo removal:
  - 532-nm QS Nd:YAG laser is perfect for red and yellow colors
  - 1064-nm QS Nd:YAG laser is best for blue and black colors
  - QS alex or ruby laser is best for green color
  - QS alex and QS ruby lasers have a higher risk of pigmentary alterations, especially permanent hypopigmentation.

Actual Technique

Treatment techniques are similar to those used in white-skinned subjects. However, the treatment parameters are generally more conservative with lower fluences. There is no foolproof parameter. Using conservative treatment fluences are extremely important when treating dark-skinned individuals:

- Test sites may be performed at inconspicuous sites in the area to be treated.
- When treating Asian skin, additional treatment sessions may be necessary, or additional time between each treatment may be needed to allow for ample dermal healing and epidermal repigmentation.
- Sun avoidance and the use of topical sun barriers are important to minimize the appearance of PIH.
- If lesions become inflamed after treatment, we recommend the use of topical corticosteroid creams to decrease the inflammatory reaction which will also minimize the appearance of PIH.

CLINICAL PEARLS

- Pre- and posttreatment epidermal cooling can minimize the nonspecific injury to the epidermis, and reduce postoperative pain and swelling.
- As mentioned previously, treatment response of dermal pigmentation may be increased by using multiple lasers during the same treatment session.
- Application of bleaching agents prior to laser treatment to decrease epidermal pigmentation may maximize the treatment responses and minimize the risks of adverse effects.
- Treatment on scar prone areas including presternal, and deltoid areas, and back should be performed with the lowest fluence possible.

Ablative Laser Systems

The use of pulsed or scanned carbon dioxide (CO_2) lasers for ablative skin resurfacing (ASR) is a popular procedure for similar indications as dermabrasion and chemical peels. The same principles of thermal confinement used in selective photothermolysis also apply to minimizing the thermal injury from CO_2 laser vaporization. In fair-skinned patients, the most common indication for skin resurfacing is to treat chronic sun damage, wrinkles, traumatic scars, surgical scars, and acne scars. In contrast, in non-white-skinned patients, acne scarring is the most common indication for this procedure. Unfortunately, the risk of prolonged or permanent dyspigmentation, especially PIH, parallels the degree of the patient's constitutive skin color or natural pigmentation: the darker the color, the greater the potential.[124–126]

PIH, the most common complication seen following cutaneous CO_2 laser resurfacing in nonwhite patients, usually develops around the first month after treatment and becomes most significant within four months (Fig. 15.15). Various studies reported an incidence of 25% and 68% on laser resurfacing in Hispanic (skin phototypes II–V)[127] and other races with skin type IV patients,[128] respectively. This compared to a 3–7% incidence of PIH that occurs after CO_2 laser resurfacing in Caucasian patients with skin phototypes I–IV. In fact, in these studies, PIH occurred only in patients with skin phototypes III and IV.[124,125]

In contrast to PIH, which typically resolves with time, the incidence of postlaser hypopigmentation is higher with a longer follow-up period. Incidence of hypopigmentation of 16–19% was noted in an 8-month follow-up[124] and our 2-year follow-up studies,[125] respectively. This may sometimes be a near permanent complication. The incidence of hypertrophic scars and keloids is comparable to that of fair-skinned patients. These later complications are usually the results of poor technique, postoperative infection or other intrinsic patient factors.

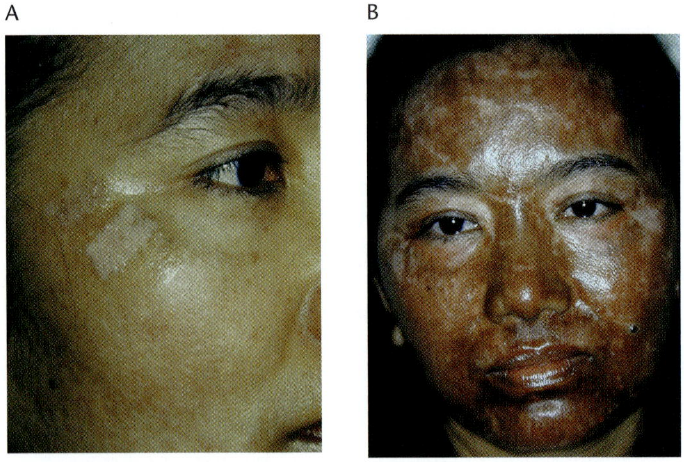

Figure 15.15 (A) Melasma in a 40-year-old skin phototype IV Thai woman, 2 weeks after test area of resurfacing with an ultrapulsed CO_2 laser. No PIH was seen. (B) Marked PIH developed 2 weeks after 2 passes of full-face CO_2 laser resurfacing. (Reprinted from Sriprachaya-Anunt S, Marchell NL et al: Lasers in Surgery and Medicine 30:90 © 2002. Reprinted with permission from Wiley-Liss, Inc., a subsidiary of John Wiley & Sons, Inc.)

We believe that the advantage of preoperative treatment is not so much in the prevention of PIH but in determining what medications a patient is sensitive to so they can be avoided in the postoperative period. A study by West and Alster[129] noted no significant difference in the incidence of post-CO_2 laser resurfacing hyperpigmentation between subjects who received pretreatment with either topical glycolic acid cream or combination tretinoin/hydroquinone creams and those who received no pretreatment regimen. In our experience, PIH may occur in spite of careful preoperative treatment. Similarly, a recent retrospective study on facial resurfacing in patients with skin type IV indicated no correlation of pretreatment or types of laser used to incidence of PIH.[128] However, PIH appears to respond to appropriate treatment once it has developed.

The application of broad-spectrum sunscreen and sun avoidance postoperatively is also beneficial in minimizing hyperpigmentation. The advantage of sun avoidance has been demonstrated in a study showing that preoperative and postoperative ultraviolet exposure on laser-treated skin resulted in a poor cosmetic appearance including, textural change and hyperpigmentation.[130]

In 1996, the introduction of the Er:YAG laser represented an alternative to the pulsed and scanned CO_2 resurfacing lasers. Er:YAG laser resurfacing requires a shorter, less painful recovery time, and causes fewer long-term adverse effects. In general, the recovery time and the incidence of adverse sequelae are proportional to the extent of tissue injury, including the total anatomic depth of necrosis, ablation and residual thermal damage.[131–133] A layer of residual thermal damage observed after a typical Er:YAG laser resurfacing procedure is less than 50 μm versus the 80–200 μm typically observed after multiple passes of pulsed CO_2 laser resurfacing.[132] Therefore, one advantage of the Er:YAG laser over the CO_2 laser is that it appears to offer a higher margin of safety when treating patients with darker complexions (skin phototypes III and higher), because the resultant inflammatory reaction caused by less extensive thermal trauma stimulates less melanocytic activity.[65]

The incidence of transient PIH following CO_2 laser resurfacing ranges from 3% to 7% for all patients and nearly 68% among those with skin type IV and higher. Although postoperative hyperpigmentation and prolonged erythema seem to occur at roughly the same rate among patients with darker skin after Er:YAG laser resurfacing, it is often less severe and resolves more quickly compared with the CO_2 laser treatment.[66] The Er:YAG laser, therefore, appears to be better suited for resurfacing of Asian skin.

With equal energy fluence and number of passes, the Er:YAG laser produces less total depth of tissue necrosis and hence less effective treatment of deeper wrinkles. The greater immediate collagen contraction effect and the hemostasis property provided by the CO_2 laser are the advantages of this laser resurfacing system over the Er:YAG laser. To combine the beneficial properties of these two systems, Goldman and Manuskiatti[134] successfully developed a resurfacing technique using the combined CO_2 and Er:YAG lasers in the same treatment session. By using the Er:YAG laser to vaporize a portion of the layer of residual thermal damage created by the CO_2 laser, one can achieve a better cosmetic response and get faster healing time, shorter duration of postlaser erythema and hence a decreased incidence of adverse sequelae. The favorable result of this combined treatment method has also been confirmed by a study on treatment of atrophic scars in Korean patients with skin phototypes IV–V.[135]

The single pass CO_2 or Er:YAG laser has been performed to help lessen the risks associated with multiple-pass CO_2, Er:YAG, or combination techniques of laser skin resurfacing.[136–138] Ruiz-Esparza & Gomez[136] evaluated 15 Hispanic patients after one-pass CO_2 laser resurfacing for a follow-up period of 18 months. All patients were re-epithelialized by 7 days, and continued clinical improvement of rhytides was observed throughout the length of the study. However, the near universal incidence of transient postoperative hyperpigmentation has still been observed in patients with dark skin tones after CO_2 single-pass resurfacing. Although superficial resurfacing is definitely safer than deep resurfacing, it is no guarantee that postinflammatory hyperpigmentation will not develop.

Studies on CO_2[139–141], Er:YAG,[65,66,142,143] and combined CO_2 and Er:YAG[135,144] lasers resurfacing on Asian skin (skin phototypes III–V) have shown that these procedures can be performed effectively and safely when proper preoperative and postoperative management is implemented. Pre- and postoperative treatment regimens are necessary to achieve optimum results and may reduce the incidence of postinflammatory hyperpigmentation.[145,146] In addition to topical retinoic acid applied each night, patients with skin phototypes III–VI are given topical preparations of hydroquinone, kojic acid, azelaic acid or vitamin C to be used for 1–2 months preoperatively. Although an arbitrary minimum preoperative treatment time of 2 weeks is often recommended, achieving maximum benefit requires months of use. These agents are restarted as soon as possible postoperatively (2–4 weeks). Reinstitution of these topical preparations too early may induce inflammation on the newly regenerated treated skin and should be avoided.[147]

Inflammation in the postoperative period is a normal cascade of the healing process, but prolonged inflammation is not. Clinically, persistent postoperative erythema is a strong predictor of delayed-onset hyperpigmentation. Consequently, inflammation in darker-skinned individuals leads to hyperpigmentation and, if long-standing, may cause permanent depigmentation. All factors producing tissue inflammation during the healing process should be minimized or eliminated in these patients to reduce the risk of pigmentary alterations. Mechanical trauma (excessive rubbing of the tissue between laser passes), irritants, chemical causing an allergic contact dermatitis, and prolonging inflammation from an opportunistic infection should be prevented.

In brief, ASR is effective in treating photodamaged skin and acne scars in Asian patients with skin phototypes III–V. However, it must be performed with great caution, together with proper preoperative and postoperative treatment regimens, and sun avoidance. A test patch may be used when considering skin resurfacing for this group of patients. However, this is not always a reliable predictor of postoperative complications.

Another application which the CO_2 laser offers definite advantage is in vaporization of selected epidermal and dermal lesions. In current practice, we successfully use the CO_2 laser to remove epidermal growth such as seborrheic keratosis or verruca vulgaris, and benign nevomelanocytic nevi with low risk of adverse complications. The definite advantages of the CO_2 laser for removal of these lesions are the extreme precision in depth of ablation, leaving minimal damage to adjacent normal tissue, the speed of the treatment of multiple lesions, and near-bloodless field.

Clinical use of the CO_2 laser for this application must be guided by close attention to laser–tissue interaction during the procedure. The lesion is vaporized layer by layer by moving a defocused beam of the CW CO_2 laser with a spot size of 3-mm at 3–5 watts across the surface of the lesion at a speed of approximately 1 cm per second. With thick lesions, several passes over the same area are necessary. A cotton-tipped applicator soaked in saline solution is used to remove vaporized debris after each pass. The endpoint of treatment is when the lesion is removed or a chamois yellow appearance is seen (Fig. 15.16). Treat-

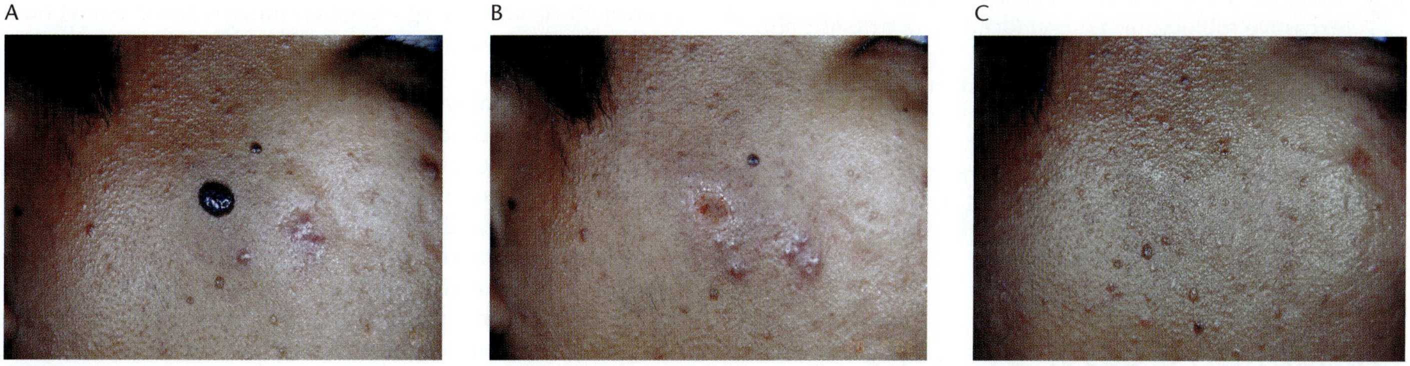

Figure 15.16 (A) A compound melanocytic nevus in a Thai man with skin photoype IV, before treatment. (B) Immediately after ablation with three passes of CW CO_2 laser with a 3-mm spot size at 3 W. (C) Two years after one treatment with CO_2 laser vaporization.

ment can be repeated at 4- to 6-week intervals if the lesion recurs.

When laser is used to remove nevomelanocytic nevi, several concerns should be judged. First, for Asians, the use of this technique should be avoided if there is any other risk of melanoma, including previous history or family history of melanoma, and clinical evidence of atypia. Second, for Caucasians, such use should be considered as the last resort of treatment. Third, recurrence of the treated nevus may show histologically atypical cells, termed pseudomelanoma.[148]

Clinical Technique

Patient Selection

- Patients with conditions amenable to skin resurfacing treatment such as photoaged facial skin, acne scars, etc. (see Chapter 7).
- Patients who understand treatment protocol and risks.
- Patients with realistic expectations of the laser resurfacing procedure.
- Patients who will comply with advised postoperative skin care and follow-up.
- Patients with skin phototype VI skin should be avoided.
- For patients with no well-demarcated area between the photodamaged skin and non- or less-photodamaged skin, it will be difficult to blend treated to untreated areas.

Choice of Laser

- Er:YAG laser.

Actual Technique

- Treatment techniques are similar to those used in white-skinned individuals. However, the treatment parameters are generally more conservative.
- Avoid excessive rubbing of the tissue between laser passes.
- If an Er:YAG laser is not available only single pass treatment using the CO_2 laser is advised.

CLINICAL PEARLS

- Pre- and postoperative treatment regimens are necessary to achieve optimum results and to reduce the incidence of PIH.
- All factors producing tissue inflammation during the healing process, including mechanical trauma (excessive rubbing of the resurfaced skin), irritants, and chemicals causing an allergic contact dermatitis, and prolonged inflammation from an opportunistic infection, should be minimized or eliminated.
- Use of topical corticosteroid ointment from days 3–10 at night will help to decrease inflammation. We recommend using an ointment that does not contain any stabilizing agents. We use fluocinolone ointment in petrolatum.

Nonablative Laser Systems

Despite the favorable results seen with CO_2 and Er:YAG laser resurfacing, the enthusiasm for these systems has been limited by the prolonged recovery time, long-lasting erythema and dyspigmentation (hypo- and hyperpigmentation). To overcome the problems associated with ASR procedures, so-called nonablative dermal remodeling (NDR) techniques have recently emerged.[149–152] The NDR technique involves the use of a cooling device to protect the epidermis, and in doing so allows high-energy laser light in the infrared spectrum to be delivered to the dermis. NDR induces formation of new dermal collagen by creation of a dermal wound without disruption to the epidermis and repairs of tissue defects related to photoaging.

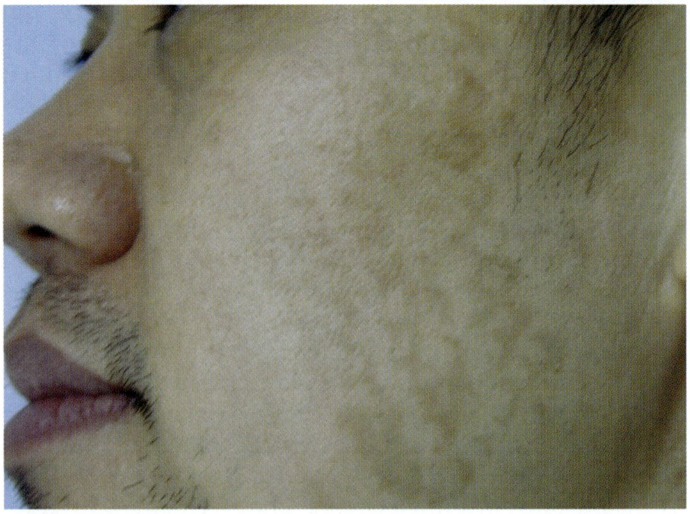

Figure 15.17 Persistence of hyperpigmented rings 3 months after a treatment with the 1450-nm diode laser equipped with a tetrafluoroethane spray cooling for nonablative dermal remodeling in a 36-year-old Thai man with skin phototype IV.

Although NDR lasers are not yet capable of results comparable with those of ablative laser systems, they have been shown to improve mild to moderate atrophic scars, rhytides, pigmentation and telangiectasia. These NDR devices may be particularly suited to Asian patients because photoaging in Asians tends to have fewer wrinkles but higher pigmentary disorders.[3] Furthermore, the adverse effects that are associated with ablative laser resurfacing systems, such as erythema and postinflammatory hyperpigmentation, are particularly common and problematic in Asian skin.

Recent studies on the use of these nonablative laser devices in Asian patients have confirmed the effectiveness and safety of this technique.[57,153,154] One important concern is the occurrence of prolonged or permanent skin dyspigmentation that might result from an improper parameter selection of a cryogen cooling device coupled to some nonablative laser systems or from an improper positioning of the laser handpiece, not from the thermal injury of laser light (Fig. 15.17).[155,156] Unfortunately, Asians with a higher epidermal melanin content are known to have an associated higher risk of PIH after skin injury which, although transient, is associated with a significant degree of patient dissatisfaction. Another more important concern is laser-induced hypopigmentation that can be prolonged or even permanent, particularly in pigmented Asian skin.

Nonablative laser skin remodeling is a relatively new treatment modality and, although several systems have been shown to effect improvement in rhytides and atrophic scars, they still do not approximate the improvement typically seen after ablative laser treatment. In addition, none of these light systems has yet emerged as being clearly superior. With further technological refinement, coupled with the relative lack of recovery and minimal morbidity, nonablative dermal remodeling will continue to be a popular treatment of choice for patients seeking noninvasive rejuvenation.

While the absence of epidermal damage in NDR techniques significantly decreases the severity and duration of the treatment-related adverse effects, the major drawback of these techniques is their limited efficacy. More recently, a new concept of cutaneous remodeling called fractional photothermolysis (FP) has been introduced.[157] Skin restoration by FP is achieved by applying an array of microscopic treatment zones (MTZ) of thermal injury to the skin. Clinical efficacy of FP for skin resurfacing depends in part on the dermal remodeling phase of MTZ repair. MTZs are intentionally designed to be small so that they can hardly be seen, if at all, without magnification. The macroscopic treatment effect of FP is characterized by both the arrangement and shape of these MTZs within the skin.

Thirty subjects with photoaged skin on the periorbital area receiving four FP treatments over a period of two to three weeks were evaluated in a clinical pilot study. Linear tissue shrinkage of 2.1% was measured 3 months after the last treatment. The wrinkle score improved 18% at 3 months after the last treatment. These results are similar to those reported with the CoolTouch and SmoothBeam lasers. Reepithelialization was fast (within 1 day) due to a small wound and short migratory paths for keratinocytes. Side effects following FP treatment included mild but noticeable erythema that persisted in the Caucasian population studied for up to 1 week. No evidence of hyper- or hypopigmentation was noted in any of these Caucasion subjects. Further clinical studies are ongoing to refine the optimum parameters and to explore the use of FP in dark-skinned individuals.

Clinical Technique

Patient Selection

- Ideal candidates for nonablative skin remodeling lasers are similar to those described in White individuals with a mild degree of photoaged skin or scars. (see Chapter 8).

Choice of Laser

- Most nonablative laser systems work equally well with Asian skin (see Chapter 8).

Actual Technique

- Treatment techniques are similar to those used in white-skinned subjects except that more conservative treatment fluences are used on Asian skin.
- When the IPL is used, the following should be applied to minimize epidermal injury:
  - use a longer-wavelength cutoff filter (590- or 640-nm)
  - apply proper epidermal cooling with an active cooling device and/or cooled gel
  - use lower fluence over bony prominence and periorbital skin
  - increase the delay time between the pulses to 30–40 ms (10–15 ms is the usual delay time when used on Caucasian skin)
- When a laser with a cryogen spray cooling is used:
  - avoid using an aggressive spray duration. An improper parameter selection of a cryogen cooling device coupled to some nonablative laser systems or an improper positioning of the laser handpiece may lead to skin dyspigmentation.

Laser Hair Removal

The use of laser and pulsed light sources for hair removal is increasing because the treatment is relatively safe and effective in removing large areas of unwanted hair. Although it has been well documented that the ideal patients for this procedure are individuals with dark hair and fair skin, unwanted or excess hair is also a cosmetic concern for the Asian population.

Most of the available laser and light source systems with wavelengths in the red and near-infrared regions have been designed to cause selective photothermal damage to pigmented hair follicles. Improved efficacy is accomplished by the high specificity and selectivity contributed by the accurate selection of an appropriate wavelength and pulse duration to maximize follicular damage and minimize unwanted injury to the epidermis. To target the follicle, these lasers and light sources count on either endogenous melanin within the follicular epithelium or hair shaft.

When using light to target these endogenous chromophores, there is also risk of epidermal injury when laser light penetrates the target. Melanin-containing structures, including melanocytes, melanosome-containing keratinocytes, or nevus cells may also be thermally injured when irradiated by red and near-infrared lasers. Consequently, epidermal injury due to the absorption of laser energy by epidermal melanin may occur to a certain degree during the laser impacts.

Most clinical studies on the efficacy of laser and intense-pulsed light systems in removing unwanted hair have been performed in fair-skinned individuals because it was theoretically postulated that a larger amount of epidermal melanin in Asian and nonwhite individuals may result in a decrease in clinical efficacy and cause an increase in the incidence of adverse effects, especially pigmentary and textural changes, and scarring. Currently, several reports on these light-assisted hair removal systems performed on darker skinned persons have shown comparable results to those of fair-skinned persons with a slightly increased risk of complications.[158–165] In addition, laser and pulsed light hair-removal systems have been proven to be safe and effective in treating some follicular-related disorders in dark-skinned patients including pseudofolliculitis barbae[166] and trichostasis spinulosa.[167]

It is difficult to compare the efficacy and side effects of light-assisted hair removal systems because of the variability in the treated anatomical sites and in the types, pulse widths, spot sizes and repetition rates of the light sources used, as well as differences in the treatment regimens. All laser and intense pulsed light systems have been shown to temporarily remove hair. Reduction of hair growth occurs in all hair colors and at all fluences. Blonde-, red- or white-haired individuals are unlikely to experience permanent hair reduction, but hair loss in these persons can be sustained by treatment at approximately 3-month intervals.[168] We note a similar response rate when treating Asian and black patients. Studies have demonstrated that in the ideal patients with fair skin and dark hair, the possibility for long-term hair reduction after a single treatment is approximately 80%.

A critical threshold fluence is needed to obtain efficacy. This fluence is determined as the lowest fluence that can produce perifollicular swelling and erythema appearing a few minutes after laser irradiation. When treating individuals with skin types IV–VI, we carefully select the endpoint that produces slight perifollicular swelling and erythema. If there is a sign of acute epidermal injury including whitening, blistering, or Nikolsky's sign (forced epidermal separation), the fluence should be reduced. Generally, the treatment fluence should be at 75% of the Nikolsky's threshold fluence.[168] A 2-year follow-up study on the efficacy of normal-mode ruby laser hair removal noted that sites treated with highest fluence (60 J/cm^2) obtained the greatest hair reduction (64.3%).[169]

Epidermal injury is an anticipated consequence when treating a darker complexioned patient. Whereas the goal of light-assisted hair removal is permanent follicular destruction, there is also a risk of epidermal damage during hair removal, especially in nonwhite individuals whose epidermis contains larger amounts of melanin. When treating this group of patients, in order to be able to use the highest tolerable fluence to achieve better hair reduction while minimizing epidermal damage, three important considerations, including wavelength and pulse duration of the light sources, and epidermal cooling methods, should be taken into account.

The first important determinant is wavelength of the light source. The ideal laser wavelength for hair removal is a wavelength that is preferentially absorbed by melanin but not by surrounding tissue. Lasers emitting longer wavelengths have the advantage of being able to penetrate deeper into the dermis, minimizing the possibility of absorptive interference by epidermal melanin.[170] Color contrast between epidermis and the hair shaft (and bulb) is crucial in determining the optimal wavelength. For high contrast (dark hair, light skin), the low range of the wavelength (650–700 nm) can be employed without risking serious injury to the epidermis (and subsequent hypo- and hyperpigmentation). For lighter hair and darker skin, the longer wavelength (800 nm and greater) should be applied.[171]

Studies in patients with skin phototype III–V have shown that temporary hair reduction after treatment with normal-mode ruby (694 nm) laser,[158,172,173] long-pulsed ruby (694 nm) laser,[174,175] long-pulsed alexandrite (755 nm) laser,[159,164,176] diode (810 and 940 nm) laser,[163,177] long-pulsed Nd:YAG (1064 nm) laser[160,161] and intense pulsed light[178,179] hair removal systems was comparable to that of skin phototype I–II. However, the incidence of undesirable side effects occurred more often compared with those noted in fair-skinned patients. Although most of these side effects, including treatment pain, erythema, edema, blistering, crusting, erosion, purpura, folliculitis and pigmentary changes (hypopigmentation and hyperpigmentation), were transient and self-limited, pigmentary alterations usually required longer to resolve (>3 months). In addition, these side effects often occurred on tanned skin, in patients with skin phototype III and higher, or on sites treated with excessively high energy fluences.

In our experience, when treating subjects with dark skin, the ruby laser system is associated with higher adverse effects, especially transient hyper- and hypopigmentation. This results from the melanin interface of the 694-nm light pulse of the ruby lasers. However, the alexandrite, diode, and long-pulsed 1064-nm Nd:YAG lasers, and the intense pulsed light source operating at longer wavelength and longer pulse widths, have been used to treat these patients safely when combined with cooling devices. Permanent pigmentary alterations (Fig. 15.18) and scarring were rare except in cases of overaggressive treatment or postoperative infection. A retrospective study of the side effects of laser-assisted hair removal treatment in skin phototypes I–V found that the Q-switched Nd:YAG laser resulted in the fewest side effects, whereas the long-pulsed ruby and the long-pulsed alexandrite lasers produced equivalent adverse effects but greater efficacy than that of Q-switched 1064-nm Nd:YAG laser.[174] Long-term adverse sequelae and scarring were not observed with any of the laser systems under study. Although it caused the fewest side effects, the 1064-nm Q-switched Nd:YAG system does not typically

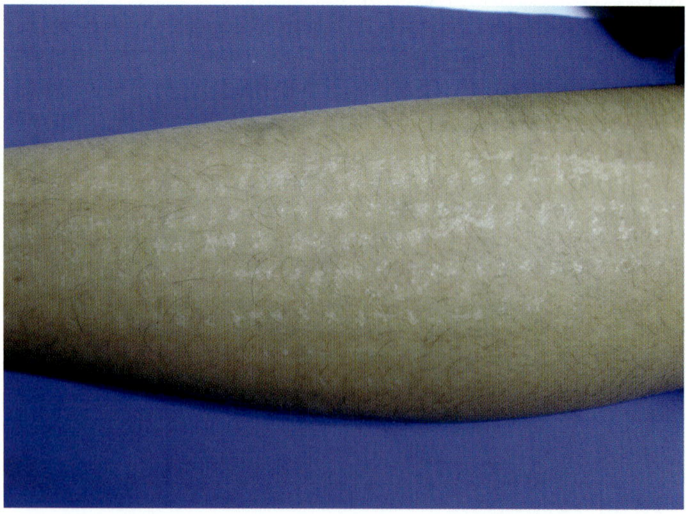

Figure 15.18 A 24-year-old Thai woman with skin phototype IV developed persistent postinflammatory hypopigmentation 8 months after one treatment with an 800-nm diode laser hair removal with a sapphire contact-cooling tip using a fluence of 30 J/cm^2 with a 30-ms pulse duration.

produce long-term hair reduction because of its very low absorption by melanin and the use of low treatment energy fluences.[180]

As anticipated, lasers with longer wavelengths produce fewer adverse effects. A hair removal study comparing the efficacy and complications of diode and long-pulsed 1064-nm Nd:YAG lasers in Chinese patients with skin phototypes IV or V noted no pigmentary or textural changes after treatment, even in skin phototype V patients.[161] However, the disadvantage of the long-pulsed Nd:YAG hair removal system is that the absorption of this laser light by melanin is decreased compared with that of the ruby laser, such that absorption by the competing chromophore, oxyhemoglobin, is substantially increased.

Pulse duration of hair removal light sources is the second important parameter for effective hair removal without epidermal injury.[181] A pulse duration of approximately 10 to 50 ms will damage hair follicles with less epidermal injury. However, caution should be exercised when using very long pulse widths to treat dense hair areas because of thermal conduction between closely adjacent hair follicles.

The last important factor to be considered is epidermal cooling. Integrating surface cooling into the delivery configuration is one way to protect the epidermis and consequently prevents or minimizes the adverse sequelae of the procedure. Presently, five types of cooling are used in conjunction with lasers and intense pulsed light systems: (1) passive cooling with a chilled aqueous gel; (2) active cooling with water encased in a glass housing; (3) active conductive cooling with water encased in a sapphire window; (4) dynamic active cooling with a cryogenic spray; and (5) air cooling with a refrigerated air stream. These cooling configurations can provide epidermal preservation compared with no surface cooling.[171,182]

In conclusion, in Asian patients, laser- and pulsed light hair removal systems provide comparable clinical efficacy to that of white-skinned patients. Treatment parameters must be individualized for each patient and with each device. When performing this procedure in darker skin individuals, a range of test fluences should be performed in an inconspicuous area prior to performing complete treatment. A delay of at least 1 hour should elapse prior to evaluation of test spots. In our practice, darker skin tones can be safely and effectively treated using a light source with a longer wavelength than that of a ruby laser (>694 nm) with a pulse duration of 10 to 50 ms and an adequate cooling device.

Clinical Technique

Patient Selection

- Ideal candidates for laser hair removal are similar to those described in white-skinned individuals (see Chapter 5).

Choice of Laser

- Most laser and light sources for hair removal coupled with an epidermal cooling device work fine with Asian skin except the long-pulsed ruby laser.

Actual Technique

- Treatment techniques are similar to those used in white-skinned subjects. Using conservative treatment fluences that create slight perifollicular edema and erythema is extremely important when treating Asian skin.
- Always start with the lowest effective fluence on the first treatment session.
- Test spots should be done as an aid to select safe and efficient parameters. These test spots should be performed on similar sun-exposed skin as the treatment site. Waiting for the laser–tissue response is imperative. Tissue response after laser irradiation on dark skin may take longer to evaluate (30 minutes to 1 hour) in comparison with white skin.
- Avoid doing pulse stacking or more than 15% of overlapping.
- When a laser with a contact-cooling hand piece is used, the contact surface should be wiped clean every five to ten pulses to remove debris.

CLINICAL PEARLS

Application of bleaching agents such as hydroquinone or azelaic acid on the treatment site 2–4 weeks prior to laser treatment may allow the use of a higher fluence and minimize the risk of adverse effects following laser hair removal.

Prevention and Management of Complications

Various attempts have been made to reduce the occurrence of side effects of laser treatment in Asian skin. These include sun avoidance, the use of preoperative and postoperative treatment regimens and proper techniques for epidermal cooling.

Sun Avoidance

UV exposure prior to laser treatment has been shown to interfere with laser treatment by increasing epidermal melanin pigmentation and epidermal thickness leading to a change in the optical property of the skin.[183] UV exposure may also interfere with the posttreatment healing process,[184,185] altering the treatment outcome, and occurrence of side effects. Moreover, laser exposure may influence the carcinogenic potential of UV radiation, which serves as a complete carcinogen, as both tumor initiation and promotion are induced by UV.[186] Nonetheless, results from a recent experimental study conclude that CO_2 laser treatment does not have a carcinogenic potential in itself nor does CO_2 laser treatment influence UV-induced carcinogenesis.[187]

In our practice, several recommendations to minimize the effects of UV light have been suggested. From a practical standpoint, it is not easy to avoid sun exposure when living in tropical countries. Most laser treatments are elective surgeries. Thus, surgery may be postponed during summer months. Topical sunscreens protecting against both UVA and UVB – usually zinc oxide based – should be applied regularly at least 6 weeks prior to the treatment to obtain the optimal outcome.[188] Patients should not visit tanning booths or go sunbathing, although the influence of acquired pigmentation compared with constitutional pigmentation for the development of adverse effects remains unidentified.

Preoperative and Postoperative Treatment Regimen

Although the advantage of preoperative treatment regimens with various topical bleaching agents remains controversial, in current practice we regularly pretreat our patients with a minimal two-week course of topical retinoic acid[189,190] each night, combined with any of the following topical preparations including hydroquinone,[191] kojic acid,[192] azelaic acid,[193] arbutin,[194] licorice[195] or vitamin C.[196] On the postoperative visit, these topical preparations are started as soon as possible (2–4 weeks), depending on the individual healing response. However, we often observe that PIH occurred even with careful preoperative treatment, and this complication resolved spontaneously without using any topical preparations other than a broad-spectrum sunscreen and sun avoidance.

Epidermal Cooling

Selective epidermal cooling during laser surgery provides great benefits, allowing the use of higher fluences, permitting treatment of darker skin tones and decreasing procedure discomfort. For treating pathology that is situated beneath either the epidermis or superficial dermis, it may often be necessary to use higher fluences to deliver sufficient photons to the intended target. This applies especially to laser surgery for Asian patients, in whom higher epidermal levels of melanin effectively decrease the number of photons reaching the dermis. Because scarring is related to the generation of excessive heat, which is greatest at or near the skin surface, methods that cool the superficial compartment of the skin should permit the safe use of higher fluences when necessary and minimize epidermal injury when it occurs (Fig. 15.19). When the epidermis and/or superficial dermis are selectively cooled either immediately before or during laser exposure, the peak temperature reached at these sites is insufficient to cause irreversible thermal damage. However, targets that are situated more deeply and that are, therefore, not cooled are able to reach the thermal threshold necessary for successful treatment.

Lowering the temperature of the skin's surface is therefore a method for selectively controlling the depth at which heat is produced in the skin by lasers or light sources. The effect of epidermal cooling has been shown to enhance clinical efficacy and minimize epidermal damage caused by the laser treatment process.[27,197–199] The

A B

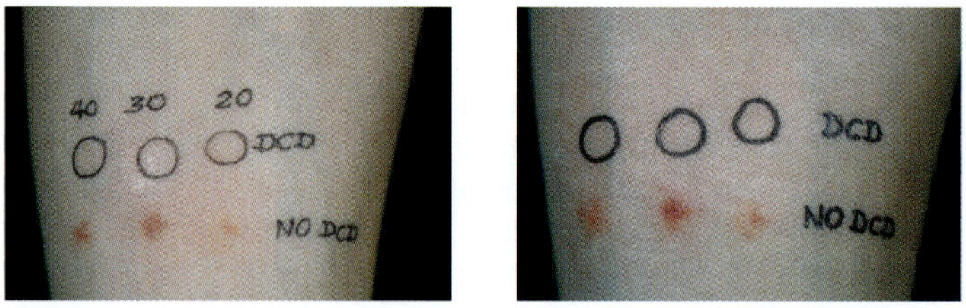

Figure 15.19 (A) Immediate reaction after a 595-nm pulse dye laser irradiation on a skin type IV subject at a fluence of 10 J/cm^2 and pulse duration of 20, 30 and 40 ms, with and without epidermal cooling using dynamic cooling device (DCD). The epidermis was well protected when cooled. (B) 24 hours after laser irradiation.

increased efficacy is a consequence of an increase in the depth of penetration[200] and an allowance of higher energy fluence used.[201]

When not using a dynamic cooling device, the depth to which skin cooling protects the skin from excessive superficial heat injury is largely determined by the temperature and contact time of the handpiece or cryogen with the skin. An appropriate cooling time and technique permit heat extraction from the epidermis before, during and after each laser pulse. Thus epidermal damage/heating can be minimized. In contrast, an overcooled epidermis may cool down the dermal target and result in a decrease in the desired clinical response. The commercial cooling methods/devices include passive cooling with aqueous gel, active cooling with water or refrigerated air and dynamic active cooling with cryogen spray. Most of these cooling devices have been used in conjunction with vascular lasers, intense pulsed light systems and laser hair removal.

In a less technically sophisticated manner, we find that precooling and postcooling the skin with an ice pack or ice cube can also be performed. This method, like water cooling at 0°C with a glass window, will decrease the dermal–epidermal junction temperature, depending on application time. However, because it is done manually, the efficacy of this method may be unpredictable. Studies comparing cooling systems suggest that cryogen spray cooling (CSC) and contact cooling with water encased in a sapphire window provide the most effective/efficient epidermal preservation followed by cold air, water encased in a glass housing and finally cold gel or ice.[171,202]

Conclusions

The majority of laser treatments on Asian skin can be performed effectively. However, this treatment must be approached with caution. Epidermal pigmentation is perhaps the most fundamental limitation because it diminishes laser light reaching the dermis and causes unwanted thermal damage to the epidermis. Thorough patient counseling regarding the risks of cutaneous laser treatment remains an essential part of therapy. Careful preoperative and postoperative treatment programs should be used as well as a prudent selection of types of lasers suited to a patient's treatment purposes. Laser parameters (wavelength, pulse duration, and fluence) can be tailored for specific cutaneous applications to effect maximal target destruction with minimal collateral thermal damage. Epidermal cooling is a useful method to minimize undesired epidermal damage. Finally, when treating an Asian individual with any laser, a conservative approach is the best.

References

1. Berardesca E, Maibach HI. Racial differences in skin pathophysiology. J Am Acad Dermatol 1996;34:667–72.
2. Richards GM, Oresajo CO, Halder RM. Structure and function of ethnic skin and hair. Dermatol Clin 2003; 21:595–600.
3. Chung JH. Photoaging in Asians. Photodermatol Photoimmunol Photomed 2003;19:109–21.
4. Alaluf S, Atkins D, Barrett K, Blount M, Carter N, Heath A. Ethnic variation in melanin content and composition in photoexposed and photoprotected human skin. Pigment Cell Res 2002; 15:112–18.
5. Taylor SC. Skin of color: biology, structure, function, and implications for dermatologic disease. J Am Acad Dermatol 2002; 46:S41–62.
6. McCurdy JA. Cosmetic surgery of the Asian face: Theime Medical; 1990.
7. Astner S, Anderson RR. Skin phototypes 2003. J Invest Dermatol 2004; 122:xxx–xxxi.
8. Lancer HA. Lancer Ethnicity Scale (LES) [letter]. Lasers Surg Med 1998; 22:9.
9. Wolbarsht ML, Urbach F. The Lancer Ethnicity Scale [letter]. Lasers Surg Med 1999; 25:105–6.
10. Goldman MP. Universal classification of skin type. Cosmetic Dermatol 2002; 15:53–7.
11. Tanzi EL, Lupton JR, Alster TS. Lasers in dermatology: four decades of progress. J Am Acad Dermatol 2003; 49:1–31.
12. Anderson RR, Parrish JA. Selective photothermolysis: precise microsurgery by selective absorption of pulsed radiation. Science 1983; 220:524–7.
13. Anderson RR, Parrish JA. The optics of human skin. J Invest Dermatol 1981; 77:13–19.
14. Ashinoff R, Geronemus RG. Treatment of a port-wine stain in a black patient with the pulsed dye laser. J Dermatol Surg Oncol 1992; 18:147–8.
15. Tan OT, Kerschmann R, Parrish JA. The effect of epidermal pigmentation on selective vascular effects of pulsed laser. Lasers Surg Med 1986; 4:365–74.
16. Tong AKF, Tan OT, Boll J, Parrish JA, Murphy GF. Ultrastructure: effect of melanin pigment on target specificity using a pulsed dye laser (577 nm). J Invest Dermatol 1987; 88:747–52.
17. Fitzpatrick RE, Lowe NJ, Goldman MP, Borden H, Behr KL, Ruiz-Esparza J. Flashlamp-pumped pulsed dye laser treatment of port-wine stains. J Dermatol Surg Oncol 1994; 20:743–8.
18. Haedersdal M, Wulf HC. Pigmentation-dependent side effects to copper vapor laser and argon laser treatment. Lasers Surg Med 1995; 16:351–8.
19. Haedersdal M, Wulf HC. Risk assessment of side effects from copper vapor and argon laser treatment: the importance of skin pigmentation. Lasers Surg Med 1997; 20:84–9.
20. Haedersdal M, Gniadecka M, Efsen J, Bech-Thomsen N, Keiding J, Wulf HC. Side effects from the pulsed dye laser: the importance of skin pigmentation and skin redness. Acta Derm Venereol 1998; 78:445–50.
21. Haedersdal M, Wulf HC. Pigmentation dependent, short time skin reactions to copper vapour laser and argon laser treatment. Burns 1994; 20:195–9.
22. Ho WS, Chan HH, Ying SY, Chan PC. Laser treatment of congenital facial port-wine stains: long-term efficacy and complication in Chinese patients. Lasers Surg Med 2002; 30:44–7.
23. Sommer S, Sheehan-Dare RA. Pulsed dye laser treatment of port-wine stains in pigmented skin. J Am Acad Dermatol 2000; 42:667–71.
24. Chan HH, Chan E, Kono T, Ying SY, Wai-Sun H. The use of variable pulse width frequency doubled Nd:YAG 532 nm laser in the treatment of port-wine stain in Chinese patients. Dermatol Surg 2000; 26:657–61.
25. Chang CJ, Kelly KM, Van Gemert MJ, Nelson JS. Comparing the effectiveness of 585-nm vs 595-nm wavelength pulsed dye laser treatment of port wine stains in conjunction with cryogen spray cooling. Lasers Surg Med 2002; 31: 352–8.
26. Greve B, Raulin C. Prospective study of port wine stain treatment with dye laser: comparison of two wavelengths (585 nm vs. 595 nm) and two pulse durations (0.5 milliseconds vs. 20 milliseconds). Lasers Surg Med 2004; 34:168–73.
27. Chang CJ, Nelson JS. Cryogen spray cooling and higher fluence pulsed dye laser treatment improve port-wine stain clearance while minimizing epidermal damage. Dermatol Surg 1999; 25:767–72.
28. Chiu CH, Chan HH, Ho WS, Yeung CK, Nelson JS. Prospective study of pulsed dye laser in conjunction with cryogen spray cooling for treatment of port wine stains in Chinese patients. Dermatol Surg 2003; 29:909–15; discussion 915.
29. Ho WS, Ying SY, Chan PC, Chan HH. Treatment of port wine stains with intense pulsed light: a prospective study. Dermatol Surg 2004; 30:887–91.
30. Dover JS, Arndt KA. New approaches to the treatment of vascular lesions. Lasers Surg Med 2000; 26:158–63.
31. Groot D, Rao J, Johnston P, Nakatsui T. Algorithm for using a long-pulsed Nd:YAG laser in the treatment of deep cutaneous vascular lesions. Dermatol Surg 2003; 29:35–42.
32. Alster TS, Williams CM. Treatment of keloid sternotomy scars with 585 nm flashlamp-pumped pulsed-dye laser. Lancet 1995; 345:1198–200.
33. Goldman MP, Fitzpatrick RE. Laser treatment of scars. Dermatol Surg 1995; 21:685–7.
34. Wittenberg GP, Fabian BG, Bogomilsky JL et al. Prospective, single-blind, randomized, controlled study to assess the efficacy of the 585-nm flashlamp-pumped pulsed-dye laser and silicone gel sheeting in hypertrophic scar treatment. Arch Dermatol 1999; 135:1049–55.
35. Manuskiatti W, Fitzpatrick RE, Goldman MP. Energy density and numbers of treatment affect response of keloidal and hypertrophic sternotomy scars to the 585-nm flashlamp-pumped pulsed-dye laser. J Am Acad Dermatol 2001; 45:557–65.
36. Chan HH, Wong DS, Ho WS, Lam LK, Wei W. The use of pulsed dye laser for the prevention and treatment of hypertrophic scars in Chinese persons. Dermatol Surg 2004; 30:987–94.
37. McDaniel DH, Ash K, Zukowski M. Treatment of stretch marks with the 585-nm flashlamp-pumped pulsed dye laser. Dermatol Surg 1996; 22:332–37.
38. Ash K, Kauver A, Lord J et al. Long term results of treatment of stretch marks with the 585 nm flashlamp-pumped pulsed dye laser, a follow-up study. Lasers Surg Med 1998; 10(suppl):41.

39. Nehal KS, Levine VJ, Ashinoff R. Treatment of mature striae with the pulsed dye laser. Lasers Surg Med 1998; 10 (suppl): 41.
40. Nouri K, Romagosa R, Chartier T, Bowes L, Spencer JM. Comparison of the 585 nm pulse dye laser and the short pulsed CO_2 laser in the treatment of striae distensae in skin types IV and VI. Dermatol Surg 1999; 25:368–70.
41. Polla LL, Margolis RJ, Dover JS et al. Melanosomes are a primary target of Q-switched ruby laser irradiation in guinea pig skin. J Invest Dermatol 1987; 89:281–6.
42. Anderson RR, Margolis RJ, Watanabe S, Flotte T, Hruza GJ, Dover JS. Selective photothermolysis of cutaneous pigmentation by Q-switched Nd:YAG laser pulsed at 1064, 532, and 355 nm. J Invest Dermatol 1989; 93:28–32.
43. Ohshiro T, Maruyama Y. The ruby and argon lasers in the treatment of naevi. Ann Acad Med Singapore 1983; 12:388–95.
44. Alster TS, Williams CM. Café-au-lait macule in type V skin: successful treatment with a 510 nm pulsed dye laser. J Am Acad Dermatol 1995; 33:1042–3.
45. Kunachak S, Kulapraditharom B, Kunachak S, Leelaudomniti P, Leopairut J. Copper vapor laser treatment of café-au-lait macules. Br J Dermatol 1996; 135:964–8.
46. Li YT, Yang KC. Comparison of the frequency-doubled Q-switched Nd : YAG laser and 35% trichloroacetic acid for the treatment of face lentigines. Dermatol Surg 1999; 25:202–4.
47. Suh DH, Han KH, Chung JH. The use of Q-switched Nd : YAG laser in the treatment of superficial pigmented lesions in Koreans. J Dermatolog Treat 2001; 12:91–6.
48. Ashinoff R, Geronemus RG. Q-switched ruby laser treatment of labial lentigos. J Am Acad Dermatol 1992; 27:809–11.
49. Murphy MJ, Huang MY. Q-switched ruby laser treatment of benign pigmented lesions in Chinese skin. Ann Acad Med Singapore 1994; 23:60–6.
50. Shimbashi T, Kamide R, Hashimoto T. Long-term follow-up in treatment of solar lentigo and café-au-lait macules with Q-switched ruby laser. Aesthetic Plast Surg 1997; 21:445–8.
51. Jang KA, Chung EC, Choi JH, Sung KJ, Moon KC, Koh JK. Successful removal of freckles in Asian skin with a Q-switched alexandrite laser. Dermatol Surg 2000; 26:231–4.
52. Dover JS, Smoller BR, Stern RS, Rosen S, Arndt KA. Low-fluence carbon dioxide laser irradiation of lentigines. Arch Dermatol 1988; 124:1219–24.
53. Huang YL, Liao YL, Lee SH, Hong HS. Intense pulsed light for the treatment of facial freckles in Asian skin. Dermatol Surg 2002; 28:1007–12; discussion 1012.
54. Kilmer SL, Goldman MP, Fitzpatrick RE. Treatment of benign pigmented cutaneous lesions. 1 vol. 2nd ed. St Louis: Mosby; 1999.
55. Hruza GJ, Dover JS, Flotte TJ, Goetschkes M, Watanabe S, Anderson RR. Q-switched ruby laser irradiation of normal human skin. Histologic and ultrastructural findings. Arch Dermatol 1991; 127:1799–805.
56. Chan HH, Fung WK, Ying SY, Kono T. An in vivo trial comparing the use of different types of 532 nm Nd : YAG lasers in the treatment of facial lentigines in Oriental patients. Dermatol Surg 2000; 26:743–9.
57. Negishi K, Wakamatsu S, Kushikata N, Tezuka Y, Kotani Y, Shiba K. Full-face photorejuvenation of photodamaged skin by intense pulsed light with integrated contact cooling: initial experiences in Asian patients. Lasers Surg Med 2002; 30:298–305.
58. Taylor CR, Anderson RR. Treatment of benign pigmented epidermal lesions by Q-switched ruby laser. Int J Dermatol 1993; 32:908–12.
59. Grossman MC, Anderson RR, Farinelli WA, Flotte TJ, Grevelink JM. Treatment of café au lait macules with lasers: a clinicopathlogic correlation. Arch Dermatol 1995; 131: 1416–20.
60. Tse Y, Levine VJ, McClain SA, Ashinoff R. The removal of cutaneous pigmented lesions with the Q-switched ruby laser and the Q-switched neodymium:yttrium-aluminum-garnet laser. A comparative study [see comments]. J Dermatol Surg Oncol 1994; 20:795–800.
61. Grekin RC, Shelton RM, Geisse JK, Frieden I. 510-nm pigmented lesion dye laser. Its characteristics and clinical uses. J Dermatol Surg Oncol 1993; 19:380–7.
62. Taylor CR, Anderson RR. Ineffective treatment of refractory melasma and postinflammatory hyperpigmentation by Q-switched ruby laser [see comments]. J Dermatol Surg Oncol 1994; 20:592–7.
63. Negishi K, Kushikata N, Tezuka Y, Takeuchi K, Miyamoto E, Wakamatsu S. Study of the incidence and nature of 'very subtle epidermal melasma' in relation to intense pulsed light treatment. Dermatol Surg 2004; 30:881–6.
64. Wang CC, Hui CY, Sue YM, Wong WR, Hong HS. Intense pulsed light for the treatment of refractory melasma in Asian persons. Dermatol Surg 2004; 30:1196–200.
65. Manaloto RMP, Alster T. Laser resurfacing for refractory melasma. Dermatol Surg 1999; 25:121–3.
66. Polnikorn N, Goldberg DJ, Suwanchinda A, Ng SW. Erbium:YAG laser resurfacing in Asians. Dermatol Surg 1998; 24:1303–7.
67. Nouri K, Bowes L, Chartier T, Romagosa R, Spencer J. Combination treatment of melasma with pulsed CO_2 laser followed by Q-switched alexandrite laser: a pilot study. Dermatol Surg 1999; 25:494–7.
68. Angsuwarangsee S, Polnikorn N. Combined ultrapulse CO_2 laser and Q-switched alexandrite laser compared with Q-switched alexandrite laser alone for refractory melasma: split-face design. Dermatol Surg 2003; 29:59–64.
69. Minwalla L, Zhao Y, Le Poole IC, Wickett RR, Boissy RE. Keratinocytes play a role in regulating distribution patterns of recipient melanosomes in vitro. J Invest Dermatol 2001; 117:341–7.
70. Hidano A, Kajima H, Ikedea S, Mizutani H, Miyasato H, Nimura M. Natural history of nevus of Ota. Arch Dermatol 1967; 95:187–95.
71. Halasa A. Malignant melanoma in a case of bilateral nevus of Ota. Arch Ophthalmol 1970; 84:176–8.
72. Sang DN, Albert SM, Sober AJ. Nevus of Ota with contralateral cerebral melanoma. Arch Ophthalmol 1977; 95:1820–4.
73. Geronemus RG. Q-switched ruby laser therapy of nevus of Ota. Arch Dermatol 1992; 128:1618–22.
74. Taylor CR, Flotte TJ, Gange RW, Anderson RR. Treatment of nevus of Ota by Q-switched ruby laser. J Am Acad Dermatol 1994; 30:743–51.
75. Watanabe S, Takahashi H. Treatment of nevus of Ota with the Q-switched ruby laser. N Engl J Med 1994; 331:1745–50.
76. Alster TS, Williams CM. Treatment of nevus of Ota by the Q-switched alexandrite laser. Dermatol Surg 1995;21: 592–6.
77. Kang W, Lee E, Choi GS. Treatment of Ota's nevus by Q-switched alexandrite laser: therapeutic outcome in relation to clinical and histopathological findings. Eur J Dermatol 1999; 9:639–43.
78. Suh DH, Hwang JH, Lee HS, Youn JI, Kim PM. Clinical features of Ota's naevus in Koreans and its treatment with Q-switched alexandrite laser. Clin Exp Dermatol 2000; 25:269–73.

79. Chan HH, King WW, Chan ES et al. In vivo trial comparing patients' tolerance of Q-switched Alexandrite (QS Alex) and Q-switched neodymium:yttrium-aluminum-garnet (QS Nd: YAG) lasers in the treatment of nevus of Ota. Lasers Surg Med 1999; 24:24–8.
80. Chan HH, Ying SY, Ho WS, Kono T, King WW. An in vivo trial comparing the clinical efficacy and complications of Q-switched 755 nm alexandrite and Q-switched 1064 nm Nd:YAG lasers in the treatment of nevus of Ota. Dermatol Surg 2000; 26:919–22.
81. Ueda S, Isoda M, Imayama S. Response of naevus of Ota to Q-switched ruby laser treatment according to lesion colour. Br J Dermatol 2000; 142:77–83.
82. Chan HH, Leung RS, Ying SY et al. A retrospective analysis of complications in the treatment of nevus of Ota with the Q-switched alexandrite and Q-switched Nd:YAG lasers. Dermatol Surg 2000; 26:1000–6.
83. Kono T, Nozaki M, Chan HH, Mikashima Y. A retrospective study looking at the long-term complications of Q-switched ruby laser in the treatment of nevus of Ota. Lasers Surg Med 2001; 29:156–9.
84. Kono T, Chan HH, Ercocen AR et al. Use of Q-switched ruby laser in the treatment of nevus of Ota in different age groups. Lasers Surg Med 2003; 32:391–5.
85. Teekhasaenee C, Ritch R, Rutnin U, Leelawongs N. Glaucoma in oculodermal melanocytosis. Ophthalmology 1990; 97: 562–70.
86. Sun CC, Lu YC, Lee EF, Nakagawa H. Naevus fusco-caeruleus zygomaticus. Br J Dermatol 1987; 117:545–53.
87. Kunachak S, Leelaudomlipi P, Sirikulchayanonta V. Q-Switched ruby laser therapy of acquired bilateral nevus of Ota-like macules. Dermatol Surg 1999; 25:938–41.
88. Manuskiatti W, Sivayathorn A, Leelaudomlipi P, Fitzpatrick RE. Treatment of acquired bilateral nevus of Ota-like macules (Hori's nevus) using a combination of scanned carbon dioxide laser followed by Q-switched ruby laser. J Am Acad Dermatol 2003; 48:584–91.
89. Lam AY, Wong DS, Lam LK, Ho WS, Chan HH. A retrospective study on the efficacy and complications of Q-switched alexandrite laser in the treatment of acquired bilateral nevus of Ota-like macules. Dermatol Surg 2001; 27:937–41; discussion 941–2.
90. Kunachak S, Leelaudomlipi P. Q-switched Nd:YAG laser treatment for acquired bilateral nevus of Ota-like maculae: a long-term follow-up. Lasers Surg Med 2000; 26:376–9.
91. Polnikorn N, Tanrattanakorn S, Goldberg DJ. Treatment of Hori's nevus with the Q-switched Nd:YAG laser. Dermatol Surg 2000; 26:477–80.
92. Suh DH, Han KH, Chung JH. Clinical use of the Q-switched Nd:YAG laser for the treatment of acquired bilateral nevus of Ota-like macules (ABNOMs) in Koreans. J Dermatolog Treat 2001; 12:163–6.
93. Kopera D, Hohenleutner U, Landthaler M. Quality-switched ruby laser treatment of solar lentigines and Becker's nevus: a histopathological and immunohistochemical study. Dermatology 1997; 194:338–43.
94. Grevelink JM, Gonzalez S, Bonoan R, Vibhagool C, Gonzalez E. Treatment of nevus spilus with the Q-switched ruby laser. Dermatol Surg 1997; 23:365–9; discussion 369–70.
95. Milgraum SS, Cohen ME, Auletta MJ. Treatment of blue nevi with the Q-switched ruby laser. J Am Acad Dermatol 1995; 32:307–10.
96. Vibhagool C, Byers HR, Grevelink JM. Treatment of small nevomelanocytic nevi with a Q-switched ruby laser. J Am Acad Dermatol 1997; 36:738–41.
97. Grevelink JM, van Leeuwen RL, Anderson RR, Byers HR. Clinical and histological responses of congenital melanocytic nevi after single treatment with Q-switched lasers. Arch Dermatol 1997; 133:349–53.
98. Nelson JS, Kelly KM. Q-Switched ruby laser treatment of a congenital melanocytic nevus. Dermatol Surg 1999; 25: 274–6.
99. Duke D, Byers HR, Sober AJ, Anderson RR, Grevelink JM. Treatment of benign and atypical nevi with the normal-mode ruby laser and the Q-switched ruby laser: clinical improvement but failure to completely eliminate nevomelanocytes. Arch Dermatol 1999; 135:290–6.
100. Ueda S, Imayama S. Normal-mode ruby laser for treating congenital nevi. Arch Dermatol 1997; 133:355–9.
101. Imayama S, Ueda S. Long- and short-term histological observations of congenital nevi treated with the normal-mode ruby laser. Arch Dermatol 1999; 135:1211–18.
102. Nanni CA, Alster TS. Treatment of a Becker's nevus using a 694-nm long-pulsed ruby laser. Dermatol Surg 1998; 24: 1032–4.
103. Gold MH, Foster TD, Bell MW. Nevus spilus successfully treated with an intense pulsed light source. Dermatol Surg 1999; 25:254–5.
104. Manuskiatti W, Fitzpatrick RE, Goldman MP. Treatment of facial skin using combinations of CO_2, Q-switched alexandrite, flashlamp-pumped pulsed dye, and Er:YAG lasers in the same treatment session. Dermatol Surg 2000; 26:114–20.
105. Park SH, Koo SH, Choi EO. Combined laser therapy for difficult dermal pigmentation: resurfacing and selective photothermolysis. Ann Plast Surg 2001; 47:31–6.
106. Momosawa A, Yoshimura K, Uchida G et al. Combined therapy using Q-switched ruby laser and bleaching treatment with tretinoin and hydroquinone for acquired dermal melanocytosis. Dermatol Surg 2003; 29:1001–7.
107. Kono T, Ercocen AR, Chan HH, Kikuchi Y, Nozaki M. Effectiveness of the normal-mode ruby laser and the combined (normal-mode plus q-switched) ruby laser in the treatment of congenital melanocytic nevi: a comparative study. Ann Plast Surg 2002; 49:476–85.
108. Kono T, Nozaki M, Chan HH, Sasaki K, Kwon SG. Combined use of normal mode and Q-switched ruby lasers in the treatment of congenital melanocytic naevi. Br J Plast Surg 2001; 54:640–3.
109. Kono T, Ercocen AR, Kikuchi Y, Isago T, Honda T, Nozaki M. A giant melanocytic nevus treated with combined use of normal mode ruby laser and Q-switched alexandrite laser. J Dermatol 2003; 30:538–42.
110. Kilmer SL, Anderson RR. Clinical use of the Q-switched ruby and the Q-switched Nd:YAG (1064 nm and 532 nm) lasers for treatment of tattoos. J Dermatol Surg Oncol 1993; 19:330–8.
111. Fitzpatrick RE, Goldman MP. Tattoo removal using the alexandrite laser. Arch Dermatol 1994; 130:1508–14.
112. Zelickson BD, Mehregan DA, Zarrin AA et al. Clinical, histologic, and ultrastructural evaluation of tattoos treated with three laser systems. Lasers Surg Med 1994; 15:364–72.
113. Alster TS. Q-switched alexandrite laser treatment (755 nm) of professional and amateur tattoos. J Am Acad Dermatol 1995; 33:69–73.
114. Taylor CR, Gange RW, Dover JS et al. Treatment of tattoos by Q-switched ruby laser. Arch Dermatol 1990; 126: 893–9.
115. Kilmer SL, Lee MS, Grevelink JM, Flotte TJ, Anderson RR. The Q-switched Nd: YAG laser effectively treats tattoos. Arch Dermatol 1993; 129:971–8.

116. Grevelink JM, Duke D, van Leeuwen RL, Gonzalez E, DeCoste SD, Anderson RR. Laser treatment of tattoos in darkly pigmented patients: efficacy and side effects. J Am Acad Dermatol 1996; 34:653–6.
117. Jones A, Roddey P, Orengo I, Rosen T. The Q-switched ND:YAG laser effectively treats tattoos in darkly pigmented skin. Dermatol Surg 1996; 22:999–1001.
118. Suzuki H. Treatment of traumatic tattoos with the Q-switched neodymium:YAG laser. Arch Dermatol 1996; 132: 1226–9.
119. Lim Y, Choi H, Myung K. Effects of treatment according to tattoo color, site and duration with the Q-switched alexandrite laser. Kor J Dermatol 1998; 36:844–9.
120. Chang SE, Choi JH, Moon KC, Koh JK, Sung KJ. Successful removal of traumatic tattoos in Asian skin with a Q-switched alexandrite laser. Dermatol Surg 1998; 24:1308–11.
121. Moreno-Arias GA, Casals-Andreu M, Camps-Fresneda A. Use of Q-switched alexandrite laser (755 nm, 100 nsec) for removal of traumatic tattoo of different origins. Lasers Surg Med 1999; 25:445–50.
122. Sherwood KA, Murray S, Kurban AK, Tan OT. Effect of wavelength on cutaneous pigment using pulsed irradiation. J Invest Dermatol 1989; 92:717–20.
123. Anderson RR. Laser–tissue interactions. 1 vol. 2nd ed. St Louis: Mosby; 1999.
124. Bernstein LJ, Kauvar ANB, Grossman MC, Geronemus RG. The short- and long-term side effects of carbon dioxide laser resurfacing. Dermatol Surg 1997; 23:519–25.
125. Manuskiatti W, Fitzpatrick RE, Goldman MP. Long-term effectiveness and side effects of carbon dioxide laser resurfacing for photoaged facial skin. J Am Acad Dermatol 1999; 40:401–11.
126. Nanni CA, Alster TS. Complications of carbon dioxide laser resurfacing. An evaluation of 500 patients. Dermatol Surg 1998; 24:315–20.
127. Ruiz-Esparza J, Barba Gomez JM, Gomez de la Torre OL, Huerta Franco B, Parga Vazquez EG. UltraPulse laser skin resurfacing in Hispanic patients. A prospective study of 36 individuals. Dermatol Surg 1998; 24:59–62.
128. Sriprachya-anunt S, Marchell NL, Fitzpatrick RE, Goldman MP, Rostan EF. Facial resurfacing in patients with Fitzpatrick skin type IV. Lasers Surg Med 2002; 30:86–92.
129. West TB, Alster TS. Effect of pretreatment on the incidence of hyperpigmentation following cutaneous CO_2 laser resurfacing. Dermatol Surg 1999; 25:15–17.
130. Haedersdal M, Bech-Thomsen N, Poulsen T, Wulf HC. Ultraviolet exposure influences laser-induced wounds, scars, and hyperpigmentation: a murine study. Plast Reconstr Surg 1998; 101:1315–22.
131. Clark RAF. Cutaneous tissue wound repair. J Am Acad Dermatol 1985; 13:701–25.
132. Khatri KA, Ross V, Grevelink JM, Magro CM, Anderson RR. Comparison of erbium:YAG and carbon dioxide lasers in resurfacing of facial rhytides. Arch Dermatol 1999; 135: 391–7.
133. Alster TS. Cutaneous resurfacing with Er:YAG lasers. Dermatol Surg 2000; 26:73–5.
134. Goldman MP, Manuskiatti W. Combined laser resurfacing with the 950-Msec pulsed CO_2 + Er:YAG lasers. Dermatol Surg 1999; 25:160–3.
135. Cho SI, Kim YC. Treatment of facial wrinkles with char-free carbon dioxide laser and erbium: YAG laser. Kor J Dermatol 1999; 37:177–84.
136. Ruiz-Esparza J, Barba Gomez JM. Long-term effects of one general pass laser resurfacing. A look at dermal tightening and skin quality. Dermatol Surg 1999; 25:169–73; discusion 174.
137. Alster T, Hirsch R. Single-pass CO_2 laser skin resurfacing of light and dark skin: extended experience with 52 patients. J Cosmet Laser Ther 2003; 5:39–42.
138. Avram DK, Goldman MP. The safety and effectiveness of single-pass erbium:YAG laser in the treatment of mild to moderate photodamage. Dermatol Surg 2004; 30:1073–6.
139. Ho C, Nguyen Q, Lowe NJ, Griffin ME, Lask G. Laser resurfacing in pigmented skin. Dermatol Surg 1995; 21:1035–7.
140. Kim JW, Lee JO. Skin resurfacing with laser in Asians. Aesthetic Plast Surg 1997; 21:115–17.
141. Song MG, Park KB, Lee ES. Resurfacing of facial angiofibromas in tuberous sclerosis patients using CO_2 laser with flashscanner. Dermatol Surg 1999; 25:970–3.
142. Kye YC. Resurfacing of pitted facial scars with a pulsed Er:YAG laser. Dermatol Surg 1997; 23:880–3.
143. Jeong JT, Kye YC. Resurfacing of pitted facial acne scars with a long-pulsed Er:YAG laser. Dermatol Surg 2001; 27:107–10.
144. Cho SI, Kim YC. Treatment of atrophic facial scars with combined use of high-energy pulsed CO_2 laser and Er:YAG laser: a practical guide of laser techniques for the Er:YAG laser. Dermatol Surg 1999; 25:959–64.
145. Lowe NJ, Lask G, Griffin ME. Laser skin resurfacing: Pre- and posttreatment guidelines. Dermatol Surg 1995; 21:1017–19.
146. Fitzpatrick RE. Laser resurfacing of rhytides. Dermatol Clin 1997; 15:431–47.
147. Fitzpatrick RE, Goldman MP. Skin resurfacing with carbon dioxide and erbium lasers. 1 vol. 2nd ed. St Louis: Mosby; 1999.
148. Trau H, Orenstein A, Schewach-Miller M, Tsur H. Pseudomelanoma following laser therapy for congenital nevus. J Dermatol Surg Oncol 1986; 12:984–6.
149. Ang P, Barlow RJ. Nonablative laser resurfacing: a systematic review of the literature. Clin Exp Dermatol 2002; 27: 630–5.
150. Alam M, Hsu TS, Dover JS, Wrone DA, Arndt KA. Nonablative laser and light treatments: histology and tissue effects – a review. Lasers Surg Med 2003; 33:30–9.
151. Sadick NS. Update on non-ablative light therapy for rejuvenation: a review. Lasers Surg Med 2003; 32:120–8.
152. Goldberg DJ. Nonablative dermal remodeling: does it really work? Arch Dermatol 2002; 138:1366–8.
153. Negishi K, Tezuka Y, Kushikata N, Wakamatsu S. Photorejuvenation for Asian skin by intense pulsed light. Dermatol Surg 2001; 27:627–31; discussion 632.
154. Chan HH, Lam LK, Wong DS, Kono T, Trendell-Smith N. Use of 1,320 nm Nd:YAG laser for wrinkle reduction and the treatment of atrophic acne scarring in Asians. Lasers Surg Med 2004; 34:98–103.
155. Anderson RR. Fire and ice. Arch Dermatol 2003; 139:787–8.
156. Kelly KM, Svaasand LO, Nelson JS. Optimization of laser treatment safety in conjunction with cryogen spray cooling. Arch Dermatol 2003; 139:1372–3.
157. Manstein D, Herron GS, Sink RK, Tanner H, Anderson RR. Fractional photothermolysis: a new concept for cutaneous remodeling using microscopic patterns of thermal injury. Lasers Surg Med 2004; 34:426–38.
158. Liew SH, Grobbelaar A, Gault D, Sanders R, Green C, Linge C. Hair removal using the ruby laser: clinical efficacy in Fitzpatrick skin types I–V and histological changes in epidermal melanocytes. Br J Dermatol 1999; 140:1105–9.
159. Garcia C, Alamoudi H, Nakib M, Zimmo S. Alexandrite laser hair removal is safe for Fitzpatrick skin types IV–VI. Dermatol Surg 2000; 26:130–4.

160. Alster TS, Bryan H, Williams CM. Long-pulsed Nd:YAG laser-assisted hair removal in pigmented skin: a clinical and histological evaluation. Arch Dermatol 2001; 137:885–9.
161. Chan HH, Ying SY, Ho WS, Wong DS, Lam LK. An in vivo study comparing the efficacy and complications of diode laser and long-pulsed Nd:YAG laser in hair removal in Chinese patients. Dermatol Surg 2001; 27:950–4.
162. Goh CL. Comparative study on a single treatment response to long pulse Nd:YAG lasers and intense pulse light therapy for hair removal on skin type IV to VI – is longer wavelengths lasers preferred over shorter wavelengths lights for assisted hair removal. J Dermatolog Treat 2003; 14:243–7.
163. Hussain M, Suwanchinda A, Charuwichtratana S, Goldberg D. A new long pulsed 940nm diode laser used for hair removal in Asian skin types. J Cosmet Laser Ther 2003; 5:97–100.
164. Hussain M, Polnikorn N, Goldberg DJ. Laser-assisted hair removal in Asian skin: efficacy, complications, and the effect of single versus multiple treatments. Dermatol Surg 2003; 29:249–54.
165. Galadari I. Comparative evaluation of different hair removal lasers in skin types IV, V, and VI. Int J Dermatol 2003; 42:68–70.
166. Ross EV, Cooke LM, Timko AL, Overstreet KA, Graham BS, Barnette DJ. Treatment of pseudofolliculitis barbae in skin types IV, V, and VI with a long-pulsed neodymium:yttrium aluminum garnet laser. J Am Acad Dermatol 2002; 47: 263–70.
167. Manuskiatti W, Tantikun N. Treatment of trichostasis spinulosa in skin phototypes III, IV, and V with an 800-nm pulsed diode laser. Dermatol Surg 2003; 29:85–8.
168. Dierickx CC, Alora MB, Dover JS. A clinical overview of hair removal using lasers and light sources. Dermatol Clin 1999; 17:357–66.
169. Dierickx CC, Grossman MC, Farinelli WA, Anderson RR. Permanent hair removal by normal-mode ruby laser. Arch Dermatol 1998; 134:837–42.
170. Dierickx CC, Grossman MC, Farinelli WA et al. Comparison between a long pulsed ruby laser and a pulsed, infrared laser system for hair removal. Lasers Med Surg 1998; 10(suppl):42.
171. Ross EV, Ladin Z, Kreindel M et al. Theoretical considerations in laser hair removal. Dermatol Clin 1999; 17:333–55.
172. Haedersdal M, Egekvist H, Efsen J, Bjerring P. Skin pigmentation and texture changes after hair removal with the normal-mode ruby laser. Acta Derm Venereol 1999; 79:465–8.
173. Omi T, Honda M, Yamamoto K et al. Histologic effects of ruby laser hair removal in Japanese patients. Lasers Surg Med 1999; 25:451–5.
174. Nanni CA, Alster TS. Laser-assisted hair removal: side effects of Q-switched Nd:YAG, long-pulsed ruby, and alexandrite lasers. J Am Acad Dermatol 1999; 41:165–71.
175. Campos VB, Dierickx CC, Farinelli WA, Lin TY, Manuskiatti W, Anderson RR. Ruby laser hair removal: Evaluation of long-term efficacy and side effects. Lasers Surg Med 2000; 26:177–85.
176. Cho S, Kim Y, Baek R. Removal of unwanted hair using the long pulse alexandrite laser. J Kor Soc Laser Med 1999; 3:8–10.
177. Campos VB, Dierickx CC, Farinelli WA, Lin TY, Manuskiatti W, Anderson RR. Hair removal with an 800-nm pulsed diode laser. J Am Acad Dermatol 2000; 43:442–7.
178. Manuskiatti W, Fitzpatrick RE, Goldman MP, Detwiler SP. Effects of long pulse duration and short interval retreatment on the efficacy of hair removal using broad-band, intense pulsed light system. Dermatol Cosmet 2000; 10:67–75.
179. Schroeter CA, Groenewegen JS, Reineke T, Neumann HA. Hair reduction using intense pulsed light source. Dermatol Surg 2004; 30:168–73.
180. Nanni CA, Alster TS. Optimizing treatment parameters for hair removal using a topical carbon-based solution and 1064-nm Q-switched neodymium:YAG laser energy. Arch Dermatol 1997; 133:1546–9.
181. Grossman MC, Dierickx C, Farinelli W, Flotte T, Anderson RR. Damage to hair follicles by normal-mode ruby laser pulses. J Am Acad Dermatol 1996; 35:889–94.
182. Duque V, Dierickx CC, Lin D, Farinelli WA, Anderson RR. Long pulsed ruby laser for hair removal: comparison between different spot sizes, temperatures and interval between first and second treatment. Lasers Med Surg 1998; 10(suppl): 39.
183. Soter NA. Sunburn and Suntan: immediate manifestations of photodamage. 1 vol. 1st ed. Oxford: Blackwell Science; 1995.
184. Kaiser MR, Davis SC, Mertz PM. Effect of ultraviolet radiation-induced inflammation on epidermal wound healing. Wound Rep Peg 1995; 3:331–51.
185. Nordback I, Kulmala R, Jarvinen M. Effect of ultraviolet therapy on rat skin wound healing. J Surg Res 1990; 48: 68–71.
186. Baadgaard O. In vivo ultraviolet irradiation of human skin results in profound pertubation of the immune system. Arch Dermatol 1991; 127:99–109.
187. Hedelund L, Haedersdal M, Egekvist H, Heidenheim M, Wulf HC, Poulsen T. CO_2 laser resurfacing and photocarcinogenesis: An experimental study. Lasers Surg Med 2004; 35:58–61.
188. Fitzpatrick RE, Williams B, Goldman MP. Preoperative anesthesia and postoperative considerations in laser resurfacing. Semin Cutan Med Surg 1996; 15:170–6.
189. Pathak MA, Fitzpatrick TB, Kraus EW. Usefulness of retinoic acid in the treatment of melasma. J Am Acad Dermatol 1986; 15:894–9.
190. Kligman AM, Grove GL, Hirose R, Leyden JJ. Topical tretinoin for photoaged skin. J Am Acad Dermatol 1986; 15:836–59.
191. Jimbow K, Obata H, Pathak MA, Fitzpatrick TB. Mechanism of depigmentation by hydroquinone. J Invest Dermatol 1974; 62:436–49.
192. Stratigos AJ, Katsambas AD. Optimal management of recalcitrant disorders of hyperpigmentation in dark-skinned patients. Am J Clin Dermatol 2004; 5:161–8.
193. Pathak MA, Ciganek ER, Wick M, Sober AJ, Farinelli WA, Fitzpatrick TB. An evaluation of the effectiveness of azelaic acid as a depigmenting and chemotherapeutic agent. J Invest Dermatol 1985; 85:222–8.
194. Chakraborty AK, Funasaka Y, Komoto M, Ichihashi M. Effect of arbutin on melanogenic proteins in human melanocytes. Pigment Cell Res 1998; 11:206–12.
195. Yokota T, Nishio H, Kubota Y, Mizoguchi M. The inhibitory effect of glabridin from licorice extracts on melanogenesis and inflammation. Pigment Cell Res 1998; 11:355–61.
196. Kameyama K, Sakai C, Kondoh S et al. Inhibitory effect of magnesium L-ascorbyl-2-phosphate (VC-PMG) on melanogenesis in vitro and in vivo. J Am Acad Dermatol 1996; 34:29–33.
197. Hoffman WL, Anvari B, Said S et al. Cryogen spray cooling during Nd:YAG laser treatment of hemangiomas. A preliminary animal model study. Dermatol Surg 1997; 23:635–41.

198. Waldorf HA, Alster TS, McMillan K, Kauvar AN, Geronemus RG, Nelson JS. Effect of dynamic cooling on 585-nm pulsed dye laser treatment of port-wine stain birthmarks [see comments]. Dermatol Surg 1997; 23:657–62.
199. Nelson JS, Kimel S. Safety of cryogen spray cooling during pulsed laser treatment of selected dermatoses [letter]. Lasers Surg Med 2000; 26:2–3.
200. Sturesson C, Andersson-Engels S. Mathematical modelling of dynamic cooling and pre-heating, used to increase the depth of selective damage to blood vessels in laser treatment of port wine stains. Phys Med Biol 1996; 41:413–28.
201. Nelson JS, Milner TE, Anvari B, Tanenbaum BS, Svaasand LO, Kimel S. Dynamic epidermal cooling in conjunction with laser-induced photothermolysis of port wine stain blood vessels. Lasers Surg Med 1996; 19:224–9.
202. Zenzie HH, Altshuler GB, Smirnov MZ, Anderson RR. Evaluation of cooling methods for laser dermatology. Lasers Surg Med 2000; 26:130–44.

Index

B

C

I

O

P

S

T